Clinical
Research

Concepts and
Principles for
Advanced Practice
Nurses

Clinical Research

Concepts and Principles for Advanced Practice Nurses

Manfred Stommel, PhD
Associate Professor
College of Nursing
Michigan State University
East Lansing, Michigan

Celia E. Wills, PhD, BSN, MS, RN
Associate Professor
College of Nursing
Michigan State University
East Lansing, Michigan

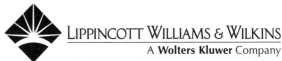

LIPPINCOTT WILLIAMS & WILKINS
A **Wolters Kluwer** Company

Philadelphia • Baltimore • New York • London
Buenos Aires • Hong Kong • Sydney • Tokyo

Acquisitions Editor: Margaret Zuccarini
Managing Editor: Helen Kogut
Editorial Assistant: Carol DeVault
Production Editor: Diane Griffith
Senior Production Manager: Helen Ewan
Managing Editor/Production: Erika Kors
Art Director: Carolyn O'Brien
Manufacturing Manager: William Alberti
Indexer: Michael Ferreira
Compositor: Peirce Graphic Services
Printer: R.R. Donnelley-Crawfordsville

9 8 7 6 5 4 3 2 1

Library of Congress Cataloging-in-Publication Data is available on request.

ISBN 0-7817-3518-1

Care has been taken to confirm the accuracy of the information presented and to describe generally accepted practices. However, the authors, editors, and publisher are not responsible for errors or omissions or for any consequences from application of the information in this book and make no warranty, express or implied, with respect to the content of the publication.

The authors, editors, and publisher have exerted every effort to ensure that drug selection and dosage set forth in this text are in accordance with the current recommendations and practice at the time of publication. However, in view of ongoing research, changes in government regulations, and the constant flow of information relating to drug therapy and drug reactions, the reader is urged to check the package insert for each drug for any change in indications and dosage and for added warnings and precautions This is particularly important when the recommended agent is a new or infrequently employed drug.

Some drugs and medical devices presented in this publication have Food and Drug Administration (FDA) clearance for limited use in restricted research settings. It is the responsibility of the health care provider to ascertain the FDA status of each drug or device planned for use in his or her clinical practice.

Dedication

Although there are just two authors who receive credit for writing this text, in reality, the content of this textbook has been substantially shaped by many years of experience in teaching research concepts to various levels of nursing students. A wise person once said, "No book ever gets written by the author(s) alone." This may well serve as a motto for this book as well. In particular, both of us would like to express our sincere appreciation to the many students enrolled in our master's level classes at Michigan State University, NUR 811, "Concepts of Research and Evaluation for Advanced Practice Nurses I," and NUR 813, "Concepts of Research and Evaluation for Advanced Practice Nurses II." The many thoughtful discussions we have had with our students have convinced us that they do indeed hunger for real understanding and are fully capable of mastering complex material if the content is presented in the right way. Some of the clinical examples we use in this textbook were originally suggested by our students as examples of research-relevant challenges in daily clinical practice. Other examples were tried out and changed over time in response to student questions. Similarly, the presentation of the more formal statistical ideas and models used in this text has been heavily influenced, for the better, by the reactions and comments of our students. While we know that the level of this text is challenging compared to other more basic textbooks available for graduate nursing research courses, we also know that it is a challenge well within the capabilities of graduate level nursing students. We truly believe that the positive payoff comes in the form of a better understanding of research, which in turn translates into a better-prepared clinician.

Having had the privilege to teach and be inspired by our students, we dedicate this book to you, our reader! We hope that we have succeeded in opening up new and highly rewarding ways of thinking about clinical practice and clinical research. We fervently hope also that you, the reader, experience some of the same excitement we have observed in our students as they gain a more satisfying conceptual understanding of nursing and health-related research concepts and methods.

Reviewers

Carol J. Cornwell, PhD, MS, RN, CS
Assistant Professor of Nursing
Georgia Southern University School of Nursing
Statesboro, Georgia

Cecily D. Cosby, PhD, RNC, FNP/PA-C, ACRN
Interim Program Director of FNP
Samuel Merritt College
Oakland, California

William P. Fehder, PhD, CRNA
Associate Professor
College of Nursing and Health Professions
MCP Hahnemann University
Philadelphia, Pennsylvania

Edna Hamera, PhD, ARNP
Associate Professor
University of Kansas Medical Center
School of Nursing
Kansas City, Kansas

Janice S. Hayes, PhD, RN
Professor
Christine E. Lynn College of Nursing
Florida Atlantic University
Davie, Florida

Maryalice Jordan-Marsh, PhD, RN, FAAN
Associate Chair, Associate Professor
USC Department of Nursing
Los Angeles, California

Jeanette H. Koshar, PhD, RN, NP
Associate Professor
Sonoma State University
Rohnert Park, California

Virginia Nehring, PhD, RN
Associate Professor
Wright State University
Dayton, Ohio

Beth L. Rodgers, PhD, RN, FAAN
Professor and Chair
Foundations of Nursing Department
University of Wisconsin
Milwaukee School of Nursing
Milwaukee, Wisconsin

Preface

INTENDED AUDIENCE AND GOALS OF THIS BOOK

Clinical Research: Concepts and Principles for Advanced Practice Nurses is intended as a research concepts and methods textbook for graduate students in nursing and others who are preparing for advanced clinical practice roles as mid-level providers. The overall goal of this textbook is to provide the learner with a thorough understanding of the methodological concepts and tools used in evidence-based clinical practice. That includes some basic skills in the use of data sets needed for the clinical management of patient populations. The coverage of topics is primarily designed to address the needs of those who will be users of research findings, but also addresses the needs of those who will generate new knowledge for clinical practice.

As might be expected, *Clinical Research: Concepts and Principles for Advanced Practice Nurses* has had a long gestation period. It represents the cumulative experience of both authors in teaching hundreds of students in the master's program at Michigan State University College of Nursing and elsewhere. We are all too familiar with the anxieties and frustrations that many students experience, especially when they are new to graduate study and are taking research or statistics courses. We are especially sympathetic to the learning needs of graduate students in nursing, who are often expert clinicians, but may have had limited exposure to the concepts and principles of empirical research. For example, we frequently talk with students who come to class or enter an online discussion in our research course after a full day of their clinical nursing work, in which they have comforted and counseled ill patients and stressed families or have otherwise provided essential health services at all levels of care. Yet these highly capable clinicians often do not present to graduate school with an educational background equivalent to that in other health-related disciplines, in which substantial exposure to mathematics, statistics, and research methods is more common. This book aims to bridge this gap between student capabilities and limited past exposure to research by offering a new approach to learning about empirical research methods.

Information Quality and the Translation of Research Evidence

We are now living in an age in which the mass media report daily on the results of clinical research, but often without providing the information necessary for well-informed decision making. Increasingly, patients ask their health care providers for additional information and advice, wanting to know the relevance of media-based information for personal health decisions. Sometimes they come with preconceived notions based on cursory media exposure, and the provider must spend some time to dispel fundamental misconceptions. Not infrequently, patients either over- or under-estimate their actual risk of developing certain health problems or undergoing treatments or health screening procedures. This is quite understandable when it is considered that the public is increasingly confronted with an overwhelming amount of information concerning the efficacy of particular health care interventions, which may, at times, lead to contradictory conclusions. For example, given the current (2002) research controversies about screening for prostate and breast cancers, a man may wonder whether or not to have PSA testing done, and a woman may be uncertain about whether or not to undergo mammography screening.

For these and many other issues, clinicians are increasingly called upon to become interpreters of research evidence for the public. Many people do not know that even the best quality evidence often entails some degree of uncertainty about the likely outcome. While media reports of research results often skip over the probabilistic nature of the results, many patients need to be assisted by clinicians to translate probability information into meaningful terms for their own decision-making. At the same time, many patients are understandably invested in finding "cures" or treatments that are "guaranteed" to help, especially for more serious illnesses, while treatment options for most health conditions have become more and more numerous. Treatment options can range from traditional medications, surgeries, non-invasive procedures, psychological counseling, and prevention and screening efforts, to emerging alternatives, such as nutritional choices (neutriceuticals), alternative/complementary, and genetic treatments. What all of these treatments share in common is that their advocates claim to be improving the human condition by curing an illness, alleviating a symptom, prolonging life, or reducing pain. In principle, all such claims are subject to testing and verification. In practice, treatments that are marketed as "effective" may or may not be validated by high-quality research evidence. In this technology and information-rich environment, it is essential that advanced practice clinicians have a solid understanding of basic research concepts and principles, including the meaning and translation of probability information, in order to assist themselves and their patients to make informed health decisions. Throughout this text, we emphasize the probabilistic (uncertain) nature of most research results and the many reasons for this.

Quality of Clinical Decision Making and Conceptual Knowledge of Research

It is our position that high-quality clinical decision making should rest on a systematic approach to evaluating research evidence in support of, or in opposition to, clinical practice decisions and subsequent actions. For example, we strongly believe that clinical practice guidelines and decision rules developed by others need to be critically evaluated by clinicians for applicability to their practice. In addition, since advanced practice clinicians perform a major teaching role, they must be able to translate the meaning of research evidence for their patients. That is to say, a clinician needs to understand the concepts and principles of empirical research well enough to be able to provide accurate explanations of research findings. In our view, these new roles and functions of an advanced practice clinician require a somewhat different and more extensive coverage of the *conceptual reasoning* underlying research methods than what has been customary in many nursing research textbooks up until now.

While the complexity and sophistication of the research literature seems to increase almost on a daily basis, few master's degree programs in nursing offer more than 3–6 credit hours for research methods and statistics. Thus, it is clear that a whole new way of thinking and learning is required to bridge this gap. First and foremost, clinicians need to understand the research principles and practices

that lead to "better" versus "lower quality" evidence. A clinician who wants to take full advantage of current research results for practice will need a solid *conceptual* (not necessarily technical) understanding of research methods and procedures, which goes beyond the more basic "primer" approach we have observed in several other research textbooks for APNs. This is where the emphasis of *Clinical Research: Concepts and Principles for Advanced Practice Nurses* lies. A number of our students have summarized the core aspects of this idea as, "We want to be good at critically thinking about research results so that we can make our own good decisions about whether or not to change our clinical practice on the basis of research findings."

What exactly do we mean by a "conceptual" versus a "technical" understanding? To a substantial extent, "critical thinking about research results" requires an understanding of the criteria and logic used to evaluate and rank-order results in terms of the underlying strength of evidence. To that end, we have striven to avoid presenting the reader with a large, seemingly unrelated collection of research techniques, or offering long lists of "rules" or "facts" for the reader to memorize. Usually such lists are soon forgotten if the content is not applied on a daily basis, and items appearing on such lists are sometimes even debatable as "truths" (e.g., a reliability coefficient such as Cronbach's alpha "should" be larger than 0.7, or clinical trials necessarily produce "superior" evidence to that provided by observational studies). Facts and rules such as these may occasionally provide useful checklists as general summaries, and their recall may indeed be tested on course examinations in research and statistics courses. But ultimately, they are not very useful to the user if he or she has no real idea or conceptual grounding in where these generalizations of fact come from. As just mentioned, we strive to provide learning experiences for clinicians to become conversant with the research world, so that there is substantial understanding of how an original clinical problem is converted into a research problem and what types of research evidence would be needed to address a clinical problem. In other words, in today's world, a good clinician must also acquire the skills of a "critical thinker" with respect to judging research results. We would want nothing less from an Advanced Practice Nurse!

Unified Treatment of Social Science and Epidemiological Concepts

Clinical Research: Concepts and Principles for Advanced Practice Nurses is unique also in that it aims to fill a significant gap among nursing research textbooks by providing a unified treatment of both social science and epidemiological concepts and terminology for research design and analysis. Until recently, nursing research textbooks have heavily emphasized social science research concepts from psychology and education. More recently, nursing research has begun to incorporate epidemiological concepts. This change in focus of nursing research is not coincidental, for epidemiological concepts are at the very heart of the current movement toward evidence-based practice. At the same time, the environment for advanced clinical practice is changing dramatically, requiring a practitioner who is also more conversant with the terminology and practices of medicine. Advanced practice nurses will need new, higher-level skills and competencies in evidence-based practice, beyond what has traditionally been provided in nursing education programs, in order to maintain viability in practice. Indeed, we believe that a solid understanding of concepts and principles for research in clinical practice has never been more essential for those who are entering advanced clinical practice roles. We hope that this text will bridge this gap in the currently available nursing research textbooks for graduate level nursing students.

APPROACH AND ORGANIZATION OF THIS BOOK

The approach taken in *Clinical Research: Concepts and Principles for Advanced Practice Nurses* is intellectually challenging, but it requires only a basic understanding of high-school-level mathematics. While high-quality clinical practice relies on statistical concepts in order to evaluate evidence, we believe that the teaching of such concepts in graduate school often leaves much to be desired, in terms of both understandability and relevance to clinical practice. The goal in this book is to provide learners with a thorough understanding of the logic of statistical reasoning as related to use of data in clinical decision making, while at the same time keeping the mathematical sophistication to a basic level.

There are several strategies we use throughout *Clinical Research: Concepts and Principles for Advanced Practice Nurses* to achieve this balance. First, the approach of this book heavily emphasizes understanding the logic of the content that is presented, as opposed to memorizing formulas (though we do not shrink from *presenting* formulas of key statistics). Numerous clinical examples are used to provide illustrations of how statistical concepts are integrated into clinical practice and research situations. In gen-

eral, our approach is to "reveal" to the learner, through commonly encountered clinical examples, how statistical concepts are integrated into clinical practice decision-making and research.

Likewise, unfamiliar concepts are explicitly linked to more familiar concepts. For example, fundamental research concepts such as controlling for the effects of extraneous variables in interventions will be illustrated using multiple 2×2 tables and focusing on the logic underlying various statistical procedures. Given the contemporary emphasis on evidence-based practice, this textbook will place considerable emphasis on the evaluation of outcome measures that can be used to assess the health status of individuals, families, or populations. Because nurses use behavioral, psychological, and physiological measures and screening tests, both psychometric and epidemiological evaluation criteria will be explained, with an emphasis on the underlying similarity of statistical reasoning in establishing the soundness or usefulness of a given measure or test.

Features

Throughout *Clinical Research: Concepts and Principles for Advanced Practice Nurses,* practical tips for conceptualizing data, and "checkpoints" with example questions or problems are posed, so that learners can assess how well they understand the concepts to that point.

Other special features to enhance the reader's learning include the following:

- A recurring feature called "Clinical Research in Action," which presents short to extended reviews of recent articles that appeared in refereed nursing, medical, and general health care journals. These reviews are meant to comprehensively illustrate and integrate the central concepts and methodological issues discussed in a chapter, referring to examples from the literature. In addition, a primary purpose of these reviews is to facilitate the reader's ability to quickly hone in on critical issues in a research article. The reader is strongly encouraged to read the reviewed articles, as this will deepen the understanding of the comments. Most importantly, if one wants to develop critical reading skills with respect to the research literature, there is no substitute for regular reading of original research articles.
- Another recurring feature labeled "Research Scenarios." Throughout *Clinical Research: Concepts and Principles for Advanced Practice Nurses,* we introduce research scenarios that often highlight how a clinical problem can be turned into a research problem. We have drawn on our extensive experience of working with

clinicians and clinically oriented students to create examples that either have or could have happened the way they are reported. One aspect of translating research into practice is also the reverse problem: of thinking about how a practical clinical problem can be turned into a workable research study. As with the "Clinical Research in Action" feature, a given research scenario is usually designed to highlight the particular methodological problem that is the focus of the chapter discussion.

- "Review Notes" that offer fresh reminders and short summaries of issues and topics dealt with at greater length in previous chapters

In addition, there are also the following features:

- Data tables and graphs providing illustrations of research and statistical concepts discussed in the text and including demonstrations of relevant calculations
- Boxes containing descriptions of clinical practice examples with research implications, vignettes of everyday experience that support the discussion of concepts, and short philosophical discussions of concepts and assumptions
- Descriptions of Web sites that have information relevant to clinical practice and clinical research, including the URLs for these sites
- Suggested activities for each chapter
- Key references and recommended readings
- A Glossary of key terms used throughout the text

connection—◡ 'Connection' Web site

Web resources to support the course will be available using the Lippincott Williams & Wilkins 'connection' Web site. (http://lww.connection.com) The site will provide interactive exercises, data analysis samples, multiple choice questions at the level of the NP Licensing Exam, and web links. These features will enhance the usability of the text in a traditional classroom setting or through an online course offering.

Acknowledgments

We wish to acknowledge our personal gratitude to several key people who have supported us in many invaluable ways during the process of writing. First, there is the staff of Lippincott Williams & Wilkins, in particular, Margaret Zuccarini and Helen Kogut. Their flexibility, expert advice, and supporting attitude were constant sources of encouragement and made the whole experience (almost!) pleasant. Manfred Stommel also would like to thank his wife, Susan, and son, Stefan, whose cheerful support and graceful endurance of late-night writing sessions made it all possible. Celia Wills wishes to thank her family and colleagues, who asked thoughtful questions, provided moral support, and were always available for an afternoon cup of tea or a walk in the beautiful gardens on the MSU campus.

Contents

▶ In this chapter, we address the importance of research concepts and skills for advanced practice nursing. We start with an overview of the current state of the health care system in the United States and other trends in Western society that result in an increased emphasis on evidence-based practice. The characteristics of the advanced practice nurse (APN) population are described, together with advanced nursing roles that rely on the APN to be a well-educated user of research findings in practice. Priorities for nursing research and the role of theory in guiding research are also discussed.

CHANGES IN HEALTH CARE AND THE ROLE OF THE ADVANCED PRACTICE NURSE

Today, the health care system in the United States continues to undergo rapid change. Both the structure and the processes of health care have been altered dramatically during the past decade, largely in response to cost but also in response to issues of access and quality of care as well as projected changes in future population needs. The emerging health care system is characterized by rapid technologic advances; including highly sophisticated, targeted treatments; and by a much more active role of third-party payers (Bodenheimer & Grumbach, 1998). It is increasingly recognized that key health problems in Western society are substantially associated with personal behavior and lifestyle choices, generating a call for a heightened emphasis on disease prevention and health promotion (Blank, 1997) within a renewed emphasis on primary care. Existing and emerging treatments are being evaluated not only by their effectiveness but also by their **cost effectiveness** (effectiveness per unit cost). Third-party payers are increasingly adopting the view that health care services must be managed not only for individuals but for whole population groups (Wilkerson, Devers, & Given, 1997). These changes, in turn, have led to a heightened emphasis on clinician accountability for treatment outcomes. Both physician and nonphysician providers are challenged, by individual patients and insurers alike, to provide sound evidence for their clinical practice decisions and to base clinical practice on well-researched, valid clinical practice guidelines (O'Neil, 1993).

Together with a renewed emphasis on primary care practice, health promotion, and disease prevention, the types and numbers of midlevel health care providers, in-

cluding advanced practice nurses and physician assistants, have proliferated. The United States remains unique among industrialized nations in that almost two thirds of all physicians are specialists, compared with the more than 50% of physicians in other countries who are generalists in primary care practice (U.S. Statistical Abstract, 2000). U.S. National discussions emphasize reducing the oversupply of specialist physicians. At the same time, the demand for the skills of APNs is expanding rapidly (Mundinger, Kane, Lenz, Totten, Tsi, Cleary, Friedewald, Siu, & Shelanski, 2000). For example, by March 2000, approximately 7.3% of the registered nurse (RN) population was prepared for one or more advanced practice roles, compared with just 6.3% of the RN population in 1996 (U.S. Department of Health and Human Services, 2001). Additional increased numbers of nonphysician clinicians are expected (Cooper, Laud, & Dietrich, 1998). The major APN roles include those of the nurse practitioner (NP), clinical nurse specialist (CNS), nurse midwife (CNM), and nurse anesthetist CRNA). APNs are more generally distinguished from other types of nurses by their advanced (graduate level) educational preparation and their advanced-level competencies and skills. More specifically, APNs are recognized as beyond-basic-level providers in their clinical judgment and decision making; their patient management; their organizational, collaborative, and independent practice; and their communication skills (Hickey, Oimette, & Venegoni, 2000).

ADVANCED PRACTICE NURSES AND RESEARCH

Although the specific activities of APNs differ depending on their role and the environment in which they work, APNs share certain competencies. These competencies include the ability to use research findings in practice, the ability to evaluate the outcomes of clinical practice, and (in some situations) the ability to conduct small-scale clinical research. Hickey et al. (2000) have also proposed that all APNs should be competent and committed "to 'evidence-based practice' and 'best practice' [and the] incorporation of evaluation into practice."

The focus of this textbook is on the research knowledge and skills needed for contemporary APN practice. In everyday language, the term **research** has many meanings, including the collection and synthesis of existing information from various sources. This book focuses on the principles and practices that underlie **empirical research,** that is, the systematic development of *new* knowledge via a process of assembling empirical (i.e., data-based) evidence. This empirical way of understanding reality[1] requires that notions, theories, assumptions, and statements about the world of practice are ultimately grounded in experiences, observations, and evidence that can be reproduced by anyone following the rules embodied in the research methods. **Nursing research** is distinguished from other types of research in that it addresses phenomena of concern to nursing.[2] The National Organization of Nurse Practitioner Faculties (NONPF; see *http://www.nonpf.com*) has described some areas of research priorities for APN practice, including those focused on the outcomes of practice (NONPF, 1998). Among these priorities are

- Assessing and comparing performance on quality of care, access, and satisfaction
- Conducting tests of theoretically driven nursing interventions and practice models
- Evaluating the match of current clinical practice to established practice guidelines
- Evaluating the cost effectiveness of practice

The NONPF research priorities reflect contemporary trends in APN practice and the health care system as a whole. In addition, other nursing organizations and key research funding agencies, such as the National Institute for Nursing Research (NINR; see *http://www.nih.gov/ninr/*), have identified research goals that are consistent with changes in advanced clinical practice and emerging population needs. For example, among the objectives for nursing research for the years 2000–2004 (see "Strategic Planning for the 21st Century, Scientific Goals and Objectives" at *http://www.nih.gov/ninr/a_mission.html*), NINR has identified leadership goals for nursing research. APNs may be involved in these and other research areas, as both users and producers of new knowledge, for the populations that are the focus of nursing care.

- Chronic illness experiences
- Cultural and ethnic considerations in health and illness (focus on decreasing health disparities)
- End-of-life/palliative care research
- Health promotion and disease prevention research
- Implications of genetic advances
- Quality of life and quality of care
- Symptom management
- Telehealth interventions and monitoring

It is clear from these priorities that APNs are interested and involved in a wide variety of health care problems. These priorities and interests may involve the treatment of specific illnesses, the maintenance of physical and psychologic well-being, and coping strategies in the face of nonreversible declines in health. In short, nursing research, regardless of the specific problem addressed, tends to emphasize the behavioral and social context of health and illness. Given the prominence of the educator's role in advanced practice nursing, nursing research has long focused on patient–provider interactions in which information (generated from research) is shared. However, it is in their role as educators and advisors to patients that APNs must become more sophisticated as purveyors of information. This is especially true for emerging areas of health-related research such as biophysiologic and genetic research.

EVIDENCE-BASED PRACTICE AND OTHER USES OF DATA IN CLINICAL PRACTICE

As defined by Cook and Levy (1998), **evidence-based practice** is "the explicit integrating of clinical research evidence with pathophysiologic reasoning, health provider experience, and patient preferences in the provision of care." In addition to understanding what information to use in practice and how to evaluate it, evidence-based practice also includes the ability to use information technology to rapidly marshal existing evidence that can address the clinical problem at hand. Evidence-based practice underpins each of the core competencies of APN practice.

---

[1] B. A. Carper has described empirics (scientific knowledge through research) as just one of four key "ways of knowing" in nursing. The other ways of knowing are esthetics, personal knowledge, and ethics. For a full discussion, see Carpenter, B. A. (1978). Fundamental patterns of knowing in nursing. *Advances in Nursing Science, 1,* 13–23.

[2] In an important article, Donaldson and Crowley define the scope of nursing research. For a full discussion, see Donaldson, S. K., & Crowley, D. M. (1978). The discipline of nursing. *Nursing Outlook, x,* 113–120.

In APN clinical practice, data are commonly used to achieve two types of objectives. First, in daily clinical practice, all APNs must be able to create and use patient records and other data for clinical decision making in the management of *individual* patients' conditions. For example, the information assembled for the record of a diabetic patient must reflect the known facts about the typical progression of the disease, the signs and symptoms to look for at various stages, and the appropriate treatments and recommended courses of action. Because clinical practice often involves the applications of tests and treatments validated in the past on other patients or patient populations, the clinician must be able to evaluate this information. For instance, the APN must understand the meaning of commonly used criteria for the validation of screening tests such as their sensitivity, specificity, and predictive values. Such knowledge is part and parcel of the clinical decision to order or not order a test for an individual patient. It should also inform patient education. This use of data involves understanding how information about *populations* can be used to inform the care of individual patients.

Second, APNs are increasingly involved in the use of data to manage care and evaluate **outcomes** (endpoints) of care in particular practice settings. Such evaluations focus not only on individual patients but also on entire patient populations. In fact, as we shall later illustrate, the effectiveness of an uncomplicated intervention (such as sending a reminder postcard 1 week before a patient's appointment with a health care provider) can be evaluated only by using population-based information. Clinical and administrative data sets generated in clinical settings can sometimes be modified and used for the evaluation of a surprising variety of clinical interventions.

This use of data to evaluate outcomes requires specific skills in the assembly of relevant data and a good sense of the analytic possibilities inherent in clinical data. Although a clinician may not need all the technical skills for analysis of such data, data should be gathered and assembled in a way that is appropriate for answering questions that inform clinical practice. Awareness that the evaluation of patient outcomes is often most useful at the group or population level is key to understanding how the data of a group or population can usefully inform clinical practice with an individual patient.

THE ROLE OF THEORY IN GUIDING RESEARCH

High-quality research on which sound clinical decisions can be based is not just a matter of gathering data. At-tempting to collect and make sense of data, without reference to some type of organizing framework to guide what is looked for, can be a daunting task. The use of theory to guide all steps of the research process involves thinking through *a priori* (in advance) what information is useful to gather for a given purpose, rather than afterward. A **theory** is essentially an organized, symbolic representation of reality that specifies relationships among key **concepts** (ideas or phenomena) of interest. As such, it provides the framework for understanding and explaining patterns found in data. Theories are frequently indispensable in guiding the research process and providing a structure for describing, explaining, or predicting outcomes of interest in clinical practice (Sidani & Braden, 1998). For example, in research and clinical practice alike, it is difficult to know how to interpret findings that differ from past experience, unless there is an idea about where to look for the solution. The use of theory allows a sound evaluation of how specific clinical actions relates to specific outcomes, because how actions should relate to outcomes can be specified in advance and tested against the predictions of theory (Fawcett, 2000; Meleis, 1997; Sidani & Braden, 1998). As expectations of accountability for care and care outcomes increase in clinical practice, reference to sound, theoretically based rationales for clinical actions is becoming essential. We shall discuss theory much more in later chapters of this book.

Suggested Activities

1. Visit the National Institute of Nursing (NINR) web site at *http://www.nih.gov/ninr/a_mission.html* to review the NINR Mission Statement and Strategic Planning for the 21st Century. Discuss with others the extent to which NINR research planning reflects changes in the health care system and population. Based on what you have reviewed and discussed, describe the implications of these changes and the information you will need for your future advanced practice role.

2. Interview several APNs about the extent to which they incorporate research evidence into their daily clinical practices. Ask these nurses to describe what they view as the benefits of, and barriers to, the use of research evidence in clinical practice. Discuss ideas for feasible approaches to working around the barriers to using research evidence.

3. Consider the type of clinical practice setting you envision yourself working in as an advanced practice provider. With others, discuss your likely role in this setting in terms of specific activities concerning the use of research and generation of new knowledge for clinical practice. Give specific examples, and include a dis-

cussion of the specific skills you will need, from your study of nursing research, to carry out these activities.

4. Identify one or two unresolved clinical problems from your clinical practice that could serve as the basis for a research project. With others, critique the importance of these problems from the perspectives of (1) the individual patient or provider, (2) the clinical care setting, and (3) the broader society. In your discussion, also consider the importance of the clinical problems in the context of changing characteristics of the health care system and population.

Suggested Readings

Hickey, J. V., Ouimette, R. M., & Venegoni, S. L. (2000). *Advanced practice nursing: Changing roles and clinical applications* (2nd ed.). Philadelphia: Lippincott.

National Organization of Nurse Practitioner Faculties (NONPF). (1998). *Research priorities for nurse practitioner education, policy and practice*. Washington, DC: Author.

References

Blank, R. H. 1997. *The price of life*. New York, NY: Columbia University Press.

Bodenheimer, T. S., & Grumbach, K. (1998). *Understanding health policy: A clinical approach*. (2nd ed.). Stamford, CN: Appleton & Lange.

Cook, D. J., & Levy, M. M. (1998). Evidence-based medicine. *Critical Care Clinics, 14,* 353–358.

Cooper, R. A., Laud, P., & Dietrich, C. L. (1998). Current and projected workforce of nonphysician clinicians. *Journal of the American Medical Association, 280,* 788–794.

Fawcett, J. (2000). *Analysis and evaluation of contemporary nursing knowledge: Nursing models and theories*. Philadelphia: F.A. Davis.

Hickey, J. V., Ouimette, R. M., & Venegoni, S. L. (2000). *Advanced practice nursing: Changing roles and clinical applications* (2nd ed.). Philadelphia: Lippincott.

Meleis, A. I. (1997). *Theoretical nursing: Development and progress* (3rd ed.). Philadelphia: Lippincott-Raven.

Mundinger, M. O., Kane, R. L., Lenz, E. R., Totten, A. M., Tsai, W. Y., Cleary, P. D., Friedewald, W. T., Siu, A. L., & Shelanski, M. L. (2000). Primary care outcomes in patients treated by nurse practitioners or physicians [online]. Available at: *http://jama.ama-assn.org/issues/v283nl/full/joc90696.html.*

National Organization of Nurse Practitioner Faculties (NONPF). (1998). *Research priorities for nurse practitioner education, policy and practice*. Washington, DC: Author.

O'Neil, E. H. (1993). *Health professions education for the future: Schools in service to the nation*. San Francisco: Pew Health Professions Commission.

Sidani, S., & Braden, C. J. (1998). *Evaluating nursing interventions: A theory-driven approach*. Thousand Oaks, CA: Sage Publications.

Statistical Abstract of the United States, 2000 (120th ed.). Washington, DC, U.S. Government Printing Office.

U. S. Department of Health and Human Services, Health Resources and Services Administration, Bureau of Health Professions, Division of Nursing. (2001, February). *The registered nurse population: National Sample Survey of Registered Nurses (March 2000): Preliminary findings*. Rockville, MD: Author. Available online at: *http://bhpr.hrsa.gov/.*

Wilkerson, J. D., Devers, K. J., & Given, R. S. (eds.) (1997). *Competitive managed care: The emerging health care system*. San Francisco: Jossey-Bass.

CHAPTER 2 The Vocabulary of Research and Overview of the Research Process

INTRODUCTION TO KEY RESEARCH TERMS: CONCEPTS, VARIABLES, THEORIES, HYPOTHESES

Any reader of the nursing and health care research literature will quickly encounter such terms as *retrospective design, hypothesis, stratified sample,* and a host of other terms that researchers routinely use to describe their research strategies and procedures. These technical terms can create a barrier to reading research reports or applying findings to clinical practice, and they often seem to have little relation to clinical problems. Yet, in a typical 10-page research report, it is not unusual for at least 3 or 4 pages to be devoted to the **research methods** (sample selection, data collection procedures, measurements, data analysis strategies) used in a research study.

Why do researchers devote so much attention to methods in their research reports? Why not just read the introductory section of a research report, determine the relevance of the clinical problem discussed, and then skip to the discussion section at the end to find out the key conclusions? Researchers usually respond, "How can the results and conclusions be trusted if the methods are not sound?" Box 2-1 gives two familiar clinical practice examples that illustrate the importance of accurate, appropriate nursing assessment and data collection for the well-being of patients. Both examples deal with conclusions that may be incorrect because of a faulty process of measurement (physiologic assessment or clinical judgment). They also illustrate a more general problem for both clinicians and researchers: Does the quality of the empirical evidence provide support for or against one's conclusions?

Empirical evidence refers to data that are gathered either directly, based on one's senses (sight, sound, touch, taste, smell), or indirectly, using instruments of measurement to substitute for direct senses. An example of the latter is the use of a stethoscope to amplify the sound of a patient's heart. Another way to think of empirical evidence is that it is the feedback received through the senses from the real world. Knowledge about any phenomenon is ultimately based on accumulating empirical evidence about that phenomenon. If the methods used to gather evidence are faulty, the ability to develop knowledge will be compromised. This is the key reason why researchers are very concerned with the adequacy of their methods.

Over many decades, researchers have developed a set of guidelines for evaluating the quality of research findings. These guidelines constitute veritable *rules of evidence.* In this book, we shall have much more to say about them: what they are and the extent to which they make sense, depending on a particular clinical problem and associated research question. For now, we turn to a discussion of some key research terms that underpin any understanding of rules of evidence. The particular terms discussed in this chapter will be used in many different places in this book, and you may find it useful to come back to them later to refresh your memory or deepen your understanding.

CONCEPTS

Essentially, a **concept** is an abstract representation of something. Consider Research Scenario 2-1, which addresses two concepts of interest to nursing: anxiety and pain. What we have here, in rudimentary form, is a **hypothesis,** or a statement about an expected outcome, if certain conditions are fulfilled. That is, *if* anxiety is reduced, *then* pain will be reduced or eliminated. More will be said about hypotheses later in this chapter. For now, we turn our focus to the nature of concepts. The term *concept* as used in research differs somewhat from its everyday meaning. Although we assume that others know what we mean when we say *anxiety* or *pain,* different people may not refer to the same underlying reality when they use these terms in conversation. This is a philosophic problem that has been around for ages. How can we make sure that apparent

---

BOX 2.1   Familiar Clinical Practice Examples

1. A patient's blood pressure reading is within the normal range. Consequently, as clinician you take no special actions. But what if the blood pressure cuff turned out to be faulty? You may conclude that your patient is doing well, when he or she actually is not.
2. Research has shown that nurses often make judgments about patients' pain levels based on their observations of patients' appearance and behavior. But this same research has also shown that observational assessment is problematic; i.e., patients who do not appear to be in pain may, in fact, be in severe pain.

agreement at the level of our words (for example, two nurses using the same terms or concepts of *anxiety* and *pain*), in fact corresponds to agreement about the *underlying reality*? To put it another way, does one nurse's picture (or conceptualization) of anxiety correspond to another nurse's conceptualization of the same term? Seemingly at odds with this situation is our understanding of science as an activity that produces objective results. Does that not, at a minimum, require that researchers use their concepts in a way that is clearly understood by everyone involved?

Research goes well beyond simple agreement on the definitions of concepts. Ultimately, researchers want to understand and explain some aspect of reality. For example, the pediatric nurse is likely to be interested in understanding how to intervene to reduce or prevent pain in children when they receive injections. However, the correspondence between concepts (used to communicate among researchers and scientists) and the true nature of reality is a key problem that demands clarity. Thus, we offer some additional considerations about the characteristics of concepts.

The Nature of Concepts

As abstractions from reality, *concepts* refer to the common properties of phenomena, which together make up reality. For example, consider the concept of a tree—an object you might see on your way to work or have growing in your yard. In everyday language, when people use the word *tree,* they refer to a variety of plants with certain properties in common. For example, many people would agree that trees generally have certain attributes or characteristics in common, such as fibrous trunks, branches, and leaves or needles. Each of these characteristics (fibrous trunks, branches, and leaves or pines) is itself a concept.

Thus, concepts are abstractions from reality in the sense that they do not describe reality exactly as it is, in all its infinite variety, right down to the atomic level. Instead, concepts concentrate on the *essential features* of something in reality. That, in turn, results in a person's understanding that she or he is looking at a tree rather than a shrub, a vine, or some other type of plant. There is a certain paradox here.[1] If reality is infinitely various, as was just emphasized, what is the source of the commonality, or the essential features, and how would we recognize it? The answer is that people group reality (phenomena) into concepts. The basis of the decision to group phenomena into concepts results entirely from the purposes for which we *invent* the concept in the first place. The same is true about the grouping of already-named phenomena.

Phenomena with common characteristics can be grouped together in several ways. For example, the concept of *wooden* is a characteristic of tables, trees, and some pencils. By contrast, the concept of *furniture* comprises diversely shaped objects (such as chairs, tables, beds) that are made of various materials (such as wood, metal, plastic), but all these objects share a common function: to facilitate living in houses. These examples illustrate the process of classifying reality through concepts. Now let's relate this to a clinical example (Research Scenario 2-2).

The concept of *arrhythmia* in this example is useful, not only in describing a particular phenomenon (the diagnosis) but also in helping the clinician consider what to do next (the treatment). In fact, the two main criteria for evaluating a concept for either clinical practice or research are the goodness and the fruitfulness of the concept. Hildyard People, considered by many to be the mother of modern psychiatric nursing, referred to the staying power of a concept as a means of evaluating its quality. A **good concept** is one that is influential for a relatively long time because of its usefulness for clinical practice or research. For example, it may be difficult to imagine work with a cardiac population without reference to the concept of arrhythmia. Researchers and clinicians alike find concepts useful to the extent that they help illuminate patterns in reality. Thus, for a researcher, a **fruitful concept** is one that allows the development of new knowledge based on the discovery of relationships that exist in reality. The more fruitful the concept, the more meaningful is the new knowledge generated from research, which uses the concept. Here is a list of concepts that have been found fruitful and are the focus of

---

[1] For a more detailed discussion of the paradox, see the writings of the very influential philosopher Ludwig Wittgenstein.

RESEARCH SCENARIO 2.2

Patient with an Irregular Heartbeat

The patient you are seeing today in clinic has an irregular heartbeat and also has been experiencing fatigue and "dizzy spells." You order a Holter monitor tracing, which reveals that there are certain times of the day that this patient has sustained runs of premature ventricular contractions (PVCs). Your diagnosis of arrhythmia for this patient is a particular concept, which subsumes what you have observed.

federally funded programs of nursing research (see Hinshawii, Fathom, & Shaver, 1999, for further reading):

- Caring
- Health promotion
- Treatment adherence
- Functional status impairment
- Management of illness symptoms, such as dyspnea, pain, incontinence, nausea and vomiting, sleep disturbance, fatigue
- Caregiving

Definition of Concepts

From the preceding discussion, it should be clear why researchers and clinicians alike spend much effort thinking about the nature and measurement of the concepts used in their research. A good conceptual definition suggests both what *is* and *is not* to be measured, eventually. For example, if an irregular heartbeat is conceptualized as an "arrhythmia," it implies that certain types of measurement may be done, such as manual auscultation of the heartbeat, or an electrocardiogram tracing of the heart rhythm. Defining a concept literally means delimiting it to a certain class of phenomena. This involves *setting boundaries in opposition to other concepts,* considering carefully the similarities and differences between the concept of interest and other concepts. For example, to what extent does the pediatric nurse consider the concepts of *anxiety* and *pain* to be both similar to, and different from, each other? Both anxiety and pain may involve unpleasant subjective experiences, but the precise natures of the experiences are somewhat different. How are concepts actually elucidated and defined? In everyday life and in research there are two broad ways of defining concepts: through a formal definition, or through usage (ostensive definition).

In a **formal definition,** already known concepts are used to define a new concept. For example, when the automobile was first invented, the concept of *automobile* was completely novel. So, to describe an automobile in terms that could be readily understood, the automobile was first known by two concepts that were familiar at the turn of the century: *horseless carriage.* Several examples of this principle are found in everyday clinical practice. For example, a hypertensive patient who is unfamiliar with the concept of *hypertension* may learn about high blood pressure by an analogy to a pressurized hose. As these examples make clear, formal definitions of concepts suffer from the fact that (at some point) they have to rely on the use of other concepts that are already understood. That is, all definitions end up with at least some terms that are not formally defined.

Concepts that are not formally defined may instead be defined ostensively. Most concepts in everyday life are defined through **ostensive definitions.** For example, a baby eventually learns the meaning of the concept *table* after having heard the word many times in contexts where other people indicate or point to a table (*ostensive* actually means "pointing to"). Sooner or later, the linking of the word *table* with a certain type of furniture acquires meaning for the child in terms of the set of phenomena to which it refers; i.e., tables tend to have four legs and smooth tops.

Although researchers often use formal definitions of concepts, the true meaning often emerges in ways quite similar to the everyday acquisition of concepts. In research, too, the meanings of concepts often derive from their use. That is to say, researchers' understanding of a concept's exact meaning is based on their ostensive experiences with it during the process of research. Concepts come to be known better and better over time through repeated exposure, through doing research that addresses and uses them. Thus, to a considerable extent, concepts can be viewed as works in progress. As more and more becomes understood about the phenomenon to which the concept refers, researchers will redefine the concept to reflect the changed understanding.

Levels of Abstraction of Concepts

Concepts can also be differentiated according to their levels of abstraction. Some concepts are so basic or concrete that knowing how to measure them comes almost automatically. For example, a person's height, weight, or temperature does not necessarily require much thought about how to measure them. These are often referred to as **observational concepts** or terms, because it is usually intuitively obvious how they can or should be measured. A second level of concepts may be referred to as **indirectly observable concepts.** This class of concepts includes all subjective experiences, many of which are of key interest in nursing and health-related research. Examples include experiences such as anger, depression, and pain. Such phenomena have a presence that cannot be directly observed but must rather be inferred from observable behaviors and other manifestations. For example, the presence of clinical depression is inferred in part on the basis of a characteristic cluster of behavioral symptoms, such as slowed motor activity and sleep disturbance.

A third level of concepts most often used by researchers is referred to as **theoretic concepts or constructs.** Key examples are found in the grand nursing theories, such as Orem's concept of *self-care agency* or King's concept of *role*. These concepts are quite abstract: often they do not refer to a set of clearly defined phenomena that can readily be measured. For example, it may be difficult to specify observable (measurable) behaviors that could be interpreted as unambiguous manifestations of a person's social role. Theoretic concepts are immensely useful for suggesting the broad scope of phenomena that might be considered together, but they become even more fruitful if they can be explicitly linked with **operationalized** (measurable) **concepts.** The latter form the basis for empirical research.

Operationalization of Concepts

The process that defines which empirical (measurable) phenomena a concept refers to is called the **operationalization** of a concept. In empirical research, it is critical to have concepts defined in such a way that they are potentially measurable (i.e., in such a manner that the properties of the phenomena can be quantified by assigning numbers to properties). For example, if a nurse wants to know whether or not a patient needs pain medication, it is important to have an objective, valid way of assessing the presence and severity of pain. The operationalization of concepts involves specifying the measurement operations for the concept. In fact, to a large degree (though not exclusively), the operational definition defines the meaning of a concept as used in a particular research project. Operational definitions are, however, almost always subject to debate and sometimes controversy (Box 2-2). Thus, it is important to keep in mind that a research article can always be critiqued on the basis of how well the researcher operationalized the key concepts of the study.

As mentioned earlier, the usefulness and fruitfulness of concepts are important criteria for evaluating their quality. But there is rarely one obviously correct way of operationalizing a concept. In general, any concept of interest can be measured in many ways. Thus, researchers also pay careful attention to the potential usefulness and merits of alternative operationalizations of concepts, or measurement procedures. These ideas have several important implications. First, it is essential for the author(s) of a research article to spell out in careful detail how the concepts were operationalized or measured. Likewise, it is equally important for the reader of research articles to be alert to the different ways in which a particular concept is measured across studies. This is especially necessary if one wishes to compare and synthesize the understanding of results from different studies, in which the same concept has been the focus. Finally, it is important to highlight how different operationalizations (or measurement procedures) can yield different conclusions about the nature of reality. For example, suppose you read two research articles on the relationship between expenditures for health care and personal health. In the first article, it is reported that there is a positive correlation (association) between people's health and how much money they spend on health care (on average, people who spend more on health care have better health), whereas the other study comes to the opposite conclusion. Why might these results contradict each other, and which study results should or should not be believed?

To begin, you would want to carefully look at the measures of "health" and "spending on health care" that were used. Suppose that you discover that the first study relied on self-reported measures of health, whereas the other used the results of physical examinations. Likewise, one study might include spending on health promotion and prevention in a person's overall spending on health care, whereas the other study might have considered only the expenses for medical care interventions for illness. If such differences are noted in your reading of a research report, the reasons for the *apparently* contradictory results may lie in the different operationalizations of the key concepts. The ability to compare results between studies depends on the concepts being measured in similar ways so that valid comparisons can be made.

A solution to the problem of differing measures of concepts is to develop standard measurement procedures for these concepts that are used by a variety of researchers across studies. A **standardized measurement procedure** (to be discussed in more detail in chapter 13) is one that yields the same results regardless of the occasion, place, or person who applies the measurement procedure. In addition,

---

BOX 2.2   Example of a Controversial Operationalization of a Concept

A recent book on intelligence by Herrnstein & Murray (1996), *The bell curve: Intelligence and class structure in american life,* sparked an enormous controversy over the role of human intelligence in explaining differences in social and economic achievements among various ethnic and racial groups. One of the principal issues in this contentious debate concerned the ability to measure the concept of human intelligence.

To examine this debate further, let's start with a purely formal, conceptual definition of intelligence like this: "Intelligence refers to a generalized capacity to solve unanticipated problems." Assuming you find this definition acceptable, how would you go about measuring a person's intelligence based on this definition? The first problem is that it is almost impossible to measure capacity. Instead, only specific instances of performance can be measured. For example, a person may well have the mental ability to solve a particular algebra problem, but poor eyesight causes the person to misread the problem, resulting in the formulation of an incorrect answer; or the person was never taught the basic rules of algebra. In other words, actual performance usually depends on a host of other physiologic and social factors, making it difficult to say to what degree a measure of performance would measure the underlying concept of intelligence in our definition.

On further reflection, you may ask yourself, why should solving a mathematics problem be taken as a valid indicator of intelligence? What about other problem-solving skills, such as the expert ability of a clinician to diagnose quickly a patient's illness, a musician's ability to recognize different rhythms or harmonies, or a carpenter's manual dexterity in using tools? Couldn't these also be signs of intelligence?

Most of the standard intelligence tests include problems that involve verbal, mathematical, and spatial-perception skills. In principle, there is nothing wrong with that, as long as one keeps in mind that one could have chosen other indicators that test different dimensions of intelligence. These other dimensions of intelligence also involve problem-solving skills, but they may or may not be highly associated with the verbal and mathematical skills measured on standardized intelligence tests.

What this example highlights is that there are different ways of operationalizing (measuring) the concept of intelligence. It depends on one's purposes as to which operational definition is most appropriate. For example, conventional academic intelligence tests are reasonably good predictors of academic failure, not-so-good predictors of academic success, and hardly-at-all good predictors of how much money you will earn in your lifetime!

---

standardized measures are often **population normed,** meaning that they provide numbers that can be directly compared to population averages. It is not difficult to see that standard measures are one important factor in aiding the progress of research in a given field of inquiry. If each researcher were to reinvent the wheel by creating completely new measurement tools, it would be very difficult to compare findings across studies, and the accumulation of knowledge about concepts would be hindered. However, many areas of research, including nursing research, lack sufficient high-quality standardized measures for key concepts. Given the central importance of measuring concepts, we shall devote several later chapters to a more detailed discussion of measurement procedures and underlying assumptions.

VARIABLES

Whereas concepts and their operationalization play a central role in all scientific research, researchers are most likely to refer to their measured concepts as variables in their daily work. A **variable** is the actual measurement outcome or the scores that represent the concept in a study. As the name implies, the variable representing the concept must vary in the study; that is, it takes on at least two values. For a **quantitative variable,** these values are numeric scores. Some familiar examples of variables include age (measured in years) and diastolic blood pressure readings (measured in mm Hg). For a **qualitative** (also known as a **nominal** or **categorical**) **variable,** the values are simply letters, words, or sometimes numbers that denote categories, such as self-reported gender (male or female) or blood type (Type A, B, or 0).

Why do researchers refer to their concepts as variables? One reason is that the concept of a variable easily incorporates the *comparative perspective* that is common to all scientific research. A fundamental principle in research is that there must be variation in the phenomena that are selected for study. In this way, phenomena can be compared with each other. More specifically, a fair amount of research is focused on showing how the variation in one variable is caused by a change (variation) in another variable(s).

Research Scenario 2-3 presents two recent examples of published studies that illustrate the central importance of having variation in phenomena. In one, an **intervention study** (Clark, Lipe, & Bilbrey, 1998), the researchers deliberately introduced and manipulated a treatment to achieve a desired effect. In the other, an **observational study** (Brown, Whittemore, & Knapp, 2000), the researchers just observed and recorded variations in attributes that were not controlled by them. Both of these studies involved specific target groups (dementia patients only, young and middle-aged adults only). Thus, in the intervention study, the type of diagnosis was held constant (the diagnosis did not vary among the study participants). In the observational study, there was some variation in the subjects' age, but it was restricted by the study design. Thus, the effects of type of diagnosis could not be studied in the first study at all (because there was no variation), and the effects of age could be studied only within the restricted age range of the study subjects.

RESEARCH SCENARIO 2.3

Music During Baths and Arm Span Measurements

1. Clark, Lipe, and Bilbrey (1998) examined the effects of recorded music on decreasing the occurrence of aggressive behaviors during the bathing of nursing home residents with dementia. These researchers deliberately introduced or withheld the playing of recorded music (the presence or absence of the stimulus is the intervention *variable:* it takes on two values) and they observed and counted the incidences of aggressive behaviors. The count of all types of aggressive behaviors, which ranged from 0 to 408 occurrences, is the outcome variable in this case.
2. Brown, Whittemore, and Knapp (2000) examined whether arm span could be used as a surrogate measure of height for patients unable to stand upright. In a sample of 90 young and middle-aged adults, they measured arm span and height and showed that the length of arm span accounted for over 90% of the variation in height. In this case, the two variables being compared and related to each other were both observed, not manipulated.

Types of Variables

Researchers distinguish many types of variables, based mainly on their causal order and their levels of measurement. Clinical research is interdisciplinary and is conducted by nurses, physicians, epidemiologists, psychologists, economists, and others. Because clinical research is interdisciplinary, and researchers have been educated in various research traditions, many different technical terms are used by researchers to refer to the same concepts. In this and subsequent chapters, we shall introduce you to the different terminologies that you are likely to encounter in nursing and other relevant health research literature.

Causal Ordering of Variables

When researchers think about the variables in their research projects, they often divide them into two broad categories: variables whose variation they want to explain, and those whose variation might explain the variation in the former. The first kind of variable is often called the **dependent variable,** and the second kind is called an **independent variable.** Usually a researcher's goal is to explain variation in the dependent variable(s) as a function of the variation in the chosen independent variable(s). Researchers use many synonyms for the terms *dependent variable* and *independent variable,* depending on which aspect of such variables they want to emphasize (Box 2-3).

Consider the two research examples in Research Scenario 2-4. In the first example, three independent variables are related to one dependent variable. In the second example, one independent variable is related to two dependent variables. Sometimes the causal ordering is more complex. For instance, a variable may function as both a dependent variable and an independent variable in the same study. If so, it is often referred to as an **intervening variable.** Take another look at the congestive heart disease (CHD) example. If the researcher were to expand the study to include two more variables (for instance, diastolic blood pressure and total serum cholesterol), both of those variables could function as dependent variables with respect to the behaviors and as independent variables with respect to the likelihood of the development of CHD. Thus, there is a causal chain of events in which subjects' behaviors (smoking, eating, physical activity) influence physiologic variables (blood pressure and total cholesterol), which in turn influence the risk of the development of CHD. In this chain-of-events example, we could view the behaviors as the original or root cause independent variables, the physiologic variables as the intervening variables, and the risk of the development of CHD as the ultimate or final dependent variable.

BOX 2.3   Synonyms for Independent and Dependent Variables

In many statistical models, independent variables are also referred to as **exogenous,** meaning that their variation is taken as given, or *generated by forces outside* of the model under investigation. In these models, dependent variables are referred to as **endogenous,** meaning that variation in these variables is viewed as explainable through other variables *within the model* under examination.

In clinical and health services research, dependent variables are often referred to as **response variables, outcomes,** or **outcome variables,** especially in studies in which the independent variable is a particular intervention.

Finally, independent variables are also referred to as **explanatory variables** because they are supposed to explain the variation in the dependent variable(s). When such independent variables are not the central focus of the study but are considered additional influences on the outcome variable of interest that must be controlled for, they are often called **confounders, confounding variables, control variables, extraneous variables,** or even **nuisance variables** (as indeed they can be!).

For example, look back at the hypothetical study of turning/lifting of immobilized patients. The frequency of the turning/lifting intervention (independent variable) varies, and the outcome variables are the incidence of pressure ulcers and recovery from effects of immobility. Here one can imagine a variety of other influences on the development of pressure ulcers and recovery from effects of immobility, other than the effects of the turning/lifting intervention: adequacy of skin care procedures, patient age, nutritional status, and so forth.

The following lists summarize various synonyms we've discussed (and some new ones) for independent and dependent variables:

Independent Variable Synonyms
Exogenous variable, experimental variable, intervention variable, treatment variable, intervention, independent factor, explanatory variable, control variable, confounder, confounding variable, extraneous variable

Dependent Variable Synonyms
Endogenous variable, outcome variable, response variable, outcome(s), effect

Variables are also distinguished by their measurement properties (often referred to as **levels of measurement**), the number of categories they comprise, and the amount of control the researcher has over them in the design of the study. We shall consider each of the distinctions in turn.

Levels of Measurement

Traditionally, researchers have distinguished measurement scales by their levels of measurement.[2] The central reason

[2] For further reading, see the seminal work by Stevens (1946).

RESEARCH SCENARIO 2.4

Coronary Heart Disease and Turning Immobilized Patients

1. A researcher wants to know how strongly smoking, physical activity, and diet are associated with coronary heart disease (CHD). In this example, variations in behaviors (independent variables) are conceptualized as influencing the likelihood of the development of CHD (dependent variable).

2. A nurse researcher is interested in how the frequency with which an immobilized person is turned affects the incidence of pressure ulcers and the recovery time from other effects of immobilization. In this example, turning frequency (independent variable) is conceptualized as affecting the likelihood of the development of pressure sores and the time of recovery from immobilization (dependent variables).

for distinguishing among levels of measurement is that they determine what types of mathematical operations are appropriate in the analysis of data. For example, it would not make sense to report an average value for gender (people are generally either male or female), but it is appropriate to report the numbers and percentages of male and female subjects in the study sample. More detailed discussion of measurement will be included in later chapters. For now, we provide brief definitions and examples. Variables may be considered nominal-level, ordinal-level, interval-level, or ratio-level, as shown in Table 2-1.

Numbers of Categories

Variables are also often distinguished in terms of the number of categories, levels, or values they can assume. For instance, a variable is called **dichotomous** (or **binary**) if it comprises only two categories. Examples are gender and survival status (dead or alive). **Polytomous** variables, by contrast, refer to variables with multiple discrete categories, such as smoker status (nonsmoker, former smoker, current smoker) or race. **Continuous** variables are those

that may have—at least in principle—an infinite number of values or gradations of values. A person's age, though usually measured discretely in years, can take on any value (such as days, seconds of life, and so forth). Many physiologic measures, such as blood pressure readings, are of this kind. These distinctions in variable categories become quite important when data are analyzed: they affect which types of statistical models and analysis strategies should or should not be used.

Finally, it is important to highlight a common area of confusion. It concerns the distinctions between a variable itself and the levels or categories of a variable. For example, suppose a researcher compares men and women who have taken different doses (5 mg, 10 mg, and 15 mg) of an experimental antihypertensive medication in order to determine the effects of the medication on reducing blood pressure. In this example, there are two independent variables: gender and medication dose. The dependent variable is the blood pressure measure. For gender, the categories (or levels) are male and female; this is an example of a nominal-level variable. Medication dose and blood pres-

TABLE 2.1	Levels of Measurement of Variables	
Level of Measurement	Description	Example
Nominal	The numerical scores assigned to each category are essentially arbitrary, but once chosen they must be applied consistently.	Assigning numbers to categories of the variable, "religious affiliation": 1 = Catholic, 2 = Jewish, 3 = Protestant, 4 = Muslim, and so forth. Note that the numbers could be shuffled around; e.g., Catholic could just as readily be coded as a 3, and so forth.
Ordinal	The numbers assigned to categories denote a sequence in rank order. However, the distance between categories (rank orderings) remains undefined/not meaningful.	A nutritionist has a patient rank order a list of 20 food items in terms of perceived tastiness. Note that the *difference* in preference for the 2nd and 4th foods cannot be interpreted as being *equally as large* as the difference between the 12th and 14th foods, for example. All we know in each comparison is which food is being preferred over another.
Interval	The numbers assigned to categories do have clearly/meaningfully interpretable distances (intervals).	The distance between points on a Celsius or Fahrenheit thermometer is meaningful; e.g., a temperature of 39° Celsius is higher (by 2°) than a temperature of 37° Celsius. The *same* difference occurs between 20 and 18° Celsius.
Ratio	The numbers assigned to categories have meaningful interpretable distances, and there is a defined zero point for the scale/variable.	Drug doses, postoperative time to recovery, out-of-pocket expenditures for health services. In these cases, we can say, for example, that dose A (30 ml) is *twice as large* as dose B (15 ml) or that expenditure C is *three times greater* than expenditure D.

sure readings are continuous variables at a ratio-level of measurement because they can, in principle, take on any values, including zero, and the distances between blood pressure levels and dosages are meaningful and interpretable. However, in the current example, dose is confined to three discrete categories, whereas blood pressure is allowed to vary from person to person.

Control Over Variables

Another distinction among variables is often made with respect to their role in the research design. Some independent variables are controlled (manipulated) by the researcher; others are not. Independent variables under the control of the researcher are often referred to as **treatment, experimental,** or **intervention variables.** For example, a researcher may control the dose of a drug given to research participants or the number of contacts with a nurse for a cognitive-behavioral intervention of smoking cessation. By contrast, independent variables not under the researcher's control are often referred to as **attribute variables.** Examples of attribute variables include age, gender, and health status of research participants.

THEORIES

In empirical research, theories often play a prominent role in organizing the researcher's thinking about concepts and directing attention to the specific relationships among them that should be investigated. **Theories** (like models) are *symbolic representations of reality* that specify how relevant variables are related to one another. In research, the ultimate goal is to understand the relationships among concepts, and it is theory that offers the explanatory model of how and why these concepts are related to one another. The explanatory model includes the **propositions** of the theory that indicate what the relationships should be. The validity of study findings from empirical research is supported to the extent that the findings mirror the propositions of the theory or theories involved. Thus, whereas empirical findings support the validity of a theory, it also works the other way around. Theories help make sense of empirical findings and validate them.

When we state that a theory must be testable against empirical evidence, we mean that it must yield behavioral predictions that are either false or true in principle. While it is not necessary that every concept used in a theory be immediately operationalized into a measurable variable, scientific theories must yield or imply hypotheses that are testable. If the empirical evidence contradicts the hypotheses derived from the theory, we are forced to reconsider or

modify the theory. Thus, when empirical researchers use the term *theory,* they use it in a sense that is often at odds with the broader, popular understanding of the term. Specifically, consider the saying "This may be true in theory, but it does not hold in practice." This saying is based on a view of theory that is *opposite* to the one held by researchers. To researchers, *any theory that is contradicted by empirical evidence is false.*

Because the theoretic world of concepts cannot be seen or measured directly, the results of research studies are often couched in language such as this: The results provide evidence in support of, or contrary to, propositions from the theoretic world. In general, the word *prove* is not often used in research reports because it is too strong a word for the information that any given study can provide to our understanding of how things really work. However, as we shall see later, even though our research designs and methods of measurement may often leave room for argument, cumulative evidence from several research studies may well be quite convincing. For a pictorial representation and summary of how the theoretic and operational worlds relate, see Figure 2-1.

It is important to recognize that nursing and other health research is not always geared toward confirming or contesting theories. Other common research goals include description, prediction, and evaluation. Although such studies may not require elaborate theories, theories often figure prominently as explanatory frameworks in their empirical findings. In a more general sense, researchers and clinicians alike always have theories about how the world works. In fact, when people purposefully enact behaviors on the basis of assumptions about how things are related to one another and how they can be changed, they are implicitly acting on the basis of theories. It is the researchers' job to make this connection explicit and to provide corroborating evidence that links findings to theoretic assumptions.

The term *theory,* as used by researchers, should also be distinguished from **conceptual framework,** such as might guide your nursing practice (Fawcett, 1995). Examples of conceptual frameworks include the **grand theories** of nursing and **general systems theory.** These frameworks can be very useful in providing an overall orientation (or language) in which to frame a problem. For example, Orem's popular concept of self-care agency has been used as a theoretic framework for understanding preventive health behaviors such as obtaining immunizations. Conceptual frameworks are useful to empirical researchers because they may provide a way of talking in an organized fashion about a subject area and may give context to the available evidence. This does not mean that conceptual

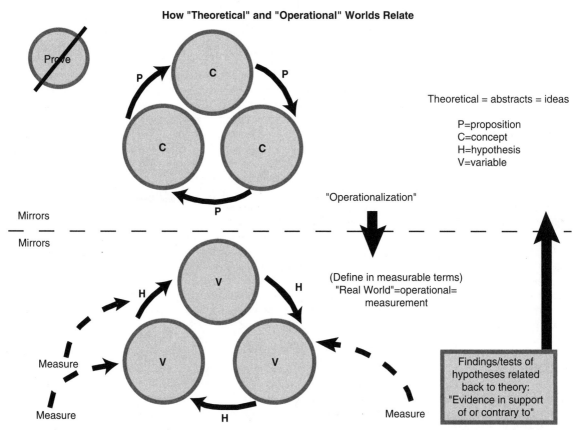

FIGURE 2.1 How the theoretical and operational worlds relate. In research, the ultimate goal is to understand the relationships between concepts, in terms of how theory indicates these concepts should relate to each other (propositions indicate what the relationships should be). The validity of study findings from real world research is directly related to how well concepts and propositions are mirrored (operationalized), in the form of variables and hypotheses that can be tested in real world research. Because the theoretical world cannot be "seen" or measured directly, the results of research studies are stated in terms of providing evidence "in support of or contrary to" propositions from the theoretical world. In general, the word "prove" is not used in reports of research because it is too strong a description of the information that any one study can provide to our understanding of how things really work, given our imperfect methods of research design and measurement.

frameworks themselves yield testable or specific hypotheses of how particular variables are related or influence each other. However, conceptual frameworks have been the basis for the development of many **middle-range theories,** such as Pender's Health Promotion Model (Pender, 1996), which do yield testable hypotheses.

In summary, empirical testability is an important criterion for assessing theories, whereas the usefulness of conceptual frameworks lies more in the generation of ideas and formally testable theories. Overall, in distinguishing a theory from a conceptual framework, it is useful to consider the following two questions: Under what condition(s) would the theory or conceptual framework be proven

wrong? What data-based evidence would lead to modification(s) in the theory or conceptual framework?

HYPOTHESES

The term hypothesis often refers to a low-level empirical implication of a theory (refer back to Figure 2-1). A theory may posit how certain variables should be related to one another, and a research study may be designed to test this relationship in the form of hypotheses specifying the relationships among variables. However, hypotheses are also formulated in research that is not explicitly theory driven but aims to solve a practical problem. Whatever its origin, a **hypothesis** is a *statement of the specific empirical findings* the researcher expects to come up with. In other words, hypotheses are formulated in such a way that they are more or less directly testable. They predict the empirical outcomes (patterns of results) that can be expected from the research.

Here are two examples of hypotheses that can be empirically tested; that is, data can be gathered and analyzed to see whether the prediction (hypothesis) is true or false:

- Functional disability increases with age.
- Depressed family caregivers are more likely to institutionalize their care-receiving relatives.

Both of the above hypotheses are **simple hypotheses.** That is, in each hypothesis, variation in only one independent variable is related to variation in only one dependent variable. For example, in the statement "functional disability increases with age," the dependent variable is functional disability, and the independent variable is age. In the second example, depression status (depressed or not depressed) is the independent variable, and likelihood of institutionalization is the dependent variable. Both of these hypotheses are also **directional hypotheses**; i.e., they specify in which direction the dependent variable changes as the independent variable changes. In the first example, the dependent variable of functional disability increases as age increases. In the second example, the presence of depression results in an increased incidence of institutionalization of care-receiving relatives.

Hypotheses can also be **complex**, relating more than one dependent and/or more than one independent variable to one another. Additionally, they can specify the conditions under which a certain relationship is expected. Finally, some hypotheses specify the functional shape of a relationship among variables. Researchers often use mathematical notations to specify a relationship.

In general, it is a good idea to be as specific as possible in formulating a hypothesis. If a researcher suspects that a relationship between a pair of variables is nonlinear, it is important to say so. If it is suspected that a specific relationship holds in one subpopulation but not in another, this too should be specified. The more concrete and specific hypotheses are, the easier it is to test them directly (Box 2-4).

Now that we are aware of the importance of stating hypotheses as specifically as possible, including the specification of the functional shape of the hypothesized relationship, let's apply this to a specific health services research example. It is well known that income and education are good predictors of mortality and morbidity in general, and that they also predict the prevalence of risk factors for heart disease in particular (Luepker, Rosamund, Murphy, Prafka, Folsom, McGovern, & Blackburn, 1993). More specifically, people with higher education and income tend to have greater longevity and to experience lower rates of morbidity. However, this relationship is not linear. See Figure 2-2 for a comparison of a linear relationship and two nonlinear relationships. To demonstrate the meaning of a linear versus nonlinear relationship between income and life expectancy, consider these hypothetical data:

Income of $20,000/year is associated with a 70-year average life expectancy.

Income of $40,000/year is associated with a 75-year average life expectancy.

Income of $60,000/year is associated with an 80-year average life expectancy.

As shown above, the form of the relationship between family income and average life expectancy is linear: For every additional $20,000 in yearly income, average life expectancy increases by a constant 5 years. But in reality, life expectancy does not increase by a given constant value for each additional $10,000 income, each additional year of schooling, or similar factor. Instead, the additional (or marginal) benefits of income gradually decline. What is being said here is that as a person's income increases from, say, $20,000 to $30,000, there are likely to

BOX 2.4   Reviewing Hypotheses Presented in Articles

An implication of the foregoing discussion for reading a research article is this: A hypothesis presented in an article should be reviewed with a critical eye. Is it formulated in such a way that it can be tested with the empirical data at hand? Does its confirmation or rejection shed light on the underlying theory, or is the connection between theory and hypothesis tenuous? Is the knowledge that is gained from the test of the presented hypothesis likely to add much to the knowledge in the field?

Examples of Three Commonly
Encountered Functional Relationships

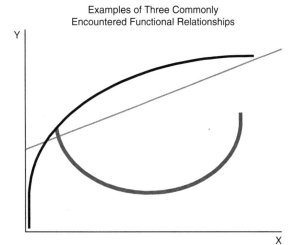

Straight line relationship, e.g., small, steady rise in blood pressure (Y) with age (X)

Logarithmic relationship, e.g., increases in overall health (Y) with increased income (X)

U-shaped relationship, e.g. depression (Y) and age (X) i.e., depression rates tend to be highest among teenagers and elderly

FIGURE 2.2 Examples of functional relationships between variables.

be real health benefits gained, in terms of the affordability of better nutrition or preventive care or access to health care providers, for example. However, if a person's income increases from $150,000 to $160,000, it is hard to see what additional health benefits may come from this increase in income. Thus, a more realistic depiction of the relationship between income and life expectancy is a curve that increases relatively rapidly at the low ranges of income, but gradually flattens out at the high ranges of income, as demonstrated by the logarithmic curve in Figure 2-2.

As this example illustrates, stating hypotheses in the form of mathematical functions will often allow clearer modeling of the expected relationship. Research in nursing, health services, and epidemiology has become increasingly sophisticated, and there are ever more examples of using mathematical and statistical tools to depict relationships among variables in a more precise manner. However, even when no sophisticated mathematical models are used, the general principle still holds: Hypotheses should be formulated so that they depict the expected relationship as precisely as possible. Here are two versions of a purely verbal statement of a hypothesis:

- Use of health care services differs among different ethnic groups.
- Use of health care services will be higher for African Americans than for European Americans. However, we hypothesize that this relationship will hold only for persons whose yearly household income from all sources is $30,000 or less. For persons with higher household incomes, we expect to find no significant differences in use of health care services among the two racial groups.

In the first example, the hypothesis does not specify the functional form of the relationship among the variables, nor is it directional. Such hypotheses are weak. Essentially, all they specify is that some variable(s) is/are related to some other variable(s). Although such a hypothesis may sometimes be appropriate for initial and very exploratory research, it does not really say very much. In other words, even if the hypothesis in its original form ends up being confirmed by the results of the study, the amount of knowledge gained is relatively small. By contrast, the second version of the hypothesis is better because it specifies directionality, tells us which ethnic group is expected to have higher or lower use of health services, and introduces a qualifying condition: The expected relationship will hold only in certain economic subgroups of the population, but not others. It is clear that this hypothesis provides much better information than the first one.

GENERAL PURPOSES OF RESEARCH

There are three general purposes or categories of research: description/exploration, prediction, and explanation. Each of these will be discussed in depth later in the book, after you become familiar with the major research designs. In this chapter, we emphasize just a few key characteristics.

First, a good **description** of a phenomenon is often a starting point for serious research. For example, consider these clinical research questions: "How does this particular rash differ from other skin irritations?" or "What characteristics distinguish people who follow a provider-recommended medical regimen from those who do not?" The essential point (and benefit) of careful description is that it orders observational data in such a way as to hint at (but not prove) causal relationships among variables. Good description is also the starting point for diagnostic reasoning (Kassirer, 1989). Clinicians often engage in an inductive process in which diagnostic hypotheses are formulated on the basis of the initial picture presented to them. The same can be said about any new subject area. The less that is known about a behavior, a disease, or a population group, the more preliminary exploration via description is necessary. Only then is it possible to formulate meaningful questions and hypotheses for more systematic study.

Second, **prediction** plays a central role in scientific research. It is the key concern in intervention studies: Will the intervention result in the desired effect? In a sense, prediction is most important for clinical practice because it answers the key question every clinician needs to know: "If I do action X, will it have the intended effect on outcome Y?" Prediction is also part of diagnostic reasoning, specifically in the hypothesis-testing phase. For instance, a patient with a sore throat, pharyngeal exudate, and swollen lymph glands could be experiencing either a minor upper respiratory infection or a strep throat infection. On the basis of these and other data, such as fever and the results of a throat culture, a clinician rules out possible diagnoses.

Finally, **explanation** and theory advancement research is focused on finding the causes of phenomena, going beyond not only knowing that something works, but also *why*. Generally, this is the most difficult goal to realize in research. It requires that the researcher can already draw on an extensive stock of existing valid theories. Given the multiple determinants of human health and illness, such theories may derive from several disciplines, ranging from pathophysiology to psychology. At this moment, the number of empirically supported theories is still limited in nursing.

Program Evaluation

Program evaluation research is designed to provide information about the success of action programs (Brink & Wood, 1998), i.e., models of practice and specific clinical interventions. This type of research is essential to policy making, which involves the allocation of resources in health care. One of the most common types of program evaluation in nursing practice involves testing the effectiveness and cost effectiveness of nursing interventions in clinical settings (Brink & Wood, 1998).

Program evaluation differs from pure research in that the goal of the research is not merely knowledge development, but involves a key focus on *evaluating effectiveness*. The effects of programs or interventions are of central interest, and the research methods reflect the real-life context of the study (Pawson & Tilly, 1997). Evaluation often incorporates description, prediction, and even explanation. One key difference from other kinds of research is the central role of stakeholders other than researchers who participate in defining the research agenda. In addition, program evaluation researchers may work with existing data sets to

evaluate the outcomes of programs, rather than designing the research from the beginning. These factors often shape the research methods that can be used, and evaluation research often involves making tradeoffs between rigorous research design and other factors in conducting an evaluation. Given the increasing importance of program evaluation in health care, the central issues involved in evaluation research will be discussed at length later in this textbook.

Basic versus Applied Research

A key emphasis in **basic research** is on generating new knowledge that may not have an immediate application to a practical problem. For example, basic research may be done to understand processes of metabolism, to accumulate knowledge for its own sake, or to test competing psychologic explanations for a set of attitudes about learning. **Applied research,** which includes most nursing research and all of program evaluation, focuses on addressing a more immediate (clinical) problem. The goal of this type of research is to produce positive change. For example, a nurse researcher may be interested in evaluating a telephone follow-up program for women in the early postpartum period. The goal of such research may be to examine whether or not the program is effective (achieves its aims) and efficient (cost effective), or what steps might be taken to improve the program in particular areas (quality improvement).

The distinction between basic and applied research is quite fluid. Ultimately, all scientific endeavors serve a practical purpose, even though basic research is often driven by theoretic questions and puzzles, the practical implications of which may not yet be fully understood. However, whether research is basic or applied, the standards of proof and methods of investigation do not differ.

THE COMPARATIVE LENS OF EMPIRICAL RESEARCH

Earlier we mentioned that scientific explanation consists of showing that the variation in one or more variables is caused by variation in another variable or variables. This principle has fundamental implications for the way in which research projects are set up (designed) to study the problems of interest. Let's consider Research Scenario 2-5, which includes some implications for how a research study might be designed. After reviewing this example, ask yourself this: Why might it *not* be sufficient to study only a sample of blind elderly people to understand the impact of blindness on social life activity? The main problem with

RESEARCH SCENARIO 2.5

Blindness and Social Life

Suppose you want to study the effects of blindness in elderly patients on their ability to maintain an active social life. You are not really interested in blindness itself, but rather in how the ability to see or not see affects people's ability to socialize. Visual ability could take on two values: 0 = blind (unable to see) and 1 = not blind (able to see). Alternatively, a researcher might decide to use finer gradations of visual ability by using some measure of visual acuity. For example, not all blind people are completely unable to see. So, instead of just two values, visual ability might take on more values: 0 = completely unable to see, 1 = can see a little (distinguish light and dark), 2 = can see somewhat (able to distinguish large objects only), and so forth. The key point of this example is that, in order to get a useful answer to the question of interest, the researcher must design a measure, so that there will be at least some variation in the visual ability variable. This means it must take on at least two values (have at least two categories, have at least two levels).

Suppose social life activity is operationalized (measured) in several ways: (1) hours of person-to-person contacts per week, (2) hours of telephone contacts per week, and (3) number of acquaintances and friends with whom the person socializes. After having obtained measures on a sample of 100 blind elderly people over the age of 64, you come up with the following findings: on average, these blind people (1) had 2.3 hours of person-to-person contacts per week; (2) had 45 minutes of telephone contacts per week, and (3) socialized with two different people during a week of observation.

this approach would be that it does not provide a comparison base (group) against which the effects of blindness, if any, can be evaluated. In other words, variations in visual capacity must be compared with variations in social life activity. An implication of this is that empirical facts take on their meaning and can be interpreted properly only in a comparative context. In fact, this can be taken as a cardinal rule of empirical research: *All research is comparative.*

Referring again to Research Scenario 2-5, it might be tempting to conclude that blindness leads to (causes) a substantial reduction on social activity (as measured through contacts), but this conclusion could be quite in error. Suppose that data were also obtained for a sample of healthy elderly people who lacked clinically significant visual impairments. Suppose further that the people without visual impairment had, on average, 1.8 hours of person-to-person contact and 25 minutes of phone contact per week and socialized with only one other person during a 1-week period of observation. Clearly, the earlier conclusion about the visually impaired elderly people now appears in a different light. Assuming that no **confounding variables** are involved (variables that could account for the observed differences in social life activity among blind versus nonblind elderly people), a more accurate interpretation of the data is that blindness may in fact help people make more social contacts. For some additional examples of the comparative approach in research, see Research Scenario 2-6. Later in this book we shall discuss in greater depth how studies can

be designed so that the necessary variation for making comparisons is achieved.

LIMITATIONS OF THE SCIENTIFIC EMPIRICAL APPROACH

So far in this chapter we have discussed the strengths of the scientific approach for research. The scientific (empirical) approach to knowledge development is also subject to certain limitations, which can be grouped as (1) general limitations, (2) specific design and measurement problems, (3) moral or ethical issues, and (4) the fact-value problem. A short discussion of each potential limitation contributes to an understanding of what the scientific approach can achieve, as well as what it cannot.

General Limitations

Probably the most important general limitation of the scientific approach is that scientific investigations are limited to phenomena about which objective empirical evidence is obtainable. Recall that objective evidence requires that the evidence can be reproduced by anyone who follows standardized, clearly documented procedures. Thus, many phenomena of interest to human beings (such as unique private experiences, conscious states, and religious beliefs) may not be amenable to scientific investigation. In addi-

Comparative Approaches to Research

If you wanted to study the often-mentioned phenomenon of a midlife crisis, you would need to compare people in their midlife years with younger and older people. Otherwise, you could not establish that people in midlife necessarily suffer from any kinds of psychologic problems that distinguish them from people in other age groups.

It has been well publicized that the initial symptoms of myocardial infarction tend to be misdiagnosed in women. This statement implies a comparison: women are misdiagnosed more often than men. To validly conclude that women are more likely to be misdiagnosed, it is important to study both men and women, comparing how they are diagnosed.

Suppose you are watching a TV ad in which one type of pain reliever is stated to be than others "better" in its pain relief properties. The validity of this type of statement cannot be assessed without a knowledge of how the pain reliever was compared with other pain relievers. Statements such as these should always be questioned: What research is there in support of the claim? More specifically, did the research design involve a comparison of pain relievers?

tion, because science is evidence based, its results and truths are, in a fundamental sense, always preliminary. Thus, although empirical evidence gives us a firm ground on which to base our beliefs and practices, nonetheless a researcher must always be willing to modify previous beliefs and practices if new evidence contradicts them. That is why what is considered best practice today may be overturned tomorrow, when better evidence comes along.

Specific Design and Measurement Problems

In addition to these general limitations, many studies also suffer from specific limitations in design and measurement, often unavoidable, which must be recognized by those who want to make use of the research findings to guide practice. Throughout this book, we shall focus much attention on critiquing research reports, with respect to what can or cannot be concluded on the basis of study procedures. Most individual research studies do not prove beyond a reasonable doubt the propositions that are being tested. This is because every research study has limitations in design or sampling or measurement, which affect what and how much can be learned, based on just that study. However, studies differ substantially in the quality of the evidence presented, and it is also important to be able to distinguish well-designed studies from poorly designed studies. For example, for reasons that will become clear later, if a researcher is interested in establishing cause-and-effect relationships, evidence from experimental studies is usually considered to be stronger than evidence from observational studies.

Studies also differ in the quality of the measurement procedures adopted. The problem of measurement in research is one of the most important challenges in enacting evidence-based practice. Measurement, together with theory and broader research design, is part of the critical foundation for the soundness of a research study. In evaluating research reports, we shall spend much time critiquing the adequacy of the measures that were used. For example, how good are measures of subjective states of patients, such as pain and satisfaction? What are the limitations to diagnostic tests in deciding what to do in clinical practice? No measure(s) used in research can be said to be without limitations. However, it is possible to establish whether an acceptable level of tradeoff between adequacy of measurement and limitations to measurement has been achieved, within the context of the purpose of the study.

Ultimately, no single study provides all the answers to a particular set of questions. Instead, scientific research usually proceeds by a series of **building blocks** (relatively small-scale studies that build progressively and sequentially on one another). A series of such studies may result in a progressively greater understanding of a phenomenon of interest. Also, greater belief can be placed in the findings of a research study if it has been **replicated,** i.e., if the same or a very similar study has been done more than once, and the same or similar findings have been reported.

Ethical Issues

Like any human activity, scientific research and conduct is subject to both legal and ethical rules that define acceptable practice. This is particularly true of clinical research involving human subjects who might be harmed by the interventions contemplated by the researcher(s). Moral and ethical issues limit the kinds of research studies that can be done. Given the central importance of ethical considerations in research involving human subjects, a separate chapter will be devoted to this topic (chapter 24). We have chosen to delay this discussion until after the reader has become familiar with many of the research strategies used in clinical studies. For instance, the specific ethical challenges of random assignment of subjects to different treatments, and the privacy issues involved in approaching patients (i.e., before their consent can be obtained), are better understood when the reader already knows the purpose and mechanisms of these procedures.

The Fact-Value Problem

The distinction between facts (assertions about what is empirically true) and values (attitudes or beliefs that are incorporated into preferences for certain actions) is important for scientific inquiry, but it is also complicated. We have already noted that objectivity in science refers primarily to the adoption of study procedures that can be replicated by others. That is, objectivity is never the property of any individual scientist but results from the social process of scientific discussion, mutual critique, and the openness of procedures to all who are competent in the field. From these discussions emerge assertions about what is empirically true. Examples of some currently accepted facts are these:

- The incidence rates for breast, colon, and lung cancers rise with age.
- Uninsured individuals have lower immunization rates.

- Skin breakdowns in bed-bound nursing home residents can largely be avoided through frequent changes of position and appropriate mattresses.

In other words, **facts** refer to statements about "what is the case," are subject to the normal process of scientific inquiry, and may change in response to new information. **Values,** by contrast, represent preferences for certain actions. For example, a voter may believe that a national health insurance system "ought to" or "should" be implemented, or that abortion should or should not remain legal. Science has no methods of objectively deciding questions of value. For instance, when a nurse or physician speaks out in favor of the legal availability of abortion, he or she is speaking on the basis of values as private citizens (see another example in Box 2-5).

Nonetheless, scientific inquiry is often relevant to our discussions of values. This is so because scientific research can investigate the consequences of holding certain values and pursuing alternative courses of action. For example, research can demonstrate the relative effectiveness in reducing teenage pregnancies of teaching abstinence, teaching contraceptive knowledge, providing contraceptives, or some combination of these strategies. The outcomes associated with the various strategies can be empirically demonstrated. The outcomes data are subject to the rules of evidence accepted in science.

Values and scientific research are also related in terms of the researcher's focus of inquiry and choice of topic. There is little question that the preferences and values of individual researchers (and funding agencies) determine what is being investigated. However, once a researcher settles on a topic, the research is conducted following rules of evidence that should be independent of the researcher's

---

BOX 2.5   Relevance of Scientific Evidence for an Ethical/Political Decision

Consider a 1998 ballot proposal in the State of Michigan: In a 1998 midterm election, Proposal B was a referendum for resident citizens to indicate their agreement or disagreement with a plan for assisted suicide. From what has been said so far, it is clear that the moral rightness or wrongness of assisted suicide legislation may be debated at length from philosophic perspectives, but the scientific method of research cannot resolve this value question directly. However, scientific research could address questions like these: What proportion of Michigan citizens support assisted suicide legislation? How many people would be likely to avail themselves of the assisted suicide option if it were legal? Does the availability of an assisted suicide option exert subtle pressures to commit suicide? All these questions refer to empirical issues that can be addressed using scientific methods. Although these questions do not directly address the moral rightness or wrongness of assisted suicide, they are relevant to such a discussion in the ways illustrated.

particular values. More to the point, it is the reproducibility of that research by other researchers, who may not share these values, that provides the objective corroboration of study findings. Thus, the term **value-free science** refers *only* to the establishment of means-and-ends or cause-and-effect relations.

As is the case in clinical practice, research involving human subjects must take into account the values and preferences of the subjects. In principle, this poses no special methodologic problems, even though it may pose ethical problems. For instance, the acceptability of treatment alternatives to human subjects surely varies depending on the cultural norms and religious convictions of the subjects. This clearly requires sensitivity and receptivity on the part of researchers and clinicians alike. However, in the basic logic of research, the researcher treats the values of subjects as given. They are, if you will, *social facts* (Durkheim, 1938). Behavioral scientists have, for many years, investigated the cultural values and convictions of certain subpopulations (e.g., Hispanics, Mormons) and related them to their actions, including their willingness to adopt recommended treatments or prevention behaviors. In this line of research, the values of subjects are treated as facts, whose relationship to health behaviors can be investigated like any other social phenomenon.

ALTERNATIVE PARADIGMS FOR NURSING SCIENCE

Many aspects of health-related and illness-related human phenomena can be studied in research. Some key foci of nursing research are biophysiology, attitudes, and behavior of individuals or groups of individuals. In the 1980s especially, nursing researchers and scholars debated the appropriateness of different **paradigms** (approaches to research based on certain assumptions about the nature of reality) for nursing research. We provide here an overview of two general paradigms for nursing research, including a discussion of the fit of scientific methods within these paradigms. These two paradigms are often referred to as **quantitative** and **qualitative** research. We think these labels are somewhat misleading. There are quantitative and statistical approaches to the analysis of qualitative and categorical data (Haberman, 1978; Haberman, 1979; Agresti, 1990), and there are qualitative and nonnumerical approaches to designing studies and analyzing data that follow the rules of evidence normally used in quantitative studies (Yin, 1994). Probably a better distinction would be between an approach to research that models itself after the natural (and quantitative social) sciences and an approach to research that sees itself in the tradition of the humanities and historical research.

Quantitative Approaches to Research

Most quantitatively oriented health and nurse researchers believe that the general principles of evidence developed in the natural sciences, particularly the experimental sciences, provide an ideal that should be emulated. Note that we mentioned general *principles* of evidence, not specific *methods* of measurement, sampling, or analysis strategies. The latter do, of course, differ from discipline to discipline. The general principles of evidence underlying the experimental sciences have been widely discussed in the philosophy of science literature, particularly in the tradition known as the philosophy of **analytic empiricism.** Variants of analytic empiricism include **logical positivism, conventionalism,** and **falsificationism.**[3]

At the heart of the empiricist philosophies are several assumptions about reality, our perception of reality, and our ability to explain it. One major assumption of empiricism is that an **objective reality** exists independently of the human observer. This assumption is more or less shared by all scientists; in this sense, scientists are philosophic realists (Popper, 1994). A second assumption is that this reality is capable of being measured and studied by the methods of scientific research. In particular, researchers and scientists in the empiricist tradition believe that numbers can be assigned to many phenomena that are being studied, resulting in quantifiable measures of the characteristics of these phenomena. Such scientists hope to be able to express the relationships among these quantified measures in terms of "laws" that are embodied in mathematically or statistically formulated equations. Although such quantification is clearly a goal of many scientists, the empiricist approach is not necessarily quantitative. There is no requirement, for instance, that outcomes of experiments be quantifiable.

Most scientists in the empiricist tradition do share the assumption that parts of a phenomenon can fruitfully be studied separately from the whole of the phenomenon. For example, a person's adjustment to (coping with) cancer may involve multiple dimensions, ranging from medical prognosis and physiologic responses to the progression of the disease and its treatment to psychologic

---

[3] An in-depth discussion of these schools of the philosophy of science is beyond the scope of this text. Interested readers are referred to the classic discussions of Nagel (1961) and Suppes (1977).

coping abilities and socially acquired views and values concerning the threat of death. In the view of scientists in the tradition of analytic empiricism, all researchers, of necessity, must always carve out some limited array of phenomena for study. For practical reasons it is not possible to design a research study that addresses everything there is to know about a given phenomenon. It may well be true that on some level "everything is connected to everything." That, however, is not a useful starting point for research. For practical reasons we must treat reality, in some respects, as "loosely coupled." In this view, social scientists can fruitfully study human organizations (such as corporations, hospitals, universities) without necessarily first studying the individual psychology of all the persons who are part of these organizations. Or, biologists can study living cells without first studying nuclear physics, and so forth. The whole of human experience can then be understood by studying different aspects at a time.

Qualitative Approaches to Research

Qualitative researchers differ in their basic philosophic views about reality and the rules of evidence to follow in research. However, certain common themes and assumptions are shared by most of them. One basic issue concerns the goals. For example, qualitative researchers do not investigate the chemical and biophysiologic processes of the human body. Instead, they concentrate on human behavior and human consciousness, which can be understood in terms of psychologic processes of the mind or the norms and preferences that arise out of the lived experience of human beings. Many qualitative researchers believe these social and psychologic processes to be historically specific and unique, and thus they reject the empirical search for laws in human behavior—an approach that is seen as ahistorical by many qualitative researchers.

It may be noted here that rejection of laws of human behavior does not necessarily entail the rejection of a search for regularities in human behavior. For instance, social norms in particular societies and population groups surely affect the regularity of human behavior. Thus, when you greet a person passing you on the street, 9 out of 10 times he or she will greet back. But such norms are group specific, whereas laws of human behavior would apply to all human beings. In any case, most empiricists implicitly or explicitly aim to uncover regularities and patterns of human behavior in the same way they look for regularities in the biochemistry and physiology of the human body to understand the causes of disease. *Thus, while quantitative researchers posit a fundamental unity of science, qualitative researchers tend to believe that the study of human behavior and consciousness requires a different approach that is historical and interpretive.*

What makes research qualitative? Traditionally, when people talk about qualitative research, they mean research that focuses on narratives and their interpretations—research that shuns the use of mathematics and statistics in the design and analysis. To some degree, these distinctions are artificial, because numerical and statistical strategies can certainly play a supporting role in interpretive analysis, as when a researcher uses a computerized program for content analysis. A more important distinction between qualitative and quantitative research derives from their respective approaches to measurement. Qualitative researchers are often skeptical of the possibility of standardized, quantitative measurement because of a concern that such approaches sacrifice context-specific information, making it more difficult or impossible to interpret the results. For instance, in a standardized depression measure like the Center for Epidemiologic Studies-Depression (CES-D), respondents are asked to indicate how often in the past 2 weeks they felt sad or were fearful. Respondents are given predetermined answer categories like "rarely or none of the time" or "almost all of the time" (Radloff, 1977). But how can we know, a qualitative researcher might ask, that being fearful means the same thing to different respondents, or that "almost all of the time" corresponds to similar actual frequencies across different subjects? As will be seen later in this book (in chapters 14 and 18), researchers in the quantitative and qualitative traditions of measurement attach different levels of importance to this question.

Beyond their shared historical or interpretive outlook, qualitative researchers tend to view the empiricist approach as inherently reductionistic. A **reductionistic** view is one that believes all human health problems can ultimately be reduced to biochemical processes and problems. Thus, if a treating clinician or researcher is able to find ways to counteract various malfunctions of the biochemical and physiologic processes in the body, any malfunction could potentially be fixed. By contrast, qualitative research approaches assert that the whole of human experience cannot be understood by studying only its constituent parts. Instead, the major emphasis in qualitative research approaches is on the **lived experience** of human beings as a subjective (not objective) reality. Reality in this view emerges in the process of interaction with those who participate in research.

There are many approaches to qualitative research, including phenomenology, grounded theory, ethnography, hermeneutics, and others.[4] A detailed discussion of these schools of thought is beyond the scope of this book.

Quantitative and Qualitative Research: Alternatives or Complements?

As researchers with backgrounds in clinical nursing and health services research, we take an eclectic approach to these methodologic and philosophic battles. Although we have strong philosophic convictions of our own, we believe that researchers need to have a pragmatic mind set. That means that research methods must be judged primarily in terms of their *adequacy in solving the problem at hand*. For instance, if you want to know whether screening for prostate cancer reduces overall mortality in men, you will need evidence from large-scale, population-based cohort studies (the characteristics of cohort studies will be discussed in detail in chapter 9). These studies inevitably use quantitative measurement and statistical analysis strategies. By contrast, if you want to know why some elderly caregivers and their care recipients reject the use of formal services even though they may be freely available, you may want to explore attitudes towards service use among caregivers. Before such attitudes can be measured in a standardized way, one would need to allow members of the target population to voice their views, concerns, and opinions freely. In that way, any instrument developed for the purpose of measuring the attitudes is more likely to truly reflect the range of opinions existing in the target population (Collins et al., 1991).

In general, we maintain that neither of the two basic paradigms in nursing research should have a lock on our attention. Instead, we see them as complementary. You will notice, however, that the primary focus of this text is on quantitative methods, because our goal is to aid the reader in understanding research that supports clinical decision making. As a clinician you need to evaluate evidence concerning the relative success or failure of different interventions. If you are responsible for a nursing home population, you may have to decide which pressure-reducing mattresses to choose for bed-bound residents. In a health maintenance organization, you may be required to monitor and guide patients with diabetes to increase their adherence to the recommended treatment plan. Working in a cardiac rehabilitation program, you may have to develop and evaluate new interventions that increase the chance that patients will remain with the rehabilitation program. As a nurse

practitioner with prescriptive authority you will need to be able to evaluate research reports on the efficacy of various drugs if you wish to go beyond taking others' opinions about the drugs at face value. In all these examples, we are dealing with the prediction of outcomes, after the introduction of some kind of intervention. It is in these areas where quantitative research has its particular strengths.

In sum, we see a strong and important role for qualitative research, particularly in the development of instruments and the exploratory phase of psychosocial interventions. However, we believe that understanding a patient's lived experience, although very important for addressing certain phenomena of concern in nursing and health care, does not offer all there is to know about patients' health or illness.

OVERVIEW OF THE RESEARCH PROCESS

Throughout this book, it will be emphasized that not all forms of evidence are equally strong. The strength of the evidence depends very much on the approach a researcher takes and, more specifically, on the decisions that are made at each step of the research process. When you read scientific, data-based articles in nursing and health-related fields, you will quickly note that the formats of such articles follow a certain formula, or generally recognizable format. In particular, most articles are divided into clearly marked sections, each focusing on one of the major steps in the research process. This enables the reader to judge more easily how the evidence was assembled to address the research questions. Each step of the research process involves many decisions by the researcher. That is, when a researcher submits his or her theories, hypotheses, or questions to testing, this is not just a passive activity of seeing what does or does not pan out. Instead, researchers are actively engaged in marshaling and shaping the evidence. The strength of that evidence depends on the appropriateness of these decisions, the adequacy of which readers must be able to judge. For now, we briefly outline the key research steps, with the intent of providing an overview that will guide much of the remaining discussion in this textbook (Figure 2-3).

Step 1: Problem Formulation

The starting point in research is the formulation of a research problem. Research problems are commonly formulated as either research question(s) or research hypotheses,

---

[4] Interested readers are referred to Guba (1990) and Streubert & Carpenter (1999).

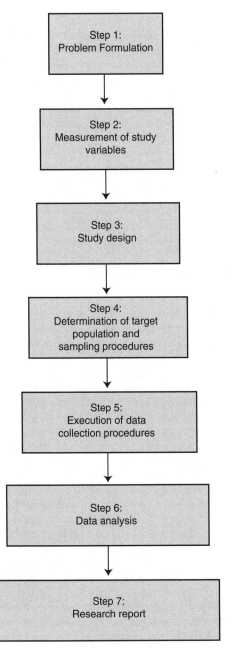

FIGURE 2.3 Flowchart illustrating the research process.

and are derived from theoretic or practical problems. As already discussed, research always takes place in some theoretic context, but this does not mean that any and all clinical problems and hypotheses must be theory driven (derived from or embedded in theories). Clinically oriented research often starts with problems encountered in clinical practice. For example, during the 1980s, nurse researchers wondered whether the site for insulin injection (e.g., arm, thigh, or abdomen) made any difference in the management of diabetes. Various experiments were designed to test how well patients did with injecting insulin in different sites. This type of research does not necessarily require justification with reference to any elaborate theory.

Step 2: Measurement of Study Variables

Once a researcher has settled on the problem as well as the concepts and variables to be investigated, the next step is to define or devise measurement procedures for the concepts in question. **Measurement** is usually defined as the assignment of numbers to objects or attributes of objects according to some sort of rule system. In some cases, the rules may be obvious or simple; e.g., the use of a ruler to measure the length of an object. Alternatively, they may be complex, such as rules involving the weighted sums of number codes to reflect questionnaire responses. This process of operationalization and measurement involves considerations of both validity and reliability. **Validity in measurement** refers to this question: Does the measurement procedure indeed get at the concept in question? For example, does a particular scale purporting to measure depression in fact measure this concept and no other related concepts, such as stress or anxiety? **Reliability** refers to the reproducibility of results when several measurements are taken of the same phenomena. In other words, do repeated measurements on different occasions, at different locations, by different observers, using alternative methods, questions, items, and so forth yield consistent results for phenomena that can be assumed to be stable and unchanging?

Step 3: Study Design

A research design is a plan that is specifically conceived and implemented to bring empirical evidence to bear on a research problem, question, or hypothesis. The design suggests what observations to make, when to make them, and how to analyze the (quantitative) representations of the observations (variables). A basic distinction between variables is that of **active** (capable of being manipulated or controlled by the researcher) and **attribute** (observable, but not able to be manipulated by the researcher) variables. Examples of active variables include interventions such as medication dosages, timing of treatments, and content of education programs. Attribute variables include things the researcher cannot control, such as a research participant's eye color or age. Note that control in research studies refers not only to the researcher's ability to manipulate treatment/independent variables but also to control over the environment in which the study takes place. Several chapters in this book will deal with design issues.

Step 4: Determination of Target Population and Sampling Procedures

Although one may consider sampling procedures to be part of the research design, the questions raised about sampling are sufficiently distinct to receive treatment as a separate step. Researchers must always ask themselves two questions. First, what is the **target population** to which the findings should ideally be generalizable? In a certain sense, researchers are never interested only in the data at hand. What they really hope to do is to make broader statements that go beyond the study context. Whatever the findings, if they pertained only to the data set under study, they would hardly be worth reporting. The whole point of doing research is to learn something that can be applied to new, future situations. Thus, the second question is always this: What confidence do we have that the findings in a particular study sample signify processes or causal relationships that hold in broader contexts as well? Or, given the sampling procedures adopted, to which population(s) can the findings actually be generalized?

Step 5: Execution of Data Collection Procedures

This step deals with quality control issues as well as the rights of human subjects that must be addressed through the study protocol and management of the data collection effort. This step is crucial to the success of any study and ultimately decides about the quality of the data obtained, yet, it remains one of the least discussed in the research literature.

Step 6: Data Analysis

In quantitative studies, data analysis relies heavily on statistical analysis tools. Particularly for studies with large study samples, the use of statistical modeling and numerical analysis is imperative because narrative analysis becomes impractical. Regardless of the types of data collected and the orientation of the researchers, data analysis always involves two steps: a summary of the results (focusing on the patterns found in the data) and interpretation.

Step 7: Research Report

The final step in the research process is the writing of the research report. In addition to reporting on the major research steps just listed, a research report provides the context for the research problem and for the interpretation of the results. This is accomplished through a literature review covering previous research on the same or related questions, discussing the critical concepts in question, and reporting on gaps in knowledge or methodologic shortcoming of previous research.

Published journal articles tend to follow a certain writing formula. Its purpose is to inform the reader about all aspects of the research process. Ideally, a research report should give the reader a good grasp of the methods and procedures followed in the conduct of research. This fulfills two major purposes: (1) to provide the reader with enough information to evaluate the strength of the research and its results and (2) to allow other researchers to reproduce the study in order to subject the hypotheses to further testing.

Suggested Activities

1. Visit the NONPF web site at *http://www.nonpg.org* to review key resources concerning research activities in advanced clinical practice.
2. Visit the National Institute for Nursing Research (NINR) web site at *http://www.nih.ninr.gov* to review key funding priorities for nursing research. To what extent do you feel that these priorities do or do not reflect what should be studied to improve clinical practice? What nursing research questions do you have that may be reflected in these priorities?
3. Do the following self-assessment check of your understanding of key content of this chapter: For each of the following statements, identify the independent and dependent variables. If possible, also identify what are *most likely* to be the levels (categories) of the variables:
   a. The purpose of the study was to test the effects of meditation versus progressive relaxation techniques on sleep pattern improvement.
   b. Nurse researchers have become increasingly concerned with the impact of smoking among teenage girls on cancer rates.
   c. This study explored the relationships between health status, career mobility, and gender.
   d. We explored the impact of age and exercise pattern on functional status improvements and depression.
   e. Little is known about why some people who smoke get COPD, while others who smoke and drink alcohol daily do not.
4. Do the following self-assessment check of your understanding of key content of this chapter: For each of the following hypotheses, identify the independent and dependent variables, whether the hypothesis is directional

or nondirectional, and whether the hypothesis is simple or complex:

a. Physicians spend less time explaining treatment options to patients compared to nurse practitioners.

b. Teenage girls are more likely to be smokers compared to middle-aged men.

c. Pain relief measures are more effective when implemented before the onset of severe pain instead of when pain is already severe.

d. Older nurses are more likely to express a need for continuing education as compared to younger nurses.

e. Depression and anxiety are significant predictors of health services utilization.

Suggested Readings

Brown, J. K., Whittemore, K. T., & Knapp, T. R. (2000). Is arm span an accurate measure of height in young and middle-aged adults? *Clinical Nursing Research, 9,* 1, 84–94.

Clark, E. M., Lipe, A. W., & Bilbrey, M. (1998). Use of music to decrease aggressive behaviors in people with dementia. *Journal of Gerontological Nursing, 24, 1,* 10–17.

Collins, C. E., Stommel, M,. & King, S. (1991). Assessment of the attitudes of family caregivers toward community services. *The Gerontologist, 31, 6,* 756–761.

Kassirer, J. P. (1989). Diagnostic reasoning. *Annals of Internal Medicine, 110, 11,* 893–900.

References

Agresti, A. (1990). *Categorical data analysis.* New York: John Wiley.

Brink, P. J., & Wood, M. J. (1998). *Advanced design in nursing research* (2nd ed.). Thousand Oaks, CA: Sage.

Brown, J. K., Whittemore, K. T., & Knapp, T. R. (2000). Is arm span an accurate measure of height in young and middle-aged adults? *Clinical Nursing Research, 9,* 1, 84–94.

Clark, E. M., Lipe, A. W., & Bilbrey, M. (1998). Use of music to decrease aggressive behaviors in people with dementia. *Journal of Gerontological Nursing, 24, 1,* 10–17.

Collins, C. E., Stommel, M,. & King, S. (1991). Assessment of the attitudes of family caregivers toward community services. *The Gerontologist, 31, 6,* 756–761.

Durkheim, E. (1938). *The rules of sociological methods.* (Translation of *Les Regles de la Methode Sociologique,* 1895). New York: Free Press.

Fawcett, J. (1995). *Analysis and evaluation of conceptual models of nursing* (3rd ed.). Philadelphia: F. A. Davis.

Guba, E. G. (1990). *The paradigm dialogue.* Newbury Park, CA: Sage.

Haberman, S.J. (1978). *Analysis of qualitative data* (Vol. 1). New York: Academic Press.

Haberman, S.J. (1979). *Analysis of qualitative data* (Vol. 2). New York: Academic Press.

Herrnstein, R. J., & Murray, C. A.. (1996). *The bell curve: Intelligence and class structure in American life.* New York: Simon & Schuster.

Hinshaw, A. S., Feetham, S. L., & Shaver, J. L. (1999). *Handbook of clinical nursing research.* Thousand Oaks, CA: Sage.

Kassirer, J. P. (1989). Diagnostic reasoning. *Annals of Internal Medicine, 110, 11,* 893–900.

Luepker, R. V., Rosamund, W. D., Murphy, R., Prafka, J. M., Folsom, A. R., McGovern, P. G., & Blackburn, H. (1993). Socioeconomic status and coronary heart disease risk factor trend: the Minnesota heart survey. *Circulation, 88,* 2171–2179.

Nagel, E. (1961). *The structure of science: Problems in the logic of scientific explanation.* New York: Harcourt, Brace & World.

Pawson, R., & Tilley, N. (1997). *Realistic evaluation.* Thousand Oaks, CA: Sage.

Pender, N.J. (1996). *Health promotion in nursing practice* (2nd ed.). Stamford, CT: Appleton & Lange.

Popper, K. M. (1994). *The myth of the framework: In defense of science and rationality.* London: Routledge.

Radloff, L. S. (1977). The CES-D Scale. A self report depression scale for research in the general population. *Applied Psychological Measurement, 1,* 385–401.

Rossi, P. H., & Freeman, H. E. (1993). *Evaluation: A systematic approach.* Thousand Oaks, CA: Sage.

Stevens, S. S. (1946). On the theory of scales of measurement. *Science, 103,* 677–680.

Streubert, H. J., and Carpenter, D. R. (1999). *Qualitative research in nursing: Advancing the humanistic imperative* (2nd ed.). Philadelphia: Lippincott.

Suppes, F. (1977). *The structure of scientific theories* (2nd ed.). Urbana, IL: University of Illinois Press.

Wittgenstein, L. (1958). *Philosophical investigations.* New York: Macmillan.

Yin, R. K. (1996). *Case study research: Design and methods* (2nd ed.). Thousand Oaks, CA: Sage.

2

The Design and Analysis of Experimental Studies (Clinical Trials)

CHAPTER 3   **The Logic of Causal Inference in Experimental Studies**

THE ROLE OF CLINICAL TRIALS AND INTERVENTION STUDIES IN CLINICAL PRACTICE

In Part II of this book, we turn to the design and analysis of **experimental** studies: studies that are conducted to examine cause-and-effect relationships between variables. For example, nurses are naturally interested in establishing whether or not nursing care (independent variable) results in (or causes) one or more positive outcomes (dependent variable), such as patients' improved self-care ability, satisfaction, or lessening of adverse health events (Box 3-1). Experimental studies are also referred to as **intervention studies** or **clinical trials** or **randomized clinical trials (RCTs)** in the medical literature. There is general agreement among scientists that experimental studies provide the best evidence about cause-and-effect relationships, for reasons that will be discussed later in this chapter.

At first blush, starting with a discussion of experimental studies seems an odd choice. A cursory review of the nursing and medical literature quickly reveals that the vast majority of studies are not experimental. True experimental studies are exacting, may interfere with the regular demands of clinical practice, may pose ethical challenges, and are resource-intensive ways of studying the effectiveness of clinical interventions (Sidani & Braden, 1998). So why begin here? Because experimental study designs provide a useful comparison point for the discussion of other, nonexperimental research designs, especially if they are used to investigate cause-and-effect relationships. But first, we set the stage with a brief discussion of the relevance of experimental studies to clinical practice.

Advanced practice nurses and other types of health care providers are concerned every day with assessment, diagnostic, planning, intervention, and evaluation activities for patients. The care of a given patient should always start with an assessment of a patient's chief (presenting) problem, the gathering of data from a physical exam, the relevant history, and an assessment of the psychosocial and cultural context. If the assessment phase concludes with a clear diagnosis of the presenting problem, a clinician will then plan and initiate some type of treatment plan (intervention), which is anticipated to be effective in improving or alleviating the patient's presenting problem.

As most clinicians are well aware, the effectiveness of an intervention is usually not assured. Many factors, both foreseen and unseen, can influence whether or not (and to what extent) the intervention actually works to produce a certain outcome. For example, a nurse practitioner may prescribe cromolyn sodium nasal spray three or four times daily to a patient with seasonal allergies (allergic rhinitis). Such a decision is based on clinical practice and knowledge of drug therapies, which in turn is based on evidence provided through RCTs. However, the prescription may or may not be effective for a particular patient. There are many reasons for such varied patient responses. In fact, even if clinical trials have shown the effectiveness of a drug beyond any reasonable doubt, such evidence tells us only what will happen *on average* or *with most patients*. It does not guarantee that any given individual will respond positively. Nonetheless, even though certainty about the effectiveness of an intervention may not be available in individual cases, it is clearly of great clinical value to know which interventions have a high probability of success and which do not.

The basic question in evaluating the effectiveness of an intervention is this: Does the chosen intervention accomplish the intended end(s)? There are additional refinements of this basic cause-and-effect question. For whom (which population groups or individuals) does the intervention

---

BOX 3.1   Variables and Levels of Variables

Because it is a frequent source of confusion, we pause here to reflect again on the relationship between variable and its categories. In the case of an experiment, the independent variable comprises all intervention or treatment modalities, including the absence of treatment or control condition. When there is only one treatment or intervention, it is compared with a control group in which no intervention takes place. In that case, the independent variable can vary between two categories or levels: absence or presence of treatment. Experiments in which several treatment levels are compared simultaneously are actually more common. For instance, in drug trials, investigators typically compare the effects of a drug given at several dosage levels. Each dosage level represents a category of the independent or intervention variable. Thus, it is the intervention or independent variable whose categories define the groups of subjects to be compared in the experimental study.

work or not work? Under what circumstances does it work or not work? When a clinician implements an intervention, he or she implicitly or explicitly assumes that a cause-and-effect relationship has already been demonstrated. For example, a nurse practitioner who prescribes cromolyn sodium for allergic rhinitis engages in causal reasoning of the following form: "If I prescribe cromolyn sodium (cause), my patient will be likely to experience a reduction in symptoms of allergic rhinitis (effect)." It follows from this and other similar examples that a clinician must always be prepared to demonstrate the effectiveness of what he or she is doing, or to make appropriate and timely adjustments to clinical practice, if new evidence on outcomes casts doubt on the effectiveness of past practice.

More recently, the connection between empirical evidence and clinical practice has become an especially critical aspect of advanced clinical practice. But how are cause-and-effect relationships best demonstrated? As it turns out, there are specific criteria for objectively establishing cause-and-effect relationships. These criteria are incorporated into various experimental study designs and, to a lesser extent, in various other types of designs that are collectively referred to as *nonexperimental*.

CRITERIA FOR ESTABLISHING CAUSALITY

Principles of causality underpin most experimental design features, many of which will be discussed in this and the following chapters. For many years, philosophers of science have debated what the specific criteria should be for inferring causality. This debate has been strongly shaped by the tradition of Western empiricist philosophy,[1] which undergirds the empirical science perspective. In turn, this perspective provides the foundation for much of the contemporary empirical research in nursing and medicine.

In more recent years, debates about causality have continued to generate strong interest and have increasingly involved practitioners of the behavioral and medical sciences (Blalock, 1964; Cook & Campbell, 1979; Susser, 1986; Kassirer & Koppelman, 1987; Susser, 1991). It is important to note that when people speak about causes in everyday language, they usually have some agent in mind that actively effects changes in some other entity: persons, events, materials, and so on. A classic example is the germ theory of disease, which views infectious diseases to be caused by the presence and activities of viruses or bacteria in the human body. Three basic ideas are incorporated in the germ theory of disease. These ideas are also common to most conceptions of causality, and they constitute criteria by which to judge the presence or absence of a cause-and-effect relationship: (1) association, (2) time-order, and (3) direction (Susser, 1991). We discuss each of these concepts in turn.

Association

Association refers to the concept that the absence and presence of a putative (presumed) cause must be associated with the parallel absence or presence of the effect. For example, consider the disease of tuberculosis (TB). The presence of *Mycobacterium tuberculosis* (presumed cause of TB) in the lung, if left untreated, coincides with the development of characteristic tubercles (rounded, gray translucent masses encircled by connective cells) in the lung. In turn, the development of these characteristic tubercles in the lung is associated with the presence of *M. tuberculosis* in the lung. Also, the absence of *M. tuberculosis* is associated with an absence of TB-characteristic tubercles.

Time-order

Time-order refers to the need for a presumed cause to precede (in time) a presumed effect. For example, as applied to TB, time-order refers to the fact that the intrusion of the bacteria into the lung occurs first, before the development of the tubercles. *M. tuberculosis* (cause of TB) must first be present in the lung before TB-characteristic tubercles can form.

Direction

Direction refers to the one-way nature of presumed cause-and-effect relationships. Applied to the TB example, direction means that the presence of *M. tuberculosis* in the lung can lead to the development of TB-characteristic tubercles, but TB-characteristic tubercles (which enclose, or serve as a storehouse for, *M. tuberculosis*) do not cause the bacteria to develop in the first place. Thus, we think of a causal relationship as an *asymmetric relationship,* in which the causes are certain events that are *necessary (needed) conditions* for other events (the effects) to happen.

Sufficient Condition

These criteria for causation need some refinement and expansion in light of the multicausal nature of most disease

---

[1] An in-depth discussion of this philosophical debate is beyond the scope of this book, but interested readers are referred to the seminal, classic writings of David Hume in the 18th century (1739–1740) and John Stuart Mill in the 19th century (1843).

processes. For example, the presence of a certain virus or bacterium may well be a necessary condition for the development of a disease, but often it is not a *sufficient condition*. Healthy people are continuously exposed to disease-causing agents, but they do not necessarily become ill because their immune systems can cope with the intruding agents. Counteracting forces (agents), such as a healthy immune system, can offset the effects of the disease-causing agents. Many disease prevention and health promotion interventions are directed toward bolstering or developing the conditions that counteract natural and artificially generated threats to health.

Deterministic versus Probabilistic Relationship

The multicausal nature of human disease and health processes is also one reason why empirical evidence concerning causal relationships is rarely, if ever, **deterministic** (certain) but instead is **probabilistic** (less than certain, subject to chance). Any exposure to a given disease-causing agent or a given therapeutic intervention usually results in *a distribution of responses in different human beings*. For example, during influenza season, some people may become ill with the flu while others may not. Influenza vaccination, a key public health intervention, is intended to increase the likelihood (probability) that fewer people will become ill with influenza. The vaccination can be seen as a counteracting agent to the cause-and-effect relationship between exposure to the influenza myxovirus and the development of influenza symptoms.

The probabilistic nature of cause-and-effect relationships applies to a wide array of processes of interest in health care. These include both biophysiologic processes (e.g., patient responses to a given amount of an analgesic) and behavioral/psychologic processes (e.g., patient responses to learning about the diagnosis of a serious illness, or adherence to professionally prescribed therapeutic regimens). For this reason, *statistical* reasoning plays a large role in medical and health care research. **Statistics** involves mathematical theories of *uncertainty* and *probability,* which are used to model the nature and strength of the relationships among variables. For example, many clinical variables, such as serum low-density lipoprotein (LDL) cholesterol readings, vary for reasons that are partly unknown. Understanding how best to intervene with patients who have elevated serum LDL levels depends on separating *systematic* relationships (such as type of diet) from *unpredictable* variation. By definition, we can establish cause-and-effect relationships only for the systematic, or predictable, part of a relationship.

Thus, research on health care interventions establishes what is likely to happen on average or in most cases, rather than what will happen for a given individual. For example, patients who regularly ingest diets that are high in saturated fat are more likely to have elevated serum LDL levels. However, for reasons that are not yet fully understood, not all patients who have diets high in saturated fat will have high LDL levels, and not all patients who have diets low in saturated fat will have low LDL levels. Data from the National Cancer Institute show that 86% of all persons with new diagnoses of invasive lung cancer will die of the disease within 5 years (National Cancer Institute, 2002). However, many individuals will beat the odds and survive longer, for reasons that are not yet fully understood.

Defining Cause-and-Effect Relationships

Given these refinements to the criteria for cause-and-effect relationships (association, time-order, and direction), Box 3-2 presents the following five (expanded) criteria as both essential and most germane to defining cause-and-effect relationships in health care practice and research.

As the last example makes clear, it is not enough to just observe an association (covariation) of two phenomena, or to observe an earlier event followed by a later event, in order to establish a causal relationship. Other factors that could account for the observed relationships between variables must be considered. In fact, a main goal in designing a research study is precisely this: *to rule out the possibility that variables, other than the ones hypothesized, caused the effect in question.* A clinical research study possesses design validity to the extent that it allows one to conclude that the intervention or treatment has indeed caused the change in the outcome, or dependent variable. Studies that possess these qualities are said to have high internal validity (Campbell & Stanley, 1966), or **design validity.**[2]

Research Design

By now, the reader may be wondering what we mean by "research design." A **research design** is a plan according to which the research must be carried out. It specifies what observations to make (which variables to focus on), how to make them (which measurement procedures to adopt), and

---

[2]We prefer the concept of *design validity* to the more commonly used concept of *internal validity,* which was introduced by Campbell and Stanley (1966). Especially when contrasted to *measurement validity,* a term introduced in later chapters, the use of the term *design validity* can reduce confusion between the two. Furthermore, we think it preferable to avoid the term *external validity* altogether and use *generalizability* instead.

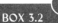

BOX 3.2   Five Essential Criteria for Defining Cause-and-Effect Relationships

Covariation (Association)

The presumed cause (X) and effect (Y) must vary together.

Example: Osteoporosis (X) is widely believed to be a major cause of functional disability (Y) in older adults. If this is so, then people with lower bone densities should have higher rates of functional disability than those with higher bone densities. In other words, different levels of bone density must vary systematically with degrees of functional ability or disability.

Temporal Order (Time-Order)

Cause-and-effect relationships assume the existence of a time order, in which the cause must precede (come before) the effect.

Example: Depression among caregivers of ill relatives is a public health concern for several reasons, including the likelihood of an ill relative eventually being institutionalized in a nursing home. If caregiver depression (X) causes more caregivers to institutionalize (Y) their dependent relative, depression (X) must be shown to occur before the decision to institutionalize (Y).

Congruity/Coherence (Direction)

Outcome changes must be logically related to the intervention and in the direction specified. This causality criterion refers to the fact that causal inference is, in part, based on theoretic, not just empirical, criteria. In other words, there must be a theoretic explanation for why the intervention would have the observed effect on the outcome. Otherwise, one has established only an empirical pattern (prediction) of the type: if X, then Y. Thus, causal relationships encompass both prediction and explanation.

*Example: In a recent study, researchers found that the daily intake of aspirin reduces a woman's chances of contracting ovarian cancer. For this finding to be taken as evidence of a causal relationship (discussed as "taking aspirin prevents ovarian cancer"), additional study (**replication**) is needed. Furthermore, this finding also needs to be explained in terms of a theoretically plausible mechanism by which aspirin affects the occurrence of ovarian cancer.*

Contiguity

The observable change in the outcome (in response to the intervention or exposure to a risk factor) comes "fairly soon" after the intervention or exposure. Strictly speaking, this is not a requirement for there to be a causal relationship, but contiguity of a cause and its effect surely makes it easier to infer causality. In general, it is much more difficult to establish causal relations when the effects are delayed.

Example: Suppose a researcher wants to find out whether providing hypertensive patients with an information booklet on hypertension and its treatment causes patient knowledge about hypertension to increase over baseline levels of knowledge. It would be important to obtain knowledge scores just before and shortly after the patient review of the booklet to provide the most convincing evidence of the effects of the booklet on knowledge. By contrast, it is much harder to establish a causal relationship between nutritional intakes (over long periods of time) on health outcomes that often occur many years after a nutritional pattern has been established.

Exclusion of Plausible Alternatives

To establish a cause-and-effect relationship between two variables (X causes Y), it must be possible to eliminate plausible alternative explanations (Q causes Y) for the observed relationship (this is also referred to as the **exclusion of rival hypotheses**).

Example: Assume that available data unequivocally (clearly) show that depressed caregivers are more likely to institutionalize the ill relatives they care for, compared with nondepressed caregivers. Even if this association and the temporal sequence (the depression is shown to occur before institutionalization) are well established, this is not sufficient evidence to show that it is the caregiver depression that "causes" caregivers to institutionalize their relative. It may, for instance, be the case that depressed caregivers are disproportionately poor and are more likely to receive Medicaid, which covers a nursing home stay for a disabled relative. If this is so, the association between caregiver depression and institutionalization is not causal per se. It is the insurance status that makes the "true" difference in whether or not a relative is placed in a nursing home.

when to make them. The research design also determines which, if any, variables will be actively manipulated by the researcher (e.g., the deliberate introduction or withholding of treatments and interventions) and how the subjects are to be selected from a target population of interest. Finally, a research design also specifies how much control will be exerted, or can be exerted, over the environment in which the study takes place. Research designs provide blueprints, or systems of rules, to be followed in the conduct of a study. Thus, the more detailed and well-specified a research plan is, the more easily can other researchers reproduce the study. Thus, well-specified research designs are key to **reproducible evidence.** From this, it follows that in designing a research study, the researcher is not simply a passive receptacle for information but an active organizer of the evidence into a coherent, meaningful pattern. Even in purely observational studies, the researcher must still make fundamental choices about the what, when, and where of the observations.

CRITICAL FEATURES OF EXPERIMENTAL STUDIES: CONTROL GROUPS AND/OR CONTROL OCCASIONS AND RANDOMIZATION

As mentioned earlier, experimental design conditions embody or incorporate principles of causality. A sound experimental research design allows strong inference (Platt, 1964) about causal relationships between variables. This can be illustrated using a non–health-related, but real-life, scenario (Research Scenario 3-1).

Bearing in mind that we have not yet discussed the key features of experimental designs, would you consider this class experiment to be a good experiment? To get a handle on this question, let's start with the fundamental problem posed here. The point of the experiment is to see how the amount of daily water addition (the independent variable) affects variation in the growth of a plant (the dependent variable). (Tip: Before you read on, make a list of all the questions you might have about this experiment. Is the experiment likely to give a satisfactory answer to the research question?)

Before anything else is discussed, you will first want to make sure that both of these key variables are measured at a reasonable level of accuracy. Are all the students instructed to use a standardized measuring cup for the water? How about the more complex problem of measuring the length of a bean sprout? Does it require pulling the plant out of the soil, laying it flat on a surface, and measuring the length from

RESEARCH SCENARIO 3.1

Water's Effects on Bean Sprouts
A high school teacher announces that the class will do an experiment to test the effects of watering on the growth of bean sprouts. She distributes 10 soybeans to each of five students in class, and she instructs them to plant the seeds in a pot at home and water them according to the following regimen: first student, no water; second student, 1 deciliter (dL) per day; third student, 2 dL per day; fourth student, 3 dL per day; fifth student, 4 dL per day. For 4 weeks after the planting, the students are asked to measure the weekly growth of the bean sprouts and to report back to the class.

the longest root tip to the tip of the tallest branch? What level of accuracy is required (centimeters or millimeters)? What measurement tool is appropriate to this task? Is the measurement procedure reliable and reproducible? In later chapters, we shall attend in much more detail to these measurement questions. For this example, we simply assume that they have been solved to a satisfactory degree.

Assume for now that the experiment goes forward, and the students report back to class after 1 week. Also assume that the results show a positive relationship between the amount of daily watering and the growth of the bean sprouts during the first week. Are these results convincing? We may not question the results in this case, because they are in line with our expectations and past experiences (remember that coherence is one criterion of causality). However, if the students' data do not confirmed the relationship, we will surely be skeptical and will ask questions about the features of the experiment itself. In particular, we will suspect that some other factors at work have somehow prevented us from showing this relationship. What might they be? For example, the growth of plants is also influenced by the amount of light to which they are exposed, the chemical composition of the soil (e.g., what amounts of which nutrients relevant to soybean growth are present in the soil), level and fluctuation in air and soil temperature, and level and fluctuation in air and soil moisture. There may well be other factors, and consideration of these issues will lead to questions about how to control for the effects of these other factors.

Control

What we mean by **control** in this study is that we want to be able to isolate the effect of varying water amounts from the effects of all the other potential causes of plant growth. These other causes are often called **confounders** or **confounding variables** because they can be reasonably discussed as possibly affecting plant growth. How is the control over the confounding variables brought about? In the bean sprout example, the experiment could be improved by specifying control mechanisms in the research design. For instance, the students could be asked to use the same size pot, to use the same commercial brand of soil packaged with the same initial soil moisture, to keep room temperatures even at 65°F, and to use blinds to avoid direct sun exposure. Although such measures help standardize the environmental conditions, it is not hard to see that they are imperfect. For example, in some homes the only room available for the experiment might face north; in another home, it might face south. The possible variations of conditions in the environment are endless, and one could quickly conclude that the best way to conduct this experiment would be to have all plants in the same room under highly controlled conditions of access to light and air.

But even that might not be enough. One principal problem to be addressed in such an experiment is this: even if environmental conditions can be controlled perfectly, there will still be variation in the characteristics of the seeds or beans themselves. That is, the same external conditions are likely to result in different growth rates of different bean sprouts because of the inevitable variations in genetic makeup of the seeds, their initial size, their age, and other factors relevant to their capacity for growth. Notice here the parallel to clinical interventions. Even if several patients receive the same treatment for a health problem, their responses are likely to vary because no two patients are genetically, physiologically, or psychologically identical. Under these conditions, how can we show the effectiveness of any treatment at all?

Control Problems in Experimental Studies

This example shows that two kinds of control problems arise in experimental studies involving living organisms:

1. Lack of *control over the environment* in which the organism lives
2. Lack of *control over the inherent variability in the organisms*, i.e., the persons being studied.

In clinical studies, the first problem—control over the environment—is often impossible to achieve unless patients are brought to live in a laboratory setting during a study. For example, where patients obtain health information, their eating habits, and life experiences during a study are examples of events that usually cannot be controlled by researchers. Even in the much simpler bean sprouts example, control over confounding variables was easier said than done. We were able to list several confounding variables that we already believed would affect the growth of the bean sprouts. By knowing what the potential confounding variables are, we can often take action to control at least some of these variables, such as standardizing room temperature or access to light. But in reality, researchers often don't know all of the potential confounders. After all, experiments are usually done because additional knowledge is needed about the causal factors in question. In addition, even if the confounding variables are known, control over them may not be easy. For instance, the proportion of CO_2 in the air affects plant growth, but it may not be easy to control. In clinical interventions that take place outside of a highly controlled laboratory, researchers often have much less prior knowledge about confounding variables. So the crucial question arises: *How can we control for variables whose confounding effects we are not even aware of?* Clearly, what we need is an all-purpose mechanism that allows us to equalize conditions and differences in inherent characteristics of the study subjects across the various experimental treatments. Such a mechanism was first suggested by Fisher (1935). It is **random assignment** (randomization) of study units or subjects to treatments or (what amounts to the same thing) of treatments to study units.

KEY FEATURES OF EXPERIMENTAL DESIGNS

Before discussing how randomization achieves the desired goal of control over confounding variables, we shall now summarize the key features of experimental designs, with reference to steps in designing an experiment.

Steps in the Design of Experimental Studies

1. The first step in designing an experimental study (depending on the discipline, experimental studies of health issues in humans are variously referred to as **intervention studies** or **clinical trials**) is to define the outcome or response variable and devise a standardized way of measuring it. Whether it is pressure on skin tissue that might lead to pressure ulcers (DeFloor & Gryp-

donck, 2000) or attitudinal/psychologic measures, such as satisfaction with a provider or with one's treatment decisions (Rothert, Holmes-Rovner, Rovner, Kroll, Breer, Talarczyk, Schmitt, Padonu, & Wills, 1997), experimental studies require **standardized outcome measures,** so that the impact of the intervention(s) in the experimental groups(s) can be compared with the impact in the control group(s).

2. The next step involves specifying the intervention(s) or treatment(s). Recall the principle discussed in the last chapter: that "all research is comparative." In the current context, that means that there must be **variation in the exposure** to the intervention or the various levels of the intervention. In that way, one can collect comparative evidence of what difference it makes whether or not a subject is exposed to the intervention or how intense the exposure is. (The latter is called the dosage problem.) In the simplest possible case, there are two levels of exposure that define the study groups: an **experimental group** that receives the intervention, (e.g., an educational intervention designed to improve acceptance of influenza vaccination) (O'Connor et al., 1996), and a **control group** from the same target population that does not receive it. In a more elaborate study, there may be more levels of exposure and therefore more comparison groups defined by the exposure pattern. For instance, Rothert et al. (1997) used three types of patient-centered decision support interventions (lecture, brochure, lecture/brochure) to assist women with decision making about menopause management options. Also, in some study designs the control "group" really consists of a control "occasion." As will be elaborated in a later chapter, **crossover designs** involve the exposure of the same group of subjects to all levels of treatment and control on different occasions. But the principle of comparing subjects after their exposure to different levels of treatment remains intact.

3. As the very word "intervention" suggests, experimental studies are deliberately engineered. In other words, intervention variables are **manipulated** by the researcher(s), not just passively observed. Outcome or response variables, by contrast, are just observed. "Manipulation of the independent variable" thus refers to deliberately varying the treatments among different (at least two) groups of study subjects, be they experimental group(s), which get some level of treatment, or the control group, which is usually defined as the one that gets no treatment. Why are independent/treatment variables manipulated in experimental studies? Recall that the overall goal in an experimental study is to show that variations in treatments lead to variations in patient outcomes. Thus, variations in the levels of treatment must be generated in the first place to see their effects. However, in most intervention studies or clinical trials, for ethical reasons the control group actually gets the usual or standard care rather than the new treatment introduced by the researcher. For many health problems that are the focus of clinical trials of experimental treatments, it is not ethical to withhold treatment completely. For example, it would not be ethically defensible to withhold cancer treatment from a cancer patient enrolled in a clinical trial of an experimental chemotherapy.

4. As we already know from the discussion of causal inference, manipulation of the intervention(s) is not sufficient for separating out the intervention effect. The researcher must also make sure that there is adequate control over the environment in which the experiment takes place. In addition, it must be possible to exclude other nonenvironmental factors, such as the variability in human beings, as alternative explanations of systematic variation in the outcome variable(s). The best mechanism through which to achieve this control is **random assignment** of subjects to the various treatment and control groups.

FROM RANDOM ASSIGNMENT TO THE SAMPLING DISTRIBUTION

NOTE: The discussion in this and the following sections may be considered quite technical, but we encourage you not to skip over it. At no point will the discussion require more than the knowledge of some simple algebra, but the rewards are likely to be high: The ideas expounded here provide the underlying logic for causal inference in all experimental studies/clinical trials, no matter how complex they are.

It is often said—and we used a similar formulation in the last section—that random assignment of subjects to treatment and control groups (or more generally: to comparison groups) achieves *preexperimental equivalence* among the comparison groups. This is actually a rather loose way of talking. In this section, we provide an example of a random assignment procedure, look at its effect on the comparison groups, and show how and why it is possible to draw causal inferences (within certain confidence limits) after random assignment has been done. For the purpose of this discussion, we offer a somewhat unrealistic example of a physical therapy intervention study of just six ($n = 6$) nursing home residents (Research Scenario 3-2). However, this

RESEARCH SCENARIO 3.2

Interventions in Assisted Living

Suppose you have been asked to serve as a consultant to an assisted living facility whose managers are interested in testing new ways to maintain or improve the functional independence of residents for activities of daily living (ADLs). The new interventions will be supervised and implemented by physical therapy staff working in the facility. The interventions under consideration range from massage to water therapy to special exercises. You recommend pilot-testing the effectiveness of these interventions as a "package" in an experimental study.

Suppose that six cognitively alert residents have volunteered to participate in this pilot study. They are Albert, Bertha, Caroline, David, Ethel, and Fred, denoted as individuals A, B, C, D, E, and F in your study. Before the physical intervention is implemented, each individual has been assessed for ADL dependencies and has been given a score that reflects how many ADL activities he or she needs assistance with. For instance, Caroline needs assistance with getting in and out of bed, walking, and dressing herself. Thus, she receives an ADL score of 3, denoting three dependencies. Similarly, Albert needs assistance only with bathing, so his score is 1. The following table shows the complete distribution of ADL scores before the planned physical therapy intervention.

Distribution of Dependencies in Activities of Daily Living (ADL) among Six Assisted Living Residents

Assisted Living Resident	A	B	C	D	E	F
ADL Dependencies	1	2	3	4	5	6

therapy intervention (treatment group), and the other three would not get this intervention (control group). To help ensure equivalence of the two groups, we randomly assign (Box 3-3) three of these cases to the treatment group and the other three to the control group. What are the *possible* outcomes from this random assignment process?

It turns out that there are 20 distinct ways of assigning, out of a total of six cases, three to one group (say, the treatment group) and the other three to the control group. Let's see why. When the first person is randomly assigned to the treatment group (by rolling a die, for instance), any one of the six individuals A through F could be chosen. For the second person, there are five possible choices among the remaining subjects, after which the last person assigned to the treatment group is chosen from the remaining four persons. The three unselected persons would automatically be assigned to the control group. How many different selection patterns are possible? There are six possible first choices, followed by five second and four third choices, or $6 \times 5 \times 4 = 120$ possible choices. However, not all of these choices result in unique subject groups. For instance, the selection of individual A followed by C and F yields the same group of people as that of C followed by F and A. Because both assignment patterns result in having individuals A, C, and F in the treatment group and individuals B, D, and E in the control group, we need not be concerned with the order in which the three individuals in the treatment group are selected. Using the same argument as before, it is easy to see that there are six different sequences or orders of selecting a given group of three individuals. Thus, for the configuration of individuals A, C, and F, we could have chosen any one of them first, followed by any two and finally the remaining third person. Thus, there are $3 \times 2 \times 1$ different orders in which the three individuals could have been chosen. If we now divide the total possible choice patterns (120) by the number of different choice patterns *within* the treatment or control groups to which we are indifferent (6), we get 20 distinct ways of randomly selecting three out of six individuals to either treatment or control group (Box 3-4).

Now, let's look at the *results* of the random assignment. In Table 3-1, the first and third columns show all the possible distinct ways in which the assisted living residents could have been assigned randomly to either the treatment group or the control group. The second and fourth columns show the resulting mean activities of daily living (ADL) scores that the random assignment can produce in the treatment and control groups. The fifth column shows the differences in mean ADL scores between the two groups that can be produced by the random assignment.

small sample size allows us to show in detail the effects of the random assignment process. How one determines whether a study sample is large enough to show an intervention effect will be discussed in Chapter 20.

Suppose that the intervention study is done with only this sample of six individuals. In the simplest possible study, three individuals would be exposed to the physical

BOX 3.3   The Role of Randomization in Experimental Studies

In the ideal study, we would like the background characteristics of members of the experimental and control groups to be as similar as possible, so that the only major difference remaining between the comparison groups is their exposure to different treatment levels. While it may be possible to do a credible job of controlling environmental conditions for the comparison groups, how do we ensure the equivalence of the group members?

One way is for the investigator to assign subjects to the comparison groups in such a manner that the group characteristics do not differ. For instance, an investigator could make sure that in a study of the effectiveness of a smoking cessation intervention, the proportion of heavy smokers (two packs of cigarettes per day) is the same in the intervention group and the control group. This process is called **matching.** However, two big problems exist with such an assignment process.

Subjects differ not only in terms of smoking habits but also according to such characteristics as age, gender, educational achievement, personality type, and susceptibility to the addictive properties of nicotine. The list of characteristics that might plausibly affect their ability to quit is quite long. Thus, one would need information on all of these variables in advance of the subject assignment process.

Furthermore, even if the information were available, matching on more than three variables is generally not feasible. Just imagine having to find pairs of subjects (one for the intervention group and one for the control group) with matching characteristics: two college-educated, 35-year-old men with depressive dispositions, and so forth. Most importantly, however, matching cannot serve as an all-purpose control mechanism: investigators often *do not know in advance* which are the most relevant variables that will affect the outcome of interest. Thus, the exclusive use of matching in subjects' assignment does not ensure that comparison groups will be identical with respect to all relevant background characteristics.

Yet, somehow a decision must be made as to which subjects will or will not be exposed to the intervention. In this situation, randomization accomplishes two major objectives. (1) The assignment process will be free of conscious or unconscious investigator bias. (2) If the comparison groups are large enough, the background characteristics of the members will be similar or **equivalent,** even in terms of factors whose effect on the outcome variables remains unknown to the investigators.

BOX 3.4   Permutations and Combinations: A Slightly More Formal Approach

The total number of ways of selecting R distinct combinations of objects from a sample of n objects, not considering the order of objects within a group, is given by the following formula (in college algebra, this is discussed under the rubric "permutations and combinations"): $n!/R!(n–R)!$, where n = number of all subjects in the sample, and R = the number of all subjects in the selected sub-group. $n!$ or $R!$ is read as ("n factorial" or "R factorial") and equals the product of $n \times (n-1) \times (n-2) \times \ldots 3 \times 2 \times 1$.

Given that we have a sample of $n = 6$ and a treatment/control group size of R = 3, the formula comes down to $6!/3!(6-3)! = 6 \times 5 \times 4 \times 3 \times 2 \times 1/3 \times 2 \times 1 \times 3 \times 2 \times 1 = 20$. In plain English, there are 20 distinct ways of selecting three cases from a sample of six cases. That is to say, if we randomly assign three cases out of six to either treatment or control group, there are only 20 different ways in which that can be done.

Note: As the sample size grows, the possibilities of randomly assigning cases to either treatment group or the control group grows exponentially. For instance, if you want to assign 10 cases from a sample of 20 to either the treatment group or the control group, there are an astonishing 184,756 distinct ways of doing it $(20!/10!(20-10)! = 184,756)$. Selecting 20 out of 40 can be done in almost 138 million different ways.

TABLE 3-1.	Twenty Possible Combinations of Assigning Three of Six Cases to Either Treatment or Control Group and Associated Mean Differences			
Cases in Treatment Group (All Possible Combinations of Randomly Assigning Cases)	Mean ADL Score in Treatment Group (Based on Distribution of ADL Score Before Intervention)	Cases in Control Group (All Possible Combinations of Randomly Assigning Cases)	Mean ADL Score in Control Group (Based on Distribution of ADL Score Before Intervention)	Sampling Distribution of Mean Differences Between Treatment and Control Groups
A, B, C	2.00	D, E, F	5.00	−3.00
A, B, D	2.33	C, E, F	4.67	−2.34
A, B, E	2.67	C, D, F	4.33	−1.66
A, B, F	3.00	C, D, E	4.00	−1.00
A, C, D	2.67	B, E, F	4.33	−1.66
A, C, E	3.00	B, D, F	4.00	−1.00
A, C, F	3.33	B, D, E	3.67	−.34
A, D, E	3.33	B, C, F	3.67	−.34
A, D, F	2.67	B, C, E	3.33	.34
A, E, F	4.00	B, C, D	3.00	1.00
B, C, D	3.00	A, E, F	4.00	−1.00
B, C, E	3.33	A, D, F	3.67	−.34
B, C, F	3.67	A, D, E	3.33	.34
B. D, E	3.67	A, C, F	3.33	.34
B, D, F	4.00	A, C, E	3.00	1.00
B, E, F	4.33	A, C, D	2.67	1.66
C, D, E	4.00	A, B, F	3.00	1.00
C, D, F	4.33	A, B, E	2.67	1.66
C, E, F	4.67	A, B, D	2.33	2.34
D, E, F	5.00	A, B, C	2.00	3.00

ADL, activities of daily living.

What can be learned from this table? Recall that the ADL scores in the study sample were originally distributed as follows: A–1, B–2, C–3, D–4, E–5, F–6. This means that if the random assignment process results in the selection of individuals A, B, and C into the treatment group (and, by default, individuals D, E, and F into the control group), then the mean ADL score in the treatment group *before the intervention* would be 2 = (1 + 2 + 3)/3, and the mean ADL score in the control group would be 5 = (4 + 5 + 6)/3. To choose another example, if individuals C, D, and F were selected into the treatment group, their mean ADL score would be 4.33 = (3 + 4 + 6)/3, and the control group mean of individuals A, B, and E would be 2.67 = (1 + 2 + 5)/3. Now, concentrate on the right-hand column in Table 3-1. It shows all the *possible mean differences* between the treatment and control groups *that could occur as the result of random assignment*. For instance, with A, B, and C in the treatment group and D, E, and F in the control group, the mean difference in ADL scores between the two groups would be 2−5 = −3. If you scan the values for the

mean differences, you will see that some values occur once, whereas others occur two or three times. All in all, there are 10 distinct mean differences, and we can collect them in the following frequency/probability distribution (Table 3-2):

NOTE: When we talk about the sampling distribution as a **probability distribution,** we mean that each of the *possible distinct outcomes,* which in this case are the mean differences listed in the first column of Table 3-2, has a certain chance of occurring. That chance of occurrence, or probability, is simply the proportion of times the assignment process produces a particular outcome among all possible outcomes. There are 20 distinct ways of assigning subjects to the two groups, as shown in Table 3-1. This means that each unique assignment configuration has a .05 (or 1/20) probability of occurrence. However, some of the assignments produce the *same outcome* in terms of the mean difference in ADL scores between treatment and control groups. For instance, three distinct subject assignments to the treatment group (A, E, F or B, D, F or C, D,

TABLE 3.2	Sampling Distribution of Mean Differences in ADL Scores Between Treatment and Control Groups

Mean Differences	Probability of Occurrence
−3.00	.05
−2.34	.05
−1.66	.10
−1.00	.15
−.34	.15
.34	.15
1.00	.15
1.66	.10
2.34	.05
3.00	.05

ADL, activities of daily living.

E) all produce the same outcome: a mean difference of 1.00. Thus, in 3 out of 20 possible random assignments (probability = .15), we get a result of +1.00 for the mean difference.

What are the implications of this example for experimental design and for nursing and health-related research? This sampling distribution shows us *what mean differences between treatment and control groups can occur purely by "chance,"* that is, as a result of random assignment. It also attaches a probability to the occurrence of various outcomes. It is this information against which we judge the significance of our results *after* the intervention. Suppose the physical therapy intervention goes forward in the treatment group, and, after one month, subjects in the treatment and control groups are again compared with respect to their mean ADL scores. Suppose further we find that the treatment group's mean ADL score is a full 4 points *lower* than the mean ADL score in the control group. Under these (highly unusual) conditions, we would actually know with certainty that the random assignment could not have produced this difference, *because a difference of −3 points is the largest that mere random assignment could have generated in this study group.* Thus, the inevitable conclusion is this (assuming the experiment/intervention study was conducted in such a way that environmental influences were sufficiently controlled): the intervention must have been effective!

In this artificial example, we could certainly draw the conclusion that differences in the background characteristics of the individual subjects alone could not explain the observed mean difference in the ADL score of −4. However, in real-world experiments, we almost never get results that are certain. Instead, we get results that indicate that a causal inference can be drawn only with greater or lesser probability of being correct (or confidence). Let us look again at Table 3-2. Assume that after the physical therapy intervention the treatment group has, on average, three fewer ADL dependencies than the control group. From our sampling distribution, we know that a difference of −3 will occur in 5% of all possible study samples *merely as a result of the random assignment process.* Now we must decide: is this evidence strong enough to conclude that the intervention causes the difference? In this case, we would have a 95% confidence that the intervention is effective. However, because in 5% of all samples, mere random assignment could have produced the observed difference, a 5% risk remains that our inference about the causal effectiveness of the intervention is wrong. This latter risk or probability of wrongly concluding that an intervention is effective, when in fact mere random assignment produced the results, is also called the **significance level** or the **Type I Error.** These formal terms will be revisited later in this chapter.

This, in a nutshell, is the logic of causal inference, on which all clinical trials are based (Fig. 3-1):

Now we can see more clearly how randomization (or random assignment) achieves control over extraneous variables. "Control" means that the effects of other confounding variables on the outcome variable are distributed between the experimental and control groups in a random fashion, thus allowing us to construct a sampling distribution. In this way, the effect of the experimental variable is isolated from the effects of all other variables. The great advantage of this technique is that it provides a mechanism for dealing with unknown confounding factors. Thus, the researcher is not required to know in advance all the possible rival factors that might also influence the outcome variable of interest.

STATISTICAL INFERENCE AND CAUSAL INTERPRETATION AFTER RANDOM ASSIGNMENT: THE LOGIC OF THE *T* TEST

The logic of random assignment fits very nicely with the statistical models that are used to analyze data from experimental studies. In this section, we shall demonstrate the congruence between the basic features of experimental

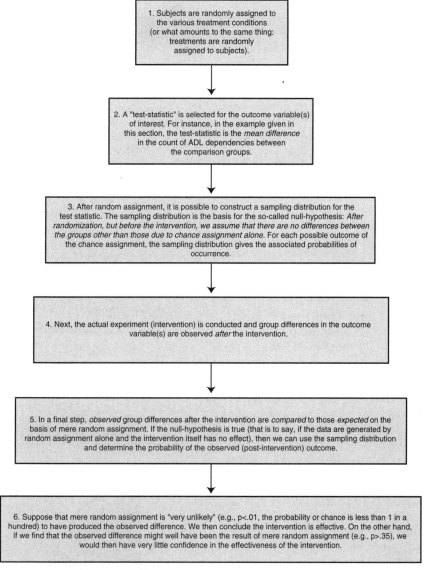

1. Subjects are randomly assigned to
the various treatment conditions
(or what amounts to the same thing:
treatments are randomly
assigned to subjects).

2. A "test-statistic" is selected for the outcome variable(s)
of interest. For instance, in the example given in
this section, the test-statistic is the *mean difference*
in the count of ADL dependencies between
the comparison groups.

3. After random assignment, it is possible to construct a sampling distribution for the
test statistic. The sampling distribution is the basis for the so-called null-hypothesis: *After
randomization, but before the intervention, we assume that there are no differences between
the groups other than those due to chance assignment alone.* For each possible outcome of
the chance assignment, the sampling distribution gives the associated probabilities of
occurrence.

4. Next, the actual experiment (intervention) is conducted and group differences in the outcome
variable(s) are observed *after* the intervention.

5. In a final step, *observed* group differences after the intervention are *compared* to those *expected* on the
basis of mere random assignment. If the null-hypothesis is true (that is to say, if the data are generated by
random assignment alone and the intervention itself has no effect), then we can use the sampling distribution
and determine the probability of the observed (post-intervention) outcome.

6. Suppose that mere random assignment is "very unlikely" (e.g., p<.01, the probability or chance is less than 1 in a
hundred) to have produced the observed difference. We then conclude the intervention is effective. On the other hand,
if we find that the observed difference might well have been the result of mere random assignment (e.g., p>.35), we
would then have very little confidence in the effectiveness of the intervention.

FIGURE 3.1 Flowchart illustrating the logic of causal inference.

studies and one popular statistical model, which is widely used in the nursing and health care literature: the *t* test.

Independent Sample and Paired Samples

The *t* test is frequently used to determine whether two mean scores should be considered equal to or different from each other. It comes in two versions. (1) The **independent-sample** (two-group) *t* test compares mean scores in two different groups (e.g., male and female patients or patients in the treatment versus the control group). (2) The **paired-samples** (dependent-samples) *t* test compares mean scores for the same group of subjects measured at two different times. (The paired *t* test will be discussed in Chapter 5.) Because both versions of the test focus on mean scores, they should be applied only to variables or measures for which it is meaningful to compute a mean. In particular, this implies that the variables in question should be measured at the interval level of measurement.[3]

Inferential Statistics

We should like to emphasize one other point here before proceeding with an example. The *t* test is an **inferential** statistical test. Thus, the comparison of means that is envisioned here involves more than the simple calculation and description of two particular sample means. That would just be a matter of simple algebra. The value of a statistical test is that it gives us a *context* in which we can interpret a particular sample result. But that context involves assumptions about how the particular data at hand were generated. Because we introduce the *t* test in the context of the analysis of data from experimental studies, we emphasize the necessity of prior random assignment of subjects to the treatment and control groups. However, a *t* test may also validly be applied to nonexperimental studies in which the random process is one of sample selection from a larger population.

Empirical Construction of a Sampling Distribution of Mean Differences After Random Assignments

Imagine the data set presented in Research Scenario 3-3 and Figure 3-2. This frequency distribution of diastolic blood pressure readings for 100 patients has a mean of 82.4, a median of 81, and a standard deviation of 9.53. Values range from a low of 68 mm Hg to a high of 113 mm Hg. (See Appendix A for detailed information on the computation of these sample statistics.) It is easy to see from the graph in Figure 3-2 that this distribution is **skewed,** with half the patients having diastolic readings of 81 or less and only 15% experiencing mild or moderate hypertension with scores of 90 mm Hg and above. A normal distribution, which is perfectly symmetric, is superimposed on the graph for comparison purposes.

Now, suppose you intend to apply the intervention to both normotensive and hypertensive patients. To control for unknown confounding variables, you divide the sample randomly into halves, with 50 patients assigned to the intervention group and 50 patients to the control group. From the previous section, we know that there are 100!/50!(100–50)!

RESEARCH SCENARIO 3.3

Blood Pressure and Nonpharmacologic Interventions

In a primary care practice, patients' blood pressure is routinely measured and recorded. As care provider you are interested in finding out whether nonpharmacologic interventions such as patient education about physical exercise at home and advice on nutrition and food preparation is at all effective in lowering blood pressure. You decide to do a study in which you intend to expose half of the participating patients to the educational intervention while the other half receives the usual care. Suppose you find 100 patients in the primary care setting willing to participate in the study. Figure 3-2 shows the distribution of the patients' diastolic blood pressure readings. Because blood pressure readings often fluctuate, we assume that each individual score is actually a mean score from three successive readings.

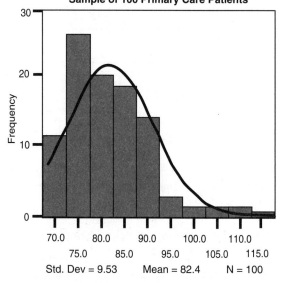

FIGURE 3.2 Diastolic blood pressure (mm Hg).

---

[3]For the mechanics of computing mean scores, see Appendix A. For a more thorough discussion of the measurement assumptions, including the conditions under which statistics for interval level variables may be applied to ordinal data, see the section on levels of measurement in Chapter 2 and the more detailed exposition in Chapter 14.

distinct ways of splitting the sample and making such assignments. There are literally trillions of different possible assignments. Even with high-speed computers, it would not be easy to actually perform all possible random splits. However, for demonstration purposes, the authors did use the computer to perform 100 random assignments (or splits) of 50 cases to the treatment group and 50 cases to the control group. For each random split, mean diastolic blood pressure readings were computed for both the prospective treatment group and the control group. Finally, all 100 mean differences between the assigned treatment and control groups were recorded. The resulting (empirically constructed) sampling distribution is shown in Figure 3-3.

Properties of the Sampling Distribution

The graph in Figure 3-3 tells a remarkable story. Recall that we have taken the same 100 patients and randomly reassigned them 100 times to two groups of 50 subjects each. Then we computed the mean difference in the diastolic blood pressure readings for each of the different splits. Because they were random splits, we would expect the process to be unbiased. That means it should be just as likely that the assigned treatment group mean exceeds the control group mean (resulting in a *positive* mean difference) as is the reverse (resulting in a *negative* mean differ-

ence). As it happens, in this particular set of 100 random splits, 51% of the mean differences were positive and 49% negative. A mere glance at the sampling distribution in Figure 3-3 should convince the reader that this distribution is, for all intents and purposes, symmetric.

One reason why this is remarkable is that the underlying data (see Fig. 3-2) on which the random splits are based do not have a symmetric distribution. In fact, had we used our computer to produce *all possible* random splits (instead of just the 100 assignments), we would have obtained a perfectly smooth and symmetric sampling distribution with a mean of zero and the shape of the normal curve. However, in practical applications of the mean difference test, the shape of the sampling distribution follows the *t* distribution instead of the normal distribution.[4]

The *t* distribution actually comprises a family of distributions shaped very similarly to that of the normal distribution (which has been superimposed on the graph in Fig. 3-2). Like the normal distribution, the *t* distributions are completely symmetric, i.e., the mean of the distribution is also the median, with 50% of the area under the curve to the right of the mean and 50% to the left of the mean. The principle difference in the normal curve is that *t* distributions for small samples are somewhat flatter in the middle and have thicker tails. The reason is that in practice, the estimate we use for the standard error comes from a single study sample. Thus, not only the estimate of the mean, but also the estimate of the standard error associated with the mean, is subject to sampling fluctuations, i.e., they differ among samples drawn from the same population. Consequently, our errors in estimation are a bit larger, resulting in a sampling distribution that is flatter than the normal curve. However, for samples larger than $n = 120$, the *t* distribution is virtually indistinguishable from the normal curve. As you can see in Figure 3-3, the empirical sampling distribution is based on random splits of a sample of 100 cases, and it already approximates the shape of the normal curve.

Why do we care about the shape of the sampling distribution? If we know that a sampling distribution is shaped like the *t* distribution, then we know for any observed outcome what proportion of random assignments would produce a value of this magnitude or larger. Let's take the graph in Figure 3-3. We can use it to answer this question: How likely is it that mere random assignment produces a *mean difference* in diastolic blood pressure readings between designated treatment and control groups of 3 mm Hg or more? If you were to measure the area represented by

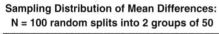

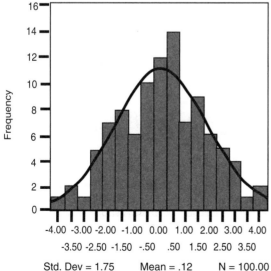

FIGURE 3.3 **Sampling distribution of mean differences.**

---

[4]The *t* distribution was so named by its inventor, William Gosset, who published it under his pen name, "Student" (1908).

the bars over the values 3, 3.5, and 4 and compared it with the total area represented by all bars, you would find that precisely 5% of all randomly produced mean differences equal or exceed the value of 3 mm Hg. This result is astonishingly close to the one you would get from using the actual *t* distribution. Before we can do that, we need to take one additional small step.

Standard Error

One other piece of information about the sampling distribution is of great importance. The randomly generated mean differences fluctuate around the average mean difference of zero, with large differences occurring less often than small differences. We can measure the spread of randomly generated mean differences around the mean of the sampling distribution by computing its standard deviation. This standard deviation of the sampling distribution goes by the special name of **standard error,** because it indicates the average error associated with the random assignment process. In Figure 3-3, our estimate of the standard error is 1.75. This is an estimate, because it is based on only 100 random splits instead of all possible random splits. This piece of information is very valuable in statistical inference. First, we can now express all deviations from the mean of the sampling distribution in terms of a standard unit. Because variables of interest to health researchers are measured in many different measurement units (e.g., mm Hg, pulse rates per minute, time to recovery from a surgery), it would be tedious to construct different sampling distributions for each measure. Instead, deviations from the mean of the sampling distribution can always be expressed in terms of the number of standard errors by which an observed value differs from the mean. Given our estimate of the standard error of 1.75 for the sampling distribution of

mean group differences in diastolic blood pressure readings, an observed mean difference of 3 in a particular split is 1.65 standard errors larger than the mean of this sampling distribution [(3−.12)/1.75 = 1.65]. Had we used the theoretical *t* distribution appropriate for a sample size of 100, we would have found that about 5.1% of all values of that *t* distribution lie beyond 1.65 standard errors.

What We Need to Apply the *t* Test

To recapitulate: In order to apply and use the *t* test, we really need three pieces of information (Box 3-5). Consider how we use this evidence to draw inferences about the effectiveness of an intervention in an experimental study. In the case of the 100 patients who have agreed to participate in an educational intervention designed to reduce blood pressure, the subjects initially show substantial individual variation with respect to their diastolic blood pressure readings and possibly other relevant characteristics. *In clinical studies, such individual variation is the norm rather than the exception.* Thus, in order to neutralize such confounding effects, subjects in experimental studies are randomly assigned to either a treatment group or a control group. Then, the intervention is implemented in the treatment group.

Outcomes

Two real outcomes are possible. (1) The first is that the intervention is indeed effective. That is our **research hypothesis** (H_r). Because human responses to almost all treatments or interventions are not uniform, an effective intervention is defined as one that results in different *average* outcomes between treatment and control groups. It is not required that every member of the treatment group

---

BOX 3.5   Required Information for Applying and Using the *t* Test

1. We need to be able to make the assumption that the sampling distribution of mean differences between two groups compared is distributed like the *t* distribution. This assumption is valid if the variable is more or less continuous, measured at the interval level, and if random assignment is used to generate the subgroup samples.
2. We need an estimate of the standard error of the sampling distribution. It was demonstrated here that such an estimate can be obtained empirically by computer generation of large numbers of random assignments. Alternatively, standard error estimates can be obtained from the sample data at hand, as any textbook in statistics will demonstrate.
3. The final piece of information is the actually observed mean difference in the sample at hand, i.e., the mean difference computed from the data.

show a positive response, only that it is effective on average. (2) The second outcome possibility is that the intervention is not effective. This is encapsulated in the **null hypothesis** (H_0) of no (systematic) difference between the treatment and the control group.

Now we must use the available evidence after the experiment to make up our minds about the effectiveness of the intervention. Suppose that 3 months after the educational intervention, the patients in the intervention group have a mean diastolic blood pressure reading of 80.33 mm Hg, and those in the control group have a mean diastolic blood pressure of 84.48 mm Hg: a difference of −4.15. Given our estimate of the standard error of 1.75, we can express this difference by saying that the two group means differ by 2.37 standard errors. If the null hypothesis is true and the intervention is not effective, then all observed differences between the treatment and the control groups are merely the result of the random assignment process. If applied repeatedly, the random assignment process will produce a sampling distribution of mean differences that follows the *t* distribution. From the *t* distribution we know that a treatment group mean that is 2.37 standard errors below the control group mean occurs randomly in less than 1% of all random assignments.

On the basis of this evidence, we would most likely argue that there is strong evidence that the intervention is effective. That is, we reject the null hypothesis that the intervention is not effective, because mere random assignment alone is unlikely to have produced the observed mean difference between the treatment and the control groups. If we adopt this stance, we would be right in 99% of all cases.

But we do not have certainty about our conclusions. In 1% of all cases, random assignment alone could have produced such observed results. Thus, the probability of drawing the wrong conclusion from the data—namely, that the intervention is effective, when in fact it is not—is 1%. As we have already learned, this probability is called the significance level, or the Type I error.

Drawing conclusions based on fallible data can also lead to another kind of error. Suppose we observe after the intervention or experiment that the treatment group's mean is .85 standard errors below the control group's mean. Normally, we would not consider that very strong evidence in favor of the effectiveness of the intervention. This is so because according to the appropriate *t* distribution, random assignment alone would produce a mean difference between the treatment and control groups of this magnitude (−.85 standard errors) in 20% of all random splits. Thus, we are likely to conclude that the observed mean difference does not warrant the conclusion that the intervention is effective. Yet, this conclusion could also be wrong. A wrong conclusion that an intervention is not effective, when in fact it is, means that a **Type II error** has been committed. We can now summarize the decision-making situation based on the evidence provided by the *t* test (Table 3-3).

Finally, consider the results from an independent-sample *t* test analysis. We continue with the example of the 100 primary care patients. Three months after the educational intervention, all 100 patients are retested, and their diastolic blood pressures are recorded. Again, in order to minimize measurement errors, this 3-month posttest (i.e., the measure *after* the intervention) is actually an average of

TABLE 3.3	Statistical Decision Making		
		True State of Affairs	
		H_0 is not true, i.e., the intervention is effective	H_0 is true, i.e., the intervention is not effective
Conclusions based on evidence from *t* test	H_0 is rejected, i.e., the observed mean difference lies outside the critical value (is statistically significant)	Correct inference (true positive)	Type I error
	H_0 is accepted, i.e., the observed mean difference lies inside the critical value (is not statistically significant)	Type II error	Correct inference (true negative)

three blood pressure readings taken within 1 hour of a clinical visit. Table 3-4 contains the results.

Take a look at the columns in this table, and you will see that the first column defines the categories of the independent variable. In this example, the independent variable takes on two levels, which define the two comparison groups: the treatment/intervention group and the control group. The second column shows the sample mean scores on the outcome variable (diastolic blood pressure) for each of the comparison groups. The third column contains the associated "95% confidence limits" for the true means. Remember that the observed sample group means of 80.33 mm Hg and 84.48 mm Hg are just *estimates of the true group means computed after a single random split* of the 100 subjects. Different random splits would likely give us somewhat different results. The 95% confidence limits tell us that there is a 95% probability that the true group means in the treatment and control groups are between 77.71 to 82.95 mm Hg and 81.68 to 87.28 mm Hg, respectively.

The fourth column reports on the observed sample mean difference between treatment and control groups, which is 4.15 = 84.48−80.33. The fifth column contains the standard error of this mean difference. Again, observed sample mean differences vary from one random split to the next. The standard error is a measure of the average variation in such mean differences among all random splits. In Figure 3-3, we provided an estimate of this standard error based on 100 random splits. Here, we provide an estimate based on the given sample data (see Appendix B for the calculations). As you can see, the estimates differ a bit, with the estimate based on the single sample being somewhat larger: 1.91 > 1.75. Such differences are to be expected with moderately sized samples, but they would be much smaller with large samples (say $n > 400$), given that sampling fluctuations decline as sample size increases.

The sixth column shows the 95% confidence limits for the mean difference: .35−7.95. Again, this indicates that the true mean difference in diastolic blood pressure between the treatment and control groups is contained, with 95% probability, within the indicated values. These confidence limits still appear quite large, but the crucial point is that they do not contain the value zero. Recall that the null hypothesis underlying this *t* test is that the educational intervention is not effective in reducing diastolic blood pressure. Because the confidence limits do not contain the value of zero, we are 95% certain that the true mean difference differs from zero. That is, we would reject the null hypothesis and accept the alternative research hypothesis that the intervention had at least some effect in reducing diastolic blood pressure.

The last two columns in Table 3-4 contain the *t* value and its associated significance level. If we divide the observed sample mean difference by its standard error, we get the *t* value: 4.15/1.908 = 2.175. Recall that if the null hypothesis is true, the mean of the sampling distribution, which is shaped like the *t* distribution, would be exactly equal to zero. (Again, some random splits lead to treatment means larger than the control means, and other random splits lead to control group means larger than the treatment group mean. If the treatment is not effective at all, and the random assignment process is conducted without bias, the average of all mean differences from random splits should be zero.) However, the observed sample difference of 4.15 is 2.175 standard errors larger than zero, as indicated by the *t* value. The significance level, or the *P* value (this term is commonly used in the medical literature), associated with this *t* value is .032. This means that the probability of observing a sample *t* value of 2.175 purely as a result of random assignment is .032, or that 32 out of 1,000 random splits would produce this result. Thus, it is quite unlikely

TABLE 3.4	Results of *t* Test Analysis (Comparison of Treatment and Control Groups After Intervention)						
Comparison Groups	Observed Sample Means	95% CI for Group Means	Observed Mean Difference	Standard Error of Mean Difference	95% CI for Mean Difference	*T* Value	Two-tailed Significance Level (*P* value)
Treatment group (n = 50)	80.33	77.71–82.95					
			4.15	1.908	.35–7.95	2.175	.032
Control group (n = 50)	84.48	81.68–87.28					

CI, confidence interval.

that the random assignment alone accounts for the observed mean difference. In fact, we are 96.8% confident $(1 - .032)$ that the intervention makes a real difference.

Earlier in this chapter, it was mentioned that the t test is a widely used statistical test in the nursing and health care literature. It is important to note, though, that t test results are often reported in different ways, not all of which are satisfactory. At a minimum, the reader of a research report containing the results from a t test should expect the following information (Box 3-6).

Notice that not all the information provided in Table 3-3 is necessary, because some of it can be recovered from other pieces of information, as was indicated above. However, just reporting a P value without giving group means or mean differences, or reporting group means without standard errors or confidence intervals, leaves the reader without critical pieces of information.

► CLINICAL RESEARCH IN ACTION
Examples of Experimental Tests of Nursing Interventions

Because the t test is discussed here in the context of analyzing experimental studies, we take a brief look at three published articles (Powell, Canterbury, & McCoy, 1998; Hayes, 1999; Naylor, Brooten, Campbell, Jacobson, Mezey, Pauly, & Schwartz, 1999). All three articles describe experimental studies in which researchers used t tests to analyze at least part of their data. In all of these studies, subjects were randomly assigned to one of two groups: an intervention group or a control group.

Powell et al. (1998) compared 48 experimental subjects (i.e., students) who viewed a faculty-generated videotape on medication administration ($=$ intervention) with 50 control group students, who received the standard in-person faculty instruction on skill performance during laboratory

practice. Hayes (1999) tested a geragogy-based medication teaching intervention with a sample of 60 elderly (aged 60 to 98 years) emergency department patients, half of whom were randomly assigned to the intervention group and the other half to the control group, which received the "usual method" of discharge instruction, namely, preprinted instructions. Naylor et al. selected a sample of 363 hospital patients, aged 65 and older, who were discharged with one of seven top ten diagnosis-related groups and were at risk for rehospitalization on the basis of such criteria as inadequate family support, a history of depression, or other chronic problems. At discharge, these patients were randomly split into two groups: 177 patients were assigned to a comprehensive discharge plan, including a home follow-up interview, and 186 patients were assigned to the usual discharge procedures used at the clinical sites.

In all three of these studies, the "control group" subjects also received a treatment, namely, whatever had been done before the proposed intervention. In general, it is therefore preferable to think about intervention studies as comparing the effects of control group treatments with those of intervention group treatments, rather than comparing the effects of absence or presence of treatments. Seen in this light, it is just as important for research reports to describe the treatment exposure of control group subjects as opposed to treatment group subjects. For instance, if the new intervention differs only slightly from the usual care intervention, it may not be surprising that no treatment effects can be detected.

Two of these studies used independent-sample t tests to gauge the effects of their interventions. Hayes (1999) used a "knowledge of medication" test and observed a mean difference of 4.45 between the intervention and control groups. This difference was statistically significant ($P \leq .016$), which means that only in 16 out of 1,000 random assignments would the random assignment alone have produced an observed difference between the treatment and

---

BOX 3.6	Information to Expect on a Research Report Containing the Results of a t Test

1. Clearly labeled comparison groups that make up the independent variable or factor
2. The number of cases in each comparison group
3. The mean scores on the dependent variable for the two comparison groups *or* the mean difference between the two groups
4. The standard error of the mean difference *or* the t value
5. The 95% confidence interval for the mean difference *or* the associated significance level

control groups of 4.45 on the knowledge score. By contrast, Powell et al. (1998) were unable to show a significant difference between intervention and control groups. The group means for the outcome variable (a knowledge test that represents a count of the right answers, ranging from 0 to 17) were 16.76 (experimental/intervention group) and 16.81 (control group). Normally, when researchers cannot reject the null hypothesis of no difference or no intervention effect, there are two possibilities: either the intervention really has had no effect, or the study sample has been too small to show the effect. The latter problem is also referred to as the problem of insufficient **statistical power.** (A fuller discussion of the power problem and how to determine appropriate sample size will be presented in Chapter 20.)

Ceiling Effect

However, in this particular case, there seems to be another problem at work. A glance at the mean knowledge scores in both comparison groups shows that the distribution of scores is extremely skewed. Out of the highest *possible* mean score of 17, both comparison groups have actual mean scores of 16.76 or above. It can be shown that among the 50 intervention group subjects, at least 38 must have scored a perfect 17. One distribution consistent with the reported mean and standard deviation in the experimental group would be 43 subjects scoring 17, 6 scoring 16, and 1 scoring 14. What is at work here is a **ceiling effect,** in this case resulting from a knowledge test that was evidently so easy that it did not discriminate among students of different ability and knowledge. It is clear that such distributions have very limited dispersion, resulting in highly restricted sampling distributions that do not resemble the t distribution. Other statistical tests can be used in such situations, for example, the Mann-Whitney test. Interested readers may consult an applied introductory statistics text, such as those by Altman (1991) and Munro (2001).

Tests of the Pre-Intervention Equivalence

In the study by Naylor et al. (1999), t tests were primarily used to show **equivalence** in the background characteristics of the subjects (such as age) between the treatment group and the control group. Recall that random assignment does not guarantee that the comparison groups have identical background characteristics. In fact, by the very nature of random assignment, occasionally differences between randomly split comparison groups can be quite large. Naylor et al. (1999) did not find any statistically sig-

nificant differences between the intervention and control groups. However, information about large differences in background characteristics, if present, would have been potentially important. Variables that show differences can be used as control variables in the comparisons of outcome scores between the treatment and control groups. This will be discussed in detail in Chapter 7.

Use of the t Test with Nonexperimental Data

Although the t test is applied in the analysis of experimental data, it is actually more common that researchers use the independent sample t test with nonexperimental/observational data to compare preexisting or self-selected groups (Cheever, 1999; Moser, Dracup, & Doering, 2000). That is, in such studies the subjects are *not* randomly assigned. For instance, in the study by Moser et al. (2000), the focus was on comparing characteristics of dropouts and completers among study participants in longitudinal clinical trials. Note that although there are legitimate uses of the t test with nonexperimental data (as when two randomly selected samples are compared), a statistically significant difference in means between two comparison groups without random assignment *does not have a causal interpretation.* Thus, a finding that study dropouts have higher mean depression scores than study completers does not necessarily imply a causal connection between dropout status and depression. Rather, in nonexperimental studies, any number of other (confounding) factors could be responsible for the observed difference.

CONCLUSION

Whenever the question arises, how effective is a clinical intervention in producing a desired outcome, the focus is on the relationship between a potential cause (the intervention) and its effect (the outcome). Over many years, researchers have developed criteria for establishing causality, chief among them covariation (association), temporal order, coherence, contiguity, and exclusion of plausible alternatives. It is generally agreed that experimental studies, also referred to as randomized clinical trials or clinical intervention studies, provide the best available causal evidence. The reason is that in such studies, study participants are randomly assigned to deliberately created treatment and control conditions. As a consequence of the random assignment, variation in exposure to treatment levels is unrelated to the study participants' background characteristics, and it thus becomes independent of other, even unknown, confounding variables. In this way, the researcher can isolate the effects of the treatment variable from those of the confounders. *Without* random assignment, there will be no basis for assuming that the effects of unknown third factors are controlled for. *With* random assignment, it can be assumed that any systematic bias that favors the intervention over the control group(s) has been removed from the experiment.

Prior random assignment is also the basis for the statistical decision rules that are used to decide whether or not experimental interventions are effective. Statistical decisions are made on the basis of the preponderance of evidence. It is important to understand that these decisions are not error free. On the contrary, the calculus of statistical decision making explicitly takes into account the probability of that certain kinds of errors will be made. In particular, when researchers have to decide whether or not to consider a tested clinical intervention effective, they are usually faced with two possible errors of inference. They may conclude that the intervention is effective when it is not (Type I error), or conclude that it is not effective when it is (Type II error). Although we demonstrated how these errors come about, using the *t* test example, the basic decision situation is general and applies to inferences based on other statistical tests. The uncertainty is the price we pay for random assignment: while it allows us to control for unknown factors, it does rob us of certainty. Yet, at the same time, the beauty of statistical decision making is that it offers *a formal means of assessing the magnitude of making wrong decisions.* Thus, after random assignment, we know how large a risk we run of drawing the wrong inferences. Consequently, we can lower the risks of both Type I and Type II errors if we deem them intolerably large. As always, there is a tradeoff: this time, the need for more resources to obtain larger study samples.

In this chapter, we introduced the basic statistical reasoning underlying causal inferences from experimental studies. Now it is time to turn to the strengths and weaknesses of specific research designs.

Suggested Activities

1. Read the three experimental studies discussed in this chapter (Powell et al., 1998; Hayes, 1999; Naylor et al., 1999).
2. For each study, list *all* interventions and experimental activities described in the articles and *all* control group activities. Then describe, as precisely as possible from the given information, how the intervention in the treatment group differs from that in the control group. Discuss to what degree you consider the differences between the treatment and control group exposures as clinically meaningful.
3. Make a list of *all* applications of *t* tests described in the three articles. Ascertain the outcome measures for which mean scores were compared, and determine their levels of measurement using the definitions provided in Table 2-4 (Chapter 2). Are all variables measured at the interval or ratio level?
4. For each example of a *t* test application in these three articles, formulate the null hypothesis and ascertain the probability of a Type I error, i.e., the probability that the rejection of the null hypothesis would yield the wrong result. Then write one or two English sentences that capture your conclusions from the *t* tests.
5. Consider a problem from your clinical practice about which you have a research question. Is your research question amenable to the use of an experimental design? Discuss why you do or do not think so, with reference to the key conditions for an experimental design.
6. Propose a study in which the evaluation of a clinical intervention of your choice can be studied by use of a simple experimental design involving a comparison of two groups. Describe the intervention you want to test, and describe the "usual" alternative, i.e., what happens to patients if they do not get the intervention. Then propose an outcome measure to test the effectiveness of your favored intervention. Describe the basic study design, and formulate your research hypothesis. What effect(s) do you expect to see?

Suggested Readings

Hayes, K. S. (1998). Randomized trial of geragogy-based medication instruction in the emergency department. *Nursing Research, 47,* 211–218.

Kassirer, J. P. (1989). Diagnostic reasoning. *Annals of Internal Medicine, 110,* 893–900.

Munro, B. H. (2001). *Statistical methods for health care research* (2nd ed.). (Chapter 5, pp.123–159) Philadelphia: Lippincott Williams & Wilkins.

Naylor, M. D., Brooten, D., Campbell, R., Jacobson, B. S., Mezey, M. D., Pauly, M. V., & Schwartz, J. S. (1999). Comprehensive discharge planning and home follow-up of hospitalized elders: A randomized clinical trial. *Journal of the American Medical Association, 281,* 613–20.

Powell, S., Canterbury, A., & McCoy, D. (1998). Medication administration: Does the teaching method really matter? *Journal of Nursing Education, 37,* 281–283.

Susser, M. (1991). What is a cause and how do we know one? A grammar for pragmatic epidemiology. *American Journal of Epidemiology, 133,* 635–648.

References

Altman, D. G. (1991). *Practical statistics for medical research*. Boca Raton, FL: Chapman & Hall/CRC.

Blalock, H. M. (1964). *Causal inference in non-experimental research*. Durham, NC: University of North Carolina Press.

Campbell, T. D., & Stanley, J. C. (1966). *Experimental and quasi-experimental designs for research*. Chicago: Rand McNally.

Cheever, K. H. (1999). Pain, analgesic use, and morbidity in appendectomy patients. *Clinical Nursing Research, 8,* 267–282.

Cook, T. D. & Campbell, D. T. (1979). *Quasi-experimentation: design and analysis issues for field settings*. Boston: Houghton Mifflin.

DeFloor, T., & Grypdonck, M. H. F. (2000). Do pressure relief cushions really relieve pressure? *Western Journal of Nursing Research, 22,* 335–350.

Fisher, R. A. (1951). *The design of experiments* (6th ed.). Edinburgh: Oliver & Boyd. (1st ed., 1935).

Hume, D. (1739/1740). *A treatise of human nature*. New York: Dutton, Everyman's Library.

Kassirer J. P., & Koppelman, R. I. (1987). Judging causality. *Hospital Practice, 22,* 43–50.

Mill, J. S. (1843). *A system of logic*. London: Routledge & Sons.

Moser, D. K., Dracup, K., & Doering, L. V. (2000). Factors differentiating dropouts from completers in a longitudinal, multi-center clinical trial. *Nursing Research, 49,* 109–116.

Munro, B. H. (2001). *Statistical methods for health care research* (2nd ed.). Philadelphia Lippincott Williams & Wilkins.

National Cancer Institute (2002). SEER Cancer Statistics Review, 1973–1998. http://seer.cancer.gov/Publications/CSR1973 1988.

Naylor, M. D., Brooten, D., Campbell, R., Jacobson, B. S., Mezey, M. D., Pauly, M. V., & Schwartz, J. S. (1999). Comprehensive discharge planning and home follow-up of hospitalized elders: A randomized clinical trial. *Journal of the American Medical Association, 281,* 613–20.

O'Connor, A. M., Pennie, R. A., et al. (1996). Framing effects on expectations, decisions, and side effects experienced: The case of influenza immunization. *Journal of Clinical Epidemiology, 49,* 1271–1276.

Platt, J. R. (1964). Strong inference. *Science, 146,* 347–353.

Powell, S., Canterbury, A., & McCoy, D. (1998). Medication administration: Does the teaching method really matter? *Journal of Nursing Education, 37,* 281–283.

Susser, M. (1991). What is a cause and how do we know one? A grammar for pragmatic epidemiology. *American Journal of Epidemiology, 133,* 635–648

Schmitt, N., Padonu, G., & Wills, C. (1997). An educational intervention as decision support for menopausal women. *Research in Nursing & Health, 20,* 377–387.

Sidani, S., & Braden, C. J. (1998). *Evaluating nursing interventions*. Thousand Oaks, CA: Sage.

Student (1908). The probable error of a mean. *Biometrika, 6,* 1–25. ("Student" is a pseudonym for W. S. Gosset.)

Susser, M. (1986). The logic of Sir Karl Popper and the practice of epidemiology. *American Journal of Epidemiology, 124,* 711–719.

Rothert, M. L., Holmes-Rovner, M., Rovner, D., Kroll, J., Breer, L., et al. (1997). An educational intervention as decision support for menopausal women. *Research in Nursing & Health, 20,* 377–387.

CHAPTER 4 The Design and Analysis of Studies With Separate Control Groups

INTRODUCTION: THREATS TO DESIGN VALIDITY

In the previous chapter, we introduced the simplest possible **between-subjects design:** a two-group comparison involving just one intervention (or treatment) group and one separate control group. In this type of study, the research subjects are randomly assigned to either the intervention group or the control group, so that any preexisting differences *among the subjects* (in their background characteristics or environments) do not generate systematic differences *between the two groups*. Suppose a nurse researcher wants to find out which of two management approaches is most effective for healing Stage III decubitus ulcers in hospitalized diabetic patients. To test the alternative approaches (interventions), patients with Stage III decubitus ulcers are *randomly* assigned to either usual care (e.g., frequent turning, skin care, use of a special mattress) or a promising new type of wound dressing, in addition to usual care. The relative effectiveness of the two interventions is then judged in terms of the *average* outcomes (say, mean time needed for the ulcers to heal) produced in the control group and the treatment group. However, this comparison is valid only if neither group is *systematically* favored over the other. With random assignment, that is precisely what happens: whatever the patient characteristics, all patients are equally likely to be assigned to either the intervention group or the control group.

Now suppose that the researcher attempts to test the same new intervention, but compares diabetic patients in two different hospital units. Such study design choices are often made on the basis of feasibility considerations. For instance, time and other resource constraints may allow for new intervention training in only one unit. Unfortunately, now the conclusion that the new intervention is superior to usual care becomes less assured, because there are several other possibilities (competing explanations other than the intervention itself) for a shorter average healing time observed in the group that gets the new intervention. Patients in that hospital unit may be younger or may be less physically debilitated, and such factors are now *viable competing explanations* for the observed differences between the two groups. Most importantly, without random assignment, there is no formal basis for constructing sampling distributions of the test statistic, and the conclusions based on significance tests are suspect.

Generally, competing explanations for an observed study finding are referred to as **threats to design validity,** which have also become known as **threats to internal validity** in the classic texts on this topic (Campbell & Stan-

ley, 1963; Cook & Campbell, 1979). While they are always an issue, threats to design (internal) validity vary depending on the features of a particular study. Thus, it is essential to anticipate them in advance of data collection, control them if possible through study design modifications, or at least address them as potential limitations to the interpretation of study findings when it is not feasible to control them. Because an understanding of design validity threats is an integral part of drawing valid causal conclusions about the effectiveness of interventions, we shall discuss the most important threats to design validity that have been identified in the literature. After that, we shall move on to a discussion of more complex research designs.

TYPES OF THREATS TO DESIGN VALIDITY

When researchers refer to **design validity** in a research report, they generally refer to all the study design features that support a causal interpretation of the relationship between treatment variable(s) and outcomes. Think back to the example of comparing patients who get usual care for decubitus ulcers versus those who get usual care plus a special wound dressing. Obviously, in this case, the researchers would like to be able to conclude that wound-healing times are shortened as a result of the application of the new wound dressing procedures. For this interpretation to be convincing, not only would researchers have to come up with the empirical evidence that wound-healing times are indeed shorter in the new intervention group; also they would have to exclude most or even all plausible alternative explanations for the observed relationship between the treatment (wound dressing) and outcome variable (wound healing time). In this section, we describe nine plausible alternative explanations (threats to design validity), together with examples for each concept. They are

1. Selection bias
2. History
3. Subject attrition
4. Maturation
5. Testing
6. Instrumentation
7. Diffusion of treatments
8. Compensatory equalization of treatments
9. Statistical regression

Which of these threats is especially germane to a given study depends very much on that study's specific design features. In selecting a study design, researchers attempt to balance their desire to eliminate threats to design validity against feasibility considerations in implementing a study.

Selection Bias

In a certain sense, selection bias is the most fundamental problem a researcher must deal with, particularly in studies that use between-subject designs. Because such studies are based on the comparison of different groups of individuals exposed to different treatment levels, the assignment of study participants to the various groups must be free of bias. Whenever there are systematic differences among the groups *before* the treatment or intervention is implemented, a **selection bias** is evident.

The example of a study comparing patients in one hospital unit, who are exposed to a new wound dressing procedure, with patients in another hospital unit, who get the usual decubitus care, is a classic example of a study design that is vulnerable to selection bias. Because there are reasons to suspect that patients in different hospital units differ with respect to a host of both biologic and social characteristics, selection bias is a real possibility. As was discussed in the previous chapter and again earlier in this chapter, the single best protection against selection bias (sometimes also referred to as **differential selection**) is random assignment of subjects to the comparison groups. However, even random assignment does not guarantee that comparison groups will be "equal" on all characteristics that could influence the outcome of an intervention. Especially in small samples, the likelihood that the assignment process yields unbiased results may not be very high (Research Scenario 4-1).

Thus, whereas random assignment avoids systematic biases in the long run, any particular division of the sample into comparison groups may turn out to be quite biased. In other words, random assignment does not guarantee equivalence of the groups to be compared. It takes fairly large samples to provide reasonable certainty that potentially important preexisting differences between the comparison groups are of limited consequences.

History

History refers to the occurrence or intrusion of other events that may interfere with the treatment or intervention to be tested. It has the potential to be a serious problem in longitudinal studies, because in such studies researchers are less able to control, over the relevant time period, the exposure of the study participants to outside events. Essentially, in an ideal experimental test of an intervention,

RESEARCH SCENARIO 4.1

Hypertension in Smokers and Nonsmokers

Suppose a researcher wants to study the effects of a new treatment for hypertension in a population in which there are both smokers and nonsmokers. The researcher plans to randomly assign smokers and nonsmokers alike to treatment (new drug therapy) and control (standard drug therapy) groups, and also estimates that about 30% of the study participants will turn out to be smokers. Because it is foreseeable that smokers will have less of a response to the new drug therapy than nonsmokers, the researcher should be reasonably sure that the proportion of smokers in each of the two **study arms,** or study groups, is about equal. Put another way, the researcher should exclude the possibility that the two groups, or arms (new drug group versus standard drug therapy group), differ systematically from each other with respect to their average smoking status (proportion of smokers versus nonsmokers). What sample size would be needed to be reasonably certain (say, with a 90% probability) that the proportion of smokers in the two study arms does not differ by more than 5%? It turns out that a total study sample of $n = 154$ (77 study participants in each arm) would be required. If a narrower difference were desired, say, no more than a 2% difference in the proportion of smokers in each study arm, a rather large sample of $n = 966$ (or 483 for each comparison group) would be needed.[1]

exposure to the different treatment levels (such as "usual care" compared with a "new treatment approach") should be the *only* factor that differs among the comparison groups. From the standpoint of research design, any other event that may occur during the intervention, or even interfere with it, is a competing **involuntary treatment.** Even events that are not group specific can pose serious problems for causal inference. For example, if *during* a smoking cessation intervention study, a local community bans smoking in all commercial establishments, that action may just provide the edge to make the intervention successful. A researcher who does not know of the smoking

---

[1]The basis for these calculations will be discussed in more detail in Chapter 20.

ban might overestimate the effectiveness of the experimental smoking cessation intervention, and a replication of the study under other circumstances might fail to show support for the intervention effectiveness.

History is of particular concern when researchers do not use random assignment but instead compare patient populations in different settings, such as communities, states, hospitals, nursing homes, and schools, some of which are exposed to an intervention. Differences in intrainstitutional histories, or histories within various geographic settings, can thus become plausible alternative explanations for the observed intervention effect. For example, over 1 year, a hospital might experience a substantial staff turnover, affecting the organizational climate and patient care processes for either better or worse. This could influence particular inpatient nursing care outcomes, which may also be considered appropriate response variables to an experimental intervention. Likewise, a researcher who uses knowledge-of-nutrition measures among community-dwelling older adults over several months to test the effectiveness of a community-based public health campaign must also consider what other events in the community (including exposure to mass media programming) might have brought about changes in nutritional knowledge. Fortunately, in studies of short to moderate duration in which fairly large samples with random assignment of subjects to study conditions are used, members of the comparison groups are likely to be exposed to similar average (home/family/work) environments.

Subject Attrition

Subject attrition, also referred to as **subject mortality,** is the loss of participants from a study at any point between enrollment and completion of the study. Study participants who are lost to a study are often referred to in the literature as **dropouts.** Even though treatment and control groups in a clinical trial may be equivalent or comparable on preexisting characteristics immediately after random assignment to study groups, loss of subjects from the study before the measurement of study outcomes can change that. In health-related research, patterns of attrition are often not random. Not surprisingly, for example, it has been found that participants who are lost from longitudinal studies of cancer caregiving are often sicker and frailer, are more often male than female, and have fewer years of formal education (Neumark, Stommel, Given, & Given, 2001). Likewise, sicker participants in a cardiovascular fitness exercise intervention may find the exercise burdensome and drop out of the intervention group but not necessarily out of the (nonexercise) control group. This causes problems in con-

cluding that an intervention is successful, especially if there is no careful analysis of the characteristics of study dropouts. The reason is that a seemingly successful intervention may reflect the fact that only the healthier individuals persevered with an intervention.

Sometimes study participants abandon a control or placebo group because they do not experience any improvement in their health (Meinert, 1986) or may not perceive that there are other meaningful benefits to their study participation. This can lead to a systematic reduction of the true difference between the treatment and control group(s), in which case the effect of the intervention is underestimated.

Subject attrition can also affect the **generalizability** of study findings. Whenever the dropouts differ in a systematic way from the study participants who remain in the study until the end, a **sampling bias** is introduced. The change in the sample composition directly affects to which population the study results can be inferred.

In summary, the key point about subject attrition is this: If any characteristic of study participants is predictive of attrition *and* is systematically related to the treatment/ intervention conditions, then inferences about the effectiveness of the intervention can be in error. Depending on the study, the error may include

1. Overestimating the benefit of the intervention
2. Underestimating the benefit of the intervention
3. Misestimating the specific effects of the intervention for a target population to which a researcher wishes to generalize study findings

Maturation

Maturation refers to all over-time changes in study participants that are not related to any particular *external* events, but instead appear to reflect *internal* changes in the study participants themselves. For certain types of studies, maturation is a plausible explanation for changes in an outcome measure, besides the intervention effects themselves. More specifically, in health-related studies, maturational change often occurs in response to time-related processes originating within the study participants. Some changes are short term, such as physiologic responses like fatigue or hunger; others may be longer term, such as general growth in knowledge or attitudes toward certain health care practices that are not directly influenced by the study intervention.

Random assignment of subjects to various treatment and control conditions provides the best protection against systematic differences in the maturation of subjects, because all comparison groups are likely to undergo, on average, similar maturation processes. However, mere random assignment of subjects may not always be sufficient, particularly for situations in which short-term maturational processes such as fatigue may strongly influence study participants' performance on research tasks. It is very important in clinical research to be aware of the particular characteristics of illnesses and treatments that may affect the study participants' responses to research tasks. For example, if a researcher wishes to survey a group of cancer chemotherapy patients as part of an experimental intervention, it would be best to schedule surveys for patients in the control and intervention groups at similar times, when energy and attentiveness are likely to be best, and when the adverse side effects of chemotherapy are minimal.

Testing

Testing effects occur when the very fact of having taken an earlier test (pretest) influences the results in subsequent test taking (posttest). This threat to design validity is of special concern in tests or measures that involve subject learning or recall. For example, suppose that a nurse wishes to track mental status changes in an elderly patient population she or he sees daily in a day treatment setting. If the nurse assesses the mental status of each patient one or two times a week, at least some patients may recall their answers from previous mental status exam assessments and repeat them for future assessments. Scores on knowledge tests often improve when the tests are taken a second time, even if there is no objective improvement in knowledge levels. Sometimes the pretest itself sensitizes study participants to an issue and, as a result, changes their responses on the posttest. For example, in an intervention study that deals with decision making about personal health actions, the study participants' completion of the pretest interview could influence their future decision making, independently of the intervention designed to improve the effectiveness of personal decision making (Rothert et al., 1997). In other words, the act of completing a pretest interview to describe one's attitudes, knowledge, or preferences may in itself be an intervention. If the same type of testing effect occurs in both the treatment and control groups, the end result may be that it is more difficult to detect the effects of the intervention that is actually being tested, particularly for interventions that are designed primarily to increase knowledge or to change attitudes.

Instrumentation

Instrumentation refers to systematic biases in the comparison of treatment and control groups that are attributable to measurement problems. One key problem is lack of sufficient **standardization** of measurement procedures. For instance, using different people to monitor outcomes in different comparison groups, when clear rules for the observational procedures are lacking, can be problematic because different observers may record the same event in different ways. For example, two nurses who are rating the skin pallor of the same patient at the same time using a 1 to 5 ordinal rating scale (1 = not at all pale; 5 = very pale) may produce different ratings. Such judgments not only are influenced by the past clinical experience of the observer, but also may be unconsciously affected by the knowledge of which study condition (control or experimental) the participant is assigned to.

One possible solution is to randomly assign all observers within each of the comparison groups, a technique that is called **blocking** (to be described in more detail later in this chapter). Another solution is to remove systematic bias in observation through the application of blinding procedures in experimental studies. A **blinding procedure** is one in which either study participants, treatment team members, or data collectors are unaware of which study participants are assigned to intervention and control study conditions. In **double-blind studies,** neither the study participants nor the data collectors/observers know which subjects are assigned to treatment and control conditions. In **triple-blind studies,** neither the study participants, the health professionals treating them, nor the persons who observe or record the outcome are aware of which subjects are assigned to treatment and control conditions.

Diffusion of Treatments

Diffusion of treatments refers to the contamination of the treatment conditions that can occur when either the participants or others involved in an intervention study have the opportunity to interact with one another and to share information about the study. For example, participants in the experimental group of a health education intervention may share information about the intervention with members of the control group, who are receiving usual care. Likewise, staff from two hospital units who are implementing the control and experimental conditions of an intervention study may interact off unit and exchange information about the study that may affect the study outcomes. If the staff who implement the new approach to managing decubitus ulcers share their perceptions with control group staff that the new approach is superior to standard care, the latter may alter their clinical practice so that the study no longer has a control group that receives care as usual. In general, teaching interventions that involve any type of knowledge or skills that can be readily shared (Powell, Canterbury, & McCoy, 1998) are particularly vulnerable to the diffusion problem. Diffusion is also more likely in studies in which subjects for all comparison groups are recruited from the same site. It is a threat to design validity against which random assignment of subjects does not provide any special protection. Usually, where diffusion threats are present, the result is comparison groups that are made more similar, thus reducing the possibility of showing the effectiveness of an intervention.

Compensatory Equalization of Treatments

This issue is really the result of an ethical dilemma. Whenever a clinical trial, in its early phases, appears to show that a new treatment is beneficial and far superior to the standard treatment given to the control group, pressures from patient groups or administrators may mount to give all subjects the benefits of the treatment. This is referred to as **compensatory equalization of treatments.** The ethical principle on which this position is based is **beneficence,** the right of people both to be free from harm and to obtain benefit from the knowledge that is gained from research. In this stance, the control group may be viewed as disadvantaged in relation to the experimental group that is receiving disproportionate benefit, so compensation occurs to the control group in the form of equalizing the control and treatment groups with respect to treatment access.

For example, suppose that, in short-term trials, a new drug is found to produce a high success rate in the treatment of an otherwise fatal disease. In that case, it may well be mandated that participants in the control group have access to the drug before the planned completion date of the treatment trial. Yet, because short-term results are not always confirmed in the long run, and unforeseen harmful side effects may reveal themselves only in more extensive trials, such midstream reversals are not without their own risks.[2] From a study design perspective, whenever compensatory equalization of treatments is present, the effect is similar to that of diffusion: It reduces the possibility of showing the effectiveness of an intervention.

Statistical Regression

Statistical regression refers to the movement of mean (average) scores between measurement points resulting from

the initial selection of participants on the basis of extreme scores. This is a subtle but very important point in clinical intervention research. For instance, patient outcomes are observed after a standard surgical procedure, and patients are most often seen to improve rapidly, regardless of any specific intervention used to help them return to baseline functioning. Thus, if a researcher recruits samples of very sick subjects, changes in health are almost certain to be observed, because the study participants' outcome scores often revert to the mean. In the case of uncomplicated illnesses and surgical procedures, the study participants' health ratings often revert to their long-run (average) health trajectory. Similarly, caregivers recruited from caregiver support groups may respond more positively to social support interventions than caregivers who are not linked to a support network. Here again, random assignment to treatment and control groups remains the best protection against mistaking regression effects for real treatment effects.

Summary

Each of these nine key design validity threats is important to consider and control for whenever possible, especially if the goal of the research is to draw accurate conclusions about causal relationships. For most potential design validity threats, random assignment of subjects to study conditions or random assignment of study conditions to subjects will either substantially reduce or eliminate the design threat. This is, however, not the case for subject attrition, diffusion of treatment(s), or compensatory equalization of treatment. These potential threats to design validity require careful consideration on the part of the researcher. This extra care includes using methods to prevent or at least reduce subject attrition and finding ways to avert exchange of information between experimental and control study conditions.

In the following sections, we present different categories of experimental studies, beyond the basic two-group control versus experimental study design we have described so far. Problems with design validity threats are discussed within the context of each experimental study design introduced.

SINGLE-FACTOR STUDIES

In a **single-factor experimental study,** only one treatment or intervention variable is deliberately varied (or manipulated) by the researcher. This independent variable must take on at least two categories (levels) but may comprise more than two levels. Typically, in two-group clinical tri-

---

[2]Chapter 24 provides an extensive discussion of the ethical dilemmas in clinical studies.

als, the treatment group receives a new intervention (either alone or in addition to usual care), and the control group receives usual care. The only requirement in a single-factor study is that the categories/groups/treatment levels defined by the independent variable must be **mutually exclusive.** This means that the levels of the independent variable must involve distinct interventions or control treatments, and subjects are assigned and exposed to only one level of the treatment. Consider the examples of single-factor experimental studies in Research Scenario 4-2.

Although there are many different ways of designing single-factor studies, our focus here is to introduce just a few key designs that exemplify the possibilities and that also constitute the vast majority of experimental designs encountered in the medical and nursing literature.[3] Between-subjects experiments, including single-factor studies, can be classified along two important dimensions. One dimension distinguishes between **completely randomized designs** and **randomized block designs;** another between **posttest only designs** and **pretest/posttest designs.**

Completely Randomized Single-Factor Studies with Control Groups

Completely randomized control group designs are frequently encountered in the literature. Often, they involve two-group comparisons of one treatment group and one control group (for examples, see Lantz, Stencil, Lippert, Beversdorf, Jaros, & Remington, 1995; Hayes, 1998; Powell et al. 1998; Overmeire, Smets, Lecoutere, Van de Broek, Weylwr, De Groote, & Langhendries, 2000), and sometimes they encompass multiple-group comparisons with more than one treatment group (see Lallemant, Jourdain, Le Couer, Kim Koetsawang, Comeau, & Phoolcharoen, 2000; Edinger, Wohlgemuth, Radtke, Marsh, & Quillian, 2001). The reason for the popularity of these designs lies both in their simplicity and in the fact that they allow for strong causal inferences. As the name implies, in a completely randomized design, randomization is the only device used to assign subjects to the comparison groups. This means that the random assignment process is rather simple.

For instance, in a two-group design, researchers might resort to a **lottery drawing,** in which some method is used to select participants for study groups in a random fashion. For example, if the research plan calls for a total sample of 80 people to be evenly divided between intervention and control groups, a researcher could prepare a

RESEARCH SCENARIO 4.2

Control and Comparison Groups
1. Naylor et al. (1999) tested an intervention consisting of comprehensive discharge planning and a home follow-up protocol designed to reduce rehospitalization among elderly patients recruited for study participation during hospitalization. The control group received routine hospital discharge planning.
2. Single-factor studies also include multiple-group trials, in which the groups are defined as different levels of the same independent variable or factor. For instance, Sutter et al. (2000) conducted a multicenter clinical trial to evaluate the responses of infants in developing countries to four different poliovirus vaccine formulations. Here, varying the type of polio vaccine formulation resulted in four comparison groups.

bowl filled with 40 red and 40 white balls, all manufactured to the same specifications of weight and size. Each time a new subject is enrolled (agrees to participate) in the study, a ball is drawn from the bowl after thorough mixing. If the ball is red, the subject is assigned to the intervention group; if it is white, the subject is assigned to the control group. It is easy to see that this procedure can be extended to three or more groups. One would just have to ensure that the bowl contains balls of three or more different colors.

In Table 4-1, two completely randomized designs are featured: one that does not include a pretest (Part A) and one that does include a pretest (Part B). The **posttest-only design** in Part A of Table 4-1 shows that it is not difficult to see why it is a strong design with respect to drawing valid causal conclusions about the effectiveness of treatments. Because subjects are randomly assigned to the comparison groups, selection bias is not a major threat to design validity. Neither are history, maturation, or testing effects. Subject attrition may occur after the random assignment but before the measurement of outcomes. If it does occur, the particular problem with a posttest-only design is that the effects of subject attrition may be difficult to assess. Without baseline data, one simply may not know whether the subjects lost were typical of (representative of) the group as a whole, or not. However, attrition problems are usually more common in longer-lasting studies with

---

[3]For a thorough treatment of different research designs, it is still worthwhile to read the classic text by Cochran & Cox (1957).

TABLE 4.1	Completely Randomized Designs

Part A: Posttest Only Randomized Control Group Design

Random Assignment of Subjects to Comparison Groups	Manipulation of Independent Variable	Observation of Outcomes
Treatment/intervention group	New intervention	Posttest measure
Control/usual care group	Usual intervention	Posttest measure

Part B: Pretest/Posttest Randomized Control Group Design

Random Assignment of Subjects to Comparison Groups	Observation of Outcomes Before Treatment	Manipulation of Independent Variable	Observation of Outcomes
Treatment/intervention group	Pretest measure	New intervention	Posttest measure
Control/usual care group	Pretest measure	Usual intervention	Posttest measure

several follow-up measures. Possibly the single biggest threat to validity of this design in clinical studies is the diffusion of treatment, i.e., the inability of researchers to keep treatment and control subjects separate and to avoid spillover or contamination effects. Because random assignment of individual subjects requires that it be done within all the clinical sites for the clinical trial, subjects recruited at the same site can and will be enrolled in different arms of the same study. This circumstance makes a clinical study vulnerable to diffusion, especially when the interventions are educational, involving learning behaviors on the part of subjects. However, if diffusion and attrition problems can be contained, posttest-only designs have a strong claim to delivering causal evidence.

Table 4-1, Part B depicts a **randomized pretest/posttest design.** The principal feature of this design is the addition of a baseline assessment of study subjects *before* the interventions or treatments take place. The use of study designs with pretests and posttests is quite common in health care research. Such studies possess undeniable attractions over posttest-only studies. For instance, pretest/posttest designs do not simply rely on the rather abstract notion that random assignment balances out the differences among study subjects. Instead, they provide direct baseline estimates of how similar subjects in the comparison groups score on the outcome measures *before* the intervention(s). In addition, when both pretest and posttest measures are available, it is possible to measure the change effected by the interventions or treatments. This is intuitively appealing because it provides a vivid example of how the presumed cause effects a change in the outcome variable. From an analysis

point of view, even more important is the fact that pretest/posttest designs improve the efficiency of a study. The reason is that the availability of pretest scores allows one to "subtract out" individual differences. This point is illustrated in Research Scenario 4-3.

RESEARCH SCENARIO 4.3

Oat Bran and Cholesterol
Suppose that a researcher conducts an experiment to investigate the extent to which the consumption of oat bran, instead of corn flakes, lowers low-density lipoprotein (LDL) cholesterol among adult primary care patients. Assume that only six study participants are randomly assigned either to the oat bran ($n_1 = 3$) or the corn flake group ($n_2 = 3$). In both groups, participants agree to consume 8 ounces of cereal every morning for 3 months. After 3 months, a mean (average) LDL cholesterol reading of 4.4 mg/dL is observed in the oat bran group, and the three scores averaged to obtain the mean are 3.8, 4.5, and 4.8 mg/dL. In the corn flakes group, the mean is 4.5 mg/dL, with individual scores of 4.0, 4.6, and 5.0 mg/dL. Based on these data, including the mean level difference between the two groups of −.1 (oat bran group mean minus corn flakes group mean), how convincing is the evidence that oat bran reduces serum cholesterol?

These data do not look particularly convincing as evidence for the cholesterol-reducing properties of oat bran. The main reason why the small mean difference of $-.1$ is not convincing evidence is that there is so much variation in scores among the individuals in the groups (referred to more formally as **between-subjects variation**) that we might well expect that a different outcome of the random assignment process would easily give us different results.

But now suppose that the researcher had obtained the following low-density lipoprotein cholesterol scores *before* the nutrition intervention was implemented. In the oat bran group, the subjects' initial scores were 4.0, 4.7 and 5.0 mg/dL, whereas in the corn flakes group, the subjects showed no change, having pretest scores identical to their posttest scores. If the pretest scores are subtracted from the posttest scores, there is a consistent difference of $-.2$ mg/dL for each member of the oat bran group, whereas there is a difference of 0 mg/dL for each member of the corn flakes group. This example illustrates how using a *mean change* score subtracts out all the individual differences in scores *between subjects*. Thus, the between-subjects variability that obscured the treatment (oat bran) effect in the posttest-only design has been removed from the comparison, and oat bran is revealed as having cholesterol-lowering properties.

Advantages and Disadvantages of Randomized Pretest/Posttest Designs

If pretest/posttest designs have such clear advantages, why don't researchers always opt for them? One reason is that comparable pretests are not available for some interventions. This would be the case for outcome measures that gauge the effectiveness of hospital discharge planning interventions, such as the number of rehospitalizations after initial discharge, the number of revisits to the emergency department, or compliance with medication regimens. By contrast, pretests are feasible and useful in the comparison of knowledge scores before and after an educational intervention, or of routine biophysiologic measures such as blood tests and blood pressure readings (for an example, see Edinger et al., 2001).

The addition of a pretest also does not add any new problems for causal inference. Just as with the posttest-only design, random assignment minimizes most threats to design validity. Note that history, maturation, testing effects, and instrumentation do not constitute a threat because, after random assignments, these effects should operate more or less the same way in both the experimental group and the control group. Selection bias is also not a major issue. As for subject attrition, there is an advantage in having pretest scores: They at least allow the researcher

to examine the random or systematic nature of the attrition. Thus, only diffusion of treatment remains a credible threat to design validity.

All in all, the **randomized pretest/posttest design** is one of the most enduring experimental designs because of its combination of simplicity and power in providing good causal inference. If there is any weakness in this design, it is one that most likely occurs in psychologic/attitude types of studies: **the interaction of testing and experimental stimulus.** This refers to the reaction to the experimental stimulus being different for people exposed to the pretest than in people not exposed to the pretest. If this occurs, then the results from pretested individuals cannot be generalized to individuals who were not pretested but were exposed to the same stimulus. This problem is most likely to occur in studies in which subjects can learn from the pretests. For example, knowledge tests may not only assess what a person already knows but also provide some additional knowledge. In addition, study participants may be influenced by the test in the sense that they discern (or believe to discern) what is "expected" of them in providing later responses. Similarly, a study participant who has been exposed to a knowledge pretest may react differently to an educational intervention because the pretest has sensitized the subject, who now views the meaning of the educational intervention in a different light. The best way to gauge the magnitude of this interaction of pretesting and experimental stimulus is to combine the two previously described designs into a single-study design, an example of which is called the **Salomon four-group design.**

The Salomon Four-Group Design

Table 4-2 depicts the **Salomon four-group design,** which combines the features of a posttest-only with a pretest/posttest design. Its advantage is that it allows a researcher to disentangle the effects of exposure to a pretest from the effects of exposure to the main intervention. Even though this design is effective and appealing, it is not often used in practice. The reasons include the four-group comparison's complexities as well as the fact that it is costlier to undertake.

For example, suppose that a workshop (intervention) for primary care clinic staff is designed to change staff beliefs and attitudes about work with primary care patients who are experiencing mental illness. In that context, exposure to a pretest measure of beliefs and attitudes about the mentally ill could act as an intervention itself, aside from the effects of the workshop. Thus, the researchers decide to create four staff groups with the following exposure patterns: (1) pretest and workshop participation, (2) pretest without workshop participation, (3) no pretest and workshop participation, and (4) neither pretest nor workshop

TABLE 4.2	The Salomon Four-Group Design		
Random Assignment of Subjects to Comparison Groups	Observation of Outcomes Before Treatment	Manipulation of Independent Variable	Observation of Outcomes
Treatment/intervention group	Pretest measure	New intervention	Posttest measure
Control/usual care group	Pretest measure	Usual intervention	Posttest measure
Treatment/intervention group	No pretest measure	New intervention	Posttest measure
Control/ usual care group	No pretest measure	Usual intervention	Posttest measure

participation. After collecting attitude scores in all four groups, the researchers will be able to make two kinds of comparisons. First, the mean (average) attitude scores of Groups 1 and 3 can be pooled (combined) and compared with the pooled mean attitude scores of Groups 2 and 4. This will give an estimate of the treatment (workshop participation) effect. Similarly, the pooled mean attitude scores of Groups 1 and 2 compared with those of Groups 3 and 4 will provide an estimate of the effect of having taken a pretest.

Randomized Block Designs

In the previous section, a simple lottery was described as a possible means of randomly assigning subjects to intervention and control groups. In some situations, however, the outcome of such a simple lottery may not be desirable. Recall that random selection and assignment do not guarantee any particular distribution of cases. Thus, it is possible, in theory, that as a result of random assignment, the first 40 subjects enrolled in the study all end up in the intervention group, with the remaining 40 subjects in the control group.[4]

It is considerably more likely that random assignments produce unbalanced results, such as long strings of newly enrolled cases consecutively assigned to the treatment group. In clinical trials in which subjects are often enrolled sequentially over extended periods of time, this may be undesirable. Suppose, for instance, that there was a gradual shift in the characteristics of patient populations over time, or a change in the standard treatments to which the new interventions are compared. In these possible situations, researchers usually want to ensure that enrollment in both

arms of the trial (intervention and control group) is balanced with respect to the time of enrollment. Otherwise, the comparison of intervention and control groups may also entail an unacknowledged comparison of (predominantly) late and early enrollees. To avoid this problem, subjects can be enrolled in **blocks.** Take a look at the assignment process in Box 4-1, and contrast it to the simple randomization via lottery.

This simple scheme involves **blocks** of two subjects, and the random assignment occurs within each block. Thus, even if the trial were to be interrupted, both comparison groups would contain the same number of subjects, as long as the total number is even. Sometimes a study may be stopped because time or money runs out before the sample reaches its targeted size, in which case a blocking scheme for assigning participants to conditions can be

BOX 4.1	Assigning Study Subjects to Groups

All enrolled subjects are numbered sequentially from 1 to *n*, as they are enrolled. *n* refers to the total sample size and would be an even number in a two-group comparison that is to produce equal sized groups. Next, the *n* subjects are divided into *n*/2 consecutive dyads or pairs. For instance, subjects 1 and 2 form the first dyad, followed by 3 and 4, 5 and 6, and so forth. Finally, using a table of random numbers (see Appendix C), the researchers assign the first member of a dyad to the intervention group (and the second member to the control group) if the random number is even. If the random number is odd, the assignment of the first and second members of a dyad is reversed.

[4]The probability of this occurrence is, however, infinitesimally small: $p = (40! \times 40!)/80! = 9.302 \times 10^{-23}$, a number that can, for all practical purposes, be treated as zero.

quite helpful to avoid imbalances in the data already obtained. For instance, there would also be an exact balance of early and late enrollees in each arm of the study. If desired, blocks can easily be enlarged, say to four or six subjects for each block, or to uneven numbers, if the number of comparison groups is uneven.

Assigning subjects randomly within predetermined blocks is actually a form of stratified random assignment. Whereas **blocked randomization** usually refers to stratification by time, **stratified randomization** refers to stratification on the basis of other factors (Friedman, Furberg, & DeMets, 1996). However, we treat them here together because the underlying logic of the procedure is the same. As we have seen, random assignment provides an all-purpose mechanism for dealing with confounding or nuisance variables (Kirk, 1992). However, there are sometimes more effective ways of controlling for known confounders. In particular, stratified randomization is used to guarantee equality of comparison groups with respect to a few key variables. The only additional requirement compared with time blocking is that subjects can be correctly identified when they are randomly assigned. That is, information on the stratification variable(s) must be easily accessible. Now consider examples of stratified random assignment processes in Research Scenario 4-4.

If more precision were desirable, the level-of-education blocking variable could be subdivided into finer educational achievement groupings. The stratified randomization guar-

antees that both the treatment group and the control group contain 60% subjects with higher and 40% subjects with lower educational credentials. This would eliminate the education variable as an explanation of between-group differences. In addition, because educational achievement is now an identifiable independent variable in the study, its effect on the outcome can be completely separated from the intervention effect during the analysis.

In summary, blocked and stratified randomizations operate in the same way. They guarantee that subjects within each block are divided among the comparison groups at a fixed ratio, resulting in each stratum being represented in the comparison groups according to its overall strength. Another way of saying this is that the blocking or grouping factor is, as a matter of design, not correlated with the treatment variable. That is why it cannot account for any observed differences among the groups.

As another example, assume that researchers conducting a clinical trial to reduce depression among post-myocardial infarction patients have stratified their sample by gender. By design, both treatment and control groups would have the same proportions of female and male subjects. With an identical gender composition, observed differences in treatment outcomes between treatment and control groups cannot be attributed to gender. However, gender is now an additional explanatory variable that accounts for some of the variation in the outcomes, i.e., the depression scores. This reduces **error variance** (portion of

RESEARCH SCENARIO 4.4

Random Assignment

1. In a recent study, Sloan et al. (1998) compared over-time completion rates on four quality-of-life measures among advanced colorectal cancer patients, who were resistant to 5FU and underwent a clinical trial studying the effectiveness of hydrazine sulfate. The random assignment to the different quality-of-life measures was undertaken during an ongoing clinical trial. To insure equal proportions of patients from treatment and control groups for all instruments, randomization followed prior stratification.

2. Suppose you are interested in studying the effectiveness of an educational intervention among patients. You are aware that there is considerable evidence that prior educational achievement generally has a large effect on patients' comprehension of complex information. You are aware that randomly assigning the study participants (regardless of their educational background) to either the intervention group or the control group may not be very effective, because random assignment does not guarantee equivalence of the comparison groups with respect to education. You have $n = 40$ participants who have a high school education or less, and $n = 60$ participants who have at least some college education. In this situation, it may be appropriate to consider a stratification of the sample based on educational level. For example, you might divide the study participants by whether or not they have a high school degree or less, versus those with at least some college, and then randomly assign the participants within each educational group to either the control or the intervention study groups.

outcomes that cannot be explained by the intervention variable) and thus increases the efficiency of the design, improving the ability of the researcher to draw conclusions about what does and does not influence outcomes.

FACTORIAL DESIGNS

Single-factor experiments do have their limitations. Chief among them is their inefficiency, often including the inability to explain much of the variation in the outcome variable. For each new set of mutually exclusive interventions that make up the independent variable or factor, a new study has to be planned, a new sample of subjects enrolled, the intervention(s) carried out, and the outcomes observed. As an alternative, researchers sometimes opt for simultaneously examining the joint effects of two or more independent variables or factors in a single experiment. That way, not only is there a gain in efficiency from obtaining information about multiple treatments in a single trial or experiment, but also there is an added ability to answer a new kind of question: Does the effectiveness of one kind of treatment depend on (or is it modified by) variations in another type of treatment?

The classic example for this kind of **multifactorial approach** is the investigation of drug interactions. For instance, HIV-positive patients often take a drug "cocktail" of several different drugs designed to control the HIV virus. The recommendation for such a drug regimen to patients should not rely only on a series of single-factor experiments that test the efficacy of each drug in the cocktail (Byar, Schoenfeld, Green, Amato, Davis, Gruttola, Finkelstein, et al., 1990). Instead, researchers must also show that the simultaneous use of several drugs does not alter the effectiveness of any individual drug, or does not cause harm to the patient by the possible toxicity of the drugs taken in combination with one another. Such possible outcomes are unobservable in separate experiments in which one drug at a time is examined.

2 × 2 Factorial Design Illustration

A clinical trial that uses a **factorial design** is an experimental study that involves the simultaneous manipulation of two or more independent variables (or factors). Its key advantage is that one cannot test only for the **main effects** of the independent variables but also tests for their **interactions,** i.e., the joint effects of the independent variables on the outcomes. Let's look at an example of how this might play out. We present the classic 2 × 2 (pronounced

RESEARCH SCENARIO 4.5

Testing Two Treatments Simultaneously

Suppose a researcher has just received funding from the National Institutes of Health to study the efficacy of two treatments (zinc inhalers and superpotent chicken broth) to improve recovery time from viral upper respiratory infections, a commonly encountered problem in primary care settings. A body of research literature already provides some support for the effectiveness of both interventions in reducing recovery time from viral infections. However, the research findings are mixed and are primarily based on observational studies. In addition, there is some suggestion in the literature that the effects of the interventions may reinforce each other, but this is less clear.

"two-by-two") factorial design for a hypothetical clinical problem in need of research. However, the logic can readily be extended to factorial designs with more factors or more categories (treatment levels) per factor. Let's look at the hypothetical example in Research Scenario 4-5.

This research problem is well suited for a randomized clinical trial based on a factorial design. The treatments can be easily manipulated—at least, the treatment recommendations can be. It is worth noting, though, that implementation in terms of actual use of zinc inhalers and consumption of super-potent chicken broth requires the cooperation of study participants in following through with the treatments. However, in this kind of study we do not have to assume that *all* study participants in fact follow through with the treatments, only that enough subjects comply to have an effect on the *average* outcome in the intervention group. The major outcome variable (recovery time) is amenable to measurement both by self-report and by follow-up primary care visits.

Assignment of Subjects to Treatment Combinations

As always in an experimental study, the treatment variables must be manipulated (varied) to show how they affect the outcome. In the simplest case, patients are asked to either use a zinc inhaler or not to use it. That is treatment

TABLE 4.3	Assignment of 200 Study Subjects to One of Four Conditions		
	No Zinc Inhaler	Zinc Inhaler	Total
No chicken broth	$n = 50$	$n = 50$	$n = 100$
Chicken broth	$n = 50$	$n = 50$	$n = 100$
Total	$n = 100$	$n = 100$	$n = 200$

These four conditions constitute all possible combinations of the two-level variables in a **fully-crossed factorial design** (cells contain numbers of research participants).

variable/factor No. 1. Similarly, patients are also asked to either consume the special chicken broth or not consume it. That is treatment variable/factor No. 2. Their combination creates four distinct categories, including a "pure" (no treatment) control group, in which subjects get neither zinc inhaler nor chicken soup. In this situation, the inclusion of a no-treatment control group could pose an ethical problem, unless the researcher defines the interventions as occurring in addition to usual care. While the usual care for upper respiratory infections consists of symptom relief measures, contingencies would also need to be built into the study protocol to allow for the use of antibiotics as part of usual care—for any study participants in whom a secondary bacterial infection develops, for example. For this illustration, we assume that no subjects receive antibiotic therapy during the course of the study. In addition, we assume that the researcher has sufficient resources to restrict patient eligibility to primary care patients who have only beginning-stage upper respiratory infections and do not have secondary bacterial infections.

As subjects consent to participate and are enrolled into the study, they are randomly assigned to one of the four possible treatment combinations created by crossing the two treatment variables. The study design is illustrated in Table 4-3. A total enrollment of 200 subjects is assumed.[5] Random assignment can be achieved fairly easily using blocks of four subjects each. Every time four new subjects are accumulated, each is assigned a random number, with the numbers chosen consecutively from a random number table (see Appendix C). Then, a simple decision rule is adopted. The subject with the lowest random number will

be assigned to the zinc inhaler and chicken soup group, the subject with the second lowest random number will be assigned to the zinc inhaler–only group. The two subjects with the larger random numbers go to the chicken soup–only group and the control group, respectively. Because the probability of drawing any of these four random numbers is the same, each subject will have the same chance of being chosen into one of the four comparison groups.

Main Effects and Interaction Effects

It was asserted above that factorial designs not only offer the advantage of efficiency but also allow for the investigation of the joint effects of the factors involved. In particular, in the investigation of the effects (if any) that the independent factors may exert on the outcome variable, two types of effects can be distinguished: **main effects** and **interaction effects.** A main effect is simply the effect of a single independent variable or factor on a dependent variable *regardless of the effect of the other factor(s).* An interaction effect occurs when effects of one variable are different depending on the levels of another variable. In Table 4-4, hypothetical numbers for mean (average) recovery time (in hours) are entered in each of the four cells representing the four experimental conditions. Because each of the four cells represents the mean score of the same number of patients ($n = 50$), we can simply average these means to get the marginal means (row or column totals).

Part A of Table 4-4 shows a hypothetical example of a main-effects-only outcome. The 100 patients who used a zinc inhaler, on average, recovered after 64 hours; the 100 patients who did not use it took, on average, 76 hours to recover (see column totals). Thus, the average effect of using the zinc inhaler is to shorten recovery time by 12 hours ($64 - 76 = -12$). Similarly, the average or main effect of consuming super-potent chicken broth is to shorten recovery time by 8 hours (see row totals).

Part B of Table 4-4 shows again some hypothetical results, this time adding an interaction. First, notice that the main effects have not changed at all. If one disregards the consumption of chicken broth, the average effect of using a zinc inhaler is still to shorten recovery time by 12 hours. Also as before, the consumption of chicken broth shortens recovery time, on average, by 8 hours. Yet, if one holds one of the factors constant and examines the effects of the other factor, a new pattern emerges. In the main-effects-only example of Part A, the average effect of chicken broth consumption (an 8-hour reduction in recovery time) was the same among subjects who used or did not use a zinc in-

[5]The discussion of determining appropriate sample size will be deferred to Chapter 20.

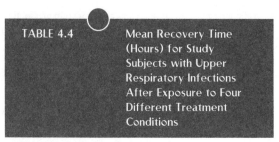

TABLE 4.4   Mean Recovery Time (Hours) for Study Subjects with Upper Respiratory Infections After Exposure to Four Different Treatment Conditions

Part A: Main Effects Only

	No Zinc Inhaler	Zinc Inhaler	Total
No chicken broth	80 hours $n = 50$	68 hours $n = 50$	74 hours $n = 100$
Chicken broth	72 hours $n = 50$	60 hours $n = 50$	66 hours $n = 100$
Total	76 hours $n = 100$	64 hours $n = 100$	70 hours $n = 200$

Part B: Main and Interaction Effects

	No Zinc Inhaler	Zinc Inhaler	Total
No chicken broth	76 hours $n = 50$	72 hours $n = 50$	74 hours $n = 100$
Chicken broth	76 hours $n = 50$	56 hours $n = 50$	66 hours $n = 100$
Total	76 hours $n = 100$	64 hours $n = 100$	70 hours $n = 200$

Cells contain means, followed by numbers of subjects.

haler. In Part B, however, we can observe that consuming chicken broth has no effect unless the zinc inhaler is also used. If it is, however, the added consumption of chicken broth leads to a recovery time that is shortened by 16 hours.

Similarly, one could discuss the same results in terms of an emphasis on the effect of zinc inhaler usage. Among subjects who do not consume chicken broth, there is a modest reduction in recovery time by 4 hours. Among the consumers of chicken broth, however, we observe an average improvement of 20 hours. Clearly, in this hypothetical example, a **synergistic effect** is present, i.e., the two treatments mutually reinforce each other. To say this in another way, the effect of one treatment variable depends on the level of the other treatment variable.

Interaction effects are common phenomena in health care, and they heighten the ability to explain outcomes.

More specifically, they limit the generality of a finding by specifying the conditions under which a certain intervention works. Not only do the effects of many interventions depend on those of other interventions, interaction effects may also involve study participant characteristics (attributes) that cannot be manipulated by the researcher. For instance, a particular educational intervention may work with adults but not with adolescents. In that case, the intervention interacts with age to produce different outcomes, depending on the subjects' age.

COMPARISON OF FACTORIAL AND STRATIFIED RANDOMIZED BLOCK DESIGNS

Comparing the **fully crossed factorial design** and the **stratified randomized (block) design** we have illustrated so far in this chapter, it is worth noticing both the similarities and the differences. In both cases, additional grouping factors such as educational level and new types of intervention are introduced that cut across the primary treatment variable. With stratified randomization, groups are formed as a result of stratifying subjects according to the categories of the blocking variable(s). Study participants are then randomly assigned to the various treatment levels of the manipulated factor *within each stratification block*. The block membership itself, however, is not manipulated or assigned to subjects and is defined in terms of attribute variables like gender or any other variable not under the control of the researcher.

By contrast, in the factorial design, at least two of the independent variables in the design can be, and are, manipulated by the researcher. Of course, there is no reason why a factorial design may not also be combined with randomized blocking. For example, in the zinc inhaler/chicken broth study, suppose the researcher had access to an "old" group of adults (55+ years) and a group of college-age adults (18–25 years). There is good evidence to suggest that the time needed to recover from an upper respiratory infection may be associated with age (on average, older adults recover more slowly than younger adults). In this case, one could stratify the sample using a $2 \times 2 \times 2$ design: two age groups (young adult versus older adult) by two zinc inhaler treatment levels (use versus no use) by two chicken broth treatment levels (use versus no use). Note that with the greater number of **cells** (mutually exclusive treatment conditions to which the subjects are assigned) generated by the factorial design, the average number of cases within each cell must inevitably decline unless total sample size is increased. For example, if we enroll 100 young and 100 old adults and stratify the initial 2×2 design by these two age groups, only 25 study participants will be available for each combination of age group, zinc inhaler, and chicken broth treatment. Again, this calls for careful planning of the factorial design to produce enough participants in each cell, so that all relevant interaction effects can be investigated with sufficient statistical power.

Salomon Four-Group Design

Finally, it is worth revisiting the **Salomon four-group design** introduced in the previous section. One way to think about this design is to view it as a 2×2 factorial design. All this requires is to reinterpret the introduction or withholding of a pretest as another factor with two treatment levels: Because in the Salomon four-group design the assignment of subjects to conditions with or without pretests occurs at random, this variable is no different from the intervention factor. As in any factorial design, we can test for the presence of interaction effects. If none exist (that is, if there are only main effects), we will not need a Salomon four-group design. Separate posttest-only or pretest/posttest designs will give us the same results. However, the presence of an interaction effect will indeed mean that the effects of the main intervention differ for pretested and not pretested subjects.

GENERALIZABILITY OF CAUSAL INTERPRETATIONS IN RELATION TO RESEARCH DESIGNS

So far, all the between-subjects designs introduced use random assignment of subjects to treatment conditions, or vice versa. This is a basic requirement for experimental research design validity. Without random assignment, we have no means of controlling unknown confounding factors, such as differences in study participant characteristics or environments, that might have unanticipated effects on the outcome variables of interest. But even if a study design delivers strong causal evidence for the efficacy of an intervention *in a particular study sample,* can this evidence be generalized toward larger target populations? The answer is clearly "not automatically." But why?

Clinical research usually relies on study participants who are available in a few clinical settings to which the researchers have access. Furthermore, truly representative samples of even these accessible clinic populations are hard to come by, because all clinical research relies on voluntary participants, who often differ systematically from eligible nonparticipants. Whereas the problems and intricacies of sampling will be discussed in detail in Chapters 19 through 21, it is important to note here that **random assignment** of subjects to various treatment conditions does *not* achieve generalizability. *The main role of random assignment is to remove systematic bias in the comparison of different treatment groups.* As we shall discuss in detail later, it is **random selection,** or random sampling from appropriate target populations, that gives us a technical means of generalizing from a particular sample to larger populations. Some study design features and decisions do, however, directly affect generalizability.

For instance, we have seen how randomized block designs can be used to build potentially confounding variables into the design. If smoking status is likely to have a strong effect on an outcome variable of interest, for example, we can simply make sure that all treatment levels are applied to groups with equal proportions of smokers, and so forth. However, this strategy may not always be feasible. If a researcher wants to control for several known confounders, stratified randomization quickly shows its limits. Suppose sex (2 categories), age (5 age groups) and smoking status (3 groups: current, former, never) need to be controlled. These three variables define 30 ($2 \times 5 \times 3$) different combinations of subject characteristics,[6] within which random assignment to various treatment groups needs to occur. The need to find within each category as many subjects as there are treatment groups (or multiples of treatment groups) is a formidable task. Instead, researchers may decide to restrict eligibility criteria for subject enrollment in order to eliminate the effects of a confounding variable by holding it constant. For example, it is highly likely that a physical therapy intervention among nursing home residents will be less successful among residents with severe cognitive limitations. In fact, in persons with advanced dementia, such interventions may not be feasible at all. Thus, the researcher may decide to limit eligibility for the intervention study to persons with certain minimal levels of cognitive functioning, as defined by a mental status assessment such as the Mini-Mental Status Exam. This strategy will result in a more homogeneous study sample, with respect not only to the subjects' cognitive standards but also to their physical functioning. This is true because mental decline is often accompanied by functional decline, i.e., mental and physical functioning are positively correlated.

The resulting greater homogeneity of subjects in both comparison groups has some clear advantages. The more

---

[6]The total possible combinations for a factorial design are calculated by multiplying the levels of all variables by one another.

the treatment and control groups are alike before the intervention, the easier it will be to discover even small differences between the two groups effected by the intervention. However, this strategy of holding confounding variables constant comes at a price. It reduces the generalizability of the findings because, by definition, nothing can be said about the effectiveness of the intervention among subject groups that were eliminated from the study. Thus, there is a clear tradeoff. *From the standpoint of being able to show the effectiveness of an intervention, homogeneous samples are desirable. From the standpoint of being able to generalize findings across larger patient population groups, heterogeneous samples are preferable.*

Traditionally, generalizability issues have been discussed under the rubric of "threats to external validity" (Campbell & Stanley, 1963; Cook & Campbell, 1979). The most important research design validity threats have already been discussed. For example, the rationale for using the Salomon four-group design is the expectation that the results of pretested groups cannot be generalized to groups that have not been pretested, even if the groups are exposed to the same stimulus. As we have discussed previously, this problem can be viewed as a case of the **interaction of pretesting and experimental stimulus.** We also just discussed issues of generalizability with respect to the representativeness of study samples. Whenever the effects documented for an intervention apply only to the specific participants in the study because of the select and unrepresentative nature of the sample, we are confronted with the problem known as the **interaction of selection and treatment**. Perhaps noteworthy in clinical research is also the **interaction of setting and treatment.** This problem occurs when the effectiveness of studied clinical interventions applies only to the setting(s) in which the study is done. Sometimes, research settings are artificial in the sense that they do not resemble the settings and environments in which the tested interventions are supposed to be applied. For instance, new clinically useful measurement instruments need to be tested in the clinical environments in which they will actually be used, rather than under idealized study conditions (Ornstein, Markert, Litchfield, & Zemp, 1988).

STATISTICAL ANALYSIS OF BETWEEN-SUBJECTS DESIGNS: BASIC PRINCIPLES OF ANALYSIS OF VARIANCE (ANOVA)

NOTE: In this section we continue with our approach of introducing you directly to the statistical language used in the analysis of data from experimental studies. We offer a brief discussion of the principles and procedures involved in the analysis of variance (ANOVA), which constitutes a rather large family of statistical models. The point of this discussion is not to provide a substitute for a statistics textbook. For a comprehensive treatment of ANOVA, see Winer, Brown, & Michels (1991); for a good, more introductory-level discussion, see Snedecor and Cochran (1988); for a less formal introduction, see Munro (2001). The point of this discussion is to show the close connection between the reasoning applied in the analysis phase and its dependence on the design phase of a study. Again, we believe that there is a large payoff in mastering a basic mathematical symbolism, because it actually simplifies the presentation of the important ideas. There are no prerequisites of knowledge here, so just plunge in and let yourself be surprised!

Although ANOVA models are often complex and may include several between-subjects and within-subjects factors, covariates, or several dependent variables, all these models are based on the same principle of decomposition of variance—hence the name "analysis of variance," or ANOVA. We shall demonstrate the basic idea of how variance is decomposed in a discussion of the simplest between-subjects model: the one-way ANOVA. This statistical model makes assumptions about the nature of the data that correspond directly to the features of a posttest-only, completely randomized design.

Our presentation is based on fictitious sample data, with numbers selected for computational convenience. We return to the physical therapy example from the previous chapter. This time, we pretend that a randomized trial of the effectiveness of a physical therapy intervention has been conducted among 10 elderly nursing home residents. Five nursing home residents are exposed to a daily hour of tailor-made exercises with a physical therapist for 3 months (intervention group). Five other nursing home residents participate daily in a card game club (control group). Assignment to either group is based strictly on the luck of the coin. In the following, we shall consider only two variables:

1. The independent variable or factor is symbolized as X_{ig} and indicates the treatment level to which a resident was exposed: i is a subscript for the case number and varies from 1 through 10; g takes on two values: 1 = intervention (physical therapy) group, 2 = control (card game) group.
2. The dependent variable Y_{ig} indicates the number of functional impairments in activities of daily living (ADLs) that these nursing home residents have at the end of the study period. In this case, 11 activities such as dressing, eating, or walking are considered. Therefore, a person's impairment score can vary from

   0 = no impairment to

   11 = need for assistance in all ADLs.

Table 4-5 contains the data and a few calculations necessary for the analysis. Our main goal is to show that the mean number of ADL impairments among residents who received physical therapy intervention is lower than the mean impairment score among residents who participated in the card-playing club. We accomplish this goal by establishing to what extent the physical therapy intervention affects the impairment scores.

As the Y values in Part A of Table 4-5 show, there are substantial differences in impairment scores among the 10

TABLE 4.5   Data on Impairment Scores (Y_{ig}) and Physical Therapy Intervention Status (X_{ig})

Part A: Total Sample of Nursing Home Residents

Case	X_{ig}	Y_{ig}	$Y_{ig} - \bar{Y}$	$(Y_{ig} - \bar{Y})^2 = 90$
1	1	1	$1 - 6 = -5$	$(-5)^2 = 25$
2	1	3	$3 - 6 = -3$	$(-3)^2 = 9$
3	1	5	$5 - 6 = -1$	$(-1)^2 = 1$
4	1	7	$7 - 6 = 1$	$(1)^2 = 1$
5	1	9	$9 - 6 = 3$	$(3)^2 = 9$
6	2	3	$3 - 6 = -3$	$(-3)^2 = 9$
7	2	5	$5 - 6 = -1$	$(-1)^2 = 1$
8	2	7	$7 - 6 = 1$	$(1)^2 = 1$
9	2	9	$9 - 6 = 3$	$(3)^2 = 9$
10	2	11	$11 - 6 = 5$	$(5)^2 = 25$
		$\Sigma\, Y_{ig} = 60$	$\Sigma\, (Y_{ig} - \bar{Y}) = 0$	$\Sigma\, (Y_{ig} - \bar{Y}..)^2 = 90$

Total sample (grand) mean: $\bar{Y} = \Sigma\, (Y_{ig})/N = 60/10 = 6$

Part B: Subjects Who Get Physical Therapy Intervention (Group 1)

Case	X_{i1}	Y_{i1}	$(Y_{ig} - \bar{Y}_{\cdot 1})$	$(Y_{i1} - \bar{Y}_{\cdot 1})^2$
1	1	1	$1 - 5 = -4$	$(-4)^2 = 16$
2	1	3	$3 - 5 = -2$	$(-2)^2 = 4$
3	1	5	$5 - 5 = 0$	$(0)^2 = 0$
4	1	7	$7 - 5 = 2$	$(2)^2 = 4$
5	1	9	$9 - 5 = 4$	$(4)^2 = 16$
		$\Sigma\, (Y_{i1}) = 25$	$\Sigma\, (Y_{ig} - \bar{Y}_{\cdot 1}) = 0$	$\Sigma\, (Y_{ig} - \bar{Y}_{\cdot 1})^2 = 40$

Group 1 Mean: $\bar{Y}_{\cdot 1} = \Sigma\, (Y_{i1})/n_1 = 25/5 = 5$

Part C: Subjects Who Participate in Card Club (Group 2)

Case	X_{i2}	Y_{i2}	$(Y_{i2} - \bar{Y}_{\cdot 2})$	$(Y_{i2} - \bar{Y}_{\cdot 2})^2$
6	2	3	$3 - 7 = -4$	$(-4)^2 = 16$
7	2	5	$5 - 7 = -2$	$(-2)^2 = 4$
8	2	7	$7 - 7 = 0$	$(0)^2 = 0$
9	2	9	$9 - 7 = 2$	$(2)^2 = 4$
10	2	11	$11 - 7 = 4$	$(4)^2 = 16$
		$\Sigma\, (Y_{i2}) = 35$	$\Sigma\, (Y_{i2} - \bar{Y}_{\cdot 2}) = 0$	$\Sigma\, (Y_{i2} - \bar{Y}_{\cdot 2})^2 = 40$

Group 2 mean: $\bar{Y}_{\cdot 2} = \Sigma\, (Y_{i2})/n_2 = 35/5 = 7$

individuals. This between-subjects variation is to be expected because each resident brings his or her own unique physical attributes and health histories to the situation. In addition, it is also unlikely that all individuals exposed to the physical therapy would show exactly the same reaction. Then there is the problem of measurement. Establishing whether or not a nursing home resident should be considered dependent in an activity like eating or walking is, to some extent, a judgment call. Thus, occasionally even well-trained observers might disagree in a particular case. For all these reasons and more, it is not surprising to find lots of between-subjects variation in ADL impairment scores. If we want to make sense out of these data, we need to find a way of distinguishing "systematic" variation in impairment scores that can somehow be attributed to the treatment levels from other "unexplained" sources of variation in impairment scores.

Total Sum of Squares (TSS)

A useful way to start is with a measure of the overall variation in the dependent variable scores. This is called the **total sum of squares** or **TSS** (see the last column of Part (a) of Table 4-5: $\Sigma (Y_{ig} - \bar{Y}..)^2 = 90$). (In words: We subtract from each observed ADL impairment score of individual i in group g the grand or overall sample mean $\bar{Y}..$, square the difference and sum over all individuals.) This TSS is always a positive number, because all individual variations from the sample mean are squared. In the limiting case, when all individuals are exactly the same, it is zero; but then, there is no variation to explain!

Next, we construct a measure that represents individual variation in Y_{ig} scores that is not accounted for by the treatment variable or factor. Because individuals within each group or factor level are exposed to the same treatment (physical therapy or card-playing club), individual variations within each group cannot have been caused by the variation between the factor levels. We thus choose the within-group sum of squares (WGSS) as our measure of individual variation unaccounted for by the factor in question. The WGSS represents the sum of all squared deviations of individual scores of Y_{i1} and Y_{i2} from their respective factor levels or group means: $\bar{Y}._1$ and $\bar{Y}._2$ (see the last columns of Part (b) and (c) in Figure 4.5):

$$\Sigma (Y_{i1} - \bar{Y}._1)^2 + \Sigma (Y_{i2} - \bar{Y}._2) = 40 + 40 = 80 = \text{WGSS}.$$

Finally, we compute the amount of variation in Y_{ig} that can be attributed to X_{ig}, also known as the between-group sum of squares (BGSS). This measure can be obtained in two ways: (1) directly, by summing the squared deviations

of the group means from the grand mean for all cases in a group:

$$\Sigma (\bar{Y}._1 - \bar{Y}..)^2 + \Sigma (\bar{Y}._2 - \bar{Y}..)^2 =$$
$$5 \times (5-6)^2 + 5 \times (7-6)^2 = 5 + 5 = 10$$

or (2) indirectly, by subtracting the WGSS (also called the *error sum of squares or* unexplained sum of squares) from the TSS: TSS−WGSS = BGSS => 90−80 = 10.

See what we have accomplished! We have divided the total variation in the scores of the outcome variables into two groups: explained and unexplained variation. The unexplained or "error" variation is directly related to the random assignment process. Because study participants in both groups were assigned randomly, we would not expect any systematic pattern in the distribution of scores within each factor level. In fact, the ANOVA model makes the assumption that scores *within factor levels* (i.e., within the groups defined by the factor) are normally distributed.

The explained variation captures the systematic differences in means across treatment levels. The more the means differ, the larger the BGSS. Because in a completely randomized design, the subjects are randomly assigned to their respective treatment levels and efforts are made to control the environment, *we are entitled to interpret the mean difference in causal terms.* In a well-designed experiment, the exposure to different treatment levels is the only systematic difference between subjects in the treatment and control groups.

There is one question we have not addressed yet. Should we consider *any difference in the group means on the outcome variable as evidence of the causal effectiveness of the treatment? From our discussion of the* t test in the previous chapter, we know that the answer is no. Recall that subjects were randomly assigned to treatment or control groups. That means we would expect some observed differences between the groups to be purely the result of chance assignment. Thus, what we need now is a test statistic, on the basis of which we can decide whether the observed differences are unlikely to be the result of mere random assignment.

In ANOVA, this test statistic is the ratio of two variances: the between-group variance divided by the within-group variance. This test statistic is also known as the F ratio, in honor of the statistician R.A. Fisher (1951), who worked it out for the first time. How do we obtain estimates of the two variance measures? In general, variances are defined as average squared deviations from a mean—in short, mean squares. We have already obtained measures of the sum of squared deviations (refer back to the computations for BGSS and WGSS); the only problem now is to divide those sum-of-squares by the appropriate numbers to get the mean squares. There is a minor difficulty here. When we estimate variances or mean squares from sample data, we divide the sum-of-squares not by n, the appropriate number of cases, but instead by a number called the **degrees of freedom.** The degrees of freedom are calculated by subtracting from the numbers of independent observations involved the linear restraints imposed on these observations. This concept has been a frequent source of confusion, but its meaning can be illustrated in a rather straightforward manner (Box 4-2).

Now we are ready to construct the test statistic, which helps us decide whether or not the observed differences in sample group means are statistically significant (Table 4-6). Our test for the mean differences in ANOVA is actually indirect. We look at the magnitude of the ratio of the systematic or between-group variance to error or within-group variance. Both variances have in their numerator the familiar sum-of-squares: BGSS and WGSS (see column entitled "mean squares"). Their denominators contain the

requisite degrees of freedom. Take a look at the between-group variance. There are k group means (in this example k = 2, because we have only one treatment group and one control group). These two group means are subject to one constraint: together they must average out to the total sample mean. Thus, the associated degrees of freedom are $k-1$ or, in the two-group case, 1.

Now look at the within-group variance. Its numerator (WGSS) actually combines two sum-of-squares calculated from data in the treatment and control groups. The computation of the WGSS for the five cases in the treatment group is subject to the constraint that their scores average out to the treatment group mean. The same constraint occurs within the control group. Consequently, the overall WGSS is subject to two constraints or, in general, to as many constraints as there are comparison groups. This leaves us with $n-k$ degrees of freedom for the WGSS. The total sum-of-squares, or TSS, is also subject to 1 constraint, because its computation already assumes a known sample mean. Its degrees of freedom are $n-1$. (Note how all the degrees of

Sum of Squares	Degrees of Freedom	Mean Squared Deviations
BGSS = $\Sigma\,(\bar{Y}_{.1} - \bar{Y}..)^2 + \Sigma\,(\bar{Y}_{.2} - \bar{Y}..)^2 = 10$	$k-1 = 2-1 = 1$	BGSS/$k-1$ = 10/1 = 10
WGSS = $\Sigma\,(Y_{i1} - \bar{Y}_{.1})^2 + \Sigma\,(Y_{i2} - \bar{Y}_{.2})^2 = 80$	$n-k = 10-2 = 8$	WGSS/$N-k$ = 80/8 = 10
TSS = $\Sigma\,(Y_{ig} - \bar{Y}..)^2 = 90$	$n-1 = 10-1 = 9$	TSS/$n-1$ = 90/9 = 10

TABLE 4.6   Analysis of Variance (ANOVA) Table for One-Factor (Two-Groups) Between-Subjects Design

F ratio = (BGSS/$k-1$)/(WGSS/$N-k$) = 10/10 = 1; F probability = .3466

n, number of cases in the sample; k, number of factor levels or group categories defined by the independent variable.

freedom for the variance components add up.) Just like TSS = BGSS + WGSS, so is $n-1 = k-1 + n-k$.

We have already emphasized the indirect nature of the ANOVA test statistic. The F ratio is the ratio of the systematic or between-group variance (BGSS/K-1) to error or within-group variance (WGSS/$n-$K). It is now clear that *the greater the differences between the group means, the larger will be the between-group variance in relation to the within-group variance*. When all group means in the sample are exactly equal, the between-group variance equals zero, and the F ratio also equals zero. Of course, under conditions of random assignment, we do not expect all the group means to be exactly equal, even if the null hypothesis is true and the intervention or treatment has no effect. The reason is, of course, that mere random distribution of cases across the comparison groups is likely to make for some observable group differences. However, if the F ratio grows larger and larger, it becomes less and less plausible to argue that mere random assignment produced it.

All we need to know now is what probabilities are attached to F ratios of a given magnitude or larger. The computation of these probabilities for the F distribution has been worked out by R.A. Fisher. On the basis of this information, we can now decide whether an observed F ratio in a particular sample is likely or unlikely to occur, *if* subjects are randomly assigned to the comparison groups *and* the intervention is not effective. These assumptions are incorporated into the null hypothesis. By convention, an F probability of $p < .05$ leads us to reject the null hypothesis; that is, an F ratio of the observed magnitude is unlikely to be the result of mere chance events.

In our example, the observed F ratio is: (BGSS/K-1)/(WGSS/$n-$K) = 10/10 = 1. The associated significance level is .347 (see Table 4-6). Thus, we conclude that the observed sample difference in group means of 2 (= 7$-$5) is well within sampling chance: almost 35% of all random assignments alone would result in F ratios of the observed magnitude or larger. Thus, in this case, we do not have strong evidence that the physical therapy intervention makes any difference. We would say that the observed differences between the groups fail to reach "statistical significance."

You might now wonder why we went through all the trouble of calculating a new and complicated test statistic, when in fact the *t* test introduced in the previous chapter could have done the job. That latter assertion is true. We could have used the *t* test, and we would have obtained the same results. In fact, it can be shown that in a two-group comparison, there is a simple relationship between the *t* statistic and the F statistic: $F = t^2$. Every other associated statistic with the *t* test or the one-way ANOVA, from *p* values to confidence intervals, is identical. However, the *t* test works only if we compare two group means (or two means of measures from the same group, taken at different times). The great virtue of the ANOVA approach is that it is perfectly general and applies to all kinds of complicated study designs. Just imagine a four-group comparison (Lallemant et al., 2000). The fundamental test of the effectiveness of the interventions is still the F statistic. Only this time, the within-group and between-group sums-of-squares are calculated from four comparison groups. The rest is the same. Larger treatment effects translate into larger observed mean differences among the comparison groups, which in turn lead to a bigger ratio of between-group variance to within-group variance (the F ratio). When F ratios become large, the probability of a mere chance effect declines, and we become more confident in our conclusion that the treatments produce real differences. This is the principle. Everything else is just elaboration.

CONCLUSION

The discussion of this chapter focused on the design and analysis of studies with separate control groups. Such studies use between-subjects designs in which the treatment effects are gauged through the comparison of different groups of individuals, some of whom are exposed to the treatments(s) and others of whom are exposed to the control condition(s). Given that the comparison of treatment and control groups also involves the comparison of different groups of individuals, one would expect there to be some group differences on account of the different group compositions alone. However, in experimental studies, differences in the compositions of comparison groups are governed by the random assignment process. That is, when we analyze data from between-subjects designs, we compare the magnitude of the observed average difference between the treatment and control groups with the magnitude of differences that could be expected on the basis of random assignment alone. In more complicated between-subjects designs, e.g., factorial designs with multiple factors or randomized designs with stratification factors, the analysis rests on a comparison of the magnitudes of systematic, between-group variation to unsystematic or random within-group variation as exemplified by the F ratio. Thus, the design features of between-subjects experiments and the logic of the ANOVA model are congruent: the designs are built around the effort to separate systematic treatment effects from mere random variation resulting from extraneous factors, and the ANOVA rests on the assumption that this separation has been accomplished.

Even with random assignment of study participants to treatment and control groups, there remain threats to design validity. In particular, subject attrition, diffusion of treatment, and compensatory equalization of treatment can seriously undermine the ability to draw causal inferences; yet, random assignment alone affords no solution to these problems. Only painstaking organizational and management effort on the part of the researcher(s) can minimize these problems, e.g., through building a "firewall" between treatment and control subjects so that they cannot communicate with each other, or through incentives to study participants not to drop out.

Suggested Activities

1. For each research situation described in the following, suggest a specific research design that would best address the research question and minimize threats to validity. Justify your selection, with reference to tradeoffs between design validity and feasibility issues:

   a. A nurse practitioner wishes to find out whether patient knowledge levels have changed as a result of attending an educational workshop on diabetes self-management.

   b. The clinical staff at a primary care clinic is interested in showing that patient telephone reminders for clinic appointments improve the rate at which patients keep their clinic appointments.

   c. A researcher obtains funding for a 2-year longitudinal intervention study to improve the quality of life among community-residing adults who have schizophrenia.

   d. A nurse researcher is interested in testing whether or not an exercise intervention is effective in improving mobility and self-esteem among residents of a nursing home.

2. Look at the descriptions of programs of research for one or two nurse researchers that are described in the following book: Hinshaw, A.S., Feetham, S.L., & Shaver, J.L.F. (Eds.). (1999). *Handbook of clinical nursing research.* Thousand Oaks, CA: Sage. What types of research designs have these researchers used to study questions of interest to nursing? With reference to the research design validity threats discussed in this chapter, what are the key strengths and limitations of the research designs that have been used in the studies conducted by these nurse researchers?

3. Select an article from a nursing or medical journal that uses an ANOVA to analyze the effects of an intervention. Identify the following, based on your review of the article you select:

   a. The main research questions/hypotheses

   b. The name or type of study design that was used

   c. The ANOVA result table(s)

   d. The specific evidence from the ANOVA results that was used to answer the questions/hypotheses

   e. The main findings with regard to the questions/hypotheses

   f. The strength of the causal conclusions about the effectiveness of the intervention examined

   g. Your overall assessment of the strengths, weaknesses, and feasible areas for improvement in the study design (assuming the study was to be redone at a future date), with reference to validity threats in research design.

Suggested Readings

Edinger, J. D., Wohlgemuth, W. K., Radtke, R. A., Marsh, G. R., & Quillian, R. E. (2001). Cognitive behavioral therapy for treatment of chronic primary insomnia. *Journal of the American Medical Society, 285, 14,* 1856–1864.

Lantz, P. M., Stencil, D., Lippert, M. T., Beversdorf, S., Jaros, L., & Remington, P. L. (1995). Breast and cervical cancer screening in a low-income managed care sample: The efficacy of physician letters and phone calls. *American Journal of Public Health, 85, 6,* 834–836.

Munro, B. H. (2001). *Statistical methods for health care research* (2nd ed.). (Chapters 6 and 7, pp.137–185) Philadelphia: Lippincott.

Ornstein, S., Markert, G., Litchfield, L, & Zemp, L. (1988). Evaluation of the DINAMAP blood pressure monitor in an ambulatory primary care setting. *The Journal of Family Practice, 26, 5,* 517–521.

References

Byar, D. P., Schoenfeld, D. A., Green, S. B., Amato, D. A., Davis, R., Gruttola, V. D., Finkelstein, D. M., et al. (1990). Design considerations for AIDS trials. *The New England Journal of Medicine, 323, 19,* 1343–1348.

Campbell, D. T., & Stanley, J.C. (1963). *Experimental and quasi-experimental designs for research.* Chicago: Rand McNally.

Cochran, W. G., & Cox, G. M. (1992). *Experimental designs.* (2nd ed.). New York: John Wiley & Sons; Wiley Classics Library, originally published in 1957.

Cook, T. D., & Campbell, D. T. (1979). *Quasi-experimentation: Design & analysis issues for field settings.* Boston: Houghton Mifflin.

Edinger, J. D., Wohlgemuth, W. K., Radtke, R. A., Marsh, G. R., & Quillian, R. E. (2001). Cognitive behavioral therapy for treatment of chronic primary insomnia. *Journal of the American Medical Society, 285, 14,* 1856–1864.

Fisher, R. A. (1951). *The design of experiments* (6th ed.). Edinburgh, UK: Oliver & Boyd. (1st ed., 1935).

Friedman, L. M., Furberg, C. D., & DeMets, D. L. (1996). *Fundamentals of clinical trials.* (3rd ed.). St. Louis, MO: Mosby.

Hayes, K. (1998). Randomized trial of geragogy-based medication instruction in the emergency department. *Nursing Research, 47, 4,* 211–218.

Lallemant, M., Jourdain, G., Le Coeur, S., Kim, S., Koetsawang, S., Comeau, A. M., Phoolcharoen, W., et al. (2000). A trial of shortened zidovudine regimens to prevent mother-to-child transmission of human immunodeficiency virus type I. *The New England Journal of Medicine, 343, 14,* 982–991.

Lantz, P. M., Stencil, D., Lippert, M. T., Beversdorf, S., Jaros, L., & Remington, P. L. (1995). Breast and cervical cancer screening in a low-income managed care sample: The efficacy of physician letters and phone calls. *American Journal of Public Health, 85, 6,* 834–836.

Meinert, C. L. (1986). *Clinical trials: Design, conduct, and analysis.* New York: Oxford University Press.

Munro, B. H. (2001). *Statistical methods for health care research* (2nd ed.). (Chapter 5, pp.123–159) Philadelphia: Lippincott.

Naylor, M. D., Brooten, D., Campbell, R., Jacobson, B. S., Mezey, M. D., Pauly, M. V., & Schwartz, J. S. (1999). *Journal of the American Medical Association, 281, 7,* 613–620.

Neumark, D. E., Stommel, M., Given, C. W. and Given, B. A. (2001). Research design and subject characteristics predicting nonparticipation in a panel survey of older families with cancer. *Nursing Research, 50, 6,* 363–368.

Ornstein, S., Markert, G., Litchfield, L, & Zemp, L. (1988). Evaluation of the DINAMAP blood pressure monitor in an ambulatory primary care setting. *The Journal of Family Practice, 26, 5,* 517–521.

Overmeire, B. V., Smets, K., Lecoutere, D., Van de Broek, H., Weylwr, J., De Groote, K., & Langhendries, J.P. (2000). A comparison of ibuprofen and indomethacin for closure of patient ductus arteriosus. *The New England Journal of Medicine, 343, 10,* 674–681.

Powell, S. S., Canterbury, M. A., & McCoy, D. (1998). Medication administration: Does the teaching method really matter? *Journal of Nursing Education, 37, 6,* 281–283.

Rothert, M. L., Holmes-Rovner, M., Rovner, D., Kroll, J., Breer, L., Talarczyk, G., Schmitt, N., Padonu, G., & Wills, C. (1997). An educational intervention as decision support for menopausal women. *Research in Nursing & Health, 20,* 377–387.

Snedecor, G. W., & Cochran, W. G. (1989). *Statistical methods.* (8th ed.). Ames, IA: Iowa State University Press.

Sloan, J. A., Loprinzi, C. L., Kuross, S. A., Miser, A. W., O'Fallon, J. R., Mahoney, M. R., Heid, I. M., et al. (1998). Randomized comparison of four tools measuring overall quality of life in patients with advanced cancer. *Journal of Clinical Oncology, 16, 11,* 3662–3673.

Winer, B. J., Brown, D. R., & Michels, K. M. (1991). *Statistical principles in experimental design.* (3rd ed.). New York: McGraw-Hill.

CHAPTER 5

The Design and Analysis of Repeated-Measures Experiments

REPEATED-MEASURES DESIGNS

Types of Repeated-Measures Studies

In studies with **repeated-measures designs,** the same variables are measured on more than one occasion, using a given sample of subjects. Such study designs are frequently encountered in the nursing and health care literature because the phenomena of concern to health care professionals often show change over time. In general, whenever a research question concerns physiologic and psychologic changes, health maintenance, growth, decline, developmental processes, adaptation, learning, maturation, or any other time-related processes that occur *within* individuals, repeated-measures designs are particularly appropriate. In many settings where health care services are provided, nursing activities often focus on health maintenance and the management of chronic diseases (Sidani & Braden, 1998; McGrath, Sullivan, Lester, & Oh, 2000; Mundinger, Kane, Lenz, Totten, Tsi, Cleary, Friedewald, Siu, & Shelanski, 2000) as well as health promotion and disease prevention. Both the observations of patient outcomes and the interventions themselves may stretch over months, if not years. For example, a nurse researcher who is interested in assessing the effects of a health promotion intervention related to diet and exercise over 24 months among a sample of adolescents may have to account for changes in attitudes and behavior that are attributable to both developmental and intervention factors. An accurate assessment of change in such a study needs to be based on a repeated-measures design capable of "capturing" the timing of projected changes in attitudes and behavior.

Not all repeated-measures studies are experimental. In Chapter 6, we shall introduce some quasi-experimental designs with repeated measures, for example, the interrupted time-series analysis. In Chapter 11, we shall look at an observational survey design with repeated measures: the panel study. In this chapter, we deal only with repeated-measures designs that are also experimental studies. In addition to the repeated observations of the study participants, experimental studies include treatments or interventions that are deliberately manipulated by the researcher, and study participants are randomly assigned to the various treatment levels.

Characteristics of Repeated-Measures Studies

As already implicit in the preceding examples, both the *timing* and the *number* of measurements provide key distinctions among different types of repeated-measures designs. Unfortunately, the terminology used to describe these designs in the nursing and health care literature can sometimes be confusing. The distinctions we make between design terms are not absolute, and there is considerable overlap in how they are used. Therefore, Table 5-1 shows a brief synopsis that focuses on the similarities and distinctions in the use of these terms.

Repeated-measures designs involve at least two measurements of the same phenomenon, using the same subjects, on separate occasions. There are no set requirements concerning the time period between the measurement occasions. The time interval(s) between measurements may vary from very short (such as minutes or hours) to very long (such as years), depending on the phenomenon being measured. In a way, then, the pretest/posttest design introduced in the previous chapter can be considered a special instance of a repeated-measures design because it meets the minimal criterion of there being at least two measures from the same subjects obtained on different occasions.

However, the purpose of a study using a pretest/posttest design is most often to evaluate the short-term effects of short-term interventions or treatments conducted within a fairly circumscribed time period. Pretest/posttest designs are often used in studies intended to evaluate the effect of an educational intervention. For example, people attending an educational conference may complete a pretest of their knowledge and attitudes before the conference, followed by a posttest assessing the stability or change in their knowledge and attitudes immediately after the conference. Pretest/posttest designs may also be used to compare groups that are exposed to different educational formats, such as comparisons of student perceptions of course content in a traditional classroom setting versus a fully web-based format (Wills & Stommel, 2002). By contrast, what are most often referred to as repeated-measures designs in the literature are those designs that involve at least three successive observations on the study participants.

It is worth restating that the timing of the measurements in a repeated-measures design may be quite variable, depending on the nature of the phenomenon. However, when change in a phenomenon is observed over a relatively long time, such as months or years, researchers often refer to their repeated-measures designs as **longitudinal study designs.** In this usage, the terms "longitudinal design" and "repeated-measures design" are essentially interchangeable, except that the use of "longitudinal design" emphasizes the long-term follow-up periods for the observation of study subjects. In addition, the term "longitudinal study" is usually applied to nonexperimental studies, such as cohort and panel designs, whereas the term "repeated-measures study"

TABLE 5.1	Key Features of Repeated-Measures Designs			
	Overlapping Repeated-Measures Design Terms Used in Literature			
	Repeated-Measures Designs	**Pretest/Posttest Designs**	**Longitudinal Designs**	**Crossover Designs**
Number of observations	Any design with two or more observations on the same subjects	Usually only two observations on the same subjects; a pretest before the intervention and a posttest after the intervention	Any design with two or more observations over time	At least two observations on the same subjects; number of observations depends on number of treatment levels to which each subject is exposed
Basic study design	Both experimental and nonexperimental/ with and without separate control groups	Mostly experimental with separate control group(s); nonexperimental: simple one-group pretest/posttest design	Usually nonexperimental with multiple (two or more) observations on the same population (trend study) or the same sample (panel study)	Randomized clinical trial with subjects exposed to more than one treatment level over time; quasi-experimental intervention study without randomization, but subjects still exposed to more than one treatment level
Timing of observations	Variable: "repeated measures" may refer to both short-term and long-term follow-ups	Almost always short-term, with pretest and posttest scheduled shortly before and after the intervention	Variable, but definitely long-term; process of change to be observed is often measured in terms of months, even years	Variable, but most cross-over studies have many observations (and prior treatments) conducted within short periods
Notes/other identifying design features	Generic term; refers to all studies with at least two observations made on the same subjects, using the same measures	Often not thought of as a repeated-measures or longitudinal design, but as single-outcome-with-baseline-information design	Generic term; can refer to all studies with more than one observation over time, but mostly applied to long-term observational studies	Use of term is confined to experimental and quasi-experimental intervention studies

is more commonly used with experimental studies that include several follow-up measures. Finally, whereas repeated-measures designs always occur in studies in which the same individuals are observed many times, "longitudinal studies" may also refer to **trend studies,** in which the same population is observed over time, but each time a different representative sample of that target population is studied. (More will be said on this topic in Chapter 11.)

As has already been mentioned, clinical researchers are often interested in longer-term effects of treatments or changes in patient states over time. For instance, high dosages of the cancer drug interferon appear to affect cognitive functioning, but such changes usually do not manifest themselves after the drug has been taken for only a short

time (Bender, Yaskp, Kirkwood, Ryan, Dunbar-Jacob, & Zullo, 2000). Likewise, with behavioral educational interventions, the key outcomes of interest are often not just short-run changes in behavior but long-run behavioral adjustments carried over into the patients' everyday life. Thus, the success of a nutritional intervention among poor women with young children needs to be measured in months, if not years, rather than weeks after the programmatic intervention (Havas, Anliker, Damron, Langenberg, Ballesteros, & Feldman, 1998). Clinically relevant educational interventions often involve repeated intervention occasions (Rothert, Holmes-Rovner, Rovner, Kroll, Breer, Talarzyck, Schmitt, Padonu, & Wills, 1997). Thus, it is only natural that outcomes are measured on repeated occasions.

Repeated-Measures Designs with Between-Subjects Factors

In each of the cited repeated-measures intervention studies, study participants were randomly assigned to two or more treatment/comparison groups and were observed, by use of the same measurement instrument(s), on three to six occasions to assess outcomes in terms of the effectiveness of the interventions. However, in all these studies, exposure to different treatments or interventions was restricted to only some of the study participants, not all of them. That means that different and separate groups of study participants were randomly assigned to different and mutually exclusive treatment levels. As was already discussed in Chapter 4, when different subject groups are exposed to different treatment levels, the treatment variable is a **between-subjects factor.** For example, participants in a study of drug efficacy may be randomly assigned to take an experimental drug, while other participants in the same study get the approved, standard drug therapy. Similarly, in testing an educational intervention, study participants may be randomly assigned to educational materials in the form of an instructional booklet only, while other participants receive an instructional booklet and the opportunity for discussion with a health educator. Again, all these examples combine a between-subjects factor with repeated outcome measures.

Crossover Studies

A **crossover design** is another kind of repeated-measures design that involves not only repeated observations or measurements but also repeated treatments. This kind of study is not necessarily focused on long-term changes in study participants, but it still involves repeated outcome measures. The crossover design is also an example of a **within-subjects design,** because all subjects are eventually exposed to all the treatment levels, which together constitute the **within-subjects factor.** Thus, in contrast to a between-subjects design, in which only some subjects are exposed to a given treatment level, a within-subjects design exposes subjects to more than one treatment level, but it retains variation in the timing of the exposure to the treatment levels. More specifically, in a crossover study, each study participant is exposed to multiple (at least two) treatment and control group episodes, followed each time by observations of the relevant outcomes. At some moment, determined in advance by the researcher, subjects experience a switch from one treatment level to the other(s). In general, when all subjects in the study sample are exposed to all treatment levels, and the assignment to the treatment

levels occurs at random, then we speak of a crossover design.[1]

The study design in Research Scenario 5-1 meets all the key requirements of an experimental study. There is a clearly operationalized, quantitative outcome variable represented by the pressure measurement. The independent variable in this study is the type of cushion or surface, which was varied/manipulated and assigned by the researchers. The researchers also maintain considerable control over the environment in which the experiment took place. For instance, all subject participants were tested in the same hospital room with room temperatures controlled and varying between the narrow limits of 18° and 20°C. In addition, a likely confounding variable—the angle between the seat of the armchair and the back—was controlled: for all study participants; it was set at 21°. Finally, the study design called for random assignment of subjects to treatments.

There is one major difference between this study design and the designs explored in the previous chapter. As we saw, in between-subjects designs, some study participants are exposed to a particular intervention or treatment level, while other study participants are exposed to different treatment levels or the control group treatment. In other words, the different treatment levels are applied to distinct subsets of study participants, who are randomly assigned to them. Naturally, under these conditions, the biggest worry in comparing outcomes after treatments is whether or not the study participants who were initially assigned to the various treatment levels are, in fact, similar in their average characteristics. By contrast, in the study of the pressure cushions, all study participants were exposed to all treatment levels. In such a situation, one no longer has to worry about similarity or equivalence of the study participants, because the groups undergoing different treatment levels are identical, i.e, composed of the same individuals, who differ only in their order of exposure to the treatment levels. In study design language, this situation is often referred to as subjects serving as their own controls. With each study participant observed after each treatment level,

---

[1]Note, however, that the term "crossover" design is sometimes used more loosely in nursing-related and health-related research to refer to quasi-experimental study designs (not just experimental), in which the timing of exposure to intervention/treatment levels varies and study participants are eventually exposed to all interventions. This situation is most likely to occur when it is impossible, for logistic reasons, to randomly vary the timing of different treatment levels for different study participants. Thus, when the term "crossover design" is seen in a research report, it is important to look carefully at the specific design that was used. It may be experimental (with random assignment) or quasi-experimental (without random assignment). For more information, see Chapter 6.

RESEARCH SCENARIO 5.1

Effects of Pressure Cushions for Relieving Pressure on the Skin

A good example of a crossover design can be found in a recent study by Defloor & Grypdonck (2000), in which the effectiveness of different types of pressure cushions was examined for relieving pressure on the skin. Although healthy volunteers were used in this study, the researchers' findings may have implications for the design of cushioning devices of hospitalized or otherwise relatively immobile people, who may sit in chairs for extended periods of time without relief of decubitus pressure points, via position changes or ambulation. The researchers examined 29 different pressure cushions (divided into six major groups like gel, foam, water, hollow fiber, air, and combination cushions) and a synthetic sheepskin (29 cushions + 1 synthetic sheepskin = 30 cushioning devices or seating surfaces). It is clear that with 30 different cushioning devices (or "treatment levels" in research design language), a between-subjects design with random assignment of different study participants to different surfaces would require a rather large study sample. Just suppose that individual variability in pressure caused by differences in weight, body shape, skin properties, and so forth were such that 20 study participants would be necessary in each group to show statistically significant pressure differences between the cushion surfaces. In that case, a total sample of 600 patients (20 subjects × 30 treatment levels) would have to be recruited. As an alternative, Defloor & Grypdonck (2000) enrolled only 20 study participants between the ages of 19 and 45, whose weights varied widely between 53.5 kg (118 pounds) and 98.5 kg (217 pounds). The study design called for each study participant to sit on all cushion surfaces, with the sequence of cushion assignments randomized. In other words, for each of the 20 study subjects, the researchers worked out a different sequence of cushions/surfaces. For example, one subject might first sit on cushion 1, then 2, then 3, and so forth, while another subject might start with cushion 5, then 7, then 1, and so forth. After establishing 20 different sequences for the 30 surfaces (there are $30! = 2.65 \times 10^{32}$ possible different ways of ordering 30 cushion surfaces), the researchers randomly assigned each of the 20 study subjects to a different sequence. Using a standardized pressure measurement tool that relied on a seat element with sensors and was inserted between the patient's body and the cushion surface, the pressure generated by the various cushion surfaces was measured after each study participant remained immobile for 1 minute on each cushion surface. Overall, the study generated 600 outcome measures (observations) from 20 subjects, each measured 30 times on the different surfaces.

there were 30 observations for each subject in the cushion study. Thus, this crossover design generated observations that could vary both between the 20 different subjects and within each subject over 30 different occasions. However, as for the effects of the different treatment levels, the key comparison in a crossover study is not among different treatment and control groups, but among different treatment occasions.

Threats to Design Validity in Crossover Designs

As described, the essential feature of a crossover design is that all study subjects are eventually exposed to all treatment levels/modalities. The sequencing of exposure to different treatment levels is varied, and subjects are randomly assigned to the various sequences. Aside from any ethical or practical considerations about the desirability of ensuring that all participants have access to an intervention that

might be shown to be beneficial, what is so useful about this study design, from a research design perspective?

Recall that in the pressure cushion study, the researchers tested the same 20 subjects sitting on 30 different surfaces. Thus, by definition, there cannot be a selection bias in the comparisons among treatment occasions. That is, the characteristics of the study participants themselves cannot account for the average observed differences in effectiveness of the cushioning devices. For example, although the subjects' weights varied substantially (ranging from 118 to 217 pounds), those between-subject differences are completely neutralized when the average pressure readings from two different cushion surfaces are compared. Furthermore, the random sequence of exposure to different surfaces means that the same surface may have been the first surface for one subject, the 12th for another, and so forth. Thus, if time of exposure to a cushioning device had a systematic effect (however unlikely), it should not have affected the comparisons among different surfaces.

For instance, if prolonged sitting in the armchairs had altered pressure readings (possibly because of more routine pressure measurements later), this could no longer explain systematic differences between different surfaces/cushions because each surface had the same chance of appearing early or late in the sequence. Not only does random sequencing of treatments exclude testing effects as plausible explanations for differences among treatment occasions, it also makes it unlikely that history, maturation, instrumentation, and even subject mortality could systematically confound the comparison of treatment occasions. This is true because any systematic change over time in subjects (like their maturation or growth or their exposure to external events) would affect different treatment levels for different study participants (because the treatment levels are randomly scheduled).

Thus, the crossover design appears to be an ideal design for a clinical experimental study, especially when one considers that it is generally more efficient with respect to sample size requirements. Recall that it took only 20 subjects to generate 600 observations on the pressure measures. However, one very important design validity issue must always be considered with crossover designs: the possible **diffusion effect** (or carryover) from one treatment level to the next.

In the pressure cushion study, the outcome variable consisted of measurements of pressure, immediately generated by the subjects sitting on the cushioning devices. However, such current pressure readings should be considered proxy indicators of the possible long-term effects of pressure from sitting. The long-term effects, such as the eventual development of pressure ulcers resulting from unrelieved pressure on pressure points, are clinically more meaningful. While it would be possible, in principle, to focus on the absence or presence of pressure ulcers as an outcome measure, such a study could not make use of a crossover design. The main reasons are the long incubation time for the development of pressure ulcers and the impossibility of a quick return to the status quo ante: the state before the ulcer developed. Last, but certainly not least, a study deliberately designed to generate pressure ulcers would also be unacceptable on ethical grounds.

In summary, the diffusion of treatment (carryover) effect constitutes the biggest threat to the design validity of crossover studies. To avoid the carryover effect, the researcher must have prior information about the probable effect periods. For instance, a comparison of the effects of different drugs using a crossover design would require that the effects of one drug be completely worn off before the next drug (or a different dosage of the same drug) is introduced. In general, any learning experiments or interventions that can be modified by the subjects' memories of previous intervention experiences are not well suited for crossover designs.

Multifactor Crossover Designs

Just as several between-subjects factors can be used simultaneously in factorial designs, researchers sometimes use several within-subjects factors simultaneously in a single crossover design. These designs are still referred to as crossover studies, but they are more complex versions of the basic design we have just discussed.

For example, in a classic study, Ornstein et al. (1988) evaluated the accuracy and reliability of an oscillometric automated blood pressure monitor, comparing it with a standard mercury sphygmomanometer in an ambulatory care setting. The study sample consisted of 80 normotensive and hypertensive patients of mixed racial and ethnic backgrounds, aged 18 years or older. Treatment levels in this measurement study were defined in terms of four factors. Each subject would be measured

1. Simultaneously on the right and the left arm
2. With the sphygmomanometer or the automated blood pressure monitor
3. Via a physician's or a registered nurse's assessment of the blood pressure
4. With measurements taken on four successive occasions

Because each of the first three factors took on two levels, their combination yielded eight ($2 \times 2 \times 2$) possibilities:

1. Physician + left arm + automated monitor
2. Nurse + left arm + automated monitor
3. Physician + right arm + automated monitor
4. Nurse + right arm + automated monitor
5. Physician + left arm + sphygmomanometer
6. Nurse + left arm + sphygmomanometer
7. Physician + right arm + sphygmomanometer
8. Nurse + right arm + sphygmomanometer

With left and right arm readings performed at the same time, there were a total of four occasions of blood pressure readings. The researchers chose to use these factor combinations in a balanced design, meaning they made sure that the same overall combination of factors applied at each occasion. The resulting design looked like this:

1. First occasion: physician/left arm/sphygmomanometer and nurse/right arm/automated monitor
2. Second occasion: physician/right arm/sphygmomanometer and nurse/left arm/automated monitor

3. Third occasion: physician/right arm/automated monitor and nurse/left arm/ sphygmomanometer
4. Fourth occasion: physician/left arm/automated monitor and nurse/right arm/ sphygmomanometer

This design was balanced with respect to every factor. At each occasion (reading), one blood pressure reading was performed by the nurse, one by the physician, one on the left arm, one on the right arm, one with the sphygmomanometer, and one with the automated monitor. Therefore, when average blood pressure readings were compared across occasions, the time effect/experience was evident, independently of all the other factors. Likewise, when the averaged physician and nurse measures were compared, each of them contributed one reading from each occasion, used the left arm twice and the right arm twice, and also used the sphygmomanometer and the automated monitor twice.[2] All of the factors were within-subjects factors, which means that they represented different occasions on which the same individual study participants were measured. Thus, with 80 subjects and $2 \times 2 \times 2 = 8$ measures per subject, this particular study generated 640 blood pressure readings (or 1,280, if one counts the systolic and diastolic readings as separate measures). Again, it is easy to see the efficiency of crossover designs with respect to the sample requirements: many observations can be generated from fairly small samples of subjects. As with other factorial designs, one could also test for possible interaction effects, say, whether the physician or nurse gets consistently different results with the sphygmomanometer but not the automatic monitor.

Mixed-Method Design

We have spent considerable time discussing crossover designs in this chapter because these designs are among the most frequently encountered types of repeated-measures experiments in the medical and nursing literature. Other repeated-measures designs deserve mention, however. When a between-subjects factor is combined with a within-subjects factor, the result is a hybrid repeated-measures design, which is often referred to as a **mixed-method design** (Ellis, 1999). For instance, in the pressure cushion study, half of the subjects could have been randomly assigned to sitting in an armchair with a 21° back angle and the other half in an armchair with a 32° back angle. In this way, the researchers would have created an additional between-subjects factor, resulting in a mixed-methods design.

Single-Subject Time Series Experiment

The **single-subject time series experiment** (Kratochwill & Levin, 1992) is yet another design variation among repeated-measures designs. Essentially, single-subject experiments represent the opposite extreme to completely randomized between-subjects designs. In the latter, all variation in the outcome variable(s) occurs among subjects, randomly assigned to different treatment levels. By contrast, in the single-subject design, all variation in the outcome measure(s) occurs between different occasions, after different treatment levels are randomly applied to a single individual. Single-subject repeated-measures designs that focus on differences in individual states over time have been used for several years in psychologic research, especially in laboratory-based "basic process" research (Ellis, 1999). However, even though clinicians are sometimes interested in individual responses to exposures of different interventions over time, such study designs remain underused in the health care literature.

PAIRED *t* TESTS

The analysis of data from repeated-measures studies, including crossover studies, is often complex, and a full discussion of the statistical methods is beyond the scope of this book.[3] However, it is worth reviewing a few basic principles for the interpretation of data from repeated-measures designs, and to introduce a statistical analysis model frequently encountered in the clinical literature: the paired *t* test.

REVIEW NOTE: In the previous discussion of the independent-sample *t*-test (Chapters 3 and 4), we introduced a statistical model that rests on a few simple assumptions. Among them is the assumption that individuals in the study sample are randomly assigned to the two comparison groups. Ideally, the only difference between the groups would be the exposure to different treatment levels, which, in a two-group experiment, means exposure to treatment or control conditions. In this model, the variation of individual scores within each group is subject to chance events because of the random assignment. In particular, any observation on one individual (*i*) is independent from an observation on any other individual (*i*). That means that knowing individual *i*'s score does not help in predicting individual *i*'s score.

---

[2]Convince yourself that the same kind of balance occurs across the two blood pressure gauges and the two arms.

[3]For a nontechnical introduction, see Munro (2001); for a more thorough introduction, see Snedecor & Cochran (1989), for a comprehensive overview and discussion, see Winer et al. (1991) or Kirk (1996).

For instance, in the independent sample *t*-test example of Chapter 3, the blood pressure readings of 50 individuals, who were randomly assigned to a nutrition intervention, were compared to the blood pressure readings of another 50 individuals, who were randomly assigned to a control group that received the usual care. There we made the assumption that the magnitude of any individual person's diastolic blood pressure reading would have no effect on the diastolic blood pressure scores of any other individual in the same group. This is a reasonable assumption after random assignment of individuals to either treatment or control group. However, when we compare diastolic blood pressure scores taken with the sphygmomanometer to those taken with the oscillometric, automated monitor, we cannot necessarily assume that the individual measures are independent or unrelated. In fact, both sets of measures are taken on the same individuals at the same time, so we can expect them to be strongly correlated since they form pairs of observations. As BP readings are a fairly stable phenomenon, these correlations should be quite high, especially when taken simultaneously. If so, the independent sample *t*-test would clearly not be an appropriate model to analyze data from repeated-measures studies, since it expressly assumes the independence of such observations.

Paired-Samples *t* Test

The **paired-samples *t* test** compares two mean scores for related or paired groups. Pairing may involve linking two different sample members as a pair, because they share some important attribute in common. For instance, in a randomized block design for a hypertension intervention trial, researchers may want to make sure that for each hypertensive female smoker aged 45 in the treatment group, there will be another individual with the same characteristics in the control group. Pairing also occurs commonly in the form of self-pairing, wherein one compares measures taken at two different times or occasions on the same group of individuals.

As already mentioned in the discussion of the independent sample *t* test, both versions of the *t* test focus on mean (average) scores. Thus, they should be applied only to variables or measures for which it is meaningful to compute means, such as interval or ratio-level variables. To demonstrate the inferential logic of the paired *t* test, we again select a simple, slightly artificial example (Research Scenario 5-2 and Table 5.2).

Intuitively, many people would point to the small sample and express skepticism about whether or not the results

RESEARCH SCENARIO 5.2

Effects of Hypertension-Reducing Drugs

Table 5-2 shows the data from a small study of six hypertensive primary care patients who are assumed to have taken a hypertension-reducing drug every day for 2 months. The table shows individual diastolic blood pressure (BP) readings taken at time 1, before the drug therapy commenced (X_{i1}), and at Time 2, 2 months into the therapy (X_{i2}). It also shows the desired descriptive statistics, including the mean diastolic BP before the start of the drug therapy ($\bar{X}_{.1} = 97$), the mean diastolic BP 2 months later ($\bar{X}_{.2} = 91$), and the difference between these two means, which represents the average decline in diastolic BP ($\bar{D} = -6$). While these descriptive results tell us the story about the cases in this particular sample, we need a context for judging the significance of this particular sample finding. Is the apparent improvement in blood pressure readings good evidence of the efficacy of the drug therapy?

would hold up. There is good reason to be skeptical. If this study were repeated, even with the same subjects, it would be unlikely to result in exactly the same mean difference in diastolic blood pressure readings of $\bar{D} = -6$. There are plenty of reasons for this. For instance, mere measurement fluctuations could account for unforeseen variation, e.g., nervousness of patients at the time of the blood pressure test, the experience of the clinicians measuring blood pressure, the pressure in the blood pressure cuffs, and so forth. If results can vary randomly from one sample to the next and from one measurement occasion to the next, we again must ask this question: is the observed sample decline in mean diastolic blood pressure so large that mere chance events are not likely to have accounted for it? To answer this question, we need an estimate of how much the blood pressure outcome measure varies from one sample to the next.

In principle, we could obtain this information by "brute force," as demonstrated earlier in Chapter 3. We would repeat the study with other samples of size six, calculate the mean difference between the before and after treatment measures for each sample, and construct the sampling distribution of these mean differences. The standard deviation of this sampling distribution, also known as the standard

Case ID	$X_{i1}(T_1)$	$X_{i2}(T_2)$	$D_i = X_{i2}-X_{i1}$	$D_i - \bar{D}$	$\Sigma(D_i - \bar{D})^2$
1	92	86	−6	0	$(0)^2 = 0$
2	94	90	−4	2	$(2)^2 = 4$
3	96	92	−4	2	$(2)^2 = 4$
4	98	92	−6	0	$(0)^2 = 0$
5	100	95	−5	1	$(1)^2 = 1$
6	102	91	−11	−5	$(-5)^2 = 25$
$n = 6$	$\bar{X}_{.1} = 97$	$\bar{X}_{.2} = 91$	$\bar{D} = -6$	$\Sigma(D_i - \bar{D}) = 0$	$\Sigma(D_i - \bar{D})^2 = 34$

TABLE 5.2 Sample Data for Paired t Test: Two Diastolic Blood Pressure Readings, Taken 2 Months Apart Before and After Drug Treatment

Standard deviation of the difference scores D_i

$$SD_{Di} = \sqrt{\frac{\Sigma(D_i - \bar{D})^2}{n-1}} = \sqrt{\frac{34}{5}} = 2.6077$$

Standard error of the mean difference score $\bar{D}$

$$SE_{\bar{D}} = SD_{Di}/\sqrt{n} = 2.6077/\sqrt{6} = 1.0646$$

t value = (sample mean difference—hypothesized population mean difference)/standard error of the mean difference score $\bar{D}$

$$t = (\bar{D} - \mu\delta)/SE_{\bar{D}} = (-6 - 0)/1.0646 = -5.636$$

Two-tailed significance level or probability (P) value associated with t value of -5.636 and 5 ($=6-1$) degrees of freedom

.002

Pearson correlation between Time 1 and Time 2 measures

.721

error, would give us the desired estimate of the average variability of results across samples. Fortunately, we do not have to go through this tedious process. Instead, we can estimate the standard error of the sample mean differences using a simple formula (for details, see Snedecor & Cochran, 1988). We take the standard deviation of the mean differences calculated from the sample (itself the square root of the sample variance of the difference scores) and divide it by the square root of the sample size:

$$SE_{\bar{D}} = SD_{Di}\sqrt{n}$$

All calculations are shown in Table 5-2. As the results indicate, the estimated standard error is 1.0646.

Applying the Paired t Test

Now we are ready to apply the paired t test. We start with the assumption that the sampling distribution of the mean differences between the two measures is distributed like the t distribution. This assumption is valid if the variable is more or less continuous, if it is measured at the interval level, and if a random process plays a role in generating the sample differences. This is not an unreasonable assumption, given the usual measurement errors associated with blood pressure readings. Also keep in mind that in a paired t test, we assume only that the random process affects the measurement procedure and thus the differences in blood pressure scores. We need not assume that the blood pressure scores at any given

| TABLE 5.3. | | Sample Data for Paired t Test: Two Diastolic Blood Pressure Readings, with 2-Month Data Changed Compared with Table 5-2 | | | |

Case ID	$X_{i1}(T_1)$	$X_{i2}(T_2)$	$D_i = X_{i2} - X_{i1}$	$D_i - \bar{D}$	$\Sigma (D_i - \bar{D})^2$
1	92	92	0	−6	$(-6)^2 = 36$
2	94	95	+1	−7	$(-7)^2 = 49$
3	96	86	−10	+4	$(4)^2 = 16$
4	98	90	−8	+2	$(2)^2 = 4$
5	100	91	−9	+3	$(3)^2 = 9$
6	102	92	−10	+4	$(4)^2 = 16$
$n = 6$	$\bar{X}_{.1} = 97$	$\bar{X}_{.2} = 91$	$\bar{D} = -6$	$\Sigma (D_i - \bar{D}) = 0$	$\Sigma (D_i - \bar{D})^2 = 130$

Standard deviation of the difference scores D_i

$$SD_{Di} = \sqrt{\frac{\Sigma (D_i - \bar{D})^2}{n - 1}} = \sqrt{\frac{130}{5}} = 5.099$$

Standard error of the mean difference score $\bar{D}$

$$SE_{\bar{D}} = SD_{Di}/ \sqrt{n} = 5.099/ \sqrt{6} = 2.0817$$

t value = (sample mean difference—hypothesized population mean difference)/standard error of the mean difference score $\bar{D}$

$$t = (\bar{D} - \mu\delta)/SE_{\bar{D}} = (-6 - 0)/2.0817 = -2.8823$$

Two-tailed significance level or probability (P) value associated with t value of -2.8823 and 5 ($=6-1$) degrees of freedom

.034

Pearson correlation between Time 1 and Time 2 measures

−.144

time among the individual subjects are distributed in a symmetric fashion. With the assumption that the sampling distribution of mean differences is shaped like a t distribution, and an estimate of its standard error from the sample data, all we need is information on the observed mean difference in the sample. With this, we are ready for the test.

Our null hypothesis is, as usual, that there is no real difference in mean diastolic blood pressure before and after the drug treatment. In other words, we assume that the true difference, which we denote by the Greek symbols $_\mu\delta$ ("mu of delta" or the population mean difference), equals 0. If that is the case, then the observed sample mean difference of

$\bar{D} = -6$ differs quite a bit from the overall population difference of $\mu\delta = 0$. In fact, we know that $\bar{D}$ is 5.636 standard errors below the hypothesized population mean of zero. This result is calculated from the available information: $t = (\bar{D} - \mu\delta)/ SE_{\bar{D}} = (-6 - 0)/1.0646 = -5.636$. All that is left now is to find the probability that a sample value of $t = -5.636$ or below would be generated as the result of mere chance events. The answer is that in a t distribution with 5 degrees of freedom (sample size minus one estimated parameter, which is the mean difference), that probability is very low, namely, $P = .002$, or less than 2 in 1,000 samples would produce this result randomly. Our conclusion would clearly be that the two diastolic blood pressure means do differ: there is a statistically significant decline in diastolic blood pressure, with an average decline of -6.

Limitations of the Paired *t* Test

Although the paired-samples *t* test is frequently encountered in the health care literature, it is important to understand its limitation. First, it allows us to evaluate change in a group mean between two occasions. It is clearly not as well adapted to estimating individual change. At the bottom of Table 5-2, we also reported the Pearson correlation between the time 1 and time 2 measures. The Pearson correlation, although it is not always reported in clinical research articles, provides valuable additional information about the change that occurred. Notice that the paired *t* test indicates only whether or not there is a *mean* change between two occasions or paired measures. To put it another way, not all individuals in the sample necessarily experience a change in the same direction.

In Table 5-3, the data for the time-2-measure (X_{i2}) were slightly altered through reshuffling of the same values. Notice that there is no change in the *mean* diastolic blood pressure for time 2. However, as the difference score shows, the first study participant (Case ID 1) now shows no change in the blood pressure score, and the second study participant (Case ID 2) shows an increase. The standard deviation of the difference scores is now a bit larger. That is to be expected. In the first sample, all subjects showed a decline, and the difference scores varied from -11 to -4. In the second sample, they varied from -11 to $+1$. Despite that, the standard error estimates remain small enough to produce significant results. The Pearson correlation, though, alerts us to the fact that the individual changes in the sample behave very differently. In the first case, a fairly strong correlation between the time 1 and time 2 measure indicates that most cases move parallel in the same direction. In the second sample, a small negative correlation indicates that there is no discernible pattern. Essentially, with a correlation close to zero, it is impossible to predict how individual members of the sample change.

It is clear that if the decline in diastolic blood pressure is the result of the drug therapy, the first situation is clinically more meaningful than the second. Even though both study samples produce the same *average* decline, in the first situation some effect is shown in all individuals, thus increasing our confidence in the generality of the effect. In the second situation, that is not the case. There is a larger issue here. Reports of results from clinical trials usually emphasize the *average* effects of an intervention or treatment. However useful that may be, clinicians also want to know something about the individual variability in the predictions. This is sometimes neglected in research reports. Even when it is presented, readers may pay little attention to such information.

Interpreting Statistical Significance

Going back to the results from Tables 5-2 and 5-3, we conclude that there is a statistically significant decline in diastolic blood pressure. Can that be interpreted in causal terms? Is it permissible to say that the significant effect shows that the drug therapy caused the diastolic blood pressure to decline? Unfortunately, the answer is "no." Recall that the setup for the paired *t* test mentioned only that we are comparing two blood pressure readings, before and after a drug treatment in a group of six hypertensive primary care patients. Clearly, this is not a true experimental design. It lacks the crucial ingredients of comparison groups and of random assignment to group or occasion. However, in the case of a simple crossover design, a paired *t* test could be used to test for the causal effectiveness of the intervention. It remains important, however, to recognize that any causal interpretation flows from the study design features and their ability to exclude confounding variables as plausible alternative explanations.

Recall again the earlier description of the crossover design for the pressure cushion study by Defloor and Grypdonck (2000). Pressure readings from any two cushions can be compared by means of the paired *t* test. If significant differences in the pressure readings exist, one can be fairly confident that these differences are attributable to the cushion surfaces. The main reason for this confidence is that plausible alternative explanations for the significant differences are hard to come by. The readings are paired, i.e., they are readings from two different occasions but from the same set of individuals. Thus, differences in background characteristics of study participants cannot be responsible for the result. In addition, unlike a simple pretest/posttest study without a comparison group, the occasions at which the pressure readings were taken were randomly assigned. Thus, no single other event (history) could explain a systematic difference in average pressure readings between two cushion surfaces. Likewise, neither maturation, testing, or instrumentation is a plausible reason for such differences. Even diffusion of treatment is not a plausible explanation for systematic differences in pressure readings between two mattresses. Whereas there might be some carryover effect in a transition from a relatively hard surface to a softer one (or vice versa), the random sequencing of the cushion surface assignments effectively undercuts the possibility of consistent transitions from one kind of cushion to the next. This makes it all but impossible for a systematic effect to develop.

Just as one-way and factorial analyses of variance are generalizations of the independent samples *t* test, so is repeated-measures analysis of variance a generalization of the paired *t* test. The former analyses test for differences between more than two different groups; the latter analysis allows for the simultaneous examination of change involving three or more measurement occasions. For more detailed discussion of these analysis techniques, the reader may consult some of the referenced literature.

▶ CLINICAL RESEARCH IN ACTION
Statistical Analysis Examples of Crossover Designs

Because crossover designs can provide compelling evidence on the efficacy of an intervention as long as the treatments do not produce diffusion problems or carryover effects, they are among the more popular experimental designs used in nursing and other health-related research. For example, nurse researchers have used them to study how the intake of iced fluids affects oral temperature taking (Cole, 1993) or how behavioral interventions versus sucrose relieve procedural pain in very–low-birthweight infants (Stevens, Johnston, Franck, Petryshen, Jack, & Foster, 1999).

One interesting example of a behavioral intervention is the recent study by Clark, Lipe, & Bilbrey (1998), briefly introduced in Chapter 2. These researchers were interested in reducing aggressive behavior among nursing home residents with dementia, especially during bathing. They devised an intervention that consisted of playing taped music thought to be soothing for the dementia patient.

Bathing to Music

1. For residents in a rural nursing home with a diagnosis of dementia and a history of aggressive behavior, but without hearing impairments, the researchers contacted relatives who had the authority to give permission for study participation.
2. Through interviews with the relatives of 18 nursing home residents, for whom agreement to participate was obtained, researchers first explored which kinds of music would be enjoyed by their residents. On the basis of this information, several tapes with selections of the preferred music (hymns, string music, big band, classical music) were made, which later served as the appropriate stimuli (intervention) in the study.
3. The study design called for 20 bathing episodes during which each of the dementia residents would be observed. These bathing episodes were split into two groups: 10 episodes without any music and 10 with tapes playing the preferred music.
4. Study participants were randomly assigned to either one of two sequences of exposure: 10 bathing episodes with music followed by 10 without music, or 10 bathing episodes without music followed by 10 with music.
5. During each episode, observers counted and independently recorded all observed instances of aggressive behavior initiated by the patient, such as hitting, biting, yelling, crying, physical resistance, spitting, or kicking. High interobserver agreement was established.

The crossover design of this study provides for fairly strong design validity. However, the researchers did make some design decisions that may have reduced the strength of the evidence. Principally, there were two areas of possible design improvement for a future study. This particular crossover design was not balanced, i.e., 6 study participants were first given the music sessions followed by bathing sessions without music, whereas 12 study participants were assigned to the reverse sequence. A balanced design would have called for a 9/9 split. This lack of balance does have the potential to affect inferences about the causal efficacy of playing music, especially when combined with the second design decision made by these researchers: to switch only once between music and no-music sessions. Instead of following 10 intervention sessions with 10 control sessions (or vice versa), it might have been desirable to randomly mix the two types of sessions. For example, assuming that at least some of the patients had the capacity to remember at least some aspects of the sessions, it is possible that repeating music (or no-music) sessions 10 times each led to a buildup of expectations by the dementia patients. This, if true, could have accounted for particularly large swings in behavior when the one-time switch in exposure occurred (figure on p. 14 in Clark et al., 1998). It is also possible that carryover effects from music to no-music sessions lasted for a while. For instance, the average number of aggressive behavior among the 6 subjects first exposed to music, then to no-music sessions, increased from about 50 to 55 in the first 10 sessions to 80 to 85 in the second 10 sessions (these figures are based on the graphs on p. 14 in Clark et al., 1998). Among the 12 subjects who first experienced no-music sessions followed by music sessions, we saw a drop from an average of 125 to 130 in the first 10 sessions to 65 to 70 in the second 10 sessions. It is clear that the differences between the two sequences of bathing sessions (a 30-point increase versus a 60-point drop) could not have influenced the overall results if the design had been balanced, because with a 9/9 split, each sequence would have carried the same weight. In summary, a completely randomized assignment of the sequencing and alternations between the two types of bathing sessions could have avoided any potential problems with habituation and carryover expectations.

As already mentioned, the outcome or criterion measures in this study for the success or failure of the music intervention were counts of specific aggressive behaviors like yelling and hitting, and one overall combined count of all aggressive behaviors. These outcome measures were time dependent, which means that the longer the observation period, the greater the chance of observing any one of the aggressive behaviors. The authors indicated that the no-music sessions lasted, on average, 2 minutes and 22 seconds longer than the music sessions, and that these differences were not statistically significant. However, they did represent a total of almost 24 minutes more observation time (16% greater) for the combined control occasions of no music. In this situation, it might have been better to time-standardize the outcome measures, by using several aggressive behaviors per hour, for instance, to reduce the potential for bias in favor of the intervention.

Clark et al. (1998) used paired *t* tests (or "*t* tests for dependent measures") for testing the main hypothesis that the playing of music reduces aggressive behavior among dementia residents during bathing episodes. To what extent did the data meet the assumptions we have discussed for use of the *t* test? All outcome variables in this study were ratio-level variables, because they were counts of activities that had meaningful zero points, i.e., the nonoccurrence of a particular activity. The comparison of behaviors after music and after no-music sessions were also paired, because they involved the same set of study participants exposed to both types of sessions. However, one concern from an analysis point of view is the extreme skewness (lopsidedness) in the distribution of the outcome variables. The researchers combined (summed, or added up) the behavior counts for all 10 music sessions and all 10 no-music sessions. Despite that, the data presented in Tables 1 and 2 of the article indicated that a few of the subjects accounted for most of the overall aggressive behavior. Using the difference scores (as in the paired *t* test) did lessen the skewness of the distribution, because the same individuals tended to be relatively more (or less) aggressive in both types of sessions. Yet, the authors reported that a single individual was responsible for 408 instances of yelling in the 10 no-music sessions and 84 instances in the music sessions (p.15): a difference of 324. The effect of such extreme outliers was that they greatly inflated the standard deviations computed from the sample, and they subsequently inflated the estimates of the standard errors used in the statistical tests. As a result, the significance tests in this study tended to be biased in a conservative direction (against the hypothesis of the beneficial effect of the music intervention), because it is difficult to show significant effects if standard errors are very large. There are alternative, nonparametric statistical tests that do not rely on the assumption of symmetric sampling distributions, such as the Wilcoxon signed-ranks test and the McNemar test. When data are highly skewed and it is difficult to maintain the assumption that the data come from a population in which the variable is normally distributed, then nonparametric alternatives to the *t* test, such as the Wilcoxon and McNemar tests, are preferable and may yield different results. For additional information, interested readers are referred to the relevant literature (e.g., Siegel & Castellan, 1988; Munro, 2001).

GENERAL ISSUES WITH CLINICAL TRIALS

One of our objectives in presenting a more detailed critique of a given article in which a repeated-measures design was used is to give the reader the sense that although a study may provide good evidence in favor of some particular hypothesis, rarely is any experimental study "perfect." That means that evidence from any single study is seldom beyond any reasonable doubt concerning the causal efficacy of the treatments or interventions tested. Clinical research often takes place under challenging, real-world conditions in which tradeoffs must be made between desired research design rigor and real-world feasibility considerations.

In Chapter 3 we stated that although experimental study designs are not the most frequently adopted study designs in the nursing and medical literature, they are nonetheless considered the "gold standard" or benchmark against which the results from other types of studies are measured. Their undeniable strength is that they offer the best causal evidence available—a fact that should be taken into account in the comparison of results from randomized clinical trials and nonrandomized studies (Ioannidis, Haidich, Pappa, Pantazis, Kokori, Tektonidou, Contopoulos-Ioannidis, & Lau, 2001; Kramer, Barr, Dagenais, Yang, Jones, Ciofani, & Jane, 2001). This does not mean that the evidence is perfect. On the contrary, randomized clinical trials do have their share of methodologic problems (Fogg & Gross, 2000). In particular, experimental studies in all their variety tend to display one or more of the following six weaknesses, which are common enough to deserve special attention.

1. **Attrition bias** or **differential dropout** (particularly in clinical trials that have repeated outcome measures with long-term follow-ups). The longer a trial goes on, the more likely are study participants to drop out; but, as stated before, study participants generally do not drop out at random (Bender et al., 1997). To be sure, there are several strategies to reduce dropout rates and increase subject retention (Motzer, Moseley, & Lewis, 1997), but it is impossible to eliminate this problem. One response to this problem has been the "intention-to-treat" approach to analysis (Newell, 1992). In this approach, the analyst attributes unchanged outcome scores to the dropout subjects. This approach is essentially conservative, because it becomes harder to show that a new treatment or intervention is effective.

2. **Identification of proper "control" conditions** (common in randomized clinical trials). As was already discussed, mostly because of the ethical problems asso-

ciated with a no-treatment or a placebo condition, researchers commonly expose their control group subjects to the usual care or treatment. This is not unproblematic. First, control group conditions are a moving target, making comparisons between studies from different settings and different times difficult. In addition, in some situations, there simply are no obvious control conditions that provide a good test of the intervention. Particularly for educational interventions, it is not always clear what the appropriate placebo condition should be (Fogg & Gross, 2000). For instance, Rothert et al. (1997) compared three decision support intervention formats, principally differentiated according to the intensity of these interventions. Although it would have been intuitively useful to include a control group, the use of a control group might have been neither feasible nor ethical for this study. For instance, women in search of information about the management of currently experienced menopausal symptoms may not accept an assignment to a "no care" (no information) group as appropriate.

3. **Nonadherence to a therapeutic regimen.** Many "interventions," including nursing interventions, rely on the patients going home and following the instructions they were given during an encounter with a health care provider. Given that many patients choose not to follow through with their therapeutic regimen (sometimes for rational reasons), and given that many clinical trials are started in institutional environments but continued within uncontrolled home environments, researchers often have no choice but to put their faith into the study participants' follow-through. True, one might argue that in large-sample, randomized trials, nonadherence is about as likely to occur in the treatment group as in the control group. But that would not be true if the trial treatment were inherently more difficult to follow, for example, producing more unwanted or adverse side effects.

4. **Random assignment of patients to alternative treatment conditions.** Even though the logic of the usefulness of random assignment in excluding systematic biases that favor particular treatments is impeccable, patients often will not (and for good reasons!) wish to be excluded from a group that has the potential to offer them a substantial benefit.[4] As Fogg and Gross (2000)

have emphasized, ". . . so long as there is voluntary consent and ethical codes that require full disclosure in research, participants will make the scientist's life more difficult by refusing to live by the random numbers table."

5. **Error.** Even in a well-designed randomized clinical trial, there is room for error. Recall that after random assignment one can calculate the risk of drawing wrong conclusions (Type I and Type II errors). Yet, while these risks can be minimized through larger samples and other study procedures like more reliable measurement, they cannot be eliminated completely. Thus, no single study, however well designed, will ever conclusively prove anything. It is the accumulation of evidence across several studies that provides the confidence that certain findings hold and are not just a fluke.

6. **Lack of statistical generalizability** (the weakest aspect of clinical experiments). Clinical studies are usually conducted with patients accessible to the researcher(s) in a particular clinic or clinics. In the chapters on sampling (Chapters 19 through 21), we shall make a distinction between **accessible** and **target** populations. It goes without saying that a single study almost never includes members of all the target populations to which the research potentially applies. Only the accumulation of evidence from different sites and different study populations can strengthen our confidence that a particular causal pattern can be considered general.

CONCLUSION

Beyond the vagaries of chance, a final point can be made about randomized trials or intervention studies. Undeniably, many health problems of great interest to clinicians cannot be studied by the clinical trial or experimental approach, because the main variable of interest cannot be manipulated. A classic example concerns the health consequences of smoking. As the public is generally aware, the tobacco industry has long denied the existence of scientific evidence linking smoking to lung cancer, other chronic lung diseases, and coronary heart disease. Of course, the definition of "scientific" in this case is rather narrow: it contends that only evidence from experimental studies provides scientific evidence. If one were to accept this definition of scientific evidence, one would indeed be in trouble to show a cause-and-effect relationship between smoking and lung disease, for instance. It is simply ethically unacceptable (and logistically impossible) to assign, say, 1,000

---

[4]It should not be forgotten that most of the experimental methods that inform health research study designs were first worked out in agricultural research (Fisher, 1935; Cochran & Cox, 1957). Manipulating agricultural treatments (e.g., different fertilizers and their random assignment to different plots) poses no ethical challenge, nor does it lead to resistance from the "study participants."

nonsmokers randomly to either a group that will adopt smoking or another group that will abstain from it for 20 years. Clearly, such a study would give us the strongest available causal evidence about the effects of smoking, but it cannot be done. What to do? As we shall see, in the case of smoking no deliberate intervention is possible, so all the evidence about smoking comes from observational studies. Nonetheless, the case for smoking as a causal agent of many diseases is very good indeed (U.S. Surgeon General, 1983), even though it is largely based on cohort studies (see Chapter 9). But judgments about how good this evidence really is start with this fundamental principle: *to what degree can these studies exclude potentially confounding explanations?* We must always ask this principal question before we draw causal conclusions.

Suggested Activities

1. Read the three experimental studies discussed in this chapter (Clark et al., 1998; Defloor & Grypdonck, 2000; Ornstein et al., 1988).
2. For each study, identify the research problem and any specific hypotheses that were tested.
3. For each study, count the number of distinct treatment levels or interventions, and describe the randomization plan in detail, using your own words. How many subjects were assigned, at how many occasions, and to how many treatment levels?
4. In all three articles, the results are reported in tables. Do the data reported in the tables speak to the research problems? That is, can you find the answers to the research questions/hypotheses that were posed by the researchers?
5. Formulate three clinical research questions that could be examined in an intervention study that appropriately uses a crossover design.
   a. State specific research hypotheses related to the three research questions.
   b. Describe the intervention you have in mind.
   c. Describe the outcome measure(s) you consider an appropriate test for the interventions.
   d. Describe the specific features of your proposed crossover design: how many treatment/intervention variables, how many treatment/intervention occasions?
6. Defend your choice of a crossover design. Given your research problem and hypotheses, why is it preferable to a between-subjects design? Can you justify that the characteristics or your interventions and outcome variables are such that treatment diffusion/carryover effects are unlikely to be a serious problem?

7. Describe the clinical setting in which you would propose to study your problem. Are there any characteristics/features of the clinical setting or its clientele that make the use of a crossover design either easy to use or unjustifiably difficult?
8. In Table 4 (p. 346) of their article, Defloor & Grypdonck (2000) list two *t* values and two 95% confidence intervals after each cushion brand. Formulate the null hypotheses underlying these tests, and interpret the meaning of the 95% confidence intervals. The two means compared in these *t* tests refer to which measures obtained from which subjects? Stevens et. al. (1999) report the main results from their crossover study in Tables 2 (p.39) and 4 (p. 40). What does the information in Table 4 add to that given in Table 2?

Suggested Readings

Clark, M. E., Lipe, A. W., & Bilbrey, M. (1998). Use of music to decrease aggressive behaviors in people with dementia. *Journal of Gerontological Nursing,* 24(7), 10–17.

Cochran, W. G. and Cox, G. M. (1992). *Experimental Designs.* (2nd ed.). New York, NY: John Wiley & Sons; Wiley Classics Library, originally published in 1957.

Defloor, T. & Grypdonck, M. H. F. (2000). Do pressure relief cushions really relieve pressure? *Western Journal of Nursing Research,* 22(3), 335–50.

Fisher, R. A. (1951). *The design of experiments (6th ed.).* Edinburgh, UK: Oliver & Boyd. (1st ed., 1935)

Newell, D. J. (1992). Intention-to-treat analysis: Implications for quantitative and qualitative research. *International Journal of Epidemiology,* 21, 837–41.

Ornstein, S., Markert, G., Litchfield, L. & Zemp, L. (1988). Evaluation of the DINAMAP blood pressure monitor in an ambulatory primary care setting. *The Journal of Family Practice,* 36(5), 517–21.

Stevens, B., Johnston, C., Franck, L., Petryshen, P., Jack, A. & Foster, G. (1999). The efficacy of developmentally sensitive interventions and sucrose for relieving procedural pain in very low birth weight neonates. *Nursing Research,* 48(1), 35–43.

References

Altman, D. G. (1991). *Practical statistics for medical research.* Boca Raton, FL: Chapman & Hall/CRC.

Bender, C. M., Yaskp, J. M., Kirkwood, J. M., Ryan, C., Dunbar-Jacob, J., & Zullo, T. (2000). Cognitive function and quality of life in interferon therapy for melanoma. *Clinical Nursing Research, 9,* 352–363.

Clark, M. E., Lipe, A. W., & Bilbrey, M. (1998). Use of music to decrease aggressive behaviors in people with dementia. *Journal of Gerontological Nursing, 2*(7), 10–17.

Cochran, W. G., & Cox, G. M. (1992). *Experimental designs.* (2nd ed.). New York: John Wiley & Sons; Wiley Classics Library, originally published in 1957.

Cole, F. L. (1993). Temporal variation in the effects of iced water on oral temperature. *Research in Nursing & Health, 16,* 107–111.

Defloor, T., & Grypdonck, M. H. F. (2000). Do pressure relief cushions really relieve pressure? *Western Journal of Nursing Research, 22,* 335–350.

Ellis, M. V. (1999). Repeated measures designs. *The Counseling Psychologist, 27,* 552–578.

Fisher, R. A. (1951). *The design of experiments* (6th ed.). Edinburgh: Oliver & Boyd. (1st ed., 1935).

Havas, S., Anliker, J., Damron, D., Langenberg, P., Ballesteros, M., & Feldman, R. (1998). Final results of the Maryland WIC 5-a-day promotion program. *American Journal of Public Health, 88,* 1161–1167.

Ioannidis, J. P. A.., Haidich, A. B., Pappa, M., Pantazis, N., Kokori, S. I., Tektonidou, M. G., Contopoulos-Ioannidis, D.G., & Lau, J. (2001). Comparison of evidence of treatment effects in randomized and non-randomized studies. *Journal of the American Medical Association, 286,* 821–830.

Kramer, M. S., Barr, R. G., Dagenais, S., Yang, H., Jones, P., Ciofani, L., & Jane, F. (2001). Pacifier use, early weaning, and cry/fuss behavior: A randomized trial. *Journal of the American Medical Association, 286,* 322–326.

McGrath, M. M., Sullivan, M. C., Lester, B. M., & Oh, W. (2000). Longitudinal neurologic follow-up in neonatal intensive care unit survivors with various neonatal morbidities. *Pediatrics, 106,* 1397–1405.

Motzer, S. A., Moseley, J. R., & Lewis, F. M. (1997). Recruitment and retention of families in clinical trials with longitudinal designs. *Western Journal of Nursing Research, 19,* 314–333.

Mundinger, M. O., Kane, R. L., Lenz, E. R., Totten, A. M., Tsai, W-Y., Cleary, P. D., Friedewald, W. T., Siu, A. L., & Shelanski, M.L. (2000). Primary care outcomes in patients treated by nurse practitioners or physicians: A randomized trial. *Journal of the American Medical Association, 283,* 59–68.

Newell, D. J. (1992). Intention-to-treat analysis: Implications for quantitative and qualitative research. *International Journal of Epidemiology, 21,* 837–841.

Ornstein, S., Markert, G., Litchfield, L., & Zemp, L. (1988). Evaluation of the DINAMAP blood pressure monitor in an ambulatory primary care setting. *The Journal of Family Practice, 36,* 517–521.

Rothert, M. L., Holmes-Rovner, M., Rovner, D., Kroll, J., Breer, L., Talarczyk, G., Schmitt, N., Padonu, G., & Wills, C. (1997). An educational intervention as decision support for menopausal women. *Research in Nursing & Health, 20,* 377–387.

Sidani, S., & Braden, C. J. (1998). *Evaluating nursing interventions: A theory-driven approach.* Thousand Oaks, CA: Sage.

Siegel, S., & Castellan, N. J. (1988). *Nonparametric statistics.* (2nd ed.). Boston: McGraw-Hill.

Snedecor, G. W., & Cochran, W. G. (1989). *Statistical methods.* (8th ed.). Ames, IA: Iowa State University Press.

Stevens, B., Johnston, C., Franck, L., Petryshen, P., Jack, A., & Foster, G. (1999). The efficacy of developmentally sensitive interventions and sucrose for relieving procedural pain in very low birth weight neonates. *Nursing Research, 48,* 35–43.

U.S. Surgeon General. (1983). *The health consequence of smoking.* Rockville, MD: U.S. Department of Health and Human Services.

Wills, C. E., & Stommel, M. (2001). Graduate nursing students' pre- and post-course perceptions and preferences concerning fully web-based courses. *Journal of Nursing Education, 41,* 193–201.

CHAPTER 6   Quasi-Experimental Studies for
Clinical Settings

INTRODUCTION: REVIEW OF EXPERIMENTAL DESIGN FEATURES

In Part II of this book, we focused on the advantages of using experimental designs for answering research questions about the effectiveness of interventions or treatments. To review, "true" experimental designs provide the strongest evidence in support of hypothesized causal relationships between variables, because they include the following basic features:

1. Researcher control or manipulation of one or more independent variables that are hypothesized to generate a change in the dependent variable(s)
2. Use of at least one control or comparison group (or occasion)
3. Random assignment of study participants to groups or study conditions defined by the independent variable(s)
4. Control over relevant environmental factors that could otherwise provide competing explanations for the seemingly effective intervention

In Part II, we included an in-depth discussion of why these features of experimental designs are so useful for examining the impact of interventions on outcomes. Among them, random assignment in particular offers a strong, all-purpose mechanism to control for both known and unrecognized confounding variables. In other words, the random assignment process makes it more credible that changes in the dependent variable (the outcome) can be attributed to the causal efficacy of the independent variable (the intervention).

It was also emphasized in Part II that studies with true experimental designs are naturally a good fit for evaluating the effectiveness of clinical interventions. This is true because interventions are often controlled (manipulated) by clinicians or researchers. At the same time, questions about the effectiveness of interventions are centrally concerned with cause-and-effect relationships. The controls included in experimental designs allow for making the strongest case scientifically; i.e., for excluding plausible rival accounts or hypotheses for the observed effects of interventions on outcomes.

SOME REAL-LIFE DESIGN CONSTRAINTS ON EXPERIMENTAL DESIGNS: EFFECTS OF A COMPANION ANIMAL INTERVENTION

Although studies using experimental designs are widely regarded as the gold standard for evaluating causal evidence, real-life feasibility and ethical considerations very often preclude the full implementation of all the basic features of experimental designs in clinical intervention studies. More often than not, nursing and other clinical research relies on study designs that deviate in some way from true experimental designs. Consider, for example, Research Scenario 6-1, which involves a personal companion animal intervention for retirement community residents. After reviewing the scenario, why, do you think, would it be difficult to implement all the features of a true experimental study for the purpose of evaluating the effectiveness of this intervention?

To begin, although the deliberate introduction of pets into a retirement community environment clearly constitutes an intervention, there are several reasons for why it might be anticipated that control over and manipulation of such an intervention could be quite limited. For example, the effects of introducing personal companion animals could not be studied by a crossover design. Not only is it likely that there are carryover effects from the intervention

RESEARCH SCENARIO 6.1

Companion Animal Scenario: Limits to Use of Experimental Design

The director of health services for a large retirement community wants to find out whether and to what extent providing companion animals to community residents will improve the residents' quality of life and functional status. Having reviewed the literature, the director believes that residents who have personal companion animals are less likely to report that they feel socially isolated or depressed and will maintain both instrumental and independent activities of daily living longer than do residents who do not have personal pets. Being mindful of the need to document outcomes of services provided, the director consults with a nurse practitioner with experience in research design on how to introduce personal companion animals into the nursing home environment and to evaluate their impact on the residents. The nurse practitioner immediately recognizes that several situational constraints would make it impossible to conduct a full experiment for evaluating the impact of a personal companion animal. Instead, to minimize disruption of the social interaction patterns and routines in the nursing home, she suggests a quasi-experiment known as the interrupted time-series design as an alternative.

time period(s) to the control time period(s), or vice versa, but the single most important obstacle to such a study design would be the unacceptability of turning the intervention on and off at random. Community residents who accept the care of companion animals could not ethically be expected to give up their pets to meet the experimental condition of researcher control of the independent variable (exposure to a companion animal). Essentially, the intervention could be introduced only once, and the researcher would not control exposure to the intervention after that point.

REVIEW NOTES If repeated-treatment designs like crossover studies are not feasible in this situation, what about between-subjects designs that use separate control groups? In Chapter 4, it was pointed out that one of the biggest threats to the design validity of a completely randomized design is the diffusion-of-treatment (contamination) problem, in which the control and experimental groups are not truly separate in their exposure to the independent variable. Recall that in an experimental study with separate control or comparison group(s), it is imperative that the control/comparison group (in the current example, the group without companion animals) and the experimental group (the group with companion animals) are truly separate in their exposure to the intervention.

To implement such separation within the same retirement community would not be an easy or even feasible task. For example, a community resident with a companion animal may well bring the animal to visit a community resident who does not have a companion animal.

The third fundamental feature of a randomized control-group design is random assignment of study participants to the various comparison groups. That too poses a problem in the personal companion animal study. As we've just mentioned, the problem of treatment diffusion is often the greatest when study subjects live in close proximity. Yet, the very nature of random assignment entails disregarding social interaction patterns, instead cutting across any socially defined barriers to control exposure to the independent variable.[1] The social obstacles to a random assignment plan are sometimes insurmountable. Any research involving human subjects must respect their personal autonomy and preferences, so a random assignment process would be feasible only if the community residents freely agreed (in an informed consent process) to the random assignment

process itself. Because many participants in a human–animal interaction study can be assumed to have a basic preference for having a companion animal, it is difficult to see how those who would be assigned to the control group would be willing to forego having a personal companion animal over the long run. Conversely, residents who dislike or even fear pet animals in the first place, or who otherwise feel unable to care for a pet, could not be required to have a pet, nor would they be likely to participate in such a study in the first place. Thus, with the limits on the manipulation of the independent variable, the difficulties in creating separate yet comparable control groups, and the inability to implement a meaningful random assignment scheme at the level of the individual study participants, a true experiment for this hypothetical study would be difficult if not impossible to implement.

Now suppose that the physical structure of the retirement community is a large high-rise apartment building; i.e., all residents live in the same building. This type of retirement community living arrangement may be common for older adults who live in urban areas. Institutional settings like these offer two main advantages for the conduct of experiments. First, because the residents probably exercise at least some choice over where they live, it can be anticipated that they share several socioeconomic traits and backgrounds, ranging from family income to education to religious affiliation or ethnicity. Such social processes of self-selection sometimes result in fairly homogeneous groups of subjects, which is an advantage in creating "comparable" intervention and control groups. The second advantage of conducting an experiment in the same building is that control over the environment is, of course, much easier in institutional settings than in less controlled community settings, such as individual homes in different geographic locations. Still, these advantages do not offset the other barriers to using a true experimental design.

OVERVIEW OF KEY TYPES OF QUASI-EXPERIMENTAL DESIGN

If an experimental design is not feasible for studies like the one assessing the effects of companion animals on health, what type of study design can be used to provide credible evidence on the effectiveness of such interventions? In this part of the book, we focus on several research designs that, though lacking some critical feature of true experiments, nonetheless offer useful alternatives for evaluating the effects of an intervention. Following the classic treatment of Cook & Campbell (1979), such research designs are

---

[1]In principle, it is possible to evaluate the efficacy of introducing companion animals in organizational settings in a study whose units of analysis ("cases") are the organizations themselves. In that case, the researcher(s) could randomize the assignment of the intervention at the level of the organizations. Of course, such a study would require substantial resources and specific skills in community-based research.

known as **quasi-experimental designs.** The term "quasi-experiment" refers to a family of research designs that have these shared characteristics:

- Goal of the research is to evaluate the causal effects of an intervention (i.e., does the intervention change an outcome?)
- Design lacks one or both of the following features of a true experimental design:
  - No random assignment of study participants to comparison groups (or occasions)
  - No separate control/comparison group

Such designs are still experiments, in the sense that they are distinct from observational-only types of studies. The hallmark of an experiment is that treatments or interventions are introduced on purpose (by design) and would not have occurred without deliberate action.[2] In this book, we refer to research designs that test causal hypotheses as quasi-experimental if they involve the deliberate introduction of a stimulus, intervention, or treatment *and* fall into either of two broad categories of designs we shall discuss in this chapter: **nonequivalent control-group designs** or **interrupted time-series designs** (Cook & Campbell, 1979). There are many examples of such studies in health-related research. *In general, the situational constraint, which most often results in the use of a quasi-experimental instead of an experimental design, is the lack of the ability (for reasons of feasibility or ethics) to assign study participants randomly to study groups, conditions, or occasions.* In studies with nonequivalent control-group designs, outcomes in intervention groups are compared with outcomes in control groups, whose equivalency in terms of their background characteristics remains in doubt. This situation is most likely to occur when it would be difficult to break up existing social groups, such as

- Clients in different community programs (Eisen, Keyser-Smith, Dampeer, & Sambrano, 2000)
- Students enrolled in courses using different teaching techniques (Freeman & Tijerina, 2000)
- Employees selected for a mentoring program (Seibert, 1999)

In studies with interrupted time-series designs, which can be considered repeated-measures quasi-experiments,

study participants are observed many times and are exposed to an intervention one or more times. However, the assignment of intervention occasions is not random, and often there is no separate control group (Hendy & Raudenbush, 2000).

Even though quasi-experiments lack one or both of the key features of true experiments (random assignment or the existence of separate control groups), how serious is the absence of these features for evaluating the causal effectiveness of an intervention? This question has no certain answer. Instead, the answer varies depending on the specific design features of a particular quasi-experiment in relation to the study questions/hypotheses. As we have emphasized in earlier chapters concerning true experimental designs, even the most carefully designed study will have at least some limitations with respect to the ability to draw causal inferences about the effects of an intervention. Thus, it is necessary to examine, for each study design, to what degree it succeeds in ruling out competing explanations for the observed changes after an intervention. In this context, it is worth emphasizing that some quasi-experimental designs can result in methodologically strong studies for testing the effects of interventions. In the following sections of this chapter, we introduce a few key quasi-experimental designs. In Chapter 7, we delve into more specific detail about the methodologic considerations and analysis of data gathered by use of a quasi-experimental design.

INTERRUPTED TIME-SERIES DESIGNS

The simplest **interrupted time-series design** is a study design in which a series of observations (repeated) is made before an intervention is implemented, followed by a series of observations (repeated) after the implementation of the intervention (Research Scenario 6-2). The observations made before the intervention are often referred to collectively as the **pretest/preintervention phase,** and the observations made after the intervention are often referred to as the **posttest/postintervention phase.** What issues would arise in drawing valid conclusions about the effectiveness of the intervention in such a study? In part, the answer depends on the pattern observed in the outcome variable.

Patterns of Results: Interrupted Time-Series Design Example

In Figure 6-1, Pattern 1 depicts a clear **discontinuity** in the *levels* of the mean depression scores after the start of the intervention. In the preintervention phase, the six consecutive mean Geriatric Depression Scores are 6.9, 7.3, 7.0, 7.2,

---

[2]It might be noted in passing that we distinguish here between a quasi-experiment and a natural experiment. A natural experiment occurs if the "intervention" is not controlled by the researcher(s) but by others, or even by situational factors. An example would be a policy change, such as the introduction of a health-labeling requirement for alcoholic beverages (Greenfield et al., 1999), which is taken by the researcher as a useful or serendipitous opportunity to study its effects on outcomes of interest. Likewise, natural disasters such as devastating hurricanes provide the opportunity to study the impact of uncontrollable life events on stress and coping.

Companion Animal Study as Interrupted Time-Series Design

Suppose the nurse practitioner in the scenario discussed in Research Scenario 6-1 decides to use this design to evaluate the effectiveness of companion animals in the nursing home population. As always, the first concern in such an evaluation study is the choice of an appropriate outcome variable or variables that can speak to the effectiveness of the intervention. In the case of the companion-animal intervention, outcomes of interest might include the community residents' relative sense of social isolation or their depression, as well as their physical functioning, expressed in terms of their ability to perform instrumental and independent activities of daily living. To illustrate this design, we assume here that the researcher decides to use only a single outcome measure: the 15-item Geriatric Depression Scale (GDS; Sheikh & Yesavage, 1986), which has been used extensively in older adult populations to screen for depression. Not only has this scale been validated for older adult populations and been shown to be sensitive to changes in depression, but also it is very easy for study participants to respond to. It contains few items, which can be answered "yes" or "no" by study participants. In addition, responses can be collected via either interview or written questionnaire. Total scales scores on the GDS represent the sum of the "yes" responses ranging from 0 to 15 points, with higher scores indicating greater depression.[3] The nurse researcher decides on a 6-month intervention study, with the depression scores of participating residents ascertained every 2 weeks. The companion animals are introduced after 3 months. In this design, there will be six preintervention-phase depression scores, and six postintervention-phase depression scores after the intervention is introduced.

6.8, and 7.4, which average to 7.1 over the six measurement occasions. The six mean scores during the postintervention phase are 6.4, 6.1, 5.9, 6.2, 5.8, and 6.3, averaging to 6.1. Clearly, the preintervention scores do not show any systematic upward or downward trend; the same can be said about the postintervention scores. In each phase, the series of mean scores fluctuates around their respective means (preintervention standard deviation, 0.237; postintervention standard deviation, 0.232) without a discernible pattern. However, there is an immediate and abrupt drop in mean scores by a full point from the preintervention to the postintervention phase. What could explain this pattern? The research hypothesis for this hypothetical study would be supported by this pattern; i.e., that the introduction of the companion animals caused the drop in scores. However, it is very important to consider also whether there are any plausible alternative explanations for the drop in scores. As it turns out, there are actually very few plausible rival hypotheses to explain this outcome pattern.

- To begin with, we can exclude testing effects as an alternative explanation. Whereas testing effects may well exist, such as some community residents remembering their previous responses to the questions on the Geriatric Depression Scale, this effect would be to make successive depression scores more alike. Thus, testing effects do not feasibly account for the sudden, one-time drop in scores after the intervention.

- In a similar vein, it does not seem plausible that instrumentation can explain the observed pattern—unless, of course, the measurement procedures were changed just at the same time when the companion animals were introduced. For instance, if the mode of data collection (interview or written questionnaire) had been changed between weeks 10 and 12, or if a new interviewer had been used at that time, this would obviously constitute a plausible rival hypothesis to explain the discontinuity in the levels of mean depression scores. Yet, such changes in instrumentation are usually under the control of the researcher (or at least somewhat under the control of the researcher).

- Selection bias is also unlikely as an explanation for the drop in scores. Although there may be some change in the resident population of the retirement community during the study period, this would be plausible as a competing explanation only if it occurred after the introduction of the companion animals.

- Similarly, attrition could lead to a change in the members of the study sample from before the intervention to afterward. However, both the accrual of new study participants and the loss of old ones are likely to be continuous processes, rather then one-time events that occur

---

[3]A detailed discussion of how to evaluate the quality and measurement properties of such multi-item scales will be presented in Chapters 13 and 14. Here we take the validity and reliability of the measurement procedures for granted.

**Mean Scores on Geriatric Depression Scale
measured every 2 weeks**

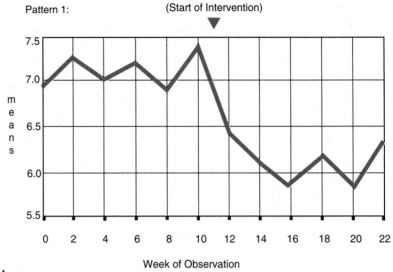

A

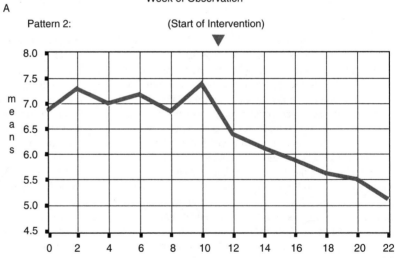

FIGURE 6.1 Mean scores on Geriatric Depression Scale measured every 2 weeks. (A) Pattern 1. (B) Pattern 2.

B

exactly at the time of the introduction of the companion animals. In addition, in the preintervention to postintervention comparisons, the researcher can always confine the analysis to only those study participants, for whom the full set of 12 observations is available.

• In a similar vein, one might argue that maturation processes are unlikely to produce sudden discontinuities coinciding with the intervention.

• Finally, statistical regression (or regression to the mean) is also not a plausible rival hypothesis. With a single preintervention observation, it would always be possible to argue that the obtained observation was unusually high or low for the long-run average, thus leading to a regression-to-the-mean phenomenon. This is not a convincing argument in the case of the outcome data shown in Pattern 1.

It seems, then, that the only serious rival hypothesis for the observed discontinuity of mean levels is history: the claim that some other important event occurred at the same time as the start of the intervention. This may be a plausible explanation for reduced depression if, for instance, a major organizational change for the better occurred in the retirement community. For example, a community intervention program with outreach to community residents who are known to be socially isolated or depressed might have been implemented around the same time as the companion animal intervention. In community-based research, it is important that researchers interpret data from intervention studies in the context of any known historical changes such as these.

The mean depression scores depicted in Pattern 2 of Figure 6-1 show another interpretable pattern. In this example, the preintervention scores are the same as those in Pattern 1 (6.9, 7.3, 7.0, 7.2, 6.8, 7.4, with an average of 7.1 over the six measurement occasions). The postintervention scores, however, show a different pattern: the six depression means are 6.4, 6.1, 5.9, 5.6, 5.5, 5.1, with an average of 5.8, but they also show a continuing decline over time. Thus, in addition to a discontinuity in the mean levels, there is also a discontinuity in the slope of the trend line. Whereas the slope for the preintervention means is flat (with no discernible tendency to increase or decrease), the slope of the postintervention means is negative, i.e., the means show an almost linear declining trend. This, then, is the other major discontinuity pattern that might occur as a result of the introduction of an intervention or treatment. Again, none of the previously discussed rival hypotheses, from testing effects to attrition to history, appear to be convincing explanations of such a pattern.

Other Issues in Interpreting Patterns of Results

The key reason for the power of the simple interrupted time-series design is that collecting multiple observations before the intervention allows us to establish a **trend line (pattern).** If there is an orderly, recognizable trend line, extrapolating this trend line into the future gives us a prediction of what observations to expect, if the process that generated these observations continues without interruption. In our example, if no companion animals were introduced (and no other salient events occurred), we would have no reason, after the first six observations, to expect any changes in average depression scores other than the usual random fluctuations. The latter might be the result of some measurement error or perhaps individual changes resulting from particular family events not shared by other

nursing home residents. Yet, the clear discontinuities observed in Patterns 1 and 2 cannot be easily explained in this way. As long as the researcher can be reasonably confident that no other salient event occurred that affected a large enough number of residents, resulting in systematic changes at the group level, the evidence for the causal efficacy of the intervention is quite convincing.

Instability in Repeated Measures

Unfortunately, the outcome patterns from interrupted time-series studies may not always be as clear as those portrayed in Figure 6-1. For one thing, the preintervention phase in the example showed a substantial stability in the mean depression scores over the six measurement times: the scores fluctuated within narrow margins from 6.8 to 7.4 on a scale of 0 to 15 (standard deviation, 0.237) with no upward or downward trend. In case of much larger fluctuations, it would have been more difficult to establish a preintervention trend line or pattern.

If trend lines are difficult to discern, so are deviations from barely recognized trend lines after the intervention.

Time-Delayed Effects

A second problem associated with interrupted time-series designs is **time-delayed intervention effects.** Essentially, in case of delayed impacts, the full impact of the intervention may not be seen until some time after the implementation of the intervention. For example, it could be argued that the series of mean depression scores shown in Pattern 2 is the result of a delayed intervention effect. At the end of the observation period (week 22), there is no indication yet that the declining depression scores have hit a floor. Thus, additional benefits may still materialize after the last observation. The downward-sloping trend in mean depression scores certainly suggests that the introduction of the companion animals sets a process in motion that generates more steam over time. Yet, in this example at least, the discontinuity appears right after the intervention is introduced. If the effects of an intervention are delayed longer, it might be more difficult to detect. Likewise, an intervention may not always produce a sudden effect; it may be gradual instead. For instance, if the six postintervention depression means showed the pattern 7.4, 7.1, 6.9, 7.0, 6.5, 6.5, one could not be confident that this pattern reveals the start of a downward trend or not. This introduces a difficulty: How would one know in advance the number of observations needed to establish trend lines in the preintervention and postintervention phases with confidence? The answer is that one does not know, unless there is prior knowledge of the natural, over-time variability of outcome scores–knowledge that can come only from previous empirical research. However, we can draw on the general principle that larger samples produce more stable results than smaller samples–a fact that results in a partial tradeoff between the study sample size and the number of required observations. With large study samples, fewer observations would be required, and vice versa. Yet, beyond such general principles, only knowledge of the particular target populations and the outcome measures in question can yield precise estimates.

Periodicity Effects

Causal interpretation of interrupted times-series designs is vulnerable to one additional possible competing hypothesis, which is unique to study designs with repeated measures. Time-series data are often subject to **periodicity effects:** effects that tend to play themselves out in fixed and repeating intervals over time. A classic example is that of the annual seasons. If the companion animal study had started in January and concluded in June, it may not be too farfetched to argue that depression scores among nursing home residents might start to decline with the advent of spring, accounting for the mean scores shown in Pattern 2 of Figure 6-1. This might be particularly viable as an alternative account for the outcomes, especially in geographic areas such as the northern United States, where seasonal affective disorder is prevalent during the fall to early spring months of the year. Likewise, a study begun in July and carried on through December could have the opposite effect of suppressing a potential positive impact of the introduction of companion animals. In other studies, periodic effects might account for changes in blood pressure during a day or changes in mortality patterns between weekdays and weekends. The best way to avoid such effects would, of course, be random assignment of treatment and control occasions over time. However, if that is not possible, the researcher must anticipate periodic effects and either time the observations to avoid period influences altogether or account for the latter in the analysis, which is possible if study participants are observed over several periods.

Other Types of Interrupted Time-Series Designs

Other, more complicated interrupted time-series designs go beyond the introduction of a single continuing treatment. For instance, a **time-series design with removed treatment** (Cook & Campbell, 1979) entails the discontinuation of the treatment. We have already commented that such a design would not be feasible for the companion animal intervention. For other treatments or interventions, like a temporary physical therapy intervention, such a design might be feasible. Given the gradual nature of most physical therapy impacts, such a design might lead one to hypothesize two discontinuities in slope effects, i.e., a gradual increase in physical functioning while the intervention lasts, followed by a gradual decrease after its discontinuation. Some drugs might be tested using interrupted **time-series designs with multiple replications,** as when a single group of study participants switches periodically between different formulae of antifungal skin lotions. As with crossover designs, repeated-treatment designs make sense only if the researcher is sure that there is no carryover or diffusion effect from one treatment period to the next.

In summary, interrupted time-series designs can provide powerful causal evidence, even though they do not involve random assignment of subjects to treatment or intervention occasions and often lack any separate control group. Such research designs may prove particularly attractive in institutional settings, in which certain outcome measures are routinely collected. For example, consider the routine gathering of vital signs on many hospital patients. If the research involves outcome measures that are regularly gathered for monitoring purposes, available past data series on current patients may be used as preintervention phase measures with future monitoring as postintervention outcome measures. Clearly, in these situations, interrupted time-series designs afford a natural fit to the institutional environment.

NONEQUIVALENT CONTROL-GROUP DESIGNS

A second type of quasi-experimental design uses **nonequivalent control groups.** Such study designs always entail the comparison of one or more study groups, including a control group. As the name implies, however, these groups may systematically differ in terms of the background characteristics of their members. This situation occurs when random assignment of subjects to comparison groups is not feasible. Thus, group members either select themselves into the comparison groups, as, for example, when students choose to enroll in parallel classes using different teaching techniques (Freeman & Tijerna, 2000), or when the comparison involves socially intact groups that already existed before a research study is undertaken (Eisen et al., 2000). The researcher(s) may be able to manipulate the intervention—hence the term "quasi-experiment" —and they may also be able to decide which of the already existing groups will be exposed to either treatment or control conditions, but control over the assignment of individual study participants is not available. The resulting nonequivalent control-group design lacks one of the key characteristics of true experiments: the random assignment of study participants to different treatment/intervention levels, or vice versa. This type of study design is commonly encountered in nursing and health-related research, because the subjects of such research are often recruited from existing groups, and the breakup of the groups for the purposes of random assignment would pose substantial obstacles.

REVIEW NOTES As discussed in Chapter 5, in addition to the logistic problems created by random assignment in clinical settings, a major reason for using intact groups in the comparison of treatment and control conditions is the threat to design validity that comes from the diffusion of treatment.

Especially with educational interventions in clinical settings, often the only way to keep treatment content from migrating across groups and contaminating the control group is through the use of separate clinical settings for the different treatment levels. Inevitably, this means that subjects in the different settings differ in known and unknown ways. Nonequivalent control group comparisons also occur in many medical studies, where the interest is in comparing outcomes for patients who did or did not get a certain clinical intervention. For instance, an obstetrician may want to compare the odds of two types of delivery (vaginal birth or cesarean section) among pregnant women treated with a cervical gel and those not so treated. Treatments like these are not assigned at random but are given on the basis of clinical judgments, which almost guarantees that the two groups of women are likely to differ in terms of several clinically relevant variables.

Finally, nonequivalent control group comparisons occur in situations where the intervention is community based rather than geared toward individual patients, as in the case of a health campaign conducted by the public health department of a particular county. In such cases, the creation of control groups within the same community that is subject to the community-wide intervention is likely to be difficult or impossible.

In all these situations, the best way to assess the effects of the intervention is to find "uncontaminated" comparison groups, which are as similar to the intervention group(s) as possible. These are either the same subjects at an earlier stage, as in the interrupted time-series design discussed in the previous section, or an entirely different set of subjects examined simultaneously, as in the nonequivalent control-group design. Such comparisons often involve different departmental populations in the same institution (e.g., a hospital, prison, or extended health care facility), but there can be no guarantee that the compared groups do not differ in some relevant way.

After the choice of more or less appropriate comparison groups from a roster of intact or preexisting groups, the only remaining decision is which group will receive the intervention and which the control condition. Of course, if the researcher(s) has access to a large number of such groups, the logic of random assignment can again be applied—this time at the group level. However, with only two groups, even a flip of the coin to determine which gets the treatment, the "law of large numbers" does not apply. Therefore, unless individual group members themselves can be reshuffled or reassigned, any systematic differences between the average characteristics of the two groups will remain intact.

Workplace Health Promotion Intervention Example

Research Scenario 6-3 presents a hypothetical example of a workplace health promotion intervention of a kind that is typically implemented at the community level. Most often, it would be very difficult if not impossible to implement this kind of health promotion program for some employees at a given site and keep it from others, especially because social interaction patterns may well cut across any group assignments made by the researcher(s). One alternative is to apply the intervention to all the personnel at one of the regional insurance offices (a preexisting intact group) and use the personnel at another site of the same insurance company as the control group. Although this approach minimizes diffusion problems,[4] it invites a host of other problems that need to be considered. To simplify the problem, we shall focus on a single criterion or outcome measure as an indicator of "success" of the health promotion: absenteeism rates during the month after the intervention. There are, of course, other useful outcome variables one could look at, such as the use of health services among employees, or smoking cessation rates among smokers. After the researcher has determined the outcome variable and accepted the fundamental principle that the comparison will be between the two sites, a host of subsidiary design decisions must still be considered.

Suppose for the sake of argument that our researcher settles on a posttest-only design. This design is identical to the completely randomized experiment described in Chapter 4, Table 4-2, Part A, except that the comparison groups are composed of the two preexisting office populations, rather than individually and randomly assigned subjects.

---

[4]There may possibly be frequent intracompany e-mail or other telecommunication exchanges between the two offices. Researchers who implement intact-group intervention studies must always check the intraorganizational communication flow in such organizations as part of the research design feasibility assessment process.

RESEARCH SCENARIO 6.3

Intact-Groups Quasi-Experimental Research Design: A Workplace Health Promotion Program

An insurance company contacts a nurse researcher who is well known for her work on designing and implementing health promotion programs in community settings. Company administrators for two regional insurance offices in different regions of a Midwestern state would like to reduce absenteeism and employee stress by providing on-site health promotion and screening activities, such as exercise, dietary enhancement, and blood pressure monitoring. The administrators are willing to pay for an on-site nurse and other resources to implement the program at each insurance company site. In addition, the administrators appreciate the need for a sound research design that makes it possible to evaluate the causal effects of the workplace intervention on the outcomes of interest. That is, the company administrators would like "solid proof" that they should continue to invest money in the program, after a reasonable test of the program's effectiveness.

Table 6-1, Part A, depicts this situation. The nurse researcher goes ahead and introduces the health promotion intervention at one of the two insurance offices but not the other. One month after the intervention, the average daily absenteeism rate at the intervention site is substantially lower than at the control site (let's assume 2% versus 8%). The problem with this finding is that it is very difficult to interpret. In a true experiment after random assignment of subjects to the comparison groups, we can construct a sampling distribution of the differences in absenteeism rates. Therefore, we would know how probable any given group difference would be, as a result of the random assignment process. If the observed difference is considered a very unlikely result of random assignment, we would conclude that the intervention produced the difference. No such benchmark is available in the case of a comparison of intact groups. For all we know, the groups may have been different from the outset. The lower absenteeism rate in the intervention group may reflect a pattern that already existed a long time ago, before the health promotion intervention was started.

For example, suppose that workers in the intervention group are older, with fewer competing family obligations, or have more attractive jobs. That could account for the lower absenteeism rates. Consequently, a simple posttest comparison of intact groups without randomization tells us next to nothing about the effectiveness of an intervention. At a minimum, we need some information about the comparison groups before the intervention took place.

Possible Patterns of Results: Nonequivalent Control-Group Design

Table 6-1, Part B, outlines a pretest/posttest design, again parallel to the design in Table 4-2, Part B, except for the absence of randomization and the substitution of the intact/preexisting comparison groups. The clear advantage of this

TABLE 6.1	Nonequivalent Control Group Designs

Part A: Posttest-Only Nonequivalent Control Group Design

Comparison of "Intact," Preexisting Groups	Manipulation of Independent Variable	Observation of Outcomes
Treatment/intervention group	New intervention	Posttest measure
Control/comparison group	Usual intervention	Posttest measure

Part B: Pretest/posttest nonequivalent control group design

Comparison of "Intact," Preexisting Groups	Observation of Outcomes Before Treatment	Manipulation of Independent Variable	Observation of Outcomes
Treatment/intervention group	Pretest measure	New intervention	Posttest measure
Control/comparison group	Pretest measure	Absence of intervention	Posttest measure

design is that the nurse researcher can now obtain information on the absenteeism rates in both office sites before the health promotion intervention is started. To what degree this additional information can be used to make sense out of the data depends partly on the outcome pattern generated by this research design. Figure 6-2 shows five different patterns. In each graph, hypothetical pretest and posttest absenteeism rates are plotted for both comparison groups.

Pattern A shows posttest absenteeism rates to be lower in the intervention group, but we know that this does not present any change from the pretests. Still, we cannot be certain that the health promotion intervention has no effect on absenteeism rates. One possible rival hypothesis is that a 4% rate represents a natural floor for this population, meaning the we could not expect a decline below this level, even though the health promotion would be effective in populations in which absenteeism rates are higher to begin with.

Pattern B, by contrast, does show a decline of the absenteeism rate from 6% to 2% in the intervention group, but no change in the control group. Is that convincing evidence? The fact that both groups had the same pretest rates certainly adds to the credibility of the inference that the health promotion intervention had some effect.

The most plausible rival hypothesis is the local history hypothesis: during that time, some other event to produce this effect occurred in the intervention group. An example would be a new chief executive officer, who is well liked and changes the climate at the work place during the health promotion intervention. In principle, a change in the way that absenteeism is recorded (instrumentation) could be responsible for the observed pattern. However, this change would again have to be local, i.e., it could occur only at the intervention site, which is unlikely because the comparison involves two local offices of the same insurance company.

Pattern C seemingly shows the same pattern as Pattern B. Again, we see a drop in the absenteeism rate of the intervention group by 4 percentage points and no change in the control group. However, the interpretation of this pattern is less certain. Especially, the pretest absenteeism rate in the intervention group appears unusually high, suggesting the possibility that the month before the health promotion was an exceptional month. If so, the decline would simply indicate a return to the more typical long-run rate for this group (**regression to the mean**). Pattern D, by contrast, does not give any indication of a regression-to-the-mean phenomenon. The fact that the absenteeism rate in the intervention group was above that of the control group before the intervention, but below it after the intervention, strengthens our conviction that the intervention is effective. The possibility of *local history* or the occurrence of

some other relevant event in the intervention group remains, of course, a viable rival hypothesis.

Finally, Pattern E is not a convincing argument for the effectiveness of the health promotion intervention. To be sure, the absenteeism rate in the intervention group falls by 4 percentage points, just as in Patterns B and D. However, absenteeism also declines in the control group by 3%. So, it looks as if some company-wide process (maybe a new incentive plan) is at work here, and the small differences in the rate of the decline could easily reflect the differences in employee composition at the two offices.

Interpretation of Results from Nonequivalent Control-Group Design

As this discussion shows, the causal interpretation of evidence from nonequivalent control-group designs is not without pitfalls, especially when there is only one pretest and one posttest measure. However, many of the rival hypotheses mentioned have some credibility, because a simple pretest/posttest design does not allow us to establish the normal trends in the comparison groups. By contrast, if the study design allows for multiple pretests, in effect producing a mix of interrupted time-series and nonequivalent control-group designs, we could know whether the immediate pretest scores are unusually high. This would, for instance, avoid the fallacy of interpreting a regression-to-the-mean effect as a causal effect of the intervention. Notice, then, that pretest/posttest designs with intact groups are not limited to just the basic form illustrated in Figure 6-2. Any number of observations can be included if the researcher has the time and resources to do so. *The key difference from the interrupted time-series design is that nonequivalent control-group designs involve comparisons of at least two groups (an intervention and control group), whose composition cannot be manipulated by the researcher.*

The most general problem in the comparison of nonequivalent intervention and control groups is the *possible interaction between differential selection and the intervention effect.* In that case, the composition of the intervention group differs from that of the control group in such a way that its members react differently to the intervention than do members of the control group, had they been exposed to the same intervention. Researchers can address this problem in two ways. In the design stage, careful attention must be paid to the selection of intervention and control groups. The general principle is to find existing groups whose average characteristics are as similar as possible. This might involve selecting two social support groups from the same area, two hospitals in neighborhoods of similar socioeconomic standing and ethnic composition, or, as in the insurance office example,

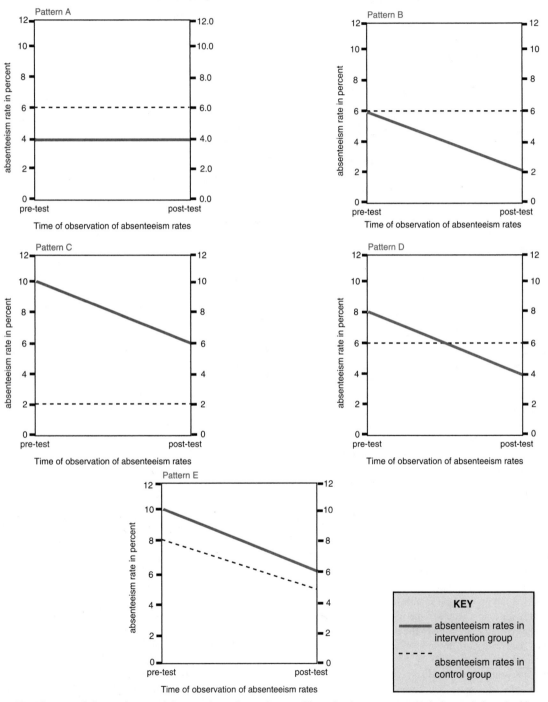

FIGURE 6.2 Patterns of absenteeism rates in intervention and control group offices of an insurance company before and after a health promotion intervention; Patterns A–E.

two branches of the same company. However, an important caveat is in order. When the study groups compared are close to each other, whether geographically or even electronically, the researcher must pay attention to possible diffusion-of-treatment problems, i.e., cross-group interactions. In an increasingly connected world, intact-group designs are becoming more challenging to implement for certain types of research questions. In a health promotion intervention that targets exercise and diet behaviors, sharing of information about an intervention can be expected to mitigate observable posttest differences. Consequently, the researcher might have to make a tradeoff between having very similar comparison groups or being unable to avoid treatment diffusion.

Potential diffusion/cross-group communication problems arise in study designs comparing departmental/ward units in hospitals, clinics, classes in schools, or offices in the same community agency, to name a few.

The only remaining strategy for dealing with non-equivalency of the comparison groups is to *control statistically* for several variables on which the comparison groups differ. How one controls for confounding variables after the data are collected will be discussed in Chapter 7.

COUNTERBALANCED DESIGNS

The third type of quasi-experimental design that is sometimes encountered in nursing and health-related research is called a **counterbalanced research design** (Campbell & Stanley, 1966). This design shares most of the features of a crossover design (see Chapter 5), a fact that sometimes leads to confusion about its name. The essential difference is that in a counterbalanced design, treatment sequences are not randomly assigned, as in a crossover design. As in the latter, study participants in a counterbalanced design are exposed to all levels of treatment and serve as their own control subjects. Again, the feasibility of such a study design depends critically on the ability to expose individual study participants to *both* intervention and control conditions at different times. That means we must be sure that there are no carryover effects from one treatment level to the next. Different from a crossover experiment, "mere" counterbalanced designs may be applied to preexisting intact groups, which marks them as subspecies of quasi-experimental designs. In a way, a counterbalanced design can be considered a cross between an interrupted time-series design and a nonequivalent control-group design, because it involves switching (interrupting) treatments among nonequivalent groups.

Table 6-2 shows an example of a counterbalanced design in Latin-square arrangement (Campbell & Stanley, 1966) for another health promotion program. Assume that the purpose of this study is to test the relative effectiveness of three different physical exercise programs in improving cardiovascular functioning among elderly residents of assisted-living facilities. The choices of month-long exercise programs performed for 30 minutes every weekday include (1) swimming, (2) brisk walking, and (3) low-impact aerobics. The program is offered in different sequences in the three facilities, as indicated in Table 6-2. At the end of each month, participants in the programs are examined with respect to their blood pressure, pulse rates before and after a 30-minute exercise, and other pertinent physiologic measures.

This particular **Latin-square design** produces nine separate outcome occasions for each measure. In each of the three comparison groups, outcomes are measured after each of three types of exercises. The sequence arrangement is also counterbalanced with respect to time, so that at each month all three types of exercises are conducted. As a result, comparisons of outcomes after swimming, walking, or aerobic dance exercises involve the same subjects, all tested at three times.

Because counterbalancing allows the participants to serve as their own control subjects, it removes the problem of accounting for preexisting differences among the nonequivalent groups, when evaluating overall differences caused by types of exercise. It also removes from the exercise comparisons the problem of cumulative improvement

TABLE 6.2	Diagrammatic Representation of a Counterbalanced Design in Latin-Square Arrangement		
	1st Month	2nd Month	3rd Month
Group A	Swimming	Brisk walking	Low-impact aerobics
Group B	Brisk walking	Low-impact aerobics	Swimming
Group C	Low-impact aerobics	Swimming	Brisk walking

in cardiovascular functioning, which is likely to result from continuous exercise of any kind. A more detailed assessment of how to analyze outcome data from a counterbalanced design will be presented in Chapter 7.

As with the other types of quasi-experimental design, there is theoretically no limit to the number of interventions or observations that can be made. The number and timing of observations depend on the purpose of the research as well as on feasibility because of the available resources and time. Although counterbalanced designs can provide strong evidence based on data from intact groups, feasibility considerations often limit the scope of this design to just a few sites or groups and intervention modes.

CLINICAL NURSING RESEARCH IN ACTION: EXAMPLES OF QUASI-EXPERIMENTAL DESIGNS

The nursing and health-related literature contains many examples of quasi-experimental research designs, although there is frequent variation in how study design terms are used in the literature. Here we present two examples from recently published research reports to illustrate the key features of the designs used, and to provide further discussion of the strengths and limitations of quasi-experimental research. In Chapter 7, both of these articles will be revisited to discuss the data analysis strategies that were used to examine the research questions and hypotheses.

Example of an Interrupted Time-Series Design

Research Scenario 6-4 discusses the management of premenstrual syndrome. Two hypotheses were examined in the Taylor (1999) study. The primary hypothesis stated that women who completed the intervention would demonstrate improvement on a variety of outcomes, including severity of premenstrual symptoms; psychologic coping measures, including personal demands and resources; and health behaviors. A secondary hypothesis stipulated that women in the waiting-for-treatment group would not show improvement on these measures during the 6-month baseline period before exposure to the intervention. It can be seen from these hypotheses that timing (of measurement) was an important part of this research, necessitating the use of repeated observations in both the preintervention and the postintervention phases.

In particular, the use of two preintervention observations, respectively spaced 1 month apart (in the early treatment group) and 6 months apart (in waiting treatment

RESEARCH SCENARIO 6.4

Management of Premenstrual Syndrome

Taylor (1999) studied the effectiveness of professional guidance and peer group support for the management of premenstrual syndrome (PMS) symptoms among women who were experiencing severe levels of such symptoms. The overall goal of the research was to examine both short- and longer-term effects of the intervention. Because long-term success in PMS symptom management was an important aspect of the research aim, a complex variation of an interrupted time series design was used. The study starts with baseline PMS symptom monitoring on two occasions prior to the intervention, followed by post-intervention monitoring of symptoms for up to 18 months on four occasions. A subsidiary feature of this study is the inclusion of two comparison groups: (1) an early treatment group (n=40), which received the intervention following a baseline of symptom monitoring during two successive menstrual cycles; and, (2) a waiting-treatment group (n=51), which received the intervention 6 months later. Study participants were randomly assigned to these two groups, but the comparison of the two groups is not the main focus of this study. Both groups were tracked at 3, 6, 12, and 18 months after their respective intervention. As far as the main comparison of the pre- and post-intervention phases is concerned, this study is a quasi-experiment, more specifically, an interrupted time series study. Table 6-3 depicts the study design.

group), allowed for a solid evaluation of outcome trends before the intervention was implemented. At the same time, for the estimation of the longer-term postintervention effects, the two groups were combined for analysis. This aspect of the study design fit most closely with an interrupted time-series design format. In Chapter 7, we shall revisit this article in greater depth, with respect to the data analyses performed to address the study hypotheses.

Example of a Nonequivalent Control-Group or Intact-Groups Design

It has already been mentioned that intact-groups study designs are among the most commonly used quasi-experimental

TABLE 6.3	Simplified Diagram of Taylor (1999) Research Design

Early Treatment Group

Preintervention Observations			Postintervention Observations			
Baseline (Menstrual Cycle 1)	Baseline (Menstrual Cycle 2)	Intervention (2 Months after Study Entry)	3 Months	6 Months	12 Months	18 Months
O_1	O_2	X	O_3	O_4	O_5	O_6

Waiting-Treatment Group

Preintervention Observations			Postintervention Observations			
Baseline (Menstrual Cycle 1)	Baseline (Menstrual Cycle 6)	Intervention (6 months after Study Entry)	3 Months	6 Months	12 Months	18 Months
O_1	O_2	X	O_3	O_4	O_5	O_6

research designs in nursing and health-related research. This is because so many questions of concern to nursing and health involve the use of preexisting groups of study participants, for which random assignment to study conditions/groups is either not possible or feasible.

KNOWLEDGE AND BELIEFS ABOUT HIV/AIDS

Carney, Werth, and Martin (1999) employed an intact groups design to study the effects of a course among nursing students of various ages. Participants in the intervention condition were students (n=29) who were enrolled in a specialized training course for increasing knowledge and improving beliefs related to the care of individuals with HIV/AIDS. The comparison group consisted of students (n=31) who were enrolled in another nursing course that did not include content related to HIV/AIDS.

Because the students were enrolled in courses to meet academic requirements, random assignment of the students to courses would not have been feasible or ethical. A pretest posttest study design was used, in which the study participants completed the pretest on the first day of course enrollment and completed the posttest one week after the end of the HIV/AIDS course. The inclusion of a pretest observation was a strength of this study, because it permitted an analysis of preexisting differences for the groups regarding the effects (on posttest outcomes) of prior knowledge and beliefs regarding HIV/AIDS. This article will be revisited

in Chapter 7, regarding data analyses that were done to assess the effect of the specialized course on HIV/AIDS knowledge and beliefs.

CONCLUSION

In this chapter, three key types of quasi-experimental designs have been presented: (1) interrupted time-series, (2) nonequivalent control-group or intact-groups, and (3) counterbalanced designs. There are many variations on these basic types of designs. In reading the literature, we suggest the following strategy for determining a specific study design used in intervention research:

1. Determine whether or not the design meets all four key criteria of a true experimental design. If so, the study should be classified as experimental.
2. If an intervention deliberately introduced and manipulated by the researcher was tested, but study participants were not randomized to intervention or control groups (or occasions), then the design is quasi-experimental. Note that study designs without manipulated interventions tested are "observational," and observational study designs will be discussed in Part IV of this book.
3. To determine what type of quasi-experimental design is used, consider carefully the following features:
   a. If only one study group is used with repeated observations both before and after the intervention, then the design is an interrupted time-series design.

b. If the design involves the comparison of two or more separate groups, whose composition is a "given," i.e., cannot be changed by the researcher, then the design belongs into the category of nonequivalent control-group or intact-groups designs.

c. If each intact group is exposed to all levels of the intervention at some point, then the study design is a counterbalanced design.

Causal interpretations of intervention effects based on quasi-experimental study designs are usually open to more challenges than causal interpretations based on true experiments. This is so because the lack of individual randomization tends to allow for more plausible alternative explanations, because it becomes more difficult to rule out that the observed effect might be due to some confounding variable(s). However, quasi-experiments often deliver solid evidence, in particular when they are combined with analysis strategies that control for some salient confounding variables. The principles underlying such statistical controls will be taken up in the next chapter.

Suggested Activities

1. After reading the Taylor (1999) and Carney, Werth, and Martin (1999) articles, try to match the features of the study design to the research questions and hypotheses that are listed by the authors. To what extent do the research designs allow the researchers to answer the questions/hypotheses posed? Be specific, and include a critique of limitations of the study designs for addressing the research questions/hypotheses.

2. Select another one or two articles from the literature that either you or the authors of the articles identify as using a quasi-experimental design. See whether you can match the features of the designs to one of the three key types of quasi-experimental design discussed in this chapter.

3. Read the following article: Foster-Fitzpatrick, L., Ortiz, A., Sibilano, H., Marcantonio, R., & Braun, L.T. (1999). The effects of crossed leg on blood pressure measurement. *Nursing Research, 48,* 105–108.

   a. Identify all the specific strategies—as described by the author—that were used in this study to control for confounding variables.

   b. On the basis of your list, to what extent are you convinced that the key finding (increased blood pressure with crossed leg position) is due to leg crossing rather than to another possible explanation for the study result?

   c. Discuss specific reasons why random assignment to study conditions would not have been feasible for this study.

Suggested Readings

Foster-Fitzpatrick, L., Ortiz, A., Sibilano, H., Marcantonio, R., & Braun, L. T. (1999). The effects of crossed leg on blood pressure measurement. *Nursing Research, 48,* 105–108.

References

Campbell, T. D., & Stanley, J. C. (1966). *Experimental and quasi-experimental designs for research.* Chicago: Rand McNally.

Carney, J. S., Werth, J. L., & Martin, J. S. (1999). The impact of an HIV/AIDS training course for baccalaureate nursing students. *Journal of Nursing Education, 38,* 39–41.

Cook, T. D., & Campbell, D. T. (1979). *Quasi-experimentation: Design and analysis issues for field settings.* Boston: Houghton Mifflin.

Eisen, M., Keyser-Smith, J., Dampeer, J., & Sambrano, S. (2000). Evaluation of substance use outcomes in demonstration projects for pregnant and postpartum women and their infants. Findings from a quasi-experiment. *Addictive Behavior, 25,* 123–129.

Freeman, V. S., & Tijerna, S. (2000). Delivery methods, learning styles, and outcomes of physician assistant students. *Physician Assistant, 24, 7,* 43–50.

Greenfield, T. K., Graves, K. L., & Kaskutas, L. A. (1999). Long-term effects of alcoholic warning labels: Findings from a comparison of the United States and Ontario, Canada. *Psychology and Marketing, 16,* 261–282.

Hendy, H. M, & Raudenbush, B. (2000). Effectiveness of teacher modeling to encourage food acceptance in preschool children. *Appetite, 34,* 61–76.

Seibert, S. (1999). The effectiveness of facilitated mentoring: A longitudinal quasi-experiment. *Journal of Vocational Behavior, 54,* 483–502.

Sheikh, J. I., & Yesavage, J. A. (1986). Geriatric depression scale (GDS): Recent findings and development of a shorter version. *Clinical Gerontologist, 5,* 165–173.

Taylor, D. (1999). Effectiveness of professional-peer group treatment: Symptom management for women with PMS. *Research in Nursing & Health, 22,* 496–511.

CHAPTER 7   The Analysis of Quasi-Experiments

STATISTICAL INFERENCE WITHOUT RANDOM ASSIGNMENT

In this chapter, we focus on several approaches commonly used to analyze data from quasi-experimental designs. In the previous chapter, quasi-experimental designs were introduced as an alternative to true experimental designs, for research situations in which the goal is to evaluate a causal question of some sort, for which a true experiment would not be ethical or feasible. One of the most common reasons for using a quasi-experimental design in place of a true experimental design is the impossibility or nonfeasibility of random assignment to study groups or conditions. For example, in Chapter 6, an example of a companion animal intervention was discussed, in which it would not be feasible to randomly assign animals to individuals because of individuals' preferences concerning personal companion animals. Similarly, ethical considerations often restrict treatment manipulations and the use of random assignment to various treatment alternatives. For example, it is not considered ethical in today's society to deliberately expose people to disease-causing agents or to withhold treatments with documented effectiveness from people with illnesses for which the treatment would be effective.

Causal Inference in the Absence of Random Assignment

The inability to use random assignment has important consequences for the analysis and interpretation of study data. Let's discuss specifically why this is so, using some key statistical concepts. The validity of causal conclusions based on data is rooted in the validity of the available statistical evidence, which in turn rests on the validity of the statistical inferences made. In any study involving a test of a causal hypothesis, statistical inference involves comparing the observed sample outcomes after an intervention with the hypothetical (hypothesized) outcomes; i.e., the actually obtained outcomes are compared with the null hypothesis. For example, a nurse researcher may posit a null hypothesis such as this: "There will be no mean level differences between the control and experimental groups in satisfaction with health care services," and then proceed to collect data on satisfaction from the control and experimental groups (after the implementation of an intervention designed to increase satisfaction with health care services) to see whether or not the null hypothesis can be rejected with a reasonable level of statistical confidence. These kinds of **expected outcomes** (or hypothesized outcomes) are derived from the **sampling distribution** of a given **test statistic,** which is constructed on the basis of the explicit assumption that the subjects were randomly assigned to the various treatment or control conditions. In the example just given, the nurse researcher might use an independent samples *t* test (see Chapter 3) to assess whether or not there are mean level differences between the control and experimental groups, and the expected outcomes would be derived from the sampling distribution of the *t* statistic.

Under the null hypothesis, it is assumed that the only source of observed differences between treatment and control groups is the random process of assigning subjects to the comparison groups.[1]

Without random assignment, the basis for causal inference is greatly diminished because any number of differences between "nonequivalent" comparison groups, other than the effects of an intervention, could have caused the observed difference in outcome. The use of research designs without random assignments of subjects to study groups/conditions poses a problem for accurate causal inferences. Thus, the key issue to be grappled with in the analysis of data from quasi-experimental designs is this: *How can we effectively control or account for differences in extraneous (confounding) variables when we compare groups that were formed on the basis of a nonrandom assignment process?*

Overview: Control of Extraneous Variables

There are several ways to control for extraneous variables in studies involving group comparisons. In Chapter 6, for example, we briefly described design strategies, such as **matching** on a few important control variables. In this chapter, we shall describe some data analysis strategies for controlling confounding variables, referred to as **statistical controls.** These strategies are used *after* the data have been collected. These techniques include a large variety of **multivariate statistical** techniques. Multivariate analysis involves the simultaneous consideration of at least three (and sometimes many more) variables and their relations to one another. Although the statistical models themselves usually do not make distinctions between independent variables that represent variation in treatment/intervention levels (as opposed to variation in confounding attributes), they can be used to separate the effects of the main treatment/intervention variable from the impact of other variables under study. The ability to separate or disentangle the effects

---

[1]To review from previous chapters, random assignment is an all-purpose form of experimental control that helps ensure that comparison groups are equivalent on variables that could affect the outcome of interest, either in place of or in addition to the intervention.

of variables from one another is exactly the main concern in the analysis of data from an intervention study. Treatment/intervention effects sometimes vary under different conditions (this is called an interaction effect; see Chapter 5), and sometimes they are completely independent of the conditions represented by the various combinations of the extraneous or confounding variables.

In this section, we review the general principles of statistical controlling for third variables that underpin the particular statistical techniques used by researchers. We then turn to a discussion of one frequently encountered specific statistical model for implementing statistical controls: the **analysis of covariance (ANCOVA).** Because statistical control via multivariate analysis occupies a central role in modern data analysis in health research, we shall demonstrate the key principles with different statistical models. Discussions in later chapters on observational studies will, for example, introduce contingency-table analysis to broaden the view of what statistical controls can and cannot accomplish.

CONTROLLING FOR CONFOUNDING VARIABLES IN THE ANALYSIS OF DATA FROM QUASI-EXPERIMENTS

Conceptualizing How Statistical Controls Work

So far, we have emphasized the idea that causal analysis requires *exclusion of plausible rival hypotheses*. This means that a researcher must be reasonably sure that variables other than the intervention (confounding variables) cannot explain the observed outcome. The most effective way to ensure this is through the features of the research design guiding the study. In particular, the ability to manipulate or fully control the interventions/treatments, coupled with random assignment of the study subjects to comparison groups (groups getting different levels of the intervention/treatment), provides the best guarantee of controlling for the influence of confounding variables. However, in quasi-experiments with at least two comparison groups, random assignment is not implemented. As a result, the comparison groups are not likely to be equivalent before the intervention, and group comparisons on outcomes after the intervention are likely to have the following problem or bias: *In addition to the differences in exposure to mutually exclusive treatment levels, comparison groups may also differ systematically with respect to a host of third variables.*

Statistical controls are aimed at either removing or adjusting for such biases. Although these aims are the same as those of achieving control through design, it is important to emphasize that the statistical controls are implemented after the data are already collected; i.e., any remaining differences or imbalances between the comparison groups can no longer be corrected, at that point, by altering the study design. As a consequence, statistical controls have some important limitations. In an ideal situation, if measures of all possible confounding variables were available, it could be possible in principle to implement a series of statistical controls to get estimates of the intervention/treatment effect(s) that are independent of the effects of all the confounding variables. The causal status of any treatment effects that could not be explained away as being the result of confounding variables would provide more credible evidence of the impact of the intervention. However, as just mentioned, statistical controls can be implemented only if information on the relevant variables is available; i.e., unmeasured variables cannot be controlled for in the data analysis stage of the study. In addition, statistical controls have other technical limitations. For instance, the more confounding variables that a researcher wishes to control for, the larger the sample size that is needed. Also, in some situations, a researcher might have to deal with the problem of **complete confounding** of the intervention effect.

For example, suppose that a study was done in which all of the study participants in the intervention groups were female, and all participants in the control group were male. In such a situation, it would be impossible to determine whether observed group differences were attributable to the effect of the intervention, to the gender difference, or to the effects of both variables. With no analytic fix available to disentangle the effects of gender from the intervention, the researchers would have to design a new study in which intervention and gender were varied independently.

In summary, when compared with the all-purpose control of random assignment in the research design stage, statistical control after the fact (in the data analysis phase) is, even in the best of circumstances, a more limited way to control for the effects of confounding variables. *There is no guarantee in this approach that all the potential confounders have been addressed and measured in the study. Thus, whatever statistical controls are implemented, there always remains the possibility that a crucial "third variable" has been left out.*

Understanding the impact of variables other than the intended intervention on outcomes is actually quite important for the development of research knowledge. For example, in many instances the results of a study do not demonstrate that an intervention is effective. Without a careful analysis of why and under what circumstances the intervention did not appear to work, the researcher will fail to develop new knowledge for clinical practice. The constellations of confounding variables at work in a study can be analyzed further to understand the specific conditions under which interventions are or are not effective.

Because the use of statistical controls relies on the researcher having obtained measures of the key confounding variables, the question arises: how can researchers anticipate which specific variables to measure in the first place? Additional data collection usually entails greater respondent burden and more resources in terms of time, money, and effort. To determine what data to collect, a researcher must consult relevant published research to shed light on possible confounders. For questions about which only limited research or no previous research has been done, it is often essential to begin with descriptive studies to obtain preliminary information about confounding variables that could affect the results of an intervention study.

Statistical Control Through Analysis of Covariance

In this section, we briefly discuss the principles of ANCOVA to show a practical example of how statistical control or statistical adjustment is implemented. For a more detailed discussion of these techniques, the reader may consult some of the already cited sources, e.g., Munro (2001), Snedecor and Cochran (1989), and Winer, Brown, & Michels (1991). ANCOVA is one of many **multivariate statistical techniques** routinely used in health research reports.

In Research Scenario 7-1, we demonstrate the multivariate approach using an ANCOVA analysis of variables that have been altered from the actual data set used in a published paper (Wills & Stommel, 2002). The numbers were modified to simplify the data presentation and to illustrate more clearly the basic principles involved in the ANCOVA approach.

For illustrative purposes, we focus on the students' responses to a question about how much they expected to enjoy, and did enjoy, the course. Response categories varied from 1 = not at all enjoyable to 5 = very enjoyable. Here, we treat these ordinal responses as interval level variables on a scale of 1 to 5.[2] Table 7-1 offers some results from the analysis of the fictitious data. Both classes are assumed to have exactly 20 students. According to the postcourse results, the students of the aging class find that class much more enjoyable than the students of the research methods

RESEARCH SCENARIO 7.1

Evaluation of Web-Based Nursing Courses

The study involved an evaluation of two web-based nursing courses comparing student perceptions about course content of a required nursing research course, versus an elective course on aging issues. While the researchers/faculty had control over the content of these courses, they did not control which students would sign up for either course; i.e., random assignment of students to courses was not possible. Different students took the (elective) aging course and the research methods course, resulting in nonequivalent comparison groups. A pretest/posttest design with intact groups (classes of students enrolled in different courses) was used to examine the effects of exposure to the content of the courses (the intervention) on students' perceptions by the end of the course (the outcome). Students in each of the courses completed surveys of their perceptions before and after taking the courses.

class. As the t test results in Table 7-1 A show, the mean class enjoyment scale score is 1.1 points higher in the aging class, a difference that is statistically significant ($P <$ .006). However, although we may consider the class contents (research versus aging issues) as alternative interventions or treatments, we should not, on the basis of the postcourse evidence alone, conclude that the different average levels of course enjoyment between the two classes of students reflect the content of these particular classes. The results in Table 7-1 B provide a hint about why such a conclusion may be premature: the t test results comparing the precourse scores on expected enjoyment for the two classes clearly indicate that these two student groups entered the classes with different sets of expectations (the mean scores differ by 1.0; $P <$ .025). Thus, a comparison of postcourse scores that speaks to the specific experience of students in these classes must somehow adjust for the differences in prior expectations.

Analysis of Covariance: Key Concepts and Example

One popular statistical model to perform such adjustments is ANCOVA, which represents a straightforward extension of the analysis of variance (ANOVA) discussed in

---

[2]The extent to which it is permissible to use statistical models appropriate for interval-level variables on ordinal-level variables will be discussed in more detail in the chapters on measurement (Chapters 13–15).

| TABLE 7.1 | Comparison of Course Enjoyment Scores from Research Methods and Aging Courses | | | | | |

Comparison Groups	Observed Enjoyment Score	Observed Mean Difference	Standard Error of Mean Difference	95% CI for Mean Difference	t Value	Significance Level (P value)
A. Comparison of Postcourse Scores						
Research methods course (n = 20)	2.45	−1.10	.377	−.34–1.86	2.921	.006
Aging course (n = 20)	3.55					
B. Comparison of Precourse Scores						
Research methods course (n = 20)	2.50	−1.00	.429	−.13–1.87	2.330	.025
Aging course (n = 20)	3.50					

CI, confidence interval.

Chapter 4. The only difference is that among the independent or explanatory variables in the model, there are not only

1. Factors that define the intervention or control groups, i.e., nominal categories like the two courses in our example, but also
2. Continuous variables like the precourse scores on the enjoyment scale.

Continuous predictor (independent) variables in the ANCOVA model are called **covariates,** hence the name "analysis of covariance." Again, from a statistical point of view, a covariate in the ANCOVA is simply another independent variable whose effect on the outcome variable is examined. Usually, the covariate(s) represent(s) confounding or nuisance variable(s) for which the researcher would like to make adjustments.

Returning to our example, we have already mentioned that it is important to adjust for the differences in expected enjoyment scores (at precourse) with respect to the influence of this variable on the outcome (postcourse scores of enjoyment). The ANCOVA accomplishes this goal by first regressing the postcourse scores on the precourse scores, thereby establishing to what degree these two sets of scores vary in common, and then by performing an ANOVA to establish whether there are systematic (mean-level) group differences in the postcourse scores *after the effects of the precourse scores have been subtracted from the postcourse scores.* The analysis is accomplished by the same method

of decomposition of variance we already encountered in the discussion of the ANOVA in Chapter 4.

Table 7-2 shows the decomposition of the sums-of-squared deviations for the ANCOVA. The results in this table indicate that a large proportion of the model sum-of-squares (i.e., the explained or between-group sum-of-squares) in the dependent (postcourse) scores is accounted for by the precourse scores. About 23.6% of the score variation (15.557/66.000) in the postcourse enjoyment scores is accounted for by the precourse expectation scores, an effect that is statistically significant (F statistic: 15.012; $P <$ .001). At the same time, the experience of having gone through one or the other course no longer has a statistically significant effect on the postcourse enjoyment scores, as indicated by the P value of .076 associated with the F statistic of 3.336. In other words, there is a 7.6% chance that the remaining score difference between the two groups (research and aging issues classes) could represent measurement error or some other random difference. The ANCOVA also allows calculation of adjusted group mean scores, taking into account the differences in precourse scores. These adjusted scores, shown at the bottom of Table 7-2, confirm the pattern: the difference between the postcourse scale scores in the two classes has now narrowed to 0.628 (3.314–2.686) from the previous unadjusted difference of 1.1 (3.55–3.45) observed in the t test. This analysis shows that the expectations that students bring to their course experiences before being exposed to the course content (the intervention) need to be taken into

TABLE 7.2.	ANOVA Table for ANCOVA with One Between-Group Factor (Two Different Courses) and One Covariate (Precourse Expectation of Enjoyment Scores)

Sum of Squares		Degrees of Freedom	F statistic	P value
Model sum-of-squares (=BGSS)	27.657	2	13.344	<.001
Pre-course score Covariate	24.300	1	23.456	<.001
Course factor	3.357	1	3.336	>.076
Error Sum-of-Squares (=WGSS)	38.373	37		
Total Sum-of-Squares (=TSS)	66.000	39		
Model F-Ratio = (BGSS/df.)/(WGSS/df.) = (27.657/2)/(38.373/37) = 3.336				

Adjusted Group Means (Postcourse Enjoyment Scores after Adjustment for Covariate (= Precourse Expected Enjoyment Scores)

	Observed Enjoyment Score	Observed Mean Difference	Standard Error of Mean Difference	95% CI for Mean Difference	F value	Significance Level (P value)
Comparison groups: research methods course (n = 20); aging course (n = 20)	2.686 3.314	.628	.436	−.25–1.51	3.336	0.76

ANOVA, analysis of variance; ANCOVA, analysis of covariance; CI, confidence interval; BGSS, between groups sum of squares; WGSS, within groups sum of squares.

account in drawing conclusions about the impact of the course content of the courses. Without the use of an analysis in which the precourse expectations scores are controlled for, it would be possible to conclude (in error) that there was an effect of exposure to specific course content on the enjoyment of the course. The data in Table 7-2 show that there is no longer a significant effect of the specific class content after controlling for precourse expectations of enjoyment.

Example of Covariate Adjustment

Figure 7-1 provides a visual illustration of how covariate adjustment works. The graph shows the simultaneous distribution of pretest and posttest scores for 100 subjects. The 100 subjects are divided into two groups; the 50 subjects in the intervention group are denoted by small circles, and the 50 subjects in the control group by larger squares. For example, the square symbol in the lower left-hand corner denotes a control group subject with a score of 1 on both the pretest and the posttest, whereas the circle in the upper right-hand corner shows a subject in the intervention group who scores 5 on both tests. The almost diagonal straight line is an example of a **regression** line. It represents the scores of the outcome/posttest variable predicted from the

covariate or pretest scores. This regression line represents the best-fitting straight line that can be drawn through the scatter of points, using the least-squares criterion. That is, if we measure the vertical distance of each point in the graph from this regression line and square it, we'll find that the regression line is drawn in such a way that the sum of these squared distances is minimized, i.e., no other straight line could be found with a smaller sum of the squared differences. For our purposes, all we want to establish is that this regression line shows quite nicely how posttest scores vary, on average, with pretest scores. It can easily be seen that subjects with higher pretest scores also tend to have higher posttest scores. In fact, this relationship is quite strong in this case, with Pearson's correlation coefficient (r) showing a value of 0.88.

The symbols in the graph convey another important piece of information. Most of the scores for subjects in the intervention group (circles) are concentrated on the upper right-hand side of the graph, and most of the control group subject scores (squares) are bunched up in the lower left side. In fact, the mean pretest score for the intervention group is 3.87, and for the control group it is 2.17. The mean posttest or outcome scores for these two groups are 3.75 and 2.18, respectively. Now it is possible to see the key point: If we simply compare the posttest or outcome

Example of Covariate Adjustment

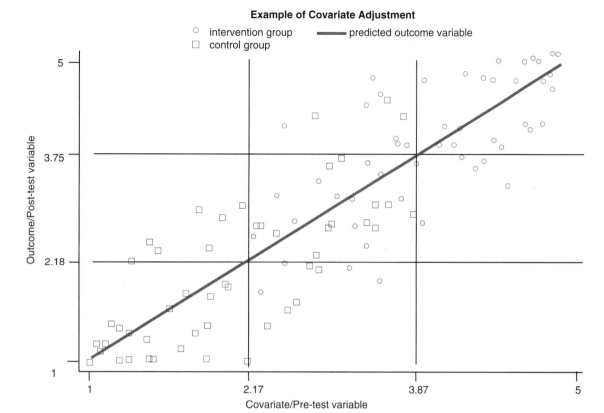

FIGURE 7.1 Example of covariate adjustment

scores in the two groups after the intervention, the independent sample *t* test indicates that the mean difference of 1.57 (3.75–2.18) between the two groups is statistically significant ($P < .001$). However, these being nonequivalent control groups, *the difference already existed at the time of the pretest*. Thus, if we subtract out or remove the impact of the pretest scores from the posttest scores, we would get a more accurate account of the effect of the intervention itself.

That is precisely what the ANCOVA accomplishes. The regression line represents the systematic covariation of posttest scores with pretest scores, but vertical variation of posttest scores *around* the regression line, also known as **deviation scores,** is variation independent of the pretest scores. The vertical variation of posttest scores occurs for given levels of the pretest scores. Thus, after we subtract out the regression line, we are left with the deviation scores that give a more accurate indication of the effect of the intervention on the posttest scores after the effect of the pretest scores has been taken into account.

Could we not have accomplished the same control effect if we had simply subtracted the pretest scores from the posttest scores, and then compared the mean change scores for intervention and control group? This is an intuitively feasible analysis strategy, but it turns out to have an important limitation. **Change score analysis** is meaningful only if the pretest and posttest are measured in the same metric. But often we want to control for other kinds of confounding variables. For example, suppose that the covariate in Figure 7-1 represents the ages of the subjects. In that case, we could not simply subtract the subjects' ages (measured in years) from the posttest/outcome scores (measured in terms of the test metric, say varying from 1 to 5). Yet, it would still be possible to estimate a regression line that shows the average change in the posttest scores with change in age. That is, ANCOVA would still accomplish the desired adjustment in the outcome scores. The other advantage of ANCOVA over a change score analysis is that we can simultaneously adjust for several covariates, or continuous confounding variables.

The purpose of this brief description of ANCOVA is to provide the reader with an understanding of the logic of statistical adjustment when the groups that are compared are "nonequivalent" with respect to their background characteristics, or their scores on a preintervention pretest. As with all statistical models, the correct application of ANCOVA also requires that the data meet several additional assumptions, among them being normally distributed error terms and a linear relationship between the covariate and the dependent variable.[3] Finally, it is worth repeating that any effort to statistically adjust for confounding variables requires the researcher to have anticipated in advance what the confounding variables are, and to have obtained measures of these variables in the data collection process. It follows that ANCOVA and similar multivariate adjustments for differences between nonequivalent control groups still do not eliminate the possibility that some other uncontrolled-for variable could have influenced the study findings. To the extent that such unrecognized confounding variables remain uncontrolled, it is still possible that the comparisons of mean outcome differences between intervention and control group(s) are biased in a systematic, if unknown fashion.

Take the example of a researcher who is trying to show the effects of a breathing intervention on reducing the pain of labor and delivery. This researcher would probably need to account for at least several potentially confounding variables in testing the effects of the intervention, such as the skill level for the intervention of the mother and labor coach, and the mother's prior experience with childbirth. The relevance of this accounting for other influences becomes heightened for quasi-experimental designs because of the inherent design limitations of quasi-experimental studies in controlling for the effects of confounding variables. Very few research studies involving the use of an intervention have effects that could not be plausibly attributed, partially or even totally, to the effects of some other confounding variable(s).

CAUSAL INFERENCES FROM REPEATED-MEASURES QUASI-EXPERIMENTS: REPEATED-MEASURES ANALYSIS OF VARIANCE

We turn now to the analysis of quasi-experimental studies with multiple consecutive observations and one or more interventions. Such studies may have no separate compari-

son group (as when a single institutional population is monitored over a long time), or, if they do, the comparison involves repeated measures in intact groups without random assignment. Such designs are often referred to as *mixed-methods designs*. As was emphasized in Chapter 6, the key to causal interpretations of data from such interrupted time-series designs is that collecting multiple observations before the intervention allows us to establish a *trend line* (pattern). The trend line need not be linear, but we can hope that it is orderly and recognizable enough to be extrapolated into the future after the intervention(s) have taken place. Inferences about the effectiveness of the intervention(s) then emerge from comparisons of predicted observations that are generated on the basis of extrapolations of the preintervention pattern, and actually observed trend lines after the intervention. Thus, if the intervention displays any causal effectiveness, we should be able to observe **discontinuities** in the pattern of means or the slopes of the trend lines before and after the intervention(s).[4]

Overview of Statistical Models and Intervention Analysis

In recent years, many new statistical models have been developed to analyze time-series/repeated-measures data (Diggle et al., 1994). Most repeated-measures studies in nursing and medicine involve relatively few repeated measurement occasions, say, between 3 and 10. Ideally, the analysis of repeated-measures designs should be able to handle missing data (a frequent occurrence in repeated-measures studies) and to model the correlations among the multiple measures of the same subjects (the within-subjects variation). More recent statistical models such as **pooled time-series** and **random-effects models** offer this flexibility, but these newer models have not yet diffused fully into nursing and other health-related research journals. Instead, **repeated-measures ANOVA,** with its more restrictive assumptions about within-subjects correlations, also known as the **compound symmetry assumption,**[5] is still the main tool for the analysis of data from repeated-measures studies in applied clinical and health-related research.

Just as one-way and factorial ANOVA are extensions of the independent-sample *t* test (ANOVAs compare mean scores for several groups; *t* tests are used for two-group

---

[3] A detailed discussion of the technical aspects of ANCOVA is beyond the scope of this book. Interested readers are referred to Munro (2001) for an introductory discussion. Comprehensive discussions can be found in Cohen and Cohen (1983) and Winer et al. (1991).

[4] However, recall also that the main rival hypothesis for an observed discontinuity of mean levels in an interrupted time-series design is **history,** i.e., the claim that some other important event occurred at the same time as the start of the intervention. In any case, how does one establish discontinuities in means over time?

[5] See Munro (2001). An extended discussion of these technical issues can be found in Winer et al. (1991).

mean comparisons), so is repeated-measures ANOVA an extension of the paired *t* test (involving more than two observations over time). In addition, repeated-measures ANOVA can also incorporate between-subjects factors, as frequently used in mixed-methods models (see Chapter 6).

For an interrupted time-series design in which the trend line is analyzed for only one group, the principal question is whether there are statistically significant differences between the group means (or between the trend lines in the group means) before and after the intervention(s). In the simplest case, a null hypothesis is posited that there are no systematic changes in the repeated measures of the outcome scores; i.e., that all the mean scores of the outcome measures do not change over time. If that is the case, individual subjects may still show some changes in their scores over time, but, on average, *no systematic group mean changes are discernible*. Thus, we get the familiar juxtaposition of systematic ("explained") mean changes in scores versus individual ("unexplained") variation in scores, and we can construct an *F* test (see discussion of ANOVA in Chapter 4). This time, however, the *F* test is calculated for the within-subjects effects. If the study uses a mixed-method design (i.e., the design involves two or more separate comparison groups), in addition to the repeated measures within each group, we can also ask additional questions about the intervention effects:

* Are the over-time trends of means identical in the comparison groups,
* Are they parallel (but different in level), or
* Do they show different trends?

The latter situation is also known as a *group-by-time interaction*.

▶ CLINICAL RESEARCH IN ACTION
Statistical Analysis of a Repeated-Measures Study

For an example of an analysis of data from a repeated-measures study, we turn back to the study of a peer group treatment of symptom management for women with premenstrual syndrome (Taylor, 1999). Recall from Chapter 6 that Taylor (1999) studied the effectiveness of professional guidance and peer group support for the management of premenstrual syndrome symptoms among women with severe levels of such symptoms. We had classified the design of this study as an example of an interrupted time-series design, because the primary hypothesis stated that women who completed the intervention would demonstrate improvement on a variety of outcomes. Because all study participants were exposed to the intervention and were observed twice before the intervention and up to four times

afterward (see Figure 6-4, Chapter 6), a test of the effectiveness of the intervention involved, in all cases, a comparison of outcome measures before and after the interventions. Taylor (1999) examined changes in eight outcome variables, including premenstrual and postmenstrual measures of premenstrual syndrome negative affect symptoms, premenstrual and postmenstrual self-esteem, depression, and total symptom severity. For our purposes, we shall concentrate on only two measures: premenstrual depression and premenstrual negative affect symptom severity. The author chose the General Contentment Scale as a measure of well-being (low scores) or depression (high scores), with possible scale scores ranging from 0 to 75.

The negative affect symptom severity measure is a subscale of the Premenstrual Assessment Form summing the scores on 11 symptom ratings (for the procedures of constructing summated rating scales, see Chapter 18). Scores can range from 0 (no symptoms reported) to 44 (extreme symptom severity for all 11 symptoms). Taylor (1999) did not report the mean scale scores for all six observations in a single table. The information for the baseline scores presented in Table 7-3 was constructed by combining (and weighting) the means for the early and waiting treatment groups (see Taylor's Table 3) because we are interested only in over-time changes in the study groups as a whole. The postintervention means are based on information provided in Taylor's Tables 4 and 5. There are some discrepancies among these tables. For instance, in Taylor's Table 4, only a single baseline mean is reported for the negative affect symptom scale with a value of 44, whereas in Taylor's Table 3, two baseline means are reported separately for both the early and the waiting treatment groups. However, all of these four means are lower than 44, so that no weighted combination could yield a value of 44. Furthermore, the reader is told that the negative affect symptom subscale has scores ranging from 0 to 44, which implies extreme baseline scores. Whatever the source of these inconsistencies, we are here interested in the use of repeated-measures ANOVA to understand the patterns of mean values in this interrupted time-series design.

In this article, some additional information is needed for a full interpretation of the mean values patterns. At first blush, the over-time pattern of means for the premenstrual negative affect symptom scale is clearly consistent with the hypothesis that the intervention (the premenstrual symptom management program) was effective. Not only is there a substantial discontinuity in the means between the last preintervention and the first postintervention scores, also there is no indication that these subjects were already on a declining trajectory during the preintervention phase. A key concern in interpreting the comparisons, however, is the amount of attrition by study participants over the course of the study. The study presents an excellent illustration of a common issue in research with people who are

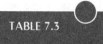

TABLE 7.3	Depression and Symptom Severity Scores for Six Observations in Taylor's (1999) PMS Intervention Study: Combined Early and Waiting Treatment Groups

Preintervention Observations			Postintervention Observations			
Baseline 1 (Menstrual Cycle 1)	Baseline 2 (Menstrual Cycle 2[a] or 6[b])	Intervention (2[a] or 6[b] Months After Study Entry)	3 Months	6 Months	12 Months	18 Months
(Premenstrual) Negative Affect Symptom Scale						
42.7 (n = 91)	43.4 (n = 79)	X	11.2 (n = 78)	10.8 (n = 70)	10.2 (n = 58)	8.6 (n = 51)
(Premenstrual) Well-Being Depression Scale						
51.6 (n = 91)	46.6 (n = 79)	X	41.7 (n = 88)	39.9 (n = 78)	36.3 (n = 65)	34.7 (n = 61)

[a]Early treatment group.
[b]Waiting treatment group.
PMS, premenstrual syndrome.

experiencing health alterations and who are monitored over time during a research study. As often occurs in repeated-measures studies like this one, researchers lose at least some study participants during the follow-up phase after the intervention. In this study, more than 40% of the participants were lost between the first preintervention measure and the last postintervention measure.

From a statistical standpoint, there is unfortunately no fully sufficient way to take account of this attrition in an ANOVA model. The within-subjects F tests reported by the author tested whether or not there were any systematic differences in the group means over time among the study participants who had complete sets of measures. Under these circumstances, it might have been better to report the scale means only for the participants with all over-time measures, on which the repeated-measures ANOVA was run, so that the inspection of the means would not confound changes in individuals (possibly because of the intervention) with attrition effects. For instance, Taylor did report that women who withdrew at various time points differed from other women on premenstrual negative affect symptom severity and depression, in such a manner that the more depressed and symptomatic women appeared more likely to drop out of the study. In an extreme case (although this was not so for this study), a pattern of declining depression and symptom scores may simply indicate greater study retention rates among the healthier subjects. To put it another way, it is possible that the systematic pattern of

study attrition (the more depressed, symptomatic women were more likely to drop out of the study) accounts better for the study findings (improved depression and symptoms) than does the intervention itself.

There is another issue to consider. The F test for the repeated measures is based on the null hypothesis that the group means do not change over time, i.e., $O_1 = O_2 = O_3 = O_4 = O_5 = O_6$. The alternative hypothesis is that at least some means are different from one another. Thus, whereas both the F test (for the premenstrual symptom and the depression scales) are statistically significant at $P < .01$, this indicates only that at least one mean scale score at one time differs from at least one mean scale score at another time. But there is no guarantee that the difference occurred between the preintervention and postintervention scores. Taylor did compare a single preintervention (baseline 1) score with each of the postintervention means separately, and found the differences statistically significant (these tests are equivalent to the paired t test). However, a better way to test the research hypothesis of the causal effectivenss of the intervention is to construct a **contrast** of preintervention and postintervention scores. This contrast compares the combined preintervention scores with the combined postintervention scores or the trend line (slope) of the preintervention means with the trend line of the postintervention means. Although visual inspection of mean scores aids in the interpretation, it is not a substitute for formal statistical tests. Only formal testing can determine whether the observed pattern in the sample data is likely to be the result of chance variation alone, or signifies a systematic pattern.

Another look at our representation of Taylor's data reveals an interesting difference in the patterns of mean scale scores for the two scales. Assuming that the reported means represent actual changes in subjects' depression and symptom scores over time (instead of being an artifact resulting from attrition), the pattern for the negative symptom scale provides stronger evidence for the causal effectiveness of the intervention than does the pattern for the depression scale. This is so even though both contrasts are statistically significant.

Recall, though, that in intervention studies without random assignments of subjects to comparison groups or measurement occasions, a finding of statistically significant differences does not in itself establish the causal effectivenss of the intervention. For instance, the two baseline measures for the depression scale indicate already a declining trend *before* the intervention. Actually, the data in the article show that this declining trend occurred only among the early treatment group but was stronger there than the subsequent intervention effect. This raises a question about whether or not it was this intervention that effected the declining depression scores, because a process of decline was already in place before the intervention began. Incidentally, this is another demonstration of the strength of interrupted time-series designs. Only from the repeated measures before and after the intervention are we able to establish a trend line, if any, to evaluate the observed changes.

CONCLUSION

In this chapter, we introduced two analysis techniques that are frequently used in the nursing and health care literature:

1. The ANCOVA
2. The repeated-measures ANOVA

Both of these statistical models can be used to analyze data from quasi-experimental designs, to adjust either for preexisting differences in nonequivalent control group designs or for the comparisons of trend lines before and after interventions in interrupted time-series designs. Both models can be used with study designs of considerable complexity, but we refer readers to other sources for more detail about these techniques.[6] It should also be kept in mind

that ANOVA (and linear regression) models are generally restricted to situations in which the outcomes are measured as continuous variables with at least interval level measurements. For dichotomous or ordered-outcome measures, there are other kinds of statistical models, some of which will be briefly introduced in later chapters. However, in this chapter we have been more concerned with the meaning and interpretation of study results that have been adjusted for preexisting differences between comparison groups. This concept of statistical control is really one of the fundamental concepts in quantitative research and is implicit in all multivariate analysis, regardless of which specific statistical model is used. Because the vast majority of published quantitative research reports make use of multivariate analysis, we shall provide additional examples of third variable controls in the next chapter, when we begin to discuss observational studies.

As a general rule, less rigorous research designs require more complicated analysis strategies if one wants to tease out causal connections among variables. Although the general reader of nursing and medical research does not need to develop a full understanding of the variety and multiplicity of multivariate analysis strategies now in use (even the "experts" can no longer master all the specific techniques and models available), a reading of the research literature is greatly facilitated if the reader is familiar with the logic of statistical significance testing and the logic of statistical controls.

Suggested Activities

1. Suppose you designed a telephone coaching intervention for the management of adult patients with moderate to severe asthma who have had at least one emergency room visit in the past year related to treatment of an acute asthma attack. A quasi-experimental study is implemented, comparing medication adherence and rates of emergency room use among convenience samples drawn from the health systems that serve two geographically separated communities. Community A is designated as the "intervention" community (study participants receive the telephone coaching intervention), and Community B is designated as the "usual care" community.
   a. Make a list of all the possible "third" or "confounding" variables that are likely to affect a comparison of participation rates between the two community populations.
   b. How would you control or account for the effects of the confounding variable(s) you identify? Be specific, with reference to the types of controls you would use, from research question to analysis phase of the proposed research.

---

[6] One of the best and most comprehensive discussions still remains that in Winer et al. (1991). A nontechnical introduction can be found in Munro (2001).

2. Suggest one or two specific and feasible ways in which the research design of the Taylor (1999) study could be improved on for future studies.
3. Select another article from the literature that either you or the authors of the articles identify as using a quasi-experimental design.
   a. List the criteria for identifying the design as quasi-experimental. Does the design in fact meet the criteria to be classified as "quasi-experimental?" Why or why not?
   b. Examine all statistical analyses reported in the article and state how, and to what extent, they served the purpose of statistically controlling for known or potential confounding variables.

Suggested Readings

Munro, B.H. (2001). *Statistical methods for health care research* (4th ed.; Chapter 8, pp. 187-200), Analysis of covariance. Philadelphia, PA: Lippincott.

Snedecor, G.W., & Cochran, W.G. (1989). Statistical Methods (8th ed.), Ames, IA: Iowa State University Press.

Taylor, D. (1999). Effectiveness of professional-peer group treatment: Symptom management for women with PMS. *Research in Nursing & Health, 22,* 496-511.

Wills, C.E., & Stommel, M. (2002). Graduate nursing students' pre- and post course perceptions and preferences concerning fully web-based courses. *Journal of Nursing Education, 40,* 193-201.

References

Cohen, J., & Cohen, P. (1983). *Applied multiple regression/correlation analysis for the behavioral sciences* (2nd ed.). Hillsdale, NJ: Lawrence Erlbaum Associates.

Diggle, P.J., Liang, K.Y., & Zeger, S.L. (1994). Analysis of longitudinal data. NY: Oxford University Press.

Hair, J. F., Anderson, R. E., Tatham, R. L., & Black, W. C. (1998). *Multivariate data analysis* (5th ed.). Upper Saddle River, NJ: Prentice-Hall.

Hendy, H. M, & Raudenbush, B. (2000). Effectiveness of teacher modeling to encourage food acceptance in preschool children. *Appetite, 34,* 61–76.

Munro, B. H. (2001). Analysis of covariance. In *Statistical methods for health care research* (4th ed., pp. 187–200). Philadelphia: Lippincott Williams & Wilkins.

Taylor, D. (1999). Effectiveness of professional–peer group treatment: Symptom management for women with PMS. *Research in Nursing & Health, 22,* 496–511.

Wills, C. E., & Stommel, M. (2002). Graduate nursing students' pre- and post course perceptions and preferences concerning fully web-based courses. *Journal of Nursing Education, 40,* 193–201.

Winer, B. J., Brown, D. R., and Michels, K. M. (1991). *Statistical principles in experimental design.* (3rd ed.). New York: McGraw-Hill.

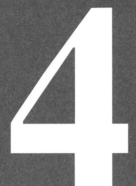

PART

The Design and
Analysis of
Observational Studies

CHAPTER 8   Introduction to Observational
Studies

THE ROLE OF OBSERVATIONAL STUDIES IN NURSING AND HEALTH CARE RESEARCH

In Part IV of this book, we turn to the design and analysis of **observational** studies. Observational studies go by many different names in the literature, including **descriptive, correlational, ex post facto,** and, most generally, **nonexperimental** studies. The defining characteristic of an observational study is that an investigator observes, records, measures, counts, or classifies events but *does nothing to actively change the course of events via a researcher-manipulated intervention or treatment.* In other words, the researcher gathers data in relation to a phenomenon of interest but does nothing to alter the phenomenon itself.[1]

Examples of Issues Addressed in Observational Studies

What exactly does it mean to observe a phenomenon for a clinically relevant study? There are many different kinds of observational methods. They include biophysiologic tests (e.g., blood pressure, blood glucose) as well as videotaped recordings of patient behavior (e.g., maternal interaction with infants during infant feeding) (Stephenson, Pridham, & Meynarczyk, 1996). They may entail highly structured interview instruments that are designed to elicit only specific, predetermined information, e.g., the Structured Clinical Interview for Diagnosis for psychiatric diagnosis (Spitzer, Williams, Gibbon, & First, 1992) or more loosely structured qualitative studies, wherein the observer, to some extent, follows events as they unfold. The latter include studies of the "lived experience" of chronic illnesses such as cancer, problematic alcohol use, or organ transplants (Karian, Jankowski, & Beal,, 1998; Thomas, 1995; Smith, 1998). Thus, **observation,** for the purposes of this chapter, refers to a broad range of methods for information gathering or data collection.

REVIEW NOTES In Chapter 2 we emphasized that health care researchers pursue many goals, not just the testing of the effectiveness of interventions and treatments or the establishment of the causes of various diseases.

In this broader context, observational studies provide vital contributions in research, especially when accurate descriptive information is a major goal. For example, many health services research and epidemiology studies focus on health and illness in populations. This type of study requires either large study samples that are representative of their target population, or the use of **population registries.** For instance, using records from managed care organizations in Tennessee, Bailey, Van Brunt, Mirvis, McDaniel, Spears, Chang, & Schaberg (1999) showed that academic managed care organizations face, on average, more patients with complicated, chronic, and high-cost conditions compared to nonacademic care organizations—a phenomenon known as *adverse selection* in the insurance literature. Such descriptive studies are often used as a basis for adjusting institutional reimbursement rates or capitation payments. As another example, consider the study conducted by Bach et al (1999). These researchers relied on the records of the Surveillance, Epidemiology, and End Results (SEER) cancer registry, linked it to Medicare inpatient discharge records, and showed that the lower survival rates among African Americans than among European Americans with diagnoses of non–small-cell lung cancer are likely to be tied to rates of surgical treatment. Both examples illustrate the importance of descriptive information and its relevance to implications for health policy decisions. However, the second study also demonstrated that questions of cause and effect (why is the survival rate and rate of surgical treatment among African Americans diagnosed with lung cancer lower than among European Americans?) are often not far behind earlier descriptive ("what is?") types of studies. Problems like these are addressed in **descriptive epidemiology** (Valanis, 1999), which is concerned with the accurate descriptions of the distribution of diseases and treatments in the population, as well as the description of the conditions under which they seem to arise. The existence of population registries like the SEER cancer registry administered by the National Cancer Institute (*http://seer.cancer.gov*) and the state registries for sexually transmitted diseases are the result of society's need for descriptive information on disease and illness.

But beyond epidemiologic studies, population-based descriptive information is needed at all levels of the health care system. For example, an individual public health nurse needs to have an accurate picture of the incidence, prevalence, and distribution of various diseases in the county population she or he is serving. Likewise, a school nurse might want to find

---

[1]There is, of course, the philosophic (and also practical) problem that measurement itself sometimes changes the very phenomenon it is intended to measure. This situation is not uncommon in behavioral research, in which subjects react to the measurement. Recall examples in earlier chapters of the "testing effect" in experimental studies and the attempt to neutralize it via study designs that contain control groups. Yet, a difference remains between unavoidable measurement effects (see Chapters 13 and 14 for a more detailed discussion of measurement issues) and the systematic effects of treatments or interventions designed to change outcomes in a predictable direction. This idea that measurement can affect a measured object has found its expression in 20th-century physics as Heisenberg's "uncertainty principle," which posits that the more precisely one tries to measure the position of an electron, the less certain one is about its momentum and vice versa. This is so because the very act of measuring the position of the electron (e.g., radiographically) influences its velocity as a result of photons colliding with the particle (Asimov, 1966).

out about the infection rates for sexually transmitted diseases among teenagers, what particular behaviors seem to increase the likelihood of these infections, and what health education content should be provided for students to reduce the spread of these diseases. A health insurance analyst may calculate average expenditures per enrollee in a certain health plan by age, to see how members of certain age groups use health plan benefits. In clinical practice, description also plays a very important role at the individual level; i.e., assessment data must be gathered before formulation of a diagnosis, planning, and intervention take place. However, population-based descriptive information is of key relevance at these levels, because it is only through aggregation across individual patients that patterns of diseases and responses to treatments become discernible. Description most often serves as the starting point for understanding how to intervene on the basis of causal hypotheses. That is, the clinician takes a patient's chief complaint and the description of his or her symptoms as her most important source of information, but when she formulates hypotheses about the cause of the chief complaint, she compares the descriptive evidence with "known" patterns of disease and illness. It is research that establishes the patterns as well as the effectiveness of the possible interventions that may provide a remedy and produce a desired effect (improvement in the chief complaint).

Classification of Nursing Research Reports in Literature by Study Designs

REVIEW NOTES Observational studies occupy a central place in the nursing and health-related literature. In the introduction to experimental study designs (Chapter 3), it was mentioned that the majority of published articles in nursing, medical, and health services research journals are reports from observational studies, as opposed to experimental or quasi-experimental studies.

To show the extent to which this generalization holds true, we reviewed all articles for the year 2000 in the three major nursing research journals in the United States: *Research in Nursing & Health,* Volume 23, *Nursing Research,* Volume 49, and the *Western Journal of Nursing Research,* Volume 22. Review articles, including reports of **meta-analyses,** and editorials were excluded, but articles containing discussions of methods or statistics were included if they presented original data. Thus, the remaining articles included only **original research** or data-based study reports. These articles or research reports were classified into four broad groups:

1. Reports on instrument development studies
2. Experimental studies

3. Quasi-experimental studies
4. Observational studies, quantitative (**cross-sectional**[2] and **longitudinal**[3]) and qualitative studies

Table 8-1 shows the results of this classification.[4] It is apparent that nonexperimental/observational research is the most common type of research in these journals, accounting for 61% of all data-based study reports. We were surprised, though, that, despite the funding priorities of the National Institutes of Health concerning longitudinal research and the frequent interest of nurse researchers in problems of change and development, only 9% of all study reports dealt with longitudinal research. It is also worth noting that in many research reports from cross-sectional studies,[5] the authors do not confine themselves to descriptive generalizations but use, either implicitly or explicitly, a causal model designed to explain the patterns found in the data. In other words, whether or not the data are experimental, researchers are often interested in using them to test theories that explicate specific causal processes.

REVIEW NOTES Although there is nothing wrong with adopting a causal model to explain patterns of correlations found in observational studies, it is worth repeating a key point from earlier chapters on experimental design: Data from observational studies do *not* provide conclusive evidence on causal relationships, for reasons that will be outlined in the next section.

CAUSAL INFERENCE FROM OBSERVATIONAL STUDIES

In the absence of a study design that is capable of testing causal inferences, it is important to be cautious in discussions of possible causal interpretations if they are based on observational study data.

▶CLINICAL RESEARCH IN ACTION
Pacifier Use and Weaning
Several recent observational (nonexperimental) studies have shown that the use of pacifiers is positively associated with early weaning. That means that mothers who regularly use pacifiers with their babies are also more likely to wean their babies from breastfeeding shortly after birth (Barros,

---

[2]Studies are called "cross-sectional" if all observations on study participants occur simultaneously at a single point in time.

[3]Studies are called "longitudinal" if they contain observations on study participants at a minimum of two different times.

[4]It may be noted in passing that in a few cases, our classifications differed from those of the authors themselves.

[5]For a discussion of qualitative research design, see Chapter 11.

TABLE 8.1	Categories of Data-Based Articles in Three Leading Nursing Research Journals (Year 2000)

	Journal			
Type of Data-Based Article	*Nursing Research,* Vol. 49	*Research in Nursing & Health,* Vol. 23	*Western Journal of Nursing Research,* Vol. 22	Total *n* (%)
Methods discussion	5	6	5	16 (12)
Instrument development/validation	7	7	3	17 (13)
Experimental design	6	4	4	14 (11)
Quasi-experimental design	1		2	3 (2)
Non-experimental/observational design				
Cross-sectional	17	10	11	38 (29)
Longitudinal	6	3	3	12 (9)
Qualitative	1	12	17	30 (23)
	43	42	45	130 (100)

Victoria, Semer, Fillno, Tomasi, & Weiderpass, 1995; Howard, Howard, Lanphear, DeBlieck, Eberly, & Lawrence, 1999). Findings like these have led the World Health Organization and the United Nations Children's Fund to support public health campaigns that discourage the use of pacifiers, based on the premise that it is likely that the use of pacifiers somehow interferes with breastfeeding (WHO/UNICEF, 1989). According to this belief, pacifier use is seen as one cause of the undesirable result of early weaning, for what may seem to be very credible reasons. For example, it may be reasonable to speculate that the underlying causal mechanism of the association between pacifier use and breastfeeding is that the use of pacifiers makes babies less demanding and fussy, which, in turn, reduces the mother's motivation for breastfeeding. This proposed causal mechanism is depicted as Pattern 1 in Table 8-2. However, when Kramer, Barr, Dagenais, Yang, Jones, Ciofani, & Jane (2001) conducted a clinical trial to test an educational intervention that combined a recommendation of avoidance of pacifier use with alternative suggestions for dealing with crying and fussing behavior, they did not find any evidence that the intervention prevented early weaning. The 140 new mothers randomly assigned to the intervention were no more likely to terminate breastfeeding within 3 months of the baby's birth than were the 141 new mothers in the control group.

Why might the above evidence be inconsistent with the findings in the prior observational studies, which documented positive, statistically significant nonzero correla-

tions between pacifier use and time of weaning?[6] The short answer is that even if a correlation/association between two variables has been demonstrated to exist, it is worth remembering the principle that "correlation does not equal causation." As discussed in Chapter 3, evidence for causality also requires one to show that (1) the presumed cause preceded the presumed effect and (2) no other variable could have produced the observed relationship. Thus, even if the finding is empirically well established that women who frequently use pacifiers also tend to wean their babies early (i.e., there are neither measurement nor sampling problems that cast reasonable doubts on the finding), it does not follow that one factor (pacifier use) is the cause of the other factor (early weaning).

To see why, it is worth looking at some of the other possible causal patterns shown in Table 8-2. For instance, Pattern 2 depicts a situation in which both pacifier use and early weaning are induced ("caused") by a *common antecedent.* Examples might include the situation of a particularly demanding baby, leading the mother to both increase her use of the pacifier and introduce the bottle early. Another possibility is that mothers who are employed may be more likely to use pacifiers and to wean the baby early.

[6]When we use the term "correlation," we refer to a statistical index of the association between two variables, the value of which can range from −1 to 1. A value of zero indicates an absence of a relationship *as defined by the correlation coefficient,* and higher numbers in either direction indicate stronger positive or negative associations.

TABLE 8.2	Possible Causal Relationships Between Pacifier Use and Early Weaning

Causal pattern 1   Pacifier use → early weaning; pacifier use → lack of crying → early weaning
Causal pattern 2   Pacifier use ← mother's employment → early weaning
Causal pattern 3   Pacifier use ← early weaning

These examples are illustrations of the classic third-variable problem we have discussed previously: Some other causal agent has an impact on *both* of the observed variables of interest (pacifier use and early weaning), and this results in a correlation. If that is the case, there are ways to demonstrate the effects of such third variables through statistical controls (see next section below).

Another possible interpretation of a correlation/association between two variables is that it indicates reverse causation. **Reverse causation** (see Pattern 3 in Table 8-2) means that instead of the assumed pattern of variable A influencing B (A ⇒ B), it is variable B that influences A (B ⇒ A). For instance, if a researcher finds in a cross-sectional, observational study that women who wean their babies within 3 months after giving birth are more likely to use pacifiers than women who continue to breastfeed their babies, this may mean that the change in breastfeeding behavior among the first group of women induces them to substitute pacifiers. Clearly, the problem of reverse causation is particularly difficult in cross-sectional studies. Recall that one of the criteria for establishing a causal relationship is the establishment of a temporal sequence: causes occur before their effects. This is inherently more difficult in cross-sectional studies. If one compares two groups of women 3 months after they have given birth, having information only on their current use of pacifiers, then one is not be in a position to decide whether pacifier use followed or preceded the decision to wean the baby. Situations in which reverse causation is possible are very common in the health care literature, because many patient groups and their family members can be identified only after a diagnosis has occurred.

For example, Stommel, Given, & Given (1990) argued that the well-established empirical relationship in cross-sectional studies between a caregiver's perceived burdens and the caregiver's depression could mean that rather than depression being the result of high caregiving demands (or burdens), depressed caregivers have a greater tendency to perceive caregiving as burdensome. If this hypothesis is true, it would be helpful to have information on a caregiver's depression before the beginning of the caregiving relationship, but for obvious feasibility reasons, it would be difficult to identify and study future caregivers, or even to measure retrospectively current caregivers' past depression.

The plausibility of reverse causation depends on the nature of the variables involved. For instance, whereas available evidence favors the conclusion that depression is more prevalent among women than among men (Weissman, Bruce, Leaf, Floria, & Holzer, 1991; Kessler, McGonagle, Swartz, Blazer, & Nelson, 1993), nobody would argue that depression determines (is a cause of) a person's gender/sex, except perhaps the tiny number of persons who have had a sex change. Even so, the correlation between gender/sex and depression only means that gender/sex is a possible cause of depression. For example, there may well be hormonal or biologic differences that account for the higher prevalence of depression among women, or there may be differences in the typical life experiences of men and women. If so, the "real" causes of higher depression rates among women may be these latter social causes, which happen to be associated with gender. From this it follows that causal interpretations based on observational data are always tentative, especially when researchers observe correlations in cross-sectional studies between variables that

1. Were measured at the same time and
2. Are subject to change over time.

► CLINICAL RESEARCH IN ACTION
Caution to Causal Interference

For example, Christopher (2000) investigated the determinants of subjective feelings of psychologic well-being among Irish immigrants, using cross-sectional survey data. The researcher used a measure of satisfaction with quality of life, resilience, and several sociodemographic descriptors as predictors of psychologic well-being. It was found that the predictors collectively accounted for 41% of the variation in psychologic well-being scores. In this case, one could also hypothesize that current levels of psychologic well-being affect current perceptions of satisfaction with quality of life. Although there may be a theoretic reason for casting one or the other variable in the role of dependent or independent variable, there is no *empirical* way with cross-sectional data to rule out an interpretation of reverse causation.

Although causal interpretations of observed cross-sectional correlations are particularly vulnerable to criticism, the third-variable problem is more general and applies to all observational studies. Thus, when we compare two groups on some variable of interest, such as mean low-density lipoprotein cholesterol levels, using an observational data set, it is always important to keep in mind the following: *Without random assignment of respondents to the comparison groups, it can never simply be assumed that the groups selected and compared in the analysis (e.g., male or female respondents, lung cancer or breast cancer patients) are truly equivalent or similar to each other in terms of their background characteristics.* Thus, we cannot know for sure which variable or factor accounts for the observed differences. The main reason is that there is no all-purpose mechanism in an observational study (such as random assignment in experimental studies) to minimize the impact of potential confounding or extraneous variables.

This does not imply that it is futile to reason and argue about causal relations among observed variables. In fact, researchers spend considerable time and energy to neutralize the effects of potential confounding variables in the analysis stage. This is particularly the case when the potential cause under investigation is an attribute variable that cannot be manipulated by the researcher, such as race, gender, or disease classifications. *What researchers can do in such situations is control for the effects of other measured variables in the analysis stage.* Whereas the logic underlying statistical controls is straightforward (see the next section), it remains important to be cautious in our causal interpretations of the effects of such attribute variables on outcomes of interest (Williams, 1994; Stommel, Given, & Given, 1998). The fundamental limitation of statistical controls is that only variables for which there are measures can be introduced in the analysis stage. Thus, there is no all-purpose mechanism such as random assignment that helps ensure that the effects of confounding variables have been neutralized.

PRINCIPLES OF STATISTICAL CONTROL

REVIEW NOTES In the previous chapter, we showed how, for data from quasi-experimental designs, the analysis of covariance is used as a means of controlling or adjusting for possible preexisting differences in nonequivalent groups.

The need for such adjustments or statistical controls is even greater in nonexperimental, or observational, studies. In fact, research articles in the nursing and medical literature, which report on observational studies with quantitative variables, routinely present their results in terms of **multivariate analyses.** As mentioned in the previous chapter, such analyses examine the simultaneous distribution of several (at least three) variables. Usually one or more variables are designated as the dependent or outcome variables, while the remaining variables are viewed as independent or predictor variables. Probably the most common form of multivariate analysis encountered in the nursing and health-related literature is multiple regression analysis, which is capable of examining the effects of two or more independent variables on a single dependent variable. In such analyses, the researchers are usually interested in showing the effect of a few focal independent variables on the outcome variable, while other independent variables in the model are considered nuisance, control, or confounding variables whose impact is to be controlled for, or accounted for. In other words, the concern is to show that whatever impact the focal independent variable has on the outcome variable can be demonstrated to be independent of the effects of the other variables. How does such statistical control actually work, and what are its limits? We discuss this by way of an example, which is conceptually similar to the example of a confounding variable impact in the previous chapter, but which expands on the role of a confounding variable. This time we use the vocabulary of observational design.

An Example of Statistical Control

To answer this question, we continue with the example of the potential impact of pacifier use on early weaning. In this example, the researcher has clearly identified pacifier use as the independent or predictor variable and weaning behavior as the dependent or outcome variable. That is, per assumption, we exclude the possibility of reverse causation, a problem that cannot be addressed with cross-sectional data. But suppose the researcher suspects that the mother's employment status is a potential confounding variable. If so, the rival hypothesis to the one that posits pacifier use as an inducement to early weaning would be depicted in Pattern 2 of Table 8-2. It only appears that pacifier use causes early weaning; the true reason for the correlation between the latter two variables is that both are influenced by the mother's employment status: Employed mothers are more likely both to use pacifiers *and* to wean their babies early. If that is the alternative rival hypothesis, and if the researcher has data on the employment status of

RESEARCH SCENARIO 8.1

Examples of Statistical Control

For illustrative purposes, we provide an example in Tables 8-3 and 8-4, which contain fictitious numbers that demonstrate the meaning of "statistical control." Suppose these numbers come from a cross-sectional study of 400 mothers who gave birth to their first child. All mothers are interviewed once, exactly 3 months after the birth of their baby. Among other information, the researchers ascertain that at the time of the interview, 230 (67.5%) of these mothers are still breastfeeding and 170 mothers (42.5%) are not breastfeeding (= early weaners). The researchers also find that at the time of the interview, 200 (50%) of the mothers use pacifiers and 200 (50%) do not. Finally, 160 (40%) mothers are again working/employed and 240 (60%) are still at home. Going back to the hypothesis mentioned earlier, namely, that pacifier use is a possible cause of early weaning, the information in Table 8-3A addresses only a preliminary, yet relevant, first question: are use of pacifiers and early weaning behavior correlated/associated with each other? As the data demonstrate, the answer is clearly yes! Over 60% of the mothers who use pacifiers have given up breastfeeding (or never started it) at the time of the interview, whereas less than 25% of the mothers who do not use pacifiers are early weaners. For 2 × 2 frequency tables like Table 8-3A, we can compute a special correlation coefficient, called phi (Φ). Its magnitude in this case equals 0.3641, and the associated significance level of $P < .001$ makes it highly unlikely that the observed sample result is due to a sampling fluke or random measurement error.[7] At first blush, this evidence seems to support the notion that pacifier use increases the likelihood that a mother becomes an early weaner. However, recall that our researcher suspects it is really the employment situation of the mother that governs both behaviors. Indeed, the data in Table 8-3B and C give a hint that this is so. Both the use of pacifiers and the practice of early weaning are correlated with the employment status of the mother. Employed mothers are far more likely to use pacifiers than are mothers staying home (80% versus 16%; $\Phi = 0.4899$, $P < .001$), and they are also much more likely to have stopped breastfeeding (87.5% versus 8.7%; $\Phi = 0.7433$, $P < .001$). Knowing that the mother's employment status is associated with both the dependent variable (early weaning or not) and the independent variable (use or no-use of pacifier) being tested, we are now in the position to test whether employment status "accounts for" the observed relationship between pacifier use and early weaning. The logic of this statistical control is straightforward: If the observed relationship between pacifier use and early weaning is an artifact of these variables being associated with employment status, then this relationship should disappear when we examine it *within* each level of employment. The data in table 8.4 tell the story. Among the group of 160 employed mothers, the percentage of early weaners is the same (87.5%), whether or not they use pacifiers. Likewise, among the 240 mothers who stayed at home, the percentage of early weaners does not change, regardless of their use of pacifiers, even though the overall level of pacifier usage is much lower (12.5%) in this group. Thus, *within each employment level,* the correlation between pacifier use and early weaning status is exactly zero.[8] In this example we were able to show that the observed correlation between pacifier use and early weaning practices in the sample as a whole can be entirely attributed to the fact that employed mothers are both more prone to use pacifiers and to discontinue breastfeeding early. In fact, the multiplicative pattern of the correlations among the variables tells the same story. Employment status of the mother correlates with pacifier use at .4899 and with early weaning practices at .7433. Multiplying the two correlations yields the originally observed correlation among pacifier use and early weaning practices (.4899 × .7433 = .3641). *Thus this observed correlation is entirely accounted for in terms of a third variable.* As introduced in the previous chapter, this is the meaning of "statistical control."

the mother, he or she can statistically control for the employment effect. Should the results show that after the statistical control, pacifier use is no longer related to early weaning behavior, then the rival hypothesis is the likely explanation for the observed correlation between pacifier use and early weaning behavior. When we statistically control for a third variable, we hold that third variable constant while examining the effect of interest. If the effect persists,

[7]Phi is computed in the following way. From the cross-product of the first and fourth cells, subtract the cross-product of the second and third cells, and divide this difference by the square root of the product of all marginal cells. For example, the following result obtains from Table 8-3, Part A: Phi (Φ) $= \frac{(121 \times 151 - 49 \times 79)}{\sqrt{170 \times 230 \times 200 \times 200}} = 0.3641$. See Munro (2001) and Snedecor & Cochran (1987).

[8]For the data on employed mothers, Phi (ϕ) $= \frac{(112 \times 4 - 28 \times 16)}{\sqrt{140 \times 20 \times 128 \times 32}} = 0.0000$; for mothers staying at home, Phi (ϕ) $= \frac{(9 \times 147 - 21 \times 63)}{\sqrt{30 \times 210 \times 72 \times 168}} = 0.0000$.

TABLE 8.3   Examples of Statistical Control

A. Relationship Between Pacifier Use and Early Weaning/Breastfeeding Patterns in a Sample of 400 Mothers 3 Months After Birth

	Early Weaning/Breastfeeding Pattern		
Phi = 0.3641; *P* < .001	Baby Weaned	Baby Breastfed	Total
Pacifier use:			
Yes	121 (60.5%)	79 (39.5%)	200 (100.0%)
No	49 (24.5%)	151 (75.5%)	200 (100.0%)
	170	230	400

B. Relationship Between Mother's Employment Status and Pacifier Use in a Sample of 400 Mothers 3 Months After Birth

	Pacifier Use		
Phi = 0.4899; *P* < .001	Yes	No	Total
Employment status of mother			
Employed	128 (80.0%)	32 (20.0%)	160 (100.0%)
Stayed at home	72 (30.0%)	168 (70.0%)	240 (100.0%)
	200	200	400

C. Relationship Between Mother's Employment Status and Early Weaning/Breastfeeding Patterns in a Sample of 400 Mothers 3 Months After Birth

	Early Weaning/Breastfeeding Pattern		
Phi = 0.7433; *P* < 0.001	Baby Weaned	Baby Breastfed	Total
Employment status of mother			
Employed	140 (87.5%)	20 (12.5%)	160 (100.0%)
Stayed at home	30 (12.5%)	210 (87.5%)	240 (100.0%)
	170	230	400

it has been shown to be independent of the variable held constant; if it vanishes, it is the third variable that accounts for the originally observed relationship among the focal independent and dependent variables. While this procedure is very useful for testing the effects of potential confounding variables, it also reveals the limits of multivariate statistical analysis when applied to observational data. The only way to test for potential confounders is to actually have data on the confounding variables and enter them into the multivariate analysis. This means the researcher must have

collected this information during the data collection phase of the observational study. Not only is it often impossible to anticipate what all the relevant confounders might be, but there are clear limitations on the amount of information that can reasonably be collected. In addition, the more variables are entered into a multivariate analysis, the larger the sample of study subjects must be to perform this analysis.

In the final analysis, although multivariate analysis of observational data and its associated statistical controls are the bread and butter of analyzing observational data, it is

TABLE 8.4	Examples of Statistical Control: Relationship between Pacifier Use and Early Weaning/Breastfeeding Patterns in a Sample of 400 Mothers 3 Months After Birth Among Employed and Not Employed Mothers

	Employment Status of Mother						
	Employed				**Stayed at Home**		
	Early Weaning/Breastfeeding Pattern				Early Weaning/Breastfeeding Pattern		
$\phi = 0.0$; $P = 1.000$	Baby Weaned	Baby Breastfed	Total	$\phi = 0.0$; $P = 1.000$	Baby Weaned	Baby Breastfed	Total
Pacifier use							
Yes	112 (87.5%)	16 (12.5%)	128 (100.0%)	Yes	9 (12.5%)	63 (87.5%)	72 (100.0%)
No	28 (87.5%)	4 (12.5%)	32 (100.0%)	No	21 (12.5%)	147 (87.5%)	168 (100.0%)
Total	140	20	160	Total	30	210	240

not a substitute for the all-purpose mechanism of controlling for third variables available in experimental studies: random assignment. At best, after multivariate analysis, we can assert that a certain relationship between two variables is independent of a few specific confounding variables, which the researcher had data on and were controlled in the analysis. Again, had we been able to show that the association between pacifier use and early weaning practices persist, even after controlling for mother's employment status, that would not have proved the causal hypothesis ("pacifier use leads to early weaning"), but it would have resulted in the exclusion of one initially plausible hypothesis. Obviously, the more such competing hypotheses can be excluded, the greater is our confidence in the causal hypothesis, but that is all there is to it.

One other form of statistical control, which is conceptually very similar to the one discussed here and has found widespread application in the health care literature, is **statistical adjustment.** In particular, **age-adjusted** or **sex-adjusted** incidence and mortality rates are often used to compare disease rates in different populations. Suppose you wished to compare the incidence rates of colon cancer among African Americans and European Americans. One problem you would encounter in such a comparison is that the age distributions in these two subpopulations differ, and cancer incidence rates are strongly correlated with age. Except for a few specific childhood cancers, cancer incidence rates tend to rise sharply after age 45. Thus, a valid comparison of overall incidence rates in these two

subpopulations would somehow have to take account of the different age distributions. The usual approach is to calculate age-adjusted incidence rates. Assuming that both populations compared had the same age distribution, we would recalculate the incidence rates based on the age-specific rates observed in these populations. A simple example of age-adjusting rates, using hypothetical mortality data, is shown in Table 8-5. This table displays, for an unspecified disease and within four broad age categories, populations at risk, observed deaths, and disease mortality rates of two populations: Population I and Population II. It also shows the overall (crude) disease mortality rate for each population. Both the age-specific mortality rates and the crude mortality rate are defined as the total number of deaths observed (in a category) divided by total population at risk in that category times 100,000. For Population II in Table 8-5, the age-specific mortality rate for persons 60 to 69 years old amounts to $(108/225,000) \times 100,000 = 48$, or 48 per 100,000. The crude death rate in the same population is computed as follows: $(496/1,000,000) \times 100,000$, or 495 deaths per 100,000. Finally, for each of the two populations, the numbers of "expected deaths" are calculated based on the assumption that the two population groups have the same age distribution as the "standard population" depicted in the right-hand column. This is accomplished by multiplying the standard population with the age-specific mortality rates. For instance, if Population I had 550,000 persons in the age group 50 to 59, we would expect to have observed 165 (= $[30/100,000] \times 550,000$)

TABLE 8.5	Computation of Age-Adjusted Mortality Rates: Example Comparing Two Populations Assumed to Have the Same Age Distribution as the Standard Reference Population

	Population I				Population II				Standard Population
Age Groups	Population At Risk	Observed Deaths Due to Disease	Age Specific Mortality Rates	Expected Deaths	Population At Risk	Observed Deaths Due to Disease	Age-Specific Mortality rates	Expected Deaths	Population At Risk
40–49	400,000	80	20	120	300,000	54	18	90	600,000
50–59	300,000	90	30	165	275,000	77	28	154	550,000
60–69	200,000	100	50	225	225,000	108	48	216	450,000
70–79	100,000	130	130	520	200,000	256	128	512	400,000
	Total population: 1,000,000	Total deaths: 400	Crude rate: 40	Adjusted rate: 51.5	Total population: 1,000,000	Total deaths: 495	Crude rate: 49.5	Adjusted rate: 48.6	Total population: 2,000,000

deaths resulting from the disease in this age group. Finally, we sum the expected deaths (for the two populations compared) by the total standard population. This yields an age-adjusted mortality rate for each of the populations. Thus, the age-adjusted incidence rates answer the question: what would be the overall population mortality rates if both subpopulations had the same age distribution as the standard population? Note the effect of the age adjustment in Table 8-5. The crude or unadjusted mortality rate for Population I equals 40 per 100,000; for Population II, it is 49.5 per 100,000. However, the age-adjusted mortality rate in Population I is higher than that in Population II: the rates are 51.5 and 48.6, respectively. How can that be? If we take a look at the age-specific mortality rates in Table 8-5, we actually see that these rates are consistently lower in Population II for each age group; for instance, 28 versus 30 per 100,000 among 50- to 59-year-old persons. However, there are relatively more older people in Population II than in Population I. For instance, 20% of Population II, but only 10% of Population I, is 70 years old or older. As a result, the crude mortality rate is higher in Population II, but once we adjust for the different age distributions, we find that mortality rates are actually higher in Population I.

Such adjustments are not without their own problems. In particular, it matters which age distribution is assumed in the reference population, but the main point is clear. Their purpose is to control for a third variable (here the age distribution) that confounds the comparison between two or more groups. For a more thoroughgoing discus-sion of the problems of age-adjusted incidence and preva-lence rates, see MacMahon and Trichopoulos (1996) and Selvin (1996).

TIMING OF OBSERVATIONS AND TYPES OF OBSERVATIONAL STUDIES

In the discussion of the experimental and quasi-experimental research designs (Parts II and III), two main distinctions were made with respect to the timing of observations. One involves the frequency of observations: outcome variables in experimental studies may be measured only once or re-peatedly. The other distinction refers to the timing of ob-servations in relation to the intervention/treatment itself. Observations may occur after intervention only, or they may be done both before and after intervention. Because there are no interventions or treatments in observational studies, the second distinction does not apply. However, the first distinction—between studies that involve only a single observation time and those that have multiple observa-tions—obviously is relevant to observational studies.

Experimental studies relying on a single observation of study participants always involve observations after the in-tervention and thus are posttest-only designs (see Chapter 4). Because observational studies confined to a single observa-tion do not entail prior interventions, they are often referred to as **cross-sectional** studies. A cross-sectional study design is most useful if the purpose of the study is to provide a snap-shot of a current situation or if the phenomenon under investigation is not expected to change very fast. Many of the large-scale sample surveys conducted by the National Center of Health Statistics (*http://www.nchs.gov*), in collaboration with the Bureau of Census (*http://www.census.gov*), provide excellent examples of such cross-sectional studies. Together with disease registries, they are the basis for estimates of disease **prevalence** in various population subgroups.[9] Cross-sectional study designs also make sense in the assessment of variations in clinical presentations of patients. For example, there is an extensive literature on the different manifestations of heart disease in men and women when they come to the emergency room (Coronado, Griffith, Geshansky, & Selker, 1997). Women's "atypical" symptoms (compared with those of men) have been held responsible for the more frequent misdiagnosis of the onset of acute myocardial infarction among women (Milner, Funk, Richards, Wilmes, Vaccarino, & Krumholz, 1999). For this type of research question, cross-sectional study designs are appropriate, because there is a central interest in the concurrent (real-time) symptom manifestations in patients, in order to obtain information about possible differences in typical symptom presentations of women and men.

Whereas cross-sectional studies involve the observation of study participants at a single point in time, **longitudinal** studies encompass multiple observations over time. A longitudinal study design is most appropriate if the phenomenon studied is either known or hypothesized to change over time. Many, if not most, health-related phenomena vary or evolve over time. For example, Knauth (2000) studied the transition to parenthood in young couples and showed how these couples adjust to their changed circumstances in terms of their family functioning, the importance they attribute to the family relationships, and their perceived parental competence. Horsburgh et al. (2000) examined the relationships between personality traits and self-care abilities of adults before and after a renal transplant. In both of these studies, a major impetus was the focus on possible changes precipitated by a signal event.

Longitudinal observational research also provides important information in the study of disease progression. For instance, much recent research has focused on changes in quality of life, physical functioning, and mental health of patients with particular chronic diseases (Given et al., 2001; Kurtz et al., 2001). Because most of these studies rely on **longitudinal surveys** of a given sample of subjects, which are also called **panel studies,** a more detailed discussion of them will be provided in the chapter on survey designs (Chapter 11).

RESEARCH SCENARIO 8.2

Example of Prospective and Retrospective Studies

Example of a prospective study: A nurse midwife is interested in studying risk factors (i.e., predictors and potential causes) of postpartum depression. From a sample of pregnant women, she obtains information on physiologic (e.g., estrogen levels), social (e.g., marital status) and behavioral (e.g., alcohol use) variables. Six weeks after birth, the women are recontacted, and depression is measured by use of a standardized inventory for postpartum depression.

Example of a retrospective study: Suppose that you are working in a primary care clinic and have become interested in the reasons why patients miss scheduled appointments for health care. Using office records about missed and kept appointments during the past year, you try to determine which patient characteristics (e.g., insurance status, sex, age, diagnosis) or which provider tend to be associated with higher rates of missed appointments.

In addition to the choice of frequency of observation, another design distinction with respect to the timing of observations is unique to observational studies. Recall that both experimental and quasi-experimental research share the characteristic that researchers must first devise a treatment/intervention and then manipulate it, before its impact on the outcome variable of interest can be measured. In other words, the outcomes from experimental and quasi-experimental studies always unfold in the future. By contrast, nonexperimental observational studies may focus entirely on events that have already occurred. When researchers study events that have already occurred and have been recorded, they use **retrospective** study designs. Because it is not possible to manipulate events that occurred in the past, the experimental requirement that the independent variable(s) must be manipulated means that experimental (and quasi-experimental) studies are always **prospective.**

In the following chapters, we shall have a lot more to say about retrospective and prospective study designs. For now, we offer two short examples of retrospective and prospective observational studies:

Some authors have advocated giving up altogether on the terminology of retrospective versus prospective study designs (MacMahon & Trichopoulos, 1996) because this terminology seems to have generated much confusion about its exact meaning. As we shall discuss in detail in Chapters 9 and 10, these terms should *not* be equated with **cohort study** as a prospective study design and **case–control study** as a retrospective design. Essentially, the terms "retrospective" and "prospective" express the researcher's position in time, relative to the events about which information is sought. If a researcher collects information on outcome variables that have already been determined (e.g., records of past treatments, physical assessments), then the study is retrospective, or looking backward. If the outcomes still lie in the future when the study begins, the study is prospective, or forward looking. Because both terms continue to be used by many authors, it remains important to discuss them, especially in contrast to cohort and case–control designs, which will be discussed in Chapters 9 and 10.

CONCLUSION

In nonexperimental or observational research studies, the role of researcher is confined to the collection and recording of observations/data. No attempt is made to deliberately change events or to intervene so as to produce a desired outcome. Such study designs make sense for several reasons:

- Even though the goal of research might be to obtain causal evidence about the relationship between two (or more) variables, the hypothesized causes (such as age or smoking) cannot be manipulated by the researcher.
- The goal of research is itself descriptive, such as showing the distribution of a phenomenon (disease, mortality, health-related behavior) in a target population of interest.
- The primary purpose of the research is to explore new areas of knowledge or to develop instruments.

If the goal is to obtain causal evidence concerning variables, which cannot be manipulated, it is important to keep in mind that any observed correlation between two variables might be **spurious,** meaning that another variable might account for it. To test this, the researcher would need to measure the third variable in order to statistically control for its effect. Although researchers usually do measure potential confounding variables, guided in their selection by past research and theoretic plausibility, there may always be other variables that could account for the study findings but were not considered and measured. For this reason, nonexperimental study results are always open to the challenge that they did not control for some important, relevant third variable.

Except for this general limitation, the strengths and weaknesses of nonexperimental research with respect to causal inference vary a lot, depending on the specific research designs adopted. In this respect, observational research studies are not different from experimental research studies, and we shall discuss several of the more common observational research designs in the following chapters: cohort studies, case–control studies, and surveys (Chapters 9–11). The strengths and weaknesses of nonexperimental research can also be judged from a different point of view. For example, how bias- and error-free are the observations? How representative are the obtained descriptions of the target populations of interest? How good are the research designs in discovering new, unanticipated information, exploring new relationships, and offering a basis for generating new hypotheses, including new causal hypotheses? These questions will be taken up in the discussion of surveys (Chapter 11) and particularly in the discussion of qualitative research design (Chapter 12).

Suggested Activities

1. Select one or more of the articles from the suggested reading or chapter references lists, in which an observational study design was used to address (a) research question(s). After reading each article, address the following questions:
   a. Was the design used truly observational? Justify your answer by reference to the definition of observational design provided in this chapter.
   b. Was there a good match between the nature of the research question and the research design that was used? Be specific, with reference to how the research design used either did or did not adequately "match up" with the research question(s) posed.
   c. How were potential or known confounding variables controlled in each study?
2. Describe one or more situations from clinical practice in which an observational study design might be used to address a research question. After describing the clinical situation(s), address the following:
   a. Formulate one to three research questions that could be addressed.
   b. Describe the design, with respect to the number and timing of observations.
   c. Describe the measures to be used at each observation point, including your rationale for selection of the measures.
   d. Describe any major confounding variables, and state

how you could control for these variables in the study design you propose.

3. Visit the web sites identified in this chapter to see what types of observational data sets are publicly available concerning national health issues.

Suggested Readings

Barros FC, Victoria CG, Semer TC, Filho ST, Tomasi E, Weiderpass E. (1995). Use of pacifiers is associated with decreased breastfeeding duration. *Pediatrics, 95,* 497-99.

Kramer MS, Barr RG, Dagenais S, Yang H, Jones P, Ciofani L, & Jane F. (2001). Pacifier use, early weaning, and cry/fuss behavior: A randomized controlled trial. *Journal of the American Medical Association, 286, 3,* 322-6.

References

Asimov, I. (1966). *Understanding physics.* London Allen & Unwin.

Bach, P. B., Cramer, L. D., Warren, J. L., & Begg, C. B. (1999). Racial differences in the treatment of early-stage lung cancer. *The New England Journal of Medicine, 342,* 1198–1205.

Bailey, J. E., Van Brunt, D. L., Mirvism D. M., McDaniel, S., Spears, C. R., Chang, C. F., & Schaberg, D. R. (1999). Academic managed care organizations and adverse selection under Medicaid managed care in Tennessee. *Journal of the American Medical Association, 282,* 1067–1072.

Barros F. C., Victoria C. G., Semer, T. C., Filho, S. T., Tomasi, E., Weiderpass, E. (1995). Use of pacifiers is associated with decreased breastfeeding duration. *Pediatrics, 95,* 497–499.

Christopher, K. A. (2000). Determinants of psychological well-being in Irish immigrants. *Western Journal of Nursing Research, 22,* 123–143.

Coronado, B. E., Griffith, J. L., Beshansky, J. R., & Selker, H. P. (1997). Hospital mortality in women and men with acute cardiac ischemia: A prospective multicenter study. *Journal of the American College of Cardiology, 29,* 1490–1496.

Given, C. W., Given, B. A., Azzouz, F., Kozachik, S., & Stommel, M. (2001). Predictors of pain and fatigue in the year following diagnosis among elderly cancer patients. *Journal of Pain and Symptom Management, 21,* 456–466.

Horsburgh, M. E, Beanlands, H., Locking-Cusolito, H., Howe, A., & Watson, D. (2000). Personality traits and self-care in adults awaiting renal transplants. *Western Journal of Nursing Research, 22,* 407–437.

Howard, C. R, Howard, F. M, Lanphear, B, DeBlieck, E. A, Eberly, S, & Lawrence, R. A. (1999). The effects of early pacifier use on breastfeeding duration. *Pediatrics, 103,* E33.

Karian, V. E., Jankowski, S. M., & Beal, J. A. (1998). Exploring the lived-experience of childhood cancer survivors. *Journal of Pediatric Oncology Nursing, 15,* 153–162.

Kendler, K. S., Thornton, L. M., & Prescott, C. A. (2001). Gender differences in the rates of exposure to stressful life events and sensitivity to their depressogenic effects. *The American Journal of Psychiatry, 158,* 587–593.

Kessler, R. C., McGonagle, K. A., Swartz, M., Blazer, D. G., & Nelson, C. B. (1993). Sex and depression in the National Comorbidity Survey I: lifetime prevalence, chronicity and recurrence. *Journal of Affective Disorders, 29,* 85–96.

Knauth, D. (2000). Predictors of parental sense of competence for the couple during the transition to parenthood. *Research in Nursing & Health, 23,* 496–509.

Kramer, M. S., Barr, R. G., Dagenais, S, Yang, H, Jones, P, Ciofani, L, & Jane, F. (2001). Pacifier use, early weaning, and cry/fuss behavior: A randomized controlled trial. *Journal of the American Medical Association, 286,* 322–326.

Kurtz, M. E., Kurtz, J. C., Stommel, M, Given, C. W., & Given, B. A. (2001). Physical functioning and depression among older persons with cancer. *Cancer Practice, 9,* 11–18.

MacMahon, B., & Trichopoulos, D. (1996). *Epidemiology: principles & methods* (2nd ed.). Boston: Little, Brown.

Milner, K. A., Funk, M., Richards, S., Wilmes, R. M., Vaccarino, V., & Krumholz, H. M. (1999). Gender differences in symptom presentation associated with coronary heart disease. *American Journal of Cardiology, 84,* 396–399.

Munro, B. H. (2001). *Statistical methods for health care research* (2nd ed., pp. 123–159). Philadelphia: Lippincott Williams & Wilkins.

Selvin, S. (1996). *Statistical analysis of epidemiologic data* (2nd ed.). New York: Oxford University Press.

Smith, B.A. (1998). The problem drinker's lived experience of suffering: An exploration using hermeneutic phenomenology. *Journal of Advanced Nursing, 27,* 213–222.

Snedecor, G. W., & Cochran, W. G. (1989). *Statistical Methods* (8th ed.). Ames, IA: Iowa State University Press.

Spitzer, R. L., Williams, J. B., Gibbon, M., & First, M. B. (1992). The structured clinical interview for DSM-III-R (SCID). I: History, rationale, and description. *Archives of General Psychiatry, 49,* 624–629.

Stephenson, G. R., Pridham, K. F., & Mlynarczyk, S. (1996). A computerized method of describing phase-related interactive events: Infant feeding as an example. *Computers in Nursing, 14,* 89–100.

Stommel, M., Given, C. W., & Given, B. A. (1990). Depression as an overriding variable explaining caregiver burdens. *Journal of Aging and Health, 2,* 80–103.

Stommel, M., Given, C. W, & Given, B. A. (1998). Racial differences in the division of labor among primary and secondary caregivers. *Research on Aging, 20,* 242–257.

Thomas, D. J. (1995). The lived experience of people with liver transplants. *Journal of Transplant Coordination, 5,* 65–71.

Valanis, B. (1999). *Epidemiology in health care* (3rd ed). Stamford, CT: Appleton & Lange.

Weissman, M. M., Bruce, M. L., Leaf, P. J., Florio, L. P., & Holzer, C. (1991). Affective disorders. In Robins, L. N., & Regier D. A. (Eds.). *Psychiatric disorders in America: The epidemiologic catchment area study* (pp. 53–80). New York: Free Press.

WHO/UNICEF. (1989). *Protecting , promoting and supporting breastfeeding: The special role of maternity services.* Geneva, Switzerland: World Health Organization.

Williams, D. R. (1994). The concept of race in health services research: 1966–1990. *Health Services Research, 29,* 261–274.

CHAPTER 9 Cohort Studies

BASIC CONCEPTS IN ANALYTIC STUDY DESIGNS

In this chapter and the next, we introduce two types of observational study designs that are commonly encountered in the health care literature: the cohort design and the case–control design. These study designs are collectively referred to as **analytic study designs** and were originally developed and refined by epidemiologists. Cohort and case–control designs have seen broad applications in medical and health services research, but until now they have been used only infrequently in nursing research. Cohort studies, in particular, are quite rare in nursing research.

Cohort and case–control studies attempt to shed light on a central problem of interest to the clinician: the causal role of exposure to a risk factor in generating changes in health or causing disease. Both study designs are observational, because researchers play no active role in, or do not determine, which subjects are or are not exposed to the suspected risk factor. This means that in contrast to experimental designs, there is no manipulation of the independent variable(s) by the researcher. Although not experimental, cohort and case–control designs are nonetheless highly structured in how the researchers select study participants to facilitate causal inference. That is why these designs are often referred to as analytic observational studies.

Features of Analytic Study Designs

Cohort Studies
One key feature of these study designs is their built-in emphasis on the time dimension involved. At least conceptually, both cohort and case–control studies are longitudinal, because they involve the comparison of measures of exposure to risk factors with measures of disease occurrence or other adverse outcomes thought to be influenced by the exposure to the risk factor(s). The principle difference between case–control studies and cohort studies lies in the way study subjects are selected. In **cohort studies,** researchers select study participants on the basis of their exposure to a risk factor of interest and then examine what, if any, diseases develop at higher rates in the exposed group than in the group not exposed. For example, a researcher might study the incidence of lung cancer in a group of workers who were exposed to high doses of a chemical suspected to cause lung cancer. .

Case–Control Studies
By contrast, in a **case–control study** (see Chapter 10), researchers select subjects who have already experienced the onset of a particular disease or adverse event of interest (cases) and work backward to find potential causes in their history of exposure to disease-causing agents. For example, a researcher might select subjects who already have diagnoses of lung cancer and compare them with other subjects in the same community without such diagnoses for the purpose of determining whether or not there are any differences between the two groups in terms of their exposure to known carcinogens.

Prospective Versus Retrospective Study Designs
This distinction between moving from exposure information to disease outcome information in the cohort study, versus moving from disease outcome to exposure causes in the case–control study, is not synonymous with the distinction between **prospective** and **retrospective** study designs that we have discussed in earlier chapters. The latter distinction refers only to the timing of observations relative to the researcher(s). Cohort studies are often conducted retrospectively (Capewell et al., 2001; Hillis, Anda, Felitti, & Marchbanks, 2001; Smith & Pell, 2001), relying on existing records to select study subjects according to their exposure status. For instance, Capewell et al. (2001) used the records of the (Scottish) National Health Service to identify all hospital admissions for coronary heart disease between 1986 and 1995; classified the admitted patients on the basis of age, sex, and socioeconomic status; and used this information to predict out-of-hospital death resulting from acute myocardial infarctions after hospital discharge.

Of course, cohort studies are also done prospectively (i.e., researchers enroll study participants with different levels of exposure to a suspected risk factor and then monitor them, often for years, to learn about disease outcomes). For example, Lee, Rexrode, Cook, Manson, & Buring (2001) monitored a cohort of 39,372 healthy professional women (aged 45+), who were divided into four groups depending on their self-rated levels of physical activity, and monitored them for as long as 7 years to ascertain their risk of experiencing coronary heart disease. Different from cohort studies, case–control studies are almost always retrospective for the simple reason that selection of subjects on the basis of information about outcomes requires that the outcomes of interest have already occurred. However, it is quite possible to conduct a case–control study prospectively, in the sense that new cases are accumulated as the subjects experience the disease in question and receive diagnoses of incident disease. Once a case is identified, the researcher would then ascertain information on the subject's history of exposure to the hypothesized/suspected risk factor.

The frequent confusion about the terminology of prospective and retrospective study designs derives from the fact that both terms are used in two different meanings. Case–control studies are backward-looking, or retrospective, in the sense that researchers start with the identification of subjects with a particular disease outcome and try to establish connection to prior exposure to a hypothesized risk factor. By contrast, in cohort studies, researchers first establish the subjects' level of exposure to a risk factor and then proceed to look for outcomes after the exposure; this may be considered a forward-looking or prospective feature of this study design. However, as just mentioned, both kinds of studies can be conducted entirely with past records (retrospective design) or may await the collection of data in the future (prospective design). It is in this latter sense that researchers usually use the terms "retrospective" and "prospective." In discussing cohort and case–control studies, there is no need to use these terms in the former sense, because the terms "cohort study" and "case–control study" already denote the distinction between the two designs. Using this terminology, it makes sense to speak of a retrospective cohort study (Hillis et al., 2001; Smith & Pell, 2001). In such studies, study participants are first selected on the basis of existing records of past exposure status. Then, a search of more recent records provides information on the outcomes of interest. Because both exposure and outcomes occurred before the start of the study, the study is retrospective, even though it retains the essential features of a cohort study.

SELECTING STUDY SUBJECTS BASED ON EXPOSURE STATUS

In cohort studies, researchers monitor individual subjects from the exposure to an illness-causing agent, state, or behavior (risk factor) to a disease outcome thought to be a consequence of the exposure to the risk factor. For example, a researcher might select a sample of smoking (exposed group) and nonsmoking (nonexposed group) men at the age of 40 and monitor them for 20 years to determine whether the incidence of lung cancer (presumed effect or outcome) differs in the two groups. It is important to note that when the subjects are enrolled, they must still be disease free (i.e., free of the adverse outcome that is hypothesized to be a consequence/effect of prolonged exposure to the suspected cause). Of course, there may be a measurement problem. In practice, "disease free" characterizes any person whose disease is in a preclinical stage and cannot (yet) be detected with conventional screening methods. If

information on exposure status and disease is unreliable, it could lead to substantial misclassification of study participants at the outset. This would be an obvious source of bias in the study. Thus, the accuracy of the information used to classify study participants in a cohort study is a major concern to researchers.

Advantages of Cohort Studies

An intuitively appealing aspect of cohort studies is that they fulfill one major criterion for causality: the time sequence of cause and effect. Once exposed and nonexposed subjects (e.g., smokers and nonsmokers) have been selected before receiving diagnoses of the disease of interest, they are monitored for a predetermined time period, not infrequently lasting several years (Kaufman & Widom, 1999; Lee et al., 2001). Given this setup, cohort studies have another advantage: researchers are not bound to the investigation of a single disease outcome but may use the same cohort of subjects to investigate several potential consequences or outcomes of risk factors in question. For instance, in the Nurses' Health Study, an ongoing cohort study of initially more than 120,000 nurses (Nurses' Health Study, 2002), such disease outcomes as coronary heart disease, breast cancer, or Type II diabetes mellitus (among many others) have been investigated (Colditz, Manson, & Hankinson, 1997; Colditz & Rosner, 2000; Fung, Willett, Stampfer, Manson, & Hu, 2001; Liu, Rexrode, Cook, Manson, & Buring, 2000).

Disadvantages of Cohort Studies

Nonetheless, cohort studies are not always the best approach to studying the effects of disease-causing agents on the occurrence of disease. First and foremost are the logistic considerations and the expense of conducting cohort studies. Cohort studies often involve the enrollment and follow-up of tens of thousands (sometimes even hundreds of thousands) of individuals who may be monitored for a long time. This is necessary because most diseases of interest are actually quite rare. For example, take a disease as common as breast cancer in women. In 1998 (National Cancer Institute, 2002), the overall age-adjusted incidence rate for breast cancer among women in the United States was 0.001181, or 118.1 newly diagnosed cases of breast cancer per 100,000 women in the population during that year. Even for women older than 64 years, the annual incidence rate in 1998 was 0.004489, or 448.9 new cases per 100,000 population. From these figures, it can easily be seen that comparing the incidence rates of a particular disease in two groups of subjects (exposed and nonexposed) may indeed require very large samples to discover any difference between the groups. Clearly, when expected disease outcomes are likely to occur in less than 1% of the population, cohort studies can be very costly. Usually, researchers have the option of conducting such studies only when they are funded for a substantial research budget for several years.

Improvement Strategies

To improve the likelihood that cohort studies will yield clinically important results, researchers have pursued several strategies. For instance, extension of the observation period to 5 years (not an uncommon time length for an R01-level research grant awarded from the National Institutes of Health) will increase the expected cumulative incidence (or risk) of disease. However, longer follow-up periods also increase the likelihood of study participants' attrition from various causes. Another strategy is to focus on high-risk subgroups in the population, among which the disease is more likely to occur. In the case of breast cancer, such **special-exposure groups** may include women with a family history of breast cancer. In general, special-exposure groups often involve individuals who are exposed to particular occupational hazards, like asbestos among factory workers or coal dust among coal miners (Finocchiaro, Lark, Keating, Ugoni, & Abramson, 1997; Raffn, Villadsen, Engholm, & Lynge, 1996; Yano, Wang, Wang, Wang, & Lan, 2001). Whereas special-exposure populations help reduce the need for very large study samples, case–control designs are generally more efficient when it comes to the study of rare outcomes (see Chapter 10).

Credibility

For cohort studies to be credible, the researchers must be able to obtain accurate information on both the exposure to the risk factor and the occurrence of the outcome in question, such as disease events or mortality. This has a direct implication on the selection of appropriate outcome variables and study samples. For instance, if the relevant outcome is the subsequent death of study participants, a researcher could use the National Death Index or state bureaus of vital statistics to get fairly complete follow-up information. For some selected diseases with population registries, such as cancer (National Cancer Institute, 2002), it may be possible to get good incidence data, at least within selected demographic areas. However, if the out-

come is not death, and if population registries are not available, follow-up information is often confined to recontacting study participants after long periods of time to obtain the requisite information on the occurrence of new diseases or health conditions. For this reason, researchers often use data from health maintenance organizations and insurance companies to track outcomes of interest. In other words, the selection of appropriate populations for cohort studies is driven just as much by practical considerations as by theoretic considerations.

Open Cohort Studies

Some of the more prominent, classic cohort studies have involved populations from which it is relatively easy to get good follow-up information, such as nurses in the Nurses' Health Study (Belanger, Hennekens, Rosner, & Speizer, 1978; Nurses' Health Study, 2002) or physicians in one of the first studies of the effects of smoking (Doll & Hill, 1964). Using health professionals helps ensure a relatively motivated, knowledgeable, and cooperative group of study participants, who also may be less likely to drop out of the study for motivational reasons. Such studies are **open cohort studies.** In these studies, when study participants are enrolled, they may not (yet) have been exposed to the risk factor in question. For instance, a study participant may not yet smoke at the time of enrollment, but may develop the habit later. Likewise, obesity related in part to dietary and lifestyle habits, as well as many other behaviorally responsive conditions, may develop only after a participant's initial enrollment into the study. That means that the identification of a case as exposed or not exposed to a particular risk factor is a variable itself, which changes over time. This clearly brings home the fact that cohort studies are observational studies. That is, researchers have no control over who is and who is not exposed to a potentially disease-causing agent or behavior. They do not randomly assign people to becoming workers in a nuclear power plant, being smokers or nonsmokers, or being physically active or inactive.

Validity of Cohort Studies

In common with other types of comparative observational study designs, the validity of a cohort comparison of exposed to nonexposed groups of individuals rests on the (relative) absence of confounding factors. Ideally, the comparison groups should be identical in their characteristics except for the defining difference of their exposure status. Practically, this may be very difficult to achieve. For instance, smokers and nonsmokers differ not only with respect to their smoking behavior but also with respect to a host of other sociodemographic and behavioral characteristics.

REVIEW NOTES By now, the reader will recognize this problem as a familiar one: the same issues of comparability or noncomparability were already discussed for the nonequivalent control group designs (see Chapter 6).

Because human subjects of research cannot ethically or feasibly be randomly assigned to their exposure status, there is no all-purpose mechanism of producing equivalent comparison groups. Thus, the best that researchers can do in this situation is to select nonexposed comparison groups that are similar to the exposed group.

One of the better ways to do this is to recruit the nonexposed group from the same population group as the exposed group. It is worth repeating that such cohort studies are very valuable and suggestive of risk factors for major diseases, but they do not establish causality in an unequivocal manner. Whereas the original study sample in the Framingham Heart Study may have been representative of town residents in 1948 who had not yet experienced heart disease or a stroke, the initial and subsequent divisions of these study participants into smokers and nonsmokers, diabetic and nondiabetic persons, hypertensive and normotensive individuals were not under the control of the researchers and surely did not occur in a random manner. As was shown in the previous chapter, in such situations, researchers use multivariate statistical analyses, i.e., they try to control statistically for several known or suspected confounding variables to increase the confidence in the validity of the findings.

►**CLINICAL RESEARCH IN ACTION**
Causes of Heart Disease and Stroke

A classic and still ongoing open cohort study is the Framingham Heart Study, originally begun in 1948 to study the general causes of heart disease and stroke. For this study, researchers initially recruited 5,209 subjects (55.2% of whom were women), who were randomly selected from the population of Framingham, Massachusetts.[1] The study participants were between 30 and 62 years of age and had not yet experienced symptoms of cardiovascular disease or a heart attack or stroke. As of 1998, 1,095 participants were known to be alive (67.8% of whom were women). Over time, the study has contributed to the discovery and identification of many of the major risk factors for cardiovascular diseases, such as high blood cholesterol, high blood pressure,

smoking, and others (National Heart, Lung, and Blood Institute, 2002; Kannel & Ellison, 1996; Sytkowski, D'Agostino, Belanger, & Kannel, 1996; Wilson, Hoeg, D'Agostino, Silbershatz, Belanger, Poehlmann, O'Leary, & Wolf, 1997).

If subjects for the nonexposed comparison group(s) cannot be directly recruited from the same population as the exposed group, researchers might improve the comparability of the extraneous comparison group through matching on a few salient criteria. Clearly, the matching procedures create socially more similar comparison groups, but that does not guarantee that there remain (delinquency-relevant) differences between the groups.

►**CLINICAL RESEARCH IN ACTION**
Childhood Victimization and Running Away

For a study of the effects of childhood victimization and running away on subsequent adolescent delinquency, Kaufman & Widom (1999) identified 908 abused children between 1967 and 1971 on the basis of court records, as well as 667 comparison children who apparently were not abused. The latter group was identified through school records from more than 100 elementary schools and was matched to the abused children on the basis of birth date, gender, race, and social class or residential neighborhood.

Risk Factors

So far we have used the language of "exposure to risk factors" without much explanation of what a risk factor is. When participants in a cohort study with special exposure groups (such as coal miners, or construction workers exposed to asbestos) are selected and enrolled, researchers usually do not have conclusive evidence about the causal effects of the **risk factor** in question. The same may be said about the subsequent division of study samples in open cohort studies into exposed and nonexposed groups. In either case, the risk factor is really a suspected or hypothesized cause of the disease or adverse outcome that the researcher is concerned with. In fact, even if the suspected risk factor proves to be predictive of the adverse outcome (e.g., workers exposed to asbestos experience more lung disease than workers not so exposed), this does not in itself provide conclusive evidence of a causal relationship between asbestos exposure and lung disease, because correlation/prediction is not a sufficient base for causal inference. Thus, it is better to think of risk factors as *predictors* of diseases and adverse outcomes, not necessarily as established causes. For instance, it is well known that diabetes mellitus is a risk factor for cardiovascular disease (Kannel, D'Agostino, Wilson, Belanger, & Gagnon, 1990); i.e., persons with di-

---

[1]Note: Random *selection* only increases the chances that the study sample is representative of the town's population at the time of the selection. It does not ensure similarity of subjects with different exposure experience. Only random *assignment* to exposure groups can accomplish that.

abetes are far more likely to experience cardiovascular disease than are persons who are not diabetic. Yet, it is far more difficult to establish to what degree there is a direct causal mechanism by which diabetes causally contributes to the development of cardiovascular disease, or to what degree being diabetic is merely associated with a host of other biologic or behavioral characteristics that, in turn, cause cardiovascular disease.

So far in our discussion of exposure status, we have relied on the simplifying assumption that exposure to a risk factor involves only two categories: being exposed or not being exposed. Obviously, in reality, exposure to a risk factor is often a matter of degree. For example, workers in nuclear power plants may have been exposed to varying degrees of radiation, the cumulative exposure to coal dust tends to vary with the length of employment as a coal miner, and among those who are categorized as obese, the extent of obesity (as measured by body mass index) also varies substantially. Even a simple classification of subjects into current smokers, ex-smokers, and nonsmokers will help to capture some of the dosage differences in exposure to the risk factor. For example, if a researcher tests the hypothesis that smoking is a contributing cause to emphysema and finds, in a cohort study with 10-year follow-up, that those who continued smoking had the highest incidence rate of emphysema, followed by the ex-smokers, followed by the study participants who never smoked, this would certainly offer supporting evidence for the causal hypothesis. A **dose–response** relationship such as this, in which variations in degrees of exposure are associated with variations in the incidence of the adverse outcome, gives greater plausibility to the causal inference, even though it remains possible that the dose–response relationship is due to a third or confounding variable.[2] In the final analysis, however, cohort studies are observational, and the case for a causal relationship between a risk factor that cannot be manipulated (such as smoking) and a disease outcome (such as emphysema) rests on an understanding of the causal mechanism and the cumulative evidence from many cohort and other observational studies.

LOSSES TO FOLLOW-UP

As with all longitudinal studies, cohort studies are vulnerable to follow-up losses. That is, study participants initially enrolled in the cohort study may move away, may refuse

participation later, may be involved in a serious accident, may die, or may later experience diseases not related to the outcome under investigation. It goes without saying that attrition of subjects is a major problem in cohort studies, especially when follow-up periods are long. There are many management strategies that researchers can (and should) adopt to keep subjects in a study (Ribisl et al., 1996). However, in clinical studies, many factors contributing to the loss of subjects (e.g., accidents, change of address, death) clearly remain beyond the control of the researcher(s). In principle, loss of subjects to follow-up need not compromise the validity of the cohort study unless the loss is correlated with either the exposure status or the outcome (See Research Scenario 9–1).

Similarly, in cohort studies involving interviews of study participants, refusal to participate is often related to how sick the study participant is or feels at the time of recontact (Neumark et al., 2001). Thus, if the study outcome is the incidence of a disease that is associated with burdensome symptoms, it may be that refusal to participate, which is one reason for loss to follow-up, masks the occurrence of the outcome of interest. Incidentally, this example points out again the desirability of having external, inde-

RESEARCH SCENARIO 9.1

Nonequivalence of Exposed and Nonexposed Groups

Suppose that a researcher identifies large numbers (say, $n > 20,000$) of smokers and nonsmokers over the age of 40 from health insurance files, and obtains their consent to track them for the next 10 years for the purpose of recording all incidences of lung disease and deaths involving lung disease. Because smoking status is not randomly assigned in a cohort study, the participating smokers and nonsmokers may differ in all sorts of unanticipated ways. Suppose the proportion of truckers, farmers and automobile workers is higher among the smokers than among the nonsmokers with whom they are compared. It might well turn out that the frequency of car and other accidents is disproportionately higher among these smokers, leading to more frequent dropouts from the exposed group in the cohort study and, therefore, to a bias in the comparison of the occurrence of lung disease between exposed and nonexposed groups.

---

[2]For instance, the study participants who remained smokers may be much more likely to work in occupational environments where they are exposed to substances that contribute to the development of emphysema.

pendent sources of information about the outcomes of interest. If the outcome is death, reliable information can be obtained from state bureaus of vital statistics or the National Death Index, although information concerning the causes-of-death classifications may be less reliable. For certain diseases and in certain geographic areas, population-based disease registries like the Surveillance, Epidemiology, and End Results (SEER) registry for cancer may be an appropriate source of information on the outcome, although such sources of information are less useful if the studied population group is highly mobile. Similarly, private insurance data on the diagnosis and treatment of new diseases in study participants may be compromised if there is high turnover among policyholders. This is certainly one reason for the popularity of using Medicare data in cohort studies. People rarely if ever quit Medicare. Of course, the tradeoff is that Medicare covers only individuals 65 years old and older. If outcome data can be obtained only through recontacting the study participant or the participant's family, then there may not always be good solutions to the bias problem resulting from differential loss to follow-up.

Sensitivity Analysis

In cohort study reports, the reader should, at the very least, expect to see information on the size (numbers and percentages) of subject attrition, as well as some analyses probing possible biases resulting from differential attrition, if such attrition occurred. If the proportion of cases lost to follow-up is not too large in comparison with the occurrence of outcome, the analysis of cohort data may also contain a form of **sensitivity analysis,** in which the results of the study are recalculated on the basis of two extreme assumptions: (1) all subjects lost to follow-up have experienced the adverse outcome under study, or (2) none of them have experienced the adverse outcome. This way, it is possible to obtain a range of estimates and a sense of the potential impact of loss to follow-up on the validity of the conclusions.

RELATIVE RISK AS A MEASURE OF ASSOCIATION

The most basic measure of association in cohort studies between exposure status as the independent variable and disease outcome as the dependent variable is the **relative risk,** defined as the ratio of two incidence rates. The incidence rate for the disease outcome in the group exposed to the risk factor is divided by the incidence rate in the nonexposed group. This definition of the relative risk includes a new term that has not yet been defined: incidence rate. This epidemiologic term is frequently used in the health care literature, but its definition is not always clearly understood. An **incidence rate** is a ratio of two quantities: the number of new (incident) cases of a particular disease within a given time period divided by the population at risk for the disease in that time period. The crucial part of this definition is that it involves both counts of events (incident disease), or persons who experience the event, and explicitly defined time periods. Thus, a rate is not simply a proportion of persons with new diagnoses of a specific disease over the total number of persons in a particular population. The denominator of the "population at risk for the disease" is the product of the number of persons exposed times their associated exposure time (See Research Scenario 9–2).

We labeled the relative risk a *measure of association*. In other words, like a correlation coefficient, it indicates the extent to which two variables (exposure status and disease outcome) are related. Different from the usual correlation measures, however, relative risk ratios have no fixed upper limit, and the value indicating absence of a relationship equals one rather than zero. The reason for this is easy to see. Suppose, among smokers, the annual incidence rate of lung cancer was 260 per 100,000 person-years, and among nonsmokers it was also 260 per 100,000 person-years. If the incidence rates of exposed (smokers) and nonexposed (nonsmokers) groups were the same, then smoker status would obviously not be related to the risk of contracting lung cancer. Just as obvious is the fact that the ratio of two equal numbers, here (260/100,000)/(260/100,000), equals 1. Thus, for exposure status to be related to the outcome risk, the relative risk ratio *must* differ from 1.

Confidence Intervals and Multivariate Statistical Techniques

When you read journal articles reporting the results of cohort studies, you will notice that in addition to the relative risk measure itself, researchers report their associated confidence intervals, most typically at the 95% level (95% CI). They also frequently use multivariate statistical techniques, such as **Cox's proportional hazard model,** showing relative risk estimates that are adjusted for other variables in the equation. The confidence intervals are interpreted in the same way as for any other parameter estimate. Remember that an observed relative risk is computed on the basis of the particular sample data available to the researcher. Thus, the usual statistical inference question arises: what confidence can we have that the observed sample values accurately reflect the values that parallel population statistics?

Incidence of Acute Myocardial Infarction

An example illustrates this definition: Suppose a researcher monitors 10 smokers and 10 nonsmokers, initially all 55 years old, for 10 years to record their first incidence of an acute myocardial infarction (AMI), if any. Over an observation period of this length, some of the study participants are quite likely be lost to follow-up (e.g., they move away, refuse further participation, or die of unrelated reasons, such as car accident). The data for this hypothetical study are in Table 9-1, which shows part of a **life table** in a simplified version. Its purpose here is to illustrate the concept of **person-time of exposure,** or "population at risk." The first column indicates the year of exposure (i.e., the year during which a person smoked or did not smoke). The second column shows the number of smokers or nonsmokers in each year who were at risk for experiencing an AMI. The third column incorporates a simplifying assumption about death or follow-up. We assume here that if a person dies or is lost to follow-up, this event always occurs exactly on the last day of the observation year, so that the person was at risk for an AMI during the entire year of observation.[3] Finally, the fourth column shows the disease outcome of interest: the first occurrence (incidence) of an AMI for a given person. Note that we defined the event of interest as the *first* occurrence of an AMI. That means once a person has had an AMI, he or she no longer is at risk for another first AMI. Because, according to the data in Table 9-1, one of the 10 smokers experienced an AMI in the first year, there are only 9 smokers left in the second year *who are at risk for a new AMI*. Similarly, at the ends of years 3, 5, and 9, 1 smoker either dies for reasons not related to an AMI or is otherwise lost to follow-up. Thus, in the immediately following years of observations, these persons are no longer at risk for experiencing their first AMI. Using the same reasoning for both smokers and nonsmokers, we see that smokers were exposed to the risk of an AMI for 72 person-years and nonsmokers for 82 person-years. With four observations of new AMIs in the smoker group and two observations in the nonsmoker group, the relative risk of experiencing an AMI is 2.3 times larger among the smokers. Note that a simple ratio of the proportions of smokers versus nonsmokers who experienced an AMI would have given us a biased estimate of the relative risk: (4/10)/(2/10) = 2. The latter ratio does not take into account that we were able to observe the nonsmokers collectively for 10 person-years more than the smokers. Thus, the relative risk should be computed as the ratio of two incidence rates, taking explicitly into account the time dimension of the observations made.

►CLINICAL RESEARCH IN ACTION
Walking and Risk of Coronary Heart Disease

For instance, Lee et al. (2001) reported that women who walk a moderate 1 to 1.5 hours per week have a relative risk of coronary heart disease of 0.37 compared with women who do not walk regularly. The associated 95% confidence interval is 0.22 to 0.62. That means that we can be 95% confident (or there is a 95% probability) that the "true" relative risk in the population lies somewhere between 0.22 and 0.62. Note that these confidence limits do not include the value 1. Thus, we can be confident that greater amounts of weekly walking are related to a lower risk of coronary heart disease. Lee et al. (2001) also provided a multivariate estimate of this relative risk adjusted, among other variables, for the age of the female subjects as well as their smoking status, alcohol consumption, menopausal status, and other factors. This adjusted relative risk is 0.49 (95% CI: 0.28–0.86). Thus, there remain differences in the risk of contracting coronary heart disease, such that moderate walking reduces the risk to about half the risk among women who do not walk.

Absolute Risks

Although this is undoubtedly an interesting and encouraging finding, the often exclusive emphasis on relative risk ratios may obscure other important information. First, as simple as it sounds, a relative risk is a relative/comparative measure, i.e., it relates risks in two comparison groups to each other. Thus, it is not a measure of the **absolute risk** of incurring a certain disease or undesired outcome. For example, the overall risk of the development of coronary heart disease during the 5-year follow-up period of this study was "only" 1.17 %. With other diseases, positive outcomes are often less frequent. Thus, a certain activity or drug or intervention may reduce the (relative) risk of an adverse event by 50% or 100%; yet, if the event's overall

---

[3]Clearly, people don't only die on the last day of a year, but we could have chosen smaller time intervals (e.g., days) to make it more realistic, or we could make the assumption that on average, deaths or losses to follow-up occur at the halfway point–an assumption that makes sense in large study populations but not with a small sample of 20 cases.

TABLE 9.1	Incidence of Acute Myocardial Infarction (AMI) Among 10 Smokers and 10 Nonsmokers During 10 Years

Start of Year	Persons at Risk for AMI During Year	New AMI	Loss to Follow-up/Death (at End of Year)
Nonsmokers			
1	10	0	0
2	10	1	0
3	9	0	0
4	9	0	1
5	8	0	0
6	8	0	0
7	8	1	0
8	7	0	0
9	7	0	1
10	6	0	0
	Total person-years at risk for AMI: 82	Total new AMIs: 2	

10-Year Incidence Rate: new AMIs/person-years at risk = 2/82 = 0.0244

Start of Year	Persons at Risk for AMI During Year	New AMI	Loss to Follow-up/Death (at End of Year)
Smokers			
1	10	1	0
2	9	0	0
3	9	0	1
4	8	0	0
5	8	1	0
6	7	0	1
7	6	0	0
8	6	1	0
9	5	0	1
10	4	1	0
	Total person-years at risk for AMI: 72	Total new AMIs: 4	

10-Year Incidence Rate: new AMIs/person-years at risk = 4/72 = 0.0556

Relative risk of AMI among smokers compared with nonsmokers: Smokers' incidence rate/nonsmokers' incidence rate = 0.0556/0.0244 ≈2.3

probability of occurrence is very low to begin with, patients (and clinicians) may still be inclined to discount the clinical significance of the finding. By contrast, even a modest (say, 30%) reduction in the risk of contracting a common ill condition (such as hypertension) may well be important enough to inspire efforts to lower exposure to known risk factors (such as unbalanced diets or lack of exercise). Thus, relative risks should also be evaluated in light of the absolute risks of adverse outcomes associated with taking no action.

In summary, it is worth repeating that relative risk ratios are measures of association; i.e., they do not, in and of themselves, establish the causal link between a risk factor and the disease outcome. Even if the relative risk is significantly different from 1, all that has been established is that the exposure status predicts the risk of an adverse outcome. Again, a risk factor is a variable that contributes to the prediction of adverse disease outcomes—no more and no less. A risk factor is not necessarily a causal agent that independently produces the adverse outcome. This remains true for all the familiar reasons. Multivariate analyses may provide some statistical adjustments for confounding factors, but they cannot guarantee the equivalence of the groups compared. Exposed and not exposed groups may always differ on an unrecognized third variable, which may account for the observed relationship. Of course, our confidence in a causal interpretation grows when multiple studies, adjusting for multiple (and different) potential confounders in different study populations, come up with similar findings concerning the relative risk. Thus, given a very large number (thousands) of studies examining the association between smoking, coronary heart disease, and lung cancer, the evidence for the causal role of smoking in lung cancer and coronary heart disease is indeed overwhelming.

Although many cohort studies address problems and issues relevant to nursing practice, traditionally nursing researchers have not conducted cohort studies, a methodology that originated in epidemiology. There are many reasons for this, including the already mentioned high costs frequently associated with conducting cohort studies that involve large samples monitored over substantial periods of time. Yet, cohort studies are designed to answer questions regarding potentially preventable public health concerns, and with the increasing focus of nursing practice on disease prevention and health promotion, cohort studies are likely to become an additional tool that proves useful to nursing researchers.

Probably the main reason for the relative underutilization of cohort studies in nursing research has been the difficulty in adapting them to the examination of questions deemed important to nursing. For example, as discussed earlier, a major challenge in large-scale cohort studies is how to obtain accurate information regarding exposure to suspected risk factors as well as the associated outcome data. Of necessity, this problem has meant heavy reliance on available data sources (such as vital statistics, disease registries, and insurance data). *These data sources typically document outcomes such as mortality much better than other outcomes, such as lifestyle behaviors, physical functioning, or mental health.* Nonetheless, behavioral outcomes and risk factors of interest to nursing have been studied on a limited basis by use of the cohort design. We present several recent examples here.

▶CLINICAL RESEARCH IN ACTION
Practical Examples of Cohort Studies

- Hillis et al. (2001) studied adverse childhood experiences (such as sexual abuse, a battered mother, or parents with criminal records) as predictors of sexual risk behavior (such as early intercourse or a large number of sexual partners). Whereas the Hillis et al. (2001) study relied on interview information from 5,060 members of a managed care organization, the information was obtained during the standard medical history in the adult health clinic and was part of the existing records of the managed care organization.

- In another retrospective cohort study (Smith & Pell, 2001), researchers relied on the Scottish Morbidity Record 2 Data Base to assemble information on all first and second births to women aged 15 to 29 who had either a live or stillborn baby weighing more than 500 grams during the years 1992 to 1998. The purpose of the study was to ascertain the relative risk of such adverse outcomes as stillbirth, neonatal death, very early (24–32 weeks) birth and early (33–40 weeks) birth, or cesarean section, based on the age of the mother (15–19 versus 20–29 years). The risks associated with the age of the mother were compared for first and second births and among smoking and nonsmoking mothers.

- In a prospective cohort study, Tsubono, Nishino, Komatsu, Hsieh, Kanemura, Tsuji, Nakatsuka, Fukao, Satoh, & Hisamichi (2001) obtained exposure data on the consumption of green tea from 31,345 residents of three Japanese municipalities representing an astounding 94% of the resident population 40 years of age or older. The questionnaires were delivered and collected by municipal health workers visiting all the residencies. Because these researchers wanted to test the hypothesis that the consumption of green tea protects against the risk of gastric cancer, they were able to use an existing cancer population registry in the three municipalities to obtain outcome data on new cancer diagnoses for 8 years after the initial interview data. Not untypical for a long-term cohort study, some 16% of the subjects were lost to follow-up; i.e., they moved away and were no longer available for the local cancer registries, but the researchers provided some evidence that loss to follow-up was not systematically related to green tea consumption. This study also provides illustrations of testing for a dose–response relationship, because the amount of green tea consumption varied substantially among study participants. Given the variability in tea consumption, the researchers decided to use four different exposure categories, varying from less than a cup a day to more than five cups a day.[4] Finally, to increase the confidence in

---

[4]As is often the case in studies involving nutritional intake, the measurement problems can be formidable. To what extent do interview data provide reliable information on nutritional intake, given the recall problems and over-time variation in behaviors; and are the original interview data reliable indicators of subsequent, continuing consumption? Such issues will be discussed in more detail in the chapters on measurement.

their finding that consumption of green tea does *not* protect against the risk of gastric cancer, their multivariate statistical model offered relative risk estimates adjusted for a host of potential confounders, including age and sex of the respondents; smoking habits; alcohol consumption; consumption of meats, vegetables, and rice; and a history of peptic ulcers. Despite the substantial sample size, none of the relative risk ratios, when the risk of higher daily green tea consumption was compared with consumption of less than a cup, differed significantly from 1, with all 95% confidence intervals for the adjusted relative risks including the value of 1.

CONCLUSION

In this chapter, we introduced the cohort design as one of the two major observational designs developed by epidemiologists, the other being the case–control design.[5] While not yet common in nursing research, cohort and case–control studies have been a mainstay of information about clinically relevant risk factors as related to altered health status of populations. The basic idea behind the cohort design is to select and enroll (usually a large number of) study participants and divide them into groups, indicating to what degree they are exposed to a suspected risk factor. If the study participants have already experienced the adverse outcome or disease in question that is supposed to result from exposure to the risk factor, they are excluded from the cohort study. The reason is simple. For such subjects it would be nearly impossible to establish the temporary sequence of exposure to risk factor followed by the outcome in question, which is the intuitively appealing aspect of the cohort design.

Prospective cohort studies often involve monitoring large numbers of subjects over long periods of time. Requirements for sample size are usually dictated by the relative frequency or infrequency of the outcome or event among subjects exposed to the risk factor. Cohort studies are also subject to several sources of bias, the most important being measurement errors resulting in misclassification of study participants in terms of exposure or outcome status and differential loss of subjects to follow-up. The fundamental measure of an exposure effect on the outcome is the relative risk, a ratio of two incidence rates comparing adverse outcome in exposed and nonexposed groups or, if there are more than two comparison groups, in two exposure categories at a time. Even though relative risks are often in-

terpreted in causal terms, the cohort design itself is observational. Because observational studies lack an all-purpose mechanism for controlling confounding variables, the causal interpretation of relative risk ratios must proceed with caution and must be based on additional evidence.

Suggested Activities

1. Select one or more of the articles from the suggested reading or reference list for this chapter, in which a cohort study design was used to provide evidence related to the research question(s). After reading each article, address the following questions:
   a. Identify the key research question(s), and describe the features of the cohort design that were used to address the question(s), with reference to exposure status and outcome(s).
   b. Was there a good match between the nature of the research question and the research design that was used?
   c. How were potential or known confounding variables controlled in each study?
   d. If information is provided in the results section about relative risk estimates, interpret the relative risk results in everyday language, such as might be used by a clinician in a clinical encounter with a patient.
   e. For a given article, to what extent could confidence be placed in the study results, based on your answers to a through d?
2. Visit the web sites identified in this chapter to see what types of data sets from cohort studies are publicly available concerning national health issues.

Suggested Readings

Belanger CF, Hennekens CH, Rosner R, & Speizer FE. (1978). The Nurses' Health Study. *American Journal of Nursing, 78,* 1039-40.

Colditz GA, Manson JE, & Hankinson SE. (1997). The Nurses' Health Study: 20-year contribution to the understanding of health among women. *Journal of Women's Health, 6, 1,* 49-62.

Hillis SD, Anda RF, Felitti VJ, & Marchbanks PA. (2001). Adverse childhood experiences and sexual risk behaviors in women: A retrospective cohort study. *Family Planning Perspectives, 33, 5,* 206-11.

Smith GCS and Pell JP. (2001). Teenage pregnancy and risk of adverse perinatal outcomes associated with first and second births: population based retrospective study. *British Medical Journal, 323,* 476-9.

Tsubono Y, Nishino Y, Komatsu S, Hsieh C-C, Kanemura S, Tsuji I, Nakatsuka H, Fukao A, Satoh H & Hisamichi S. (2001). Green tea and the risk of gastric cancer in

---

[5]The case–control design will be discussed in Chapter 10.

Japan. *The New England Journal of Medicine, 344, 9,* 632-6.

References

Belanger, C. F., Hennekens, C. H., Rosner, R., & Speizer, F. E. (1978). The Nurses' Health Study. *American Journal of Nursing, 78,* 1039–1040.

Colditz, G. A., Manson, J. E., & Hankinson, S. E. (1997). The Nurses' Health Study: 20-year contribution to the understanding of health among women. *Journal of Women's Health, 6,* 49–62.

Colditz, G. A., & Rosner, B. A. (2000). Cumulative risk of breast cancer to age 70 years according to risk factor status: Data from the Nurses' Health Study. *American Journal of Epidemiology, 152,* 950–964.

Finocchiaro, C., Lark, A., Keating, M., Ugoni, A., & Abramson, M. (1997). Does occupational exposure to brown coal dust cause a decline in lung function? *Occupational and Environmental Medicine, 54,* 642–645.

Fung, T. T., Willett, W. C., Stampfer, M. J., Manson, J. E., & Hu, F. B. (2001). Dietary patterns and the risk of coronary heart disease in women. *Archives of Internal Medicine, 161,* 1857–1862.

Hillis, S. D., Anda, R. F., Felitti, V. J., & Marchbanks, P. A. (2001). Adverse childhood experiences and sexual risk behaviors in women: A retrospective cohort study. *Family Planning Perspectives, 33,* 206–211.

Kannel, W. B., D'Agostino, R. B., Wilson, P. W. F., Belanger, A. J., & Gagnon, D. R. (1990). Diabetes, fibrinogen, and risk of cardiovascular disease: The Framingham experience. *American Heart Journal, 120,* 672–676.

Kannel, W. B., & Ellison, R. C. (1996). Alcohol and coronary heart disease: The evidence for a protective effect. *Clinica Chimica Acta, 246,* 59–76.

Kaufman, J. G., & Widom, C. S. (1999). Childhood victimization, running away, and delinquency. *Journal of Research in Crime and Delinquency, 36,* 347–370.

Lee, I.-M., Rexrode, K. M., Cook, N. R., Manson, J. A., & Buring, J. E. (2001). Physical activity and coronary heart disease in women: Is "no pain, no gain" passe? *Journal of the American Medical Association, 285,* 1447–1454.

Liu, S., Manson, J. E., Stampfer, M. J., Hu, F. B., Giovan-nucci, E., Colditz, G. A., Hennekens, C. H., & Willett, W. C. (2000). A prospective study of whole-grain intake and risk of type 2 diabetes mellitus in US women. *American Journal of Public Health, 90,* 1409–1415.

National Cancer Institute. (2002). *SEER Cancer Statistics Review, 1973–1998. http://seer.cancer.gov/Publications/ CSR1973_1998.*

Neumark, D.E., Stommel, M. Given, C.W., & Given, B.A. (2001). Research design and subject characteristics predicting nonparticipation in a panel survey of older families with cancer. *Nursing Research, 50,* 363–368.

National Heart, Lung, and Blood Institute. (2002). *Framingham Heart Study: 50 Years of Research. http://www. nhlbi.nih.gov/about/framingham/index.html.*

Nurses' Health Study. (2002). *http://www.channing.harvard. edu/nhs/index.html.*

Raffn, E., Villadsen, E., Engholm, G., & Lynge, E. (1996). Lung cancer in asbestos cement workers in Denmark. *Occupational and environmental medicine, 53,* 399–402.

Smith, G. C. S., & Pell, J. P. (2001). Teenage pregnancy and risk of adverse perinatal outcomes associated with first and second births: Population based retrospective study. *British Medical Journal, 323,* 476–479.

Sytkowski, P. A., D'Agostino, R. B., Belanger, A. J., & Kannel, W. B. (1996). Secular trends in long-term sustained hypertension, long-term treatment, and cardiovascular mortality: The Framingham Heart Study 1950 to 1990. *Circulation, 93,* 697–703.

Tsubono, Y., Nishino, Y., Komatsu, S., Hsieh, C.-C., Kanemura, S., Tsuji, I., Nakatsuka, H., Fukao, A., Satoh, H., & Hisamichi, S. (2001). Green tea and the risk of gastric cancer in Japan. *The New England Journal of Medicine, 344,* 632–636.

Wilson, P. W. F., Hoeg, J. M., D'Agostino, R. B., Silbershatz, H., Belanger, A. M., Poehlmann, H., O'Leary, D., & Wolf, P. A. (1997). Cumulative effects of high cholesterol levels, high blood pressure, and cigarette smoking on carotid stenosis. *The New England Journal of Medicine, 337,* 516–522.

Yano, E., Wang, Z. M., Wang, X. R., Wang, M. Z., & Lan, Y. J. (2001). Cancer mortality among workers exposed to amphibole-free chrysotile asbestos. *American Journal of Epidemiology, 154,* 538–543.

CHAPTER 10 Case-Control Studies

INTRODUCTION TO CASE–CONTROL STUDIES

In this chapter, we discuss the second major analytic research design originally developed for observational epidemiology, the **case–control design.** As mentioned in the previous chapter, the distinguishing features of cohort and case–control designs are based on the selection criteria that determine eligibility of study participants. In cohort studies, subjects are selected *on the basis of their exposure status* with respect to a suspected risk factor. By contrast, the study subjects in case–control studies are selected *on the basis of their outcome status,* which usually turns on the question of whether or not the subjects have experienced a disease of interest.

In **case–control studies,** researchers start by selecting study subjects who have a certain disease or illness syndrome (**case subjects**), and compare them with a group of study subjects who do not have the disease or syndrome (**control subjects**). The simplest case–control design has one group of study participants who are designated as case subjects and another group who are designed as control subjects. Once selected, the groups are then compared in terms of their *exposure* to conditions that are hypothesized to cause the disease or syndrome. In the simplest case, the exposure status is also a dichotomous variable (exposed versus not exposed). As in cohort studies, exposure status indicates whether or not the study participants engaged in certain risky behaviors, have certain physiologic markers, or live under social or economic conditions that are considered potential causes of the disease, dysfunction, or syndrome under investigation.[1]

Because the adoption of a case–control design means selecting study subjects on the basis of an outcome of interest, it follows that at the time of enrollment of a study subject, all events of interest have already occurred. Thus, the main focus of investigation in a case–control study is to unearth the study participants' histories with respect to their exposure to the suspected risk factors. Just like the cohort study design discussed in Chapter 9, the case–control design is nonexperimental; i.e., the researcher only makes observations and collects data, and does not attempt to intervene in any way to alter the phenomena of interest. But whereas cohort studies clearly establish the temporal sequence of events from risk factor exposure to the development of the disease or outcome in question, even this lim-

ited evidence in support of a causal interpretation may be difficult to establish in a case–control study. Just by virtue of the fact that in case–control studies, exposure information must be collected after the fact (retrospectively), often by relying on information from the study participants, researchers cannot always be certain that exposure to the risk factor occurred before the onset of the disease. This is particularly an issue when the subjects include both incident and prevalent cases.[2] As an observational study design that occasionally may not even allow the researcher to establish a clear temporal sequence from exposure to outcome, the case–control design produces primarily evidence of associations or correlations between outcome and exposure status. All the usual limitations to causal inference that have been discussed previously for other types of nonexperimental research designs (see Chapters 3–9) also apply to case–control study designs. Still, case–control studies can provide powerful heuristic evidence for potential cause-and-effect relationships.

In certain situations, the case–control design is the only feasible study design. In other situations, it provides the searched-for evidence for efficiently than any other study design. For instance, in the case of rare diseases like leukemia, the cohort approach of monitoring study participants from, for example, possible exposure to x rays during pregnancy to the disease outcome is simply not feasible. In the United States, the incidence rates for childhood leukemia peak at age 2 at a rate of 96 cases per million (National Cancer Institute, 2000), http://www.cancer.gov. To study risk factors for leukemia prospectively would require enrolling very large numbers of newly born babies to yield a meager sample of incident cases of leukemia, even when the subjects are accumulated over a 10-year period. This is clearly not economical. How much better to enroll case subjects known to have leukemia and to find control subjects who are similar except that they did not get leukemia. In addition, cancers like leukemia, as well as many other diseases, have long latency periods, but it is difficult and costly to monitor subjects for a long time, as would be required in a prospective study approach. In these and similar situations, case–control designs provide a much more efficient approach to studying the association between exposure status and disease outcome.

In the past, it has been mainly epidemiologists who have studied the causes of diseases and altered health states in

---

[1]As mentioned in the previous chapter, exposure often varies in strength (dose), e.g., degrees of hypertension, years of smoking. For the current purposes, it is sufficient to lump all exposed cases together.

[2]Incident cases are newly diagnosed cases, whereas prevalent cases include both newly diagnosed cases and cases of survival with the disease. For chronic diseases like hypertension and some cancers, prevalent cases include the cases of many subjects who survived several years after the onset of the disease.

populations. Increasingly, however, researchers from other disciplines (including nurses) have developed a strong interest in questions of disease etiology. For example, public health nurses and advanced practice nurses (APNs) are concerned with health issues such as the incidence and prevention of sexually transmitted diseases (STDs) (Carson, 1997; Hutchinson, 1999). Better understanding of the factors contributing to the spread of STDs can enable nurses and others to design and implement interventions, both to prevent exposure to STDs and to mitigate the spread of existing disease. Thus, a key goal of this chapter is to illustrate the usefulness of the case–control study design in addressing research questions of relevance to APNs that concern sources of disease/dysfunction and how to intervene to prevent disease/dysfunction, or how to at least control or mitigate the impact of disease/dysfunction. It is also worthwhile to mention that the case–control design is flexible enough to incorporate behavioral and social variables as measures of exposure status. A recent example can be found in a study that used case–control methods to investigate cultural values as predictors of early-stage or late-stage diagnosis of breast cancer (Lannin, Mathews, Mitchell, Swanson, Swanson, & Edwards, 1998).

To show the relevance of case–control designs in addressing questions encountered in APN clinical practice, it may be helpful to start with a real-life example of findings from case–control studies that have resulted in an important change in how young infants are cared for around the world.

▶CLINICAL RESEARCH IN ACTION
Sudden Infant Death Syndrome

For many years, researchers have tried to understand which factors contribute to sudden infant death syndrome (SIDS), the sudden and seemingly unforeseeable death of an infant during sleep that is not attributable to an identifiable disease process. Many published studies on this topic have been based on case–control designs (e.g., Ford, Mitchell, Stewart, Scragg, & Taylor, 1997; Scragg et al., 1996), and the reason is quite simple: SIDS is fortunately a rare event. Thus, studying its causal contributors prospectively would require very large study samples, although at least one prospective cohort studies has been conducted (Dwyer et al., 1991). However, the typical SIDS study has involved sampling infants who recently died of SIDS as case subjects and using a comparison sample of non-SIDS infants as control subjects. After the enrollment of study subjects, investigators often test one or more hypothesis comparing the case subjects' and control subjects' exposure rates to the suspected risk factors(s). For example, Ford et al. (1997) used a case–control design to study appropriate use of med-

ical care as a hypothesized predictor of SIDS. As always, after the identification and enrollment of case subjects and control subjects into the study, researchers begin to assemble information on possible exposure to risk factors. In the case of SIDS, researchers have conducted in-depth interviews with the mothers of deceased SIDS infants to obtain data regarding past childcare practices, possible environmental factors associated with SIDS, and so forth (for an example of this interview approach, see Scragg et al., 1996). In addition, researchers might also conduct careful reviews of prenatal and infant medical records, collected before the outcome event in question.

In essence, with case–control studies, researchers can pursue hunches and explore several plausible risk factors simultaneously, often looking for potentially modifiable variables that can be altered in some way through future interventions. In several SIDS case–control studies, it was discovered that placing infants to sleep on their backs helped prevent SIDS (Dwyer et al., 1991; Willinger, Hoffman, & Hartford, 1994). As a result, the Back to Sleep campaign, which promoted the placement of infants on their backs to sleep, was implemented in 1994. It has been associated with a 38% reduction in the incidence of SIDS between 1992 and 1996 (Willinger et al., 1998).

SELECTING STUDY SUBJECTS BASED ON OUTCOMES

Selection of Case Subjects

As already stated, in case–control studies, researchers first select the case subjects, or study participants, among whom the outcome of interest has already occurred. For example, in the previously cited SIDS studies, researchers typically began with the identification and selection of families who had recently experienced SIDS in their midst. Similarly, McKenzie & Wurr (1998) identified persons who had committed suicide after they had been discharged from mental health facilities. Lannin et al. (2001) identified early-stage and late-stage breast cancer in patients after diagnosis. Where and how does one get appropriate samples of such cases?

The identification of cases depends, in the first place, on reasonably accurate and reliable diagnostic/identification procedures. For instance, the classification of an infant death as SIDS requires a clear set of procedural definitions, involving an elaborate autopsy protocol (Scragg et al., 1996). Likewise, to classify a death as suicide is not unproblematic. McKenzie & Wurr (2001) for example, relied on inquest records and decided to include all cases identified in these records as suicide or as undetermined injury ("open verdict"). The reason why these definitions and classification decisions are important is that misclassification of cases (e.g., an accident as suicide) will make it harder, if not impossible, to discover common risk factors. For instance, if definitions of cases are very broad, as in "all cases of heart disease," one may lump together a variety of quite distinct diseases like congenital heart disease, congestive heart failure, and cardiac atrophy. If cases comprise a heterogeneous set of diseases or diagnoses, it will be difficult to detect clear patterns of exposure to risk factors, because the risk factors for the various subcategories of cases may be quite different.

By far the most common approach to selecting case subjects is to start with patients in a particular hospital, clinic, or private practice (Lannin et al., 1998). After all, that is where we find persons who have particular diseases. Although this approach is relatively convenient it has its limitations. One is a likely selection bias, in the sense that patients in a particular facility are rarely representative of all patients who have the same disease or condition. Beyond generalizability, the more important issue here is that selection bias among case subjects may result in a biased association (underestimate or overestimate) between exposure status and disease outcome. For instance, many people with hypertension do not know that they have it (Stamler, 1994). If they have no other reasons for visiting a primary care provider, they may not easily find out. Thus, hypertensive patients enrolled in primary care practices may well differ from undiscovered hypertensive individuals in ways that lead to the misidentification of risk factors.

One way to avoid selection bias is to target case subjects in a clearly defined general population, such as a community, county, or even state (Habel, Stanford, Vaughan, Rossing, Voigt, Weiss, & Daling, 1995; Beautrais, Joyce, Mulder, Fergusson, Deavoll, & Nightingale, 1996; McKenzie & Wurr, 2001). A good way to gain access to such populations of case subjects is through offices of vital statistics or disease registries, like those for cancer or STDs. Lacking such registries, it may be difficult or impossible to identify most of the new case subjects in a given area with any degree of accuracy, let alone obtain and enroll representative samples of such case subjects.

When the outcome in question is a chronic disease with many long-term survivors, selection from all cases of the disease includes both *incident* (recent diagnosis) and *prevalent* (longer-term survival) cases. This may complicate the search for risk factors, because different factors may predict incidence and long-term survival. Thus, it is preferable to enroll only incident cases, even though this may substantially reduce the pool of available cases.

Selection of Control Subjects

Whereas cases may sometimes be difficult to come by, the validity of the case–control comparison stands and falls with the selection of appropriate control subjects. As a general rule, control subjects should be as similar as possible to the case subjects except that they did not experience the disease or other outcome in question. Thus, the primary concern in selecting control subjects is not that they be representative of a larger population but that they come from a similar study base.

One common technique is to select control subjects from the same institutions or clinics where the case subjects are found (McKenzie & Wurr, 2001), thus making it more likely that the same social processes of self-selection that produced the case subjects also produced the control subjects. In addition, if information on exposure to risk factors is based on the same institutional records, an added benefit of this approach is that the recording procedures and errors are similar among both case subjects and control subjects. However, if the institution involved is a hospital or clinic, then the control subjects are also patients, albeit with different diagnoses. This may pose problems when some of these other diagnoses have similar risk factors as the disease that is the focus of the case–control study. For instance, if case subjects are defined as hospital patients admitted with an acute myocardial infarction, and control subjects include stroke patients in the same hospital, this is likely to reduce differences between case subjects and control subjects with respect to such risk factors as hypertension. Thus, if other diseases are known to have the same risk factors as the disease under study, patients with these diagnoses should be excluded.

In community-based studies, control subjects are often selected randomly from the same population **catchment area,** a specific geographic region in which a target population resides, as the case subjects (Beautrais, et al., 1996; Scragg et al., 1996). The key question in such selections is the purpose of the case–control comparisons. For instance, if a researcher were to obtain a random sample of case subjects with incident lung cancer using one of the SEER area registries, then draw a random sample of control subjects from the general population in the same area, she would find a lower average age among the general population than among the case subjects with cancer simply because age is an important risk factor for the development of this disease. Knowing that, the researcher may instead draw a stratified random sample from the area population having the same age distribution as that of the case subjects with incident cancer.[3] In this way, the control sample is no longer representative of the larger population. It is, however, more similar to the case sample, which allows for better exploration of other risk factors independently of age. What emerges here is that there may not be one ideal control group; indeed, researchers have occasionally used multiple control groups (Hurwitz, Barrett, Bregman, Gunn, & Pinsky, 1987).

DATA QUALITY IN CASE–CONTROL STUDY DESIGNS

As we have seen, case–control study designs involve the selection of study participants based on known outcomes of interests (e.g., whether or not subjects committed suicide [McKenzie & Wurr, 2001], did or did not succumb to SIDS [Scragg et al., 1996], or had late-stage or early-stage breast cancer [Lannin, et al., 1998]). After the selection of subjects, researchers then reconstruct the study participants' history of exposure to the risk factors of interest, using a variety of information sources. For a case–control study to deliver usable evidence, researchers must address several data quality issues.[4]

- Inaccurate information about case/control status
- Inaccurate/incomplete/missing information about risk factors (exposure status)
- Inaccurate/incomplete/missing information about extraneous/confounding variables

Information on Case–Control Status

In the previous section, we emphasized the importance of clear definitions and inclusion criteria for deciding whether a subject is a case subject or a control subject. Because researchers often use records from registries, hospitals, and other clinics, it is important not only to devise clear definitions but also to ascertain information about the decision rules that went into establishing the requisite data records.

For instance, reported case subjects in brain tumor registries include patients with diagnoses based on a neurologic examination and computed tomography, magnetic resonance imaging, positron emission tomography, or a biopsy. Except for a biopsy, available diagnostic tools may not always discover (early) brain tumors (Brain Tumor Society, 2002).

Similarly, information on the precise cause of death is subject to errors of classification. Furthermore, for certain types of health issues, there may not necessarily be an agreed-upon "gold standard" measure with objective criteria for reliably classifying study subjects. Such lack of agreement in disease classification has historically been a problem for psychiatric diagnosis, particularly before the development of the criteria-based third edition of the *Diagnostic and Statistical Manual for Mental Disorders* (American Psychiatric Association, 1980). When information to classify people into case subjects or control subjects is insufficient, the case–control study approach is doomed from the start.

Two situations need to be distinguished in a discussion of the effects of poor information quality concerning the case or control status of study subjects. The resulting misclassification of cases may be either random or systematic. Generally, the former is of less concern than the latter.

Suppose the determination of case subjects as having late-stage breast cancer and of control subjects as having early-stage breast cancer both occur at the same medical center according to a single set of pathology procedures. In this situation, any errors in classification should be present among both case subjects and control subjects. Thus, no bias is introduced in the comparison of the two groups, although when error rates are high, researchers will have to compensate by using much larger samples.[5] Now suppose the rate of misclassification is systematically different between case subjects and control subjects, and 90% of supposedly depressed case subjects, but only 70% of supposedly not-depressed control subjects, have accurate diagnoses. Then the estimated relationship between case–control status and exposure-to-a-risk-factor status will be biased. Systematic differences in the accuracy of classifications of study participants as case subjects or control subjects are most likely to occur if the procedures for determining case–control status vary between the two groups, e.g., a determination based on medical records in the case group and a determination based on interview screening in the control group.

---

[3]A stratified random sample is one in which a researcher first determines how many subjects to draw from the various strata (here, age groups, such as 21–30, 30–40) and then selects subjects randomly from within the population strata. In Chapter 14, we offer a detailed discussion of various sampling schemes.

[4]Many of these issues are not unique to case–control studies, but we discuss them here because they must be addressed, anticipated, and planned for in a case–control study.

[5]In Chapters 13 and 14, the effects of measurement errors on standard deviations and standard errors will be explored in more depth. Implications for sample size will be discussed in Chapter 20.

Information on Exposure Status

Overall, the more difficult data quality problem in case–control studies is to obtain accurate information on the history of exposure to the risk factors investigated. It is not uncommon for researchers to lack complete information about exposure status. One reason is that in case–control studies, researchers look back at risk factors, exposure to which must have occurred before the onset of the disease or the event that defines the case subjects or control subjects. Principally, information about past events can be obtained from the subjects directly; possibly from surrogates such as family members, as in the case of the SIDS studies; or from historical records. Historical records about study participants' exposure to risk factors have this disadvantage: the researcher does not control the methods that were used to collect the data and may no longer be able to gather additional data to refine information about exposure status. However, the big advantage of relying on records of exposure to risk factors is that they were assembled before the outcome event of interest (e.g., diagnosis of a disease, suicide). Thus, they could not possibly represent a bias based on the knowledge that a subject would become a case subject or a control subject in a later study.

►CLINICAL RESEARCH IN ACTION
Suicide After Hospital Discharge

McKenzie & Wurr (2001) used records from psychiatric hospitals assembled before the suicides investigated, and they obtained the primary discharge diagnoses as well as the handwritten diagnostic comments of the mental health professionals. They found the sheer length (not content) of these psychiatric records to be predictors of early suicide after patients' discharge from the mental hospital. Because these record entries were made without knowledge of who among the discharged patients would later commit suicide, the diagnostic information contained in them was considered uncontaminated, providing unbiased predictors of outcomes.

The situation is quite different when information about exposure status comes from the study participants themselves. In these cases, researchers must rely on the accuracy of study participants' memory concerning exposure information. Not surprisingly, this problem is greater when much time has passed between exposure and disease outcome. However, the primary threat to the validity of the case–control design does not come from a generalized memory problem but from a recall bias. **Recall bias** refers to a systematic difference in the information remembered and reported by case and control subjects. It occurs because subjects can be interviewed only after their enrollment into the study, which, in case–control studies, occurs after the

diagnosis of the disease or the occurrence of the adverse outcome. Thus, the respondent knows about the outcome and recalls exposure events in light of this knowledge.

For example, in a case–control study of potential risk factors for melanoma, people with a diagnosis of melanoma may systematically overestimate and overreport past exposure to sunlight, especially during childhood. This is particularly likely for subjects sensitized by public information and cancer prevention campaigns about the need to avoid sun exposure (Cockburn, Hamilton, & Mack, 2001). Given that case subjects have already experienced the adverse outcome and have been provided with a ready-made causal theory, they may systematically overestimate their past exposure, especially because recalling past exposure to sunlight is likely to be error prone under the best of circumstances.

Control subjects, by contrast, would not have this cognitive incentive to overreport past exposure to sunlight. In such a study, the role of sun exposure as a risk factor for melanoma would be systematically overestimated if exposure information rested exclusively on the subjects' recall. In general, recall bias can be expected to be stronger when there are long time delays between initial exposure and the development of a disease, as with malignant melanoma.

Information on Extraneous/Confounding Variables

As we have seen, case–control study designs are observational, and it is always possible that other variables, correlated with the exposure variable, may account for part or even all of the observed relationship between case or control status and exposure status. For that reason, researchers often collect additional information on suspected confounding variables so that their influence can be statistically controlled for. For instance, while Lannin et al. (1998) focused on the link between cultural beliefs and breast cancer staging at the time of diagnosis, they also controlled for known socioeconomic predictors of late-stage presentation, such as education and health insurance. If information about confounding variables is obtained from study participants after their classification into case subjects and control subjects, questions of possible recall bias need to be considered with these variables as well.

THE ODDS RATIO AS A MEASURE OF ASSOCIATION IN CASE–CONTROL STUDIES

When data from case–control studies are analyzed and presented in research reports, the examined relationship be-

TABLE 10.1	Association Between Diagnosis of Melanoma (Yes/No) and History of Exposure to High or Low Levels of Sunlight: Sample results from a Case–Control Study (Numbers and Column Percents; Odds Among Cases and Controls; Odds Ratio)	
	Cases: Study Participants With Diagnoses of Melanoma	**Controls: Study Participants Without Diagnoses of Melanoma**
Levels of past exposure to sunlight		
High levels	60 (=40%)	30 (=20%)
Low levels	90 (=60%)	120 (=80%)
Total	150 (=100%)	150 (=100%)
Odds of high-level vs. low-level exposure	60/90 = 2/3	30/120 = 1/4
Odds ratio	(60/90)/(30/120) = (60/30)/(90/120) = 2.67	
95% confidence interval for odds ratio	1.59 < odds ratio in population < 4.47	

tween subjects' case or control status and their exposure-to-a-risk-factor status is very often reported in terms of (unadjusted or adjusted) **odds ratios** (OR). This statistic is so commonly used that every serious reader of health- and illness-related research must know how to interpret results couched in terms of ORs.

Computation of Sample Odds Ratios

To illustrate, we present fictitious sample data related to the problem of melanoma and a prior history of exposure to sunlight. In the example, we take it for granted that the measurement problem of relatively accurate and unbiased information about past sun exposure has been resolved. On the basis of the information obtained, the researchers may divide all case subjects (with melanoma) and control subjects (without melanoma) into two categories of exposure: high and low sunlight exposure.[6] Table 10-1 shows the data.

The data in the columns show the two groups selected by the researcher: the subsample of case subjects and the second subsample of control subjects. The case and control subjects may be age-matched and sex-matched random samples of subjects from the same community, both resident at the time of diagnosis. Because the researchers select the subsamples, the numbers of case and control subjects in a case–control study are fixed.[7] Thus, they in no way reflect the actual prevalence of people with or without

the condition or disease in the community. As mentioned above, this is, in fact, one of the attractions of using case–control designs when the disease or outcome of interest is rare. The researcher "only" has to find a sufficient number of case subjects but is not required to find nondiseased control subjects in numbers that reflect their relative prevalence in the population. Of course, the price paid is that one cannot use such data for the estimation of true incidence rates and risks.[8]

Now we shall use the data to demonstrate (sample) how ORs are computed and interpreted. As the name indicates, an **odds ratio** is a ratio of two odds. The **odds** are themselves a ratio, namely, the number or proportion of cases in one of two mutually exclusive categories divided by the number or proportion of cases in the other category. For example, for the data in Table 10-1, we might ask this question: what are the odds among the cases that the subjects have been exposed to high levels of sunlight versus their not having been so exposed? The data show that 60 case subjects had high levels of exposure and 90 case subjects did not; thus, the odds of exposure among this group are 60/90, or 2/3. We might say: "The odds are 2 to 3 that a patient (with a diagnosis of melanoma) has a history of high-level exposure to sunlight." We would have obtained exactly the same result if we had computed the odds from the proportions. The proportion of case subjects with high exposure levels is 60/150 = 0.40 (40%); the proportion of case subjects with low exposure levels is 90/150 = 0.6 (60%). The ratio of the two proportions is 0.4/0.6, or 2/3.

[6]Remember the discussion of the dose–response problem in Chapter 9; a more sophisticated measurement procedure may well allow for finer dosage grading of exposure to the risk factor.

[7]Equal-sized comparison groups often maximize statistical power, but in other situations, researchers may prefer unequal comparison groups. A more detailed discussion can be found in Chapters 14 and 15.

[8]However, as we shall see shortly, under certain circumstances it is possible to compute the RR from case–control data.

Now, we repeat the same analysis for the control subjects. As Table 10-1 shows, among control subjects, only 30 reported high levels of past sun exposure, and 120 did not. Thus, in this group, the odds of high-level exposure are 30/120, or 1/4. In terms of proportions, we again obtain the same result: 30/150 = 0.2 and 120/150 = 0.8, resulting in 0.2/0.8, or odds of 1/4.

Knowing the odds of exposure to high levels of sunlight among *both* case subjects *and* control subjects, we are now ready to compute the OR:

- Odds of high sun exposure in childhood among subjects with diagnoses of malignant melanoma in adulthood (case subjects) = 2/3
- Odds of high sun exposure in childhood among subjects *without* diagnoses of malignant melanoma in adulthood (control subjects) = 1/4

The OR is the ratio of the odds among case subjects and the odds among control subjects:

$$(2/3)/(1/4) \cong 2.7$$

Properties of Odds Ratios

This result means that the odds of a history of high sun exposure are approximately 2.67 times higher among the case subjects than among the control subjects. In a way, then, the OR expresses the degree of association between exposure to a risk factor (history of high levels of sun exposure in childhood) and the occurrence of a disease/disorder (malignant melanoma in adulthood). Indeed, one can think of the OR as a special kind of correlation coefficient. Most correlation coefficients, like Pearson's *r*, Spearman's rho, and Phi, are normed so that they range from -1 (a perfect negative relationship) to $+1$ (a perfect positive relationship).[9] But ORs can vary from a low value of just above zero to infinity.[10] And whereas complete absence of a relationship between two variables results in a value of zero for the familiar correlation coefficients, for ORs, as for relative risk (RR) ratios, the value of 1 is what indicates this absence of a relationship. Why is this so? The answer lies in recalling the conceptual meaning of the OR, which compares the odds of exposure for case subjects with the odds for control subjects. Whatever the absolute magnitude of these odds, if they are the same in both groups, then high-level sun exposure does not differ in the two groups. In

short, an OR of 1 would indicate that case or control status is not related to levels of exposure.

The OR shares another important property with other correlation coefficients, but not with RR ratios. The OR is a symmetrical measure. That means that it has the same values whether we take the ratio of two column odds, as we have done in the previous calculations, or the ratio of two row odds. Go back to the data in Table 10-1. Suppose we first compute the odds of a subject's being a case subject, rather than a control subject, among those who were exposed to high levels of sunlight. As the data in the relevant row show, these odds are 60/30, or 2. Among subjects with a history of low-level exposure to sunlight, the parallel odds are 90/120, or 0.75. The ratio of these two odds (2/0.75) yields the same number as before: approximately 2.67. This is an important result because we have shown that one can estimate the strength of the relationship between exposure status and case or control status based on data from a case–control study. Although such data are assembled after the fact, based on the knowledge of the outcome, researchers can still answer the question they are more likely to be interested in: is the exposure to the risk factor (here, sunlight exposure) predictive of the outcome (here, development of malignant melanoma)?

Confidence Intervals for Odds Ratios

We have presented an example of how one calculates sample odds, i.e., the odds based on the data at hand. As always, researchers are interested not only in the results computed from a particular data set. They also want to be confident that the results indicate a pattern that holds up in other situations. In other words, the observed relationships should not be the result of mere sampling fluctuations, which might occur as a result of sample selection or measurement error.

REVIEW NOTES In Chapter 3, we used the example of the *t* test to show how inferences beyond the observed sample data can be made if one knows the sampling distribution of a statistic.

Applied to the ORs, this means that we need to know the shape of the sampling distribution of the ORs and its associated standard error.[11] With this information, we can

---

[9]See Munro et al. (2001) for an introductory treatment and Snedecor & Cochran (1989) for a more comprehensive treatment of correlation coefficients.

[10]Just picture odds of 2/999,998 or odds of 999,998/2.

[11]As demonstrated with the sampling distribution of mean differences in Chapter 3, the sampling distribution of ORs could also be constructed. This would require drawing thousands of samples repeatedly from the same population, computing the sample OR each time, and constructing the frequency distribution of these sample ORs. Theoretically, it can be shown that the sampling distribution of the OR follows the log-normal distribution, and its standard error can be estimated from the sample data at hand (Agresti, 1990).

estimate the 95% confidence intervals for the OR. Although it is not necessary for the reader of clinically relevant research reports to understand the derivation of these confidence intervals, she or he needs to understand their meaning to draw correct conclusions from them. Going back to the data shown in Table 10-1, we see that it contains both the computed sample OR and its estimated 95% confidence interval:

OR: 2.67, CI: 1.59 − 4.47[12]

What additional information does the confidence interval give us? On the basis of the confidence interval, we are 95% confident (i.e., the probability is 0.95) that the confidence interval of 1.59 to 4.47 contains the true OR, indicating that the relationship between risk-factor exposure and disease outcome lies somewhere between 1.59 and 4.47. Note that this confidence interval does not contain the value of 1. Thus, we are in a strong position to reject the null hypothesis of no relationship between exposure and outcome, which would mean a true OR equal to 1. We are at least 95% confident that the true OR differs from 1, and we take that as evidence that risk factor exposure and disease outcome are related.

Brief Comparison of Odds Ratios and Relative Risk Ratios

REVIEW NOTES In Chapter 9, we introduced the RR as the fundamental measure of association used in cohort studies.

In many ways, ORs and RRs seem like very similar measures. They do share two important properties in common, and it is worthwhile to mention them again.

- Both the OR and the RR are ratios of two quantities. The OR is the ratio of the odds of exposure to a risk factor among case subjects over the odds of exposure among control subjects. The RR is the ratio of the incidence rate for the disease among the exposed groups over the incidence rate among the nonexposed group.
- Both measures being ratios, a value of 1 indicates same odds or same incidence rates in the comparison groups; thus, a value of 1 indicates no relationship between exposure and disease outcome.

Nonetheless, there are also important differences between the two measures that are sometimes overlooked:

- The RR is based on the ratio of two incidence rates; i.e, the populations at risk are defined in terms of both numbers of population members and length (time) of exposure.
- ORs are based on odds, which in turn compare the proportions of exposed with nonexposed case subjects or control subjects, so no explicit time frame is attached.
- The OR is a symmetrical measure of association. Whether we divide the odds of exposure among case subjects by the odds of exposure among control subjects, or divide the odds of being a case subject among the exposed by the odds of being a case subject among the nonexposed, the resulting OR is the same.
- By contrast, the RR is not a symmetrical measure. In fact, it cannot be computed directly from case–control data, because case–control data do not yield incidence rates. To see why, revisit Table 10-1. To compute a true incidence rate of new melanomas developed after high (or low) levels of sun exposure, one would need to enroll representative samples of subjects exposed to high and low levels and see how many incident cases of melanoma develop over a specified observation period. Thus, the number of new melanoma cases observed in a cohort study is an empirical outcome recorded by the researcher. In the case–control study, it is the researcher who fixes the number of melanoma cases through sample selection. Such data cannot yield valid estimates of incidence rates.

Despite these clear, conceptual differences between ORs and RRs, we indicated earlier in Footnote 8 that there are special circumstances when case–control studies do yield a close approximation for RR. Recall first that the OR is a symmetrical measure. That is, it can be read as a measure of association that predicts odds of exposure based on outcome (case or control) status or as a measure predicting odds of case or control outcome based on exposure status. Furthermore, there is one situation in which the numerical value of the OR is very close to that of the RR. This occurs when the disease/outcome in question is relatively rare. Suppose that for a rare disease there are 20 incident cases per 100,000 exposed population at risk and 10 incident cases per 100,000 in the population not exposed. Assuming the same average exposure times in the comparison groups, the RR of development of the disease among the exposed group would be (20/100,000)/(10/100,000) = 2. The corresponding OR for these data would be (20/99,980)/(10/99,990) = 2.0002.[13] It

---

[12]In most research reports on case–control studies, this is the way the results are presented. For illustration, you may consult any of the case–control studies referred to in the readings.

[13]The reason for the closeness in the two measures is not hard to see. In the RR, the numerator in each comparison group is made up of the total population at risk; in the OR, the numerator is the population at risk *minus the patients in whom the disease developed*. If there are only a few of those, the OR will be very close to the RR.

is clear that under these circumstances, the OR provides a good approximation to the RR. Thus, if the investigator knows that a disease outcome is rare in a particular population, a case–control study can provide good estimates for the RR of exposure to the risk factor, even though incidence rates cannot be computed directly from such data.

A SHORT INTUITIVE INTRODUCTION TO LOGISTIC REGRESSION

So far, we have introduced the *unadjusted* OR as an empirical measure of association between exposure status and case/control or outcome status. This measure is akin to a simple, bivariate correlation coefficient depicting the strength of the relationship between just two variables. However, case–control studies use observational study designs, i.e., the researcher does not have the power to influence study participants' exposure or their case or control status. As always in observational studies, the next best thing a researcher can do is to control statistically for known (and measured) confounding variables that might otherwise distort the comparison of cases and controls.

The statistical technique of choice for adjusting ORs, taking into account the potential effects of confounding variables, is logistic regression analysis, which has found widespread application in the research literature of nursing and other health-related disciplines. **Logistic regression analysis** (LR) is a special type of (multivariate) regression analysis in which the dependent variable is dichotomous.[14] Because case–control studies focus on a dichotomous outcome variable—the presence or absence of a disease/disorder—a regression model that takes the odds of disease occurrence as the dependent variable and can accommodate multiple independent variables is well suited to this task. Conceptually, LR analysis is similar in many ways to linear, "regular" regression analysis after both sides of the regression equation, the dependent odds and the independent prediction equation, have been logarithmically transformed. However, for interpreting reported results, it is better to focus on the multiplicative version of the LR model, which can be depicted in the following equation:

- Odds of being a case subject = constant × OR associated with exposure variable 1 × OR associated with exposure variable 2 × OR associated with exposure variable 3, etc.; in short:

$$Y = C \times OR_1 \times OR_2 \times OR_3$$

In this model, the dependent or outcome variable can be thought of as the odds of being a case subject (having a diagnosis of melanoma) versus a being a control subject (not having melanoma). If p = the proportion of case subjects and $1-p$ is the proportion of control subjects, then $Y = p/(1-p)$, or the odds of being a case subject. Now, the crucial part is to see that these odds may change, depending on a study participant's exposure status. For instance, we know from our data in Table 10-1 that 210 study participants had low levels of exposure to sunlight, 90 of whom were case subjects and 120 of whom were control subjects. Thus, in this low-exposure group, the odds of being a case subject were $(90/210)/(120/210) = 0.75$. If we now multiply the odds of being a case subject in the low-exposure group by the OR of 2.67, we get $0.75 \times 2.67 = 2.00$. This value is exactly equal to the odds of being a case subject in the high-exposure group: $(60/90)/(30/90) = 2.00$. Thus, the OR gives us the crucial information of interest: how the odds of being a case subject change if exposure status changes. The LR generalizes this procedure to multiple predictor variables. Suppose the model contains, in addition to the variable of exposure to sunlight, the variable of race as a potential confounder: Whites are known to have a much higher risk of the development of melanoma than Blacks (American Cancer Society, 2002). Suppose the resulting equation now reads:

$$Y = C \times 2.2 \times 1.5, \text{ where C is a constant,}$$
$$OR_1 = 2.1 \text{ and } OR_2 = 8.5$$

The main difference here, compared with the original (unadjusted) OR of 2.67, is that the sunlight exposure OR (OR_1) has now been adjusted for the effects of race. The adjusted OR is now smaller (2.1 versus the original 2.67). This suggests that part of the originally estimated exposure effect was confounded by the race effect: Whites are more likely to expose themselves to the sun and incur a higher risk of contracting melanoma. However, if we hold the proportion of Whites and Blacks constant within each of the two sunlight exposure categories, the remaining exposure effect (which is independent of race) reduces to an OR of 2.1. Thus, we could say that differences in race have been accounted for, exposure to high levels of sunlight increase a person's odds of getting melanoma by a factor of 2.1, or more than 2 times. Like unadjusted ORs, adjusted ORs have their confidence limits. An example of interpreting such output from the literature follows.

▶CLINICAL RESEARCH IN ACTION
Example of a Case–Control Study
As mentioned previously, case–control and cohort study designs have a relatively long history of use in public health

---

[14]A comprehensive discussion is beyond the scope of this book. For an introductory treatment, see Munro et al. (2001); for a comprehensive treatment, see Hosmer and Lemeshow (2000).

and medicine, but only recently are these designs being recognized for their application to nursing research questions. In this section, we provide an example of a case–control study that illustrates many of the key concepts addressed in this chapter. We recommend a first-hand review of this article, including careful review of how the researchers attempted to control for extraneous/confounding variables in a retrospective analysis of medical records.

Herrinton and Husson (2001) recently published a report on a case–control study designed to test the hypothesis that girls who were tall before puberty would be at higher risk for the development of breast cancer in later life. The authors posit a causal mechanism for increasing the risk of breast cancer: it may, in part, be influenced by early puberty and the attendant earlier exposure to hormones. In turn, early puberty is a likely result of an "affluent-type" diet and lifestyle, for which height can serve as a "proxy" variable. Thus, indirectly, height during adolescence may be used as a predictor of breast cancer in later life. To test their hypothesis, the authors enrolled 214 case subjects, defined as patients using a long-term health plan, who had received diagnoses of breast cancer within a certain time interval and who were 12 years of age or younger when they joined the health plan. Also enrolled were an equal number of control subjects. These control subjects were matched with the case

subjects on (1) year of birth and (2) age of entry into the health plan. Women were excluded from the study if they reported a family history of maternal breast cancer.

The researchers gathered data about several variables, in addition to height, that could reasonably be expected to influence the development of breast cancer. These variables included demographic characteristics, presence of benign breast disease, weight, and menstrual and reproductive variables. The researchers computed the ORs for the association of breast cancer status with three height categories (short, medium, tall) based on measurements taken at each year of age. They also added a fourth category (missing) if a height measure could not be obtained from a year in that age category. The ORs were statistically adjusted for several confounding variables, which included the matched variables of birth year and age of entry into the health plan, marital status, use of alcohol, race, parity, age at first birth, and menopausal status.

The data in Table 10-2 show some of the results. The total sample consists of case subjects with diagnoses of breast cancer ($n = 214$) and control subjects who did not have a breast cancer diagnosis ($n = 214$). Among these 428 study participants, only 138 had records that indicated their height between the ages of 3 and 5. For 290 study participants (148 case subjects and 142 control subjects), records on their

TABLE 10.2	Association between Adolescent Height and Adult Breast Cancer (Expressed as Odds Ratios) Depending on Age When Height Was Achieved				
Age Category (Years)	Cases With Breast Cancer (*n*)	Controls Without Breast Cancer (*n*)	Height Category	OR	95% CI for OR
3–5	22	18	Short	1.0	Reference
	26	35	Medium	0.6	0.2, 1.4
	18	19	Tall	0.8	0.3, 1.9
	148	142	Missing	0.8	0.4, 1.7
6–8	27	29	Short	1.0	Reference
	25	29	Medium	0.8	0.4, 1.7
	33	35	Tall	0.9	0.5, 1.8
	124	119	Missing	1.0	0.6, 18
9–11	42	39	Short	1.0	Reference
	47	47	Medium	0.9	0.5, 1.7
	39	37	Tall	1.0	0.5, 1.8
	86	91	Missing	0.9	0.5, 1.5
12–14	37	37	Short	1.0	Reference
	35	56	Medium	0.6	0.4, 1.1
	77	55	Tqall	1.7	1.1, 2.8
	107	101	Missing	1.2	0.8, 2.0
15–18	22	34	Short	1.0	Reference
	37	49	Medium	1.2	0.6, 2.3
	59	42	Tall	2.2	1.1, 4.3
	96	89	Missing	1.7	0.9, 3.1

OR, odds ratio; CI, confidence interval.

Adapted with permission from Herrinton, L.J., & Husson, G. (2001). Relation of childhood height and later risk of breast cancer. *American Journal of Epidemiology, 154,* 618-623.

height during this early age were missing. The study participants with records ($n = 138$) were divided into the three height groups. For instance, 22 case subjects and 18 control subjects were classified as short when they were 3 to 5 years old, 26 case subjects and 35 control subjects were classified as medium tall when they were 3–5 years old, and so forth. Finally, for the OR comparisons, researchers compared the medium and tall height categories, as well as the case subjects without height data (missing), with the lowest height category (short). Because all other categories were compared with the lowest height category, it was called the reference category. Now, we are ready to interpret the results.

Table 10-2 shows, for example, that the odds of having breast cancer were 0.6 times lower among subjects who had attained a medium height than among subjects who had attained a short height when they were 3 to 5 years old. Because the associated 95% confidence interval includes the value of 1, we can actually not say that the odds of breast

Table 10.3.   Key Similarities and Differences Between Case–Control and Cohort Study Designs

Case–Control Study	Cohort Study
Observational/nonexperimental design	Observational/nonexperimental design
Goal: to establish an association between an antecedent, suspected risk factor ("exposure" variable) and a later disease/mortality outcome	Goal: to establish an association between an antecedent, suspected risk factor ("exposure" variable) and a later disease/mortality outcome
Focus on causal role of exposure in changes in health, disease/disorder cause	Both designs have an ultimate goal of prediction, mitigation, and/or prevention of disease/disorder
Selection of study subjects is based on disease mortality outcome: division of study sample into cases (with disease or adverse outcome) and controls (without disease/adverse outcome)	Selection of study subjects is based on exposure to risk factor: division of study sample into exposed and nonexposed study subjects (subjects must be disease free at time of study entry)
Design perspective: looks back from known outcome(s) to (multiple) potential risk factors/causes	Design perspective: look forward from known exposure to risk factors to (multiple) hypothesized disease/mortality outcomes
Timing of data collection: almost always retrospective, because outcome must be known at the time of enrollment of subjects (however, recruitment can be prospective in the sense that researchers wait for cases to be identified in the future)	Timing of data collection: both prospective and retrospective; retrospective cohort studies rely on existing records to identify study subjects based on information about past exposure; prospective cohort studies identify exposure status at the time of entry into study and monitor subjects (sometimes for years) to observe disease/mortality outcomes
Sample size: relatively small, often a few hundred study participants; sizes of cases and controls subsamples determined by researcher	Sample size: relatively large, sometimes tens of thousands of study participants (if outcomes in question are relatively rare events); sizes of exposed and nonexposed subsamples determined by researcher
Typical settings for subject recruitment: patients in individual hospitals, clients in particular clinics and community settings	Typical settings for subject recruitment: large-area populations (identified through disease registries, bureaus of vital statistics), populations enrolled in health maintenance organizations, health insurance programs, etc.
Typical data sources: to determine case/control status: both institutional records and interviews; for exposure status: mostly interviews involving recall, sometimes available institutional records	Typical data sources: for exposure status: interviews and institutional records, including disease registries, health maintenance organization and insurance databases, state community health records, vital statistics; for disease outcomes: mostly records, sometimes interviews
Methods of control over extraneous/confounding variables: matching of cases and controls during design stage; multivariate statistical controls in analysis	Methods of control over extraneous/confounding variables: matching of exposed and nonexposed special cohorts during design stage; multivariate statistical controls in analysis
Primary measure of association: odds ratio	Primary measure of association: relative risk (ratio of incidence rates)

cancer in the medium height group are different from those in the short height group. The same can be said about the tall group and the missing height group. Both appear to have the same odds of breast cancer as the short group, i.e., the reference group to which they are compared. The same pattern is repeated for height measures taken between ages 6 to 8 and 9 to 11. Differences in height at those ages do not appear to be related to the odds of having breast cancer as an adult. The picture changes only with the postadolescent measures. Women who were tall as 12- to 14-year-old girls had 1.7 time higher odds of the development of breast cancer than women who were short at the same age. This pattern is repeated and strengthened in later adolescence. Women who were tall as15- to 18-year-old girls had 2.2 times higher odds of the development of breast cancer than women who were short at the same age. In both age groups, the OR comparing tall and short girls has 95% confidence intervals that do not include the value 1. Thus, we can be reasonably confident that tallness in later adolescents is a predictor of the development of breast cancer in adulthood.

Contrary to their initial hypothesis, the authors observed the strongest association between height and breast cancer risk among girls after puberty, as opposed to before puberty. The researchers also adjusted the results for a variety of other variables, such as age of menarche, menopausal status, and maternal height, but they did not find that the results were affected by these adjustments. However, they noted other case–control differences, such as marital status, use of alcohol, and menopausal status, that may have affected the study findings but for which they had no measures.

CONCLUSION

In Chapters 9 and 10, we have presented the two main analytic/observational designs used by researchers to address possible causal relationships between hypothesized risk factors and disease/disorder/mortality outcomes: the cohort and case–control designs. Many risk factors that are investigated by use of the case–control and cohort approaches are behavioral risk factors. These are of special interest to nursing because they are, at least in principle, amenable to the types of educational interventions as well as prevention or mitigation efforts that are carried out by APNs in primary care and other community settings.

Both case–control and cohort designs represent attempts to illuminate causal relationships, even though the exposure to risk factors is not under the control of researchers and cannot be manipulated because of feasibility and ethical limitations. Nonetheless, accumulated evidence from many cohort studies and case–control studies can provide solid evidence for a causal link. The connection between smoking and lung or heart diseases is a classic case in point. No researcher has ever conducted an experiment that randomly assigned non-smokers to a regimen of 20 years of smoking versus non-smoking to see whether smoking raises the incidence rates of lung cancer, emphysema, or coronary heart disease. Yet, the evidence about the causal contribution of smoking to these diseases, gained from cohort and case–control studies, is very strong. The main reason is that so many different studies, each including samples from different target populations and statistically controlling for different sets of confounding variables, have found a significant relationship between smoking and lung and heart diseases. When this relationship can be confirmed among African Americans and European Americans; among men and women; among Japanese, South Africans, Germans, and Canadians; among vegetarians and carnivores, and among other populations, then it is time to accept a finding as convincing rather than as tentative.

Table 10-3 presents a brief summary of the key similarities and differences between the two types of study designs.

Suggested Activities

1. After reading a research article of your choice that is based on a case–control study design, address the following questions:
   a. Are there potential limitations to how the researchers classified subjects as case subjects or control subjects for the study? In your response, consider any potential issues for the reported study concerning data quality and/or diagnostic classification criteria that were used.
   b. How did the researchers ascertain information on exposure? Did they use records assembled before the outcome, or retrospective interviews conducted after the outcome or the case or control status of participants was known?
   c. If (a) significant difference(s) was/were reported between case and control groups, identify other plausible explanations for the study findings. To what extent did the researchers control for these plausible explanations in their study design? What specific control strategies did they use?
2. Describe how the concepts of OR and RR are similar to, and different from, each other. Under what specific circumstances is the OR a close estimate of RR?
3. Suppose you see in a newspaper a short summary report about a (hypothetical) study probing the health effects of exposure to certain chemicals. The report reads: "Researchers at X University compared two groups of people at Factory Y who either worked in a building where

they were exposed to Chemical A from 1990 to 1993 or worked during the same time in a different building without exposure to this chemical. On the basis of medical and insurance records, the researchers were able to detect a statistically significantly higher rate of lung cancer among the workers who were exposed to Chemical A."

a. What additional information would you want about this study, in order to interpret the study findings?

b. Does the study, as described in this newspaper excerpt, meet the criteria for a case–control study or a cohort study? Justify your answer with reference to the key features of case–control and cohort design. If you think there is not enough information to classify the design, outline the additional information that is needed to distinguish what type of design was used.

Suggested Readings

Herrinton, L.J., & Husson, G. (2001). Relation of childhood height and later risk of breast cancer. *American Journal of Epidemiology, 154,* 618-623.

References

Agresti, A. (1990). Categorical data analysis. NY: Wiley.

American Cancer Society. (2002). *Cancer facts & figures 2002. http://www.cancer.org/downloads/STT/CFF2002.pdf*

American Psychiatric Association. (1980). *Diagnostic and statistical manual of mental disorders* (3rd ed.). Washington, DC: American Psychiatric Association.

Beautrais, A. L., Joyce, P. R., Mulder, R. T., Fergusson, D. M., Deavoll, B. J., & Nightingale, S. K. (1996). Prevalence and comorbidity of mental disorders in persons making serious suicide attempts: A case–control study. *American Journal of Psychiatry, 153,* 1009–1014.

Brain Tumor Society. (2002). *http://www.tbts.org/welcome.htm*

Carson, S. (1997). Human papillomatous virus infection update: Impact on women's health. *Nurse Practitioner, 22,* 24–25, 28–30, 35–37.

Cockburn, M., Hamilton, A., & Mack, T. (2001). Recall bias in self-reported melanoma risk factors. *American Journal of Epidemiology, 153,* 1021–1026.

Dwyer, T., Ponsonby, A. L., Newman, N. M., & Gibbons, L. E. (1991). Prospective cohort study of prone sleeping position and sudden infant death syndrome. *Lancet, 337,* 1244–1247.

Ford, R. P., Mitchell, E. A., Stewart, A. W., Scragg, R., & Taylor, B. J. (1997). SIDS, illness, and acute medical care. *Archives of Disease in Childhood, 77,* 54–55.

Gibson, E., Dembofsky, C. A., Rubin, S., & Greenspan, J. S. (2000). Infant sleep position practices 2 years into the "back to sleep" campaign. *Clinical Pediatrics, 39,* 285–289.

Habel, L. A., Stanford, J. L., Vaughan, T. L., Rossing, M. A., Voigt, L. F., Weiss, N. S., & Daling, J. R. (1995). Occupation and breast cancer risk in middle-aged women. *Journal of Occupational and Environmental Medicine, 37,* 349–356.

Herrinton, L. J., & Husson, G. (2001). Relation of childhood height and later risk of breast cancer. *American Journal of Epidemiology, 154,* 618–623.

Hosmer, D. W., & Lemeshow, S. (2000). *Applied logistic regression.* (2 nd ed.). New York: John Wiley.

Hurwitz, E. S., Barrett, M. J., Bregman, D., Gunn, W. J., Pinsky, P. (1987). Public health service study on Reye's syndrome and medications: Report of the pilot phase. *Journal of the American Medical Association, 257,* 1905–1911.

Hutchinson, M. K. (1999). Individual, family, and relationship predictors of young women's sexual risk perceptions. *Journal of Obstetrics, Gynecologic & Neonatal Nursing, 28,* 60–67.

Lannin, D. R., Mathews, H. F., Mitchell, J., Swanson, M. S., Swanson, F. H., & Edwards, M. S. (1998). Influence of socioeconomic and cultural factors on racial differences in late-stage presentation of breast cancer. *Journal of the American Medical Association, 279,* 1801–1807.

McKenzie, I., & Wurr, C. (2001). Early suicide following discharge from a psychiatric hospital. *Suicide & Life-Threatening Behavior, 31,* 358–363.

Munro, B. H. (2001). *Statistical methods for health care research* (4th ed.). Philadelphia: Lippincott Williams & Wilkins.

Scragg, R. K., Mitchell, E. A., Stewart, A. W., Ford, R. P., Taylor, B. J., Hassall, I. B., Williams, S. M., & Thompson, J. M. (1996). Infant room-sharing and prone sleep position in sudden infant death syndrome. *Lancet, 347,* 7–12.

Snedecor, G. W. & Cochran, W. G. (1989). Statistical methods (8th ed.), Ames, IA: Iowa State University Press.

Stamler, J., Elliott, P., Stamler, R., Dyer, A., Marmot, M., & Kesteloot, H. (1994), Non-pharmacological treatment of hypertension. *Lancet, 344,* 884–885.

Willinger, M., Hoffman, H. J., & Hartford, R. B. (1994). Infant sleep position and risk for sudden infant death syndrome: Report of meeting held January 13 and 14, 1994, National Institutes of Health, Bethesda, MD. *Pediatrics, 93,* 814–819.

Willinger, M., Hoffman, H. J., Wu, K. T., Hou, J. R., Kessler, R. C., Ward, S. L., Keens, T. G., & Corwin, M. J. (1998). Factors associated with the transition to nonprone sleep positions of infants in the United States. *Journal of the American Medical Association, 280,* 329–335.

CHAPTER 11 Survey Studies

INTRODUCTION TO SURVEYS

This chapter focuses on a common method used to obtain data from research participants: the **survey study.** Approaches to survey studies are quite varied, but they share the core requirement that the data are based on **self-reports** of subjective perceptions and observations from human respondents. This essential element of survey studies can be contrasted, for example, with biophysiologic measurements, such as blood pressure or temperature, in which data are collected from human subjects, but the subjects do not provide self-report data. This distinction is quite important because the validity of surveys relies heavily on both the willingness and the ability of human respondents to report their perceptions accurately. As will be discussed in more detail, surveys cannot be used with persons who are unable to provide valid self-reports, for example, preverbal infants or study participants who have severe cognitive impairments. Nonetheless, when used appropriately, survey studies can provide much useful information for health-related research. As examples, consider four recently published survey studies of health- and care-related topics.

►CLINICAL RESEARCH IN ACTION
Four Examples of Survey Studies

Bradley et al. (2002) studied domestic violence issues among 1871 women who attended 22 selected general (primary care) practices in Ireland. The practices were selected to obtain variation based on the sex of the practitioner and the location and type of practice. The participating patients were asked about their experiences with various types of domestic violence, its severity, and the contexts in which it occurred. The researchers also asked about the extent to which the patients favored routine questioning about domestic violence by their practitioner.

Craft-Rosenberg, Powel, and Culp (2000) asked a convenience sample of 31 rural homeless women who lived in a shelter about their physical and mental health as well as their self-care and risk behaviors. Information obtained about health status, health needs, substance use, and access to care providers was compared with similar information for the population as a whole to determine areas of special need worthy of interventions.

Willinger et al. (1998) analyzed data from repeated cross-sectional telephone surveys conducted between 1992 and 1996. Each year, the surveys reached a nationally representative (random) sample of U.S. households in which a new baby had been born within the previous 7 months. Survey questions focused on the sleeping positions of the infant and factors associated with the transition to nonprone sleeping positions.

Using data from two panel studies, the National Longitudinal Survey of the Labor Market Experience of Youth and the Panel Study of Income Dynamics, Hofferth et al. (2001) focused on the relationship between a mother's age at the birth of her first child and how much education she receives in the end, comparing several cohorts from the early 1960s through the early 1990s.

These four recent survey studies give an indication of the variety of survey designs that are used in health care research. Surveys range from small-scale studies conducted by just one person (e.g., a nurse in an obstetrics/gynecology practice inquiring about the well-being of new mothers and their infants 3 months after birth) to large, multi-million dollar studies conducted by teams of survey specialists (e.g., a study designed to provide an accurate picture of national target populations at the National Center of Health Statistics [Box 11-1]).

Surveys have become the most commonly used tool for gathering information about life in industrialized societies. For instance, knowledge about crime and divorce rates, unemployment and inflation rates, consumer preferences (market research), and political attitudes (public opinion research) is all based on surveys. Likewise, health-related research relies heavily on surveys to obtain information about such topics as the physical frailty of and support for the elderly, the prevalence of diseases for which there are no population registries, the number and proportion of people in the population without health insurance, out-of-pocket expenditures for health care services, hospital bed occupancy rates, and so forth.

Because much of the information that is collected on the population's health and illness comes from surveys conducted at the national level, it is important for users of this information, such as advance practice nurses (APNs), to be familiar with the key advantages and limitations of survey methods. In addition, APNs are increasingly involved in the design and implementation of survey studies that are done as part of clinical practice. For example, an APN may conduct a survey study of patient satisfaction in a local or regional health care setting. Several chapters in this book address survey research methods. In this chapter, we focus our discussion on the principles of survey design, including the advantages and limitations of surveys. In subsequent chapters (chapters 16, 19, and 20), we address more practical considerations and solutions to the potential limitations of survey approaches, specifically, issues in questionnaire design (chapter 16) and sampling from target populations (chapters 19 and 20). Survey studies are sometimes considered particular types of observational, nonexperimental study *designs*. It is probably more accurate, however, to think of surveys as a particular method of *data collection* rather than as a study design. For instance, in the previous two chapters, we introduced cohort and

BOX 11.1   Examples of Longitudinal Survey Studies Conducted by the National Center for Health Statistics

The National Ambulatory Medical Care Survey. Provides data on ambulatory care delivered in physicians' offices. Conducted every 1 to 2 years since 1973.
The National Hospital Ambulatory Medical Care Survey. Provides data on ambulatory care delivered in hospital emergency rooms. Conduced every 1 to 2 years since 1992.
The National Hospital Discharge Survey. Provides data on hospital utilization in the U.S. Conducted annually since 1973.
The National Health Interview Survey. Collects data on social, demographic, and economic aspects of illness, disability, and the use of medical services for the civilian, noninstitutionalized U.S. population. Conducted every 1 to 2 years since 1957.
National Health and Nutrition Examination Survey (NHANES). Collects information about the health and diet of U.S. residents. Since 1960, eight surveys have been conducted. The latest is a continuous survey conducted since 1999, involving a sample of 5000 residents from 15 U.S. locations.
The National Long-Term Care Survey. Provides data on functional limitations and assistance patterns of the U.S. elderly population residing in the community. Conducted every 5 to 6 years since 1982.
The National Medical Expenditure Survey. Provides data on U.S. household expenditures for any kind of health care services as well as insurance coverage. Conducted infrequently since 1987.
The National Nursing Home Survey. Provides data on nursing homes in U.S. Conducted infrequently (every 5–10 years) since 1969. The latest was conducted in 1995.

case–control study designs. These designs often use survey information to assess outcomes or to screen populations for exposure to risk factors. In earlier chapters (chapters 4 and 5), we introduced intervention studies, some of which used survey methods to obtain information on psychosocial outcomes (Moser, Dracup, & Doering, 2000; Rothert, Holmes-Rovner, Rovner, Kroll, Breer, Talarczyk, Schmitt, Padonu, & Wills, 1997). Nonetheless, most of the time, when researchers refer to *surveys,* they have in mind non-experimental, observational, or descriptive research studies.[1] That is to say, the main emphasis in surveys is on their descriptive, information-gathering capacity rather than on the goal of testing causal relationships. From the point of view of study design, surveys can be divided into **cross-sectional studies,** in which information is obtained at a single point in time, and **longitudinal studies,** in which information is obtained repeatedly on two or more occasions.

PRINCIPAL FEATURES OF SURVEY STUDIES

As mentioned at the beginning of this chapter, survey studies are varied in their specific approaches to data collection,

but they all include the collection of self-report data from human respondents. In this section, we discuss the three key features of surveys:

1. Sampling of survey participants
2. Questioning of study participants
3. Standardization and quantification of survey questions

Sampling of Survey Participants

Sample Survey Versus Population Census
Typically, it is not feasible for a researcher to study each person in the target population of interest. For instance, a researcher who is interested in patients' satisfaction with health care received from nurse practitioners would not survey every living person in the United States who has ever received health care from a nurse practitioner. Instead, the researcher would rely on sampling methods to select a subset of the broader target population for study.[2] Only if the target population of interest is quite small would a researcher attempt to study all subjects in the population. For example, in educational research, it is not uncommon for researchers to study all of the students in a given grade level in an institution. Likewise, for certain types of rare diseases (e.g., an annual incidence rate of 1 in 1,000,000), a researcher may study all people who are identified as having that disease. In

---

[1]Here, we use the term *observational study* in the sense in which it was used in chapter 8, where we also used the terms *correctional, descriptive,* and *expost facto* studies. All of these terms emphasize the different aspects of the nonexperimental nature of the study design in question.

[2]A more detailed discussion of available sampling methods and procedures is provided in chapters 19, 20, and 21.

RESEARCH SCENARIO 11.1

Example of Sampling in an HMO Relocation Impact Survey

Suppose that the management of an HMO with approximately 40,000 members is interested in moving its structurally outdated central patient clinic to another location. It has been estimated that a larger, state-of-the-art facility can be built and operated at lower cost. To minimize loss of membership, the management decides to obtain information on enrollees' opinions on the proposed move. A survey researcher hired by the management counsels against a population census of HMO enrollees. He explains that, if the goal is to minimize error, with the amount of resources budgeted for the survey, it is more important to reduce other types of errors than to minimize pure sampling errors. For example, if the management wants to ensure that at least 80% of the current membership would welcome the move, a sample of 419 randomly chosen HMO members would be enough to detect, with 95% confidence, a 5% deviation from this level of satisfaction. If HMO management needs to attain greater accuracy and wants to be able to detect deviations as small as three percentage points, a random sample of 1139 members would be sufficient.* Yet, even obtaining a sample of this size is far removed from the need to survey all 40,000 HMO enrollees.

*The principles and calculations underlying these results will be presented in chapter 20.

that case, the study is a **population census** rather than a **sample survey.** However, with rare exceptions, such as when the target population of a research project is manageably small, surveys usually are, and should be, sample surveys.

A **sample**[3] is formally defined as a subset of cases from the target population. One reason for using samples of respondents is to lower the cost of conducting a sample survey. Another reason, as strange as it may seem, is that information from a well-designed sample survey can actually be more accurate than information from a population census, which is aimed at interviewing all members of a target population. Why is this so? Let's consider the example in Research Scenario 11-1.

---

[3]This definition as well as various techniques of selecting samples will be discussed in greater detail in chapters 19, 20, and 21.

Sources of Error in Surveys

The example given in Research Scenario 11-1 illustrates only one type of error, known as **sampling error.** This error occurs when the sample selection process results in a sample that does not faithfully reflect the characteristics of the target population. Yet, compared with other sources of error and bias in a survey, sampling error may actually be less important. Consider the following list of problems that may become sources of bias or error in surveys:

1. The survey questions themselves, including their formatting
2. The accuracy and interpretability of the responses
3. The consistency of the data collection procedures across survey participants
4. The accuracy of information about the membership of the target population
5. Refusal to participate among selected sample members
6. Item nonresponse by respondents participating in the survey

As this list illustrates, random sampling error is not necessarily the most important problem in designing a survey study. For instance, if the rate of nonresponse or refusal to participate in a study is high among a subgroup of the target population, it may be worthwhile to allocate more resources toward reducing barriers to study participation in the randomly selected subset of the target population as opposed to using most of the resources in a quest to contact everyone. For example, if a researcher wants to foster the participation of community-dwelling older adults in an exercise program, regardless of their household income, it may be better to obtain a smaller, but unbiased, sample by removing barriers to participation, such as transportation to and from the exercise program site. Likewise, if a question is worded awkwardly and is not understood or is misinterpreted by many survey respondents, the responses to this question are useless, even if all members of the target population provide an answer.

Good surveys, therefore, must minimize *total survey error* (Anderson, 1970; Fowler, 2002), and not just sampling error. To accomplish this goal, a survey designer and health maintenance organization (HMO) manager, as illustrated in Research Scenario 11-1, must engage in a discussion about tradeoffs between acceptable versus unacceptable errors as well as the costs and resources needed to reduce these possible errors. This action requires knowledge of both the strategies to reduce errors and the costs of the resources involved.

Sampling and Units of Analysis

When designing and interpreting results from a survey study, it is always important to distinguish between the units of analysis (such as analysis of data from patients, clinic visits, or primary care practices) and the sources of information. In all surveys, it is individual respondents who are the sources of information: they respond to written questions on questionnaires or web sites or to questions asked during telephone or personal interviews. However, this does not mean that the survey researcher is necessarily interested in questions about the individual respondents.[4] Instead, the researcher may be interested in other units of analysis, such as the health care agencies for which the respondents work. Sometimes researchers focus on multiple units of analysis within a given study, such as when they collect information on both the individual respondent and the respondent's family or household characteristics. More specifically, survey studies may be designed to seek information about one or more of the following:

- The individual respondent who participates in the survey
- Persons other than the respondents, such as caregivers providing information about care recipients
- The respondent's family or household unit, such as the head of a household giving information about household characteristics
- Organizations and agencies in which persons hold defined positions, such as managers, employees, or even customers
- Events, actions, or situations, regardless of the persons involved, such as visits to hospitals or primary care practices, regardless of whether they are repeat visits with the same patient or with different patients

When units of analysis are not identical to the individual survey respondents, researchers must consider the implications for sampling respondents. One common issue in surveys is that available databases that serve as **sampling frames**[5] for the target population may be organized on the basis of units other than those of interest to the survey researcher. For instance, hospital and insurance records are often organized on the basis of visits or services. In this case, the basic entry unit is a particular service or a bundle of services given at a particular time. If a sample were drawn from such a data file without proper adjustments, patients who have multiple visits or many services would be systematically overrepresented in the final sample. Consider a patient who, in a given calendar year, has five visits to the emergency department of a hospital and another patient who has only one visit. Sampling from records that consider each visit a *case* would mean that the first patient has a five times greater chance of being selected. It is easy enough to make the appropriate adjustments,[6] and yet these issues are often overlooked.

Questioning of Study Participants

As has been mentioned already, the questioning of study participants, with the corresponding self-reports, is a defining characteristic of surveys. This characteristic distinguishes surveys from other methods of gathering information, such as direct observations of people's behaviors, audits of certain types of administrative medical records, or biophysiologic measures. However, there are many different ways to "ask questions." They include:

- Questionnaires mailed to individual respondents
- In-person interviews
- Internet web sites that allow viewers to enter responses
- Telephone interviews

Each of these various methods of administering questionnaires has its advantages and disadvantages.[7] A key issue with any of these data collection methods is **participant nonresponse.** To some extent, all survey studies suffer from biases inherent in nonresponse of study respondents (Fowler, 2002). We will address practical strategies for reducing nonresponse in survey samples in a later chapter (chapters 19–20). Here, we focus our discussion on the definitions of and the problems associated with response rates in health-related surveys.

A survey **response rate** is defined as the following ratio:

$$\frac{\text{number of persons completing the survey interview}}{\text{number of persons eligible and approached for the survey sample}}$$

For example, if a researcher identified and contacted an eligible sample of 400 women with newly diagnosed breast cancer and succeeded in interviewing 280 of them, the re-

---

[4]The primary units of analysis may also be population subgroups. For example, current National Institutes of Health (NIH) research priorities (including priorities for nursing research; see *http://www.nih.ninr.gov*) strongly emphasize health disparities (inequalities) of subgroups in the overall U.S. population, which by definition requires at least subgroup level data analyses of survey data. However, in that case, information on the subgroups is *aggregated* from information obtained on individual members of these subgroups.

[5]The term *sampling frame* refers to a list of the members of the target population from which the research actually draws the sample, such as telephone listings, administrative records, and so forth. In chapter 19, we will consider in more detail the problems and issues associated with the use of such sampling frames.

[6]See chapter 19 for different sampling plans.

[7]For a detailed discussion, see chapter 16.

sponse rate would be 70% [(280/400) × 100]. It is clear from the definition of the response rate that its magnitude can be influenced by *both* the numerator (number of persons actually interviewed) *and* the denominator (number of persons eligible for the sample). This point is an important one in many health care studies because it is sometimes difficult to determine, with accuracy, which persons are eligible for a study without having some information available before the interview. For instance, in many clinical studies, eligibility criteria include clinical criteria (such as elevated troponin levels to identify patients with acute coronary symptoms) coupled with social criteria (such as discharge to a local cardiologist after hospitalization, the ability to speak English, or the accessibility of the discharged person via telephone for follow-up interviews). Social criteria often cannot be obtained unless this information is volunteered when the person is asked for consent to participate in the study. If the person refuses to consider the request before this information is obtained, it may not be possible to obtain a completely accurate figure on the eligible, but nonparticipating population.

Concerns about Nonresponse in Health-Related Studies

What are the specific reasons to be concerned about response rates? Even if a researcher succeeds in *approaching and contacting* a true probability sample of the eligible target population, the contacted persons who consent to participate are likely to differ systematically from those who refuse to participate. For instance, Neumark, Stommel, Given, & Given (2001) showed that among patients who were contacted within 6 weeks after the diagnosis of cancer, those with lung and colon cancer were much less likely to consent to participate, whereas those who identified a support person or caregiver were much more likely to participate. In general, there is ample evidence that persons who are or feel ill are less likely to participate in studies (Thompson et al., 1994). Because subjects for most clinical studies are patients who have various diseases or illnesses, there may be a frequent bias toward enrolling relatively "healthy" or "nonsymptomatic" subjects, at least when compared to those who refuse to give their consent to participate.

Fortunately, this general tendency can be offset by other factors. For example, research participation is often fostered by the perception of the study participants that clinical research is important to improving health and, thus, is worthwhile to support. It is not unusual that patients who are experiencing substantial health problems nonetheless are well motivated to help by volunteering information

in the hope that the research findings will benefit future patients (Aday, 1996). In addition, there are many useful strategies to increase response rates. These strategies depend on:

- The specific data collection techniques used
- The target population to be studied
- The specific study design, in particular, the cross-sectional or longitudinal nature of the study (Given).

In addition, both ethical and feasibility considerations must play a central role in any incentives used to foster study participation.

Despite available methods for improving response rates, relatively few clinically oriented survey studies achieve very high response rates (> 80%), so researchers must address the limitations to their conclusions resulting from lower response rates. In the final analysis, when response rates are lower than 80%, it is reasonable to expect that there will be some sort of bias. It is incumbent on the researchers to take steps to determine what biases might be present as well as to analyze and present information about how problematic (or unproblematic) the biases may be relative to the goals of the study. For example, readers of a research report should expect not only a clear accounting of all subjects approached and those who responded, but also some effort to analyze the nature of the bias resulting from nonresponse. Fortunately, clinical research studies conducted within health care or other organizations often provide the advantage of having at least some information available about the pool of eligible patients who chose not to participate. For example, sex, age, and insurance distributions in study samples can often be compared with those in the target population as a whole. Not all biases related to nonresponse can be identified in this way, but if no differences exist on some characteristics between the study sample and the target population, the confidence increases that the effects of nonresponse may not severely limit the interpretation of the results.

Item Nonresponse

Nonresponse is an issue not only with respect to participation in a study as a whole, but also with respect to responses to particular items or questions on the survey. Suppose that in a survey containing a total of 120 questions, the average response is about 98% to 99% per item, but two items generate more than 20% refusal or nonresponse. This kind of **item nonresponse** can also lead to bias when analyzing data involving the variables in question. Often, the reason for such disproportionate refusal is either some technical defect in the way the questions were posed or a special sensitivity that the item provoked among the survey partici-pants. For example, participants may be confused by items that are not clearly worded, or they may be reluctant to pro-vide information about socially or personally sensitive is-sues, such as drug misuse or household income. Although item nonresponse can have implications for drawing infer-ences from sample data, at its core, it is a measurement is-sue, and thus will be discussed in more depth in the chap-ter on measurement (chapter 16).

Standardization and Quantification of Survey Questions

A final key aspect of survey studies concerns the standard-ization and quantification of response options. In quantita-tive survey studies, the responses to the survey questions are usually standardized and predetermined by the re-searcher.[8] An advantage of having survey respondents choose among fixed ("closed-ended") response alterna-tives is that it is possible to attach numerical values to the response categories. For instance, the predetermined re-sponses to the question, "How satisfied are you with the services you received in this primary care clinic?" could be coded in the following way:

Very satisfied = 4
Somewhat satisfied = 3
Somewhat unsatisfied = 2
Very unsatisfied = 1

Although survey researchers rely mostly on closed-ended response formats, exploratory questions with "open-ended" response formats may also be used. Open-ended response formats are useful when the researcher wants to obtain additional information from respondents that may not be fully "captured" by fixed response options. How-ever, when samples are relatively large (N > 100), open-ended, narrative responses can be both challenging and time-consuming to analyze. In contrast, with a structured instrument, in which most response categories are prede-termined and standardized across respondents, quantifica-tion is possible. The primary advantage of quantification is that it vastly facilitates the analysis. Box 11-2 provides a summary of the main advantages and disadvantages of providing respondents with fixed versus open response options.

[8]See chapters 12 and 18 for an overview of qualitative research approaches, which often rely on nonstandardized, nonpredetermined response options.

SURVEY DESIGNS

As mentioned earlier, survey studies typically use nonex-perimental, observational study designs. From a design point of view, the main issues in survey studies are the sampling design and the timing of the observations or in-terviews for data collection. We discuss sampling issues separately in Chapters 19, 20, and 21. As far as the overall timing of the observations is concerned, the fundamental choices are similar to those in experimental studies: sur-veys are either cross-sectional or longitudinal, and the specific timing of measurements is ideally well-matched to the research questions and the phenomena that are be-ing studied.

Cross-sectional Surveys

Previously, we defined cross-sectional surveys as studies in which information is obtained at a single point in time and longitudinal surveys as studies in which information is obtained repeatedly on two or more occasions. Given the special circumstances associated with subject recruitment in many clinical studies, these definitions need to be ex-panded somewhat. The "classic" cross-sectional approach to surveys is exemplified by studies seeking to establish the prevalence of attitudes, behaviors, or health and illness events (e.g., Schwartz et al., 2000; Fischbacher et al., 2001). Typically, such studies are designed to obtain a rep-resentative sample of a clearly defined target population, with actual data collection taking place within a short pe-riod of time, such as 2 to 3 months.

However, because large samples of clinical popula-tions are not always easy to come by, it is not uncommon for the accrual of study participants in large-scale studies to take several months or longer. For example, a recent study of domestic violence involved a survey of women attending primary care practices for which subject accrual took more than a year (Bradley et al., 2002). Just the same, even though the interview in this study did not take place at a single point in time in a literal sense, the study design is still considered cross-sectional because every sample member was interviewed once and the underlying target population is unlikely to have experienced dramatic changes with respect to the phenomenon investigated: the preva-lence and severity of domestic violence.

It is important to note that the cross-sectional character of a survey is based entirely on the fact that such a study involves only one interview per survey participant. How-ever, this does not mean that the researchers' interests are confined to current events.

BOX 11.2 — Advantages and Disadvantages of Predetermined Response Categories in Survey Instruments

Advantages

- Highly structured instruments are easier to fill out and answer, reducing demands on respondents, who simply indicate agreement or disagreement with given responses.
- Predetermined response categories do not require efforts of verbal formulation from respondents. Usually, the greater the demands on respondents' verbal skills, the more likely it is that response rates will be lower and *biased* toward those in the target population who have higher literacy skills.
- Predetermined response categories clarify questions by providing a frame of reference. For example, a question about living arrangements may include categories such as *living alone, living with a spouse, living with unrelated individuals in the same household,* and so forth.
- Structured questions yield the same answer categories across responses, greatly facilitating comparison across respondents.
- Highly structured interview schedules are almost necessary for self-administered questionnaires. Requiring potential respondents to write many open-ended responses leads to relatively large-scale nonparticipation.
- Limited and standardized response categories simplify analysis. Highly structured interview schedules are necessary in studies that involve large samples (N > 100) because it is very time-consuming to analyze a large set of open-ended responses.

Disadvantages

- Although easier to analyze structured questionnaires require thorough preparation. A researcher must already know a great deal about the subjects in the target population to avoid misleading questions, ill-defined response categories that force respondents into unwanted choices, or categories that disregard distributions of characteristics in the target population. (For a discussion of structured questionnaires, see Chapter 16.)
- The main limitation of predetermined, or fixed, response categories is their limited usefulness in exploring new topic areas and learning something unanticipated about the respondents. (For a more detailed discussion of open-ended interviews, see Chapter 18).

Indeed, as we have seen in the previous chapter on case–control designs (chapter 10), such studies are sometimes conducted relying entirely on survey data, as when information about the history of exposure to a risk factor is obtained in the interviews. For example, many of the studies examining risk factors for sudden infant death syndrome (SIDS) rely on one-time interviews of parents of *cases* (babies who purportedly died of SIDS) and parents of *controls* (babies who did not die of SIDS [e.g., Scragg et al., 1996]). Thus, as long as it is reasonable to expect interviewees to answer questions accurately about past events, behaviors, observations, and so forth, cross-sectional surveys need not be confined to information about current events.

However, in many situations, respondents are unable to recall past events or emotions or physical states (Stone, Turkkan, Bachrach, Jobe, Kurtzman, & Cain, 2000), thus necessitating repeated interviews over time, if the purpose of the study is to capture changes in individual respondents or populations; hence, the need for longitudinal surveys.

Longitudinal Surveys

Longitudinal surveys can be divided into two broad categories:

1. Surveys that are primarily focused on tracking changes over time in a *population*
2. Surveys that seek information about changes in *individual respondents*

Repeated Cross-sectional Surveys

The annual National Health Interview Survey (NHIS) conducted by the National Center of Health Statistics (NCHS, 2003) is a **repeated cross-sectional survey** (since 1957) that is representative of the civilian, noninstitutionalized resident population in the United States. Each year, a different sample is chosen to reflect, among other characteristics, the changing ethnic and age composition of the U.S. resident population. Such data can be used to show trends in the population as a whole, with respect to a host of health behaviors. Other repeated cross-sectional surveys conducted by NCHS include the National Medical Care Expenditure Survey (NMCES), which tracks, for instance, changes in the health insurance coverage of the U.S. population, and the National Health and Nutrition Examination Surveys (NHANES), which combine household interview data with medical examinations performed in mobile units (NCHS, 2003). Although repeated cross-sectional surveys based on random samples allow us to track population changes, each new survey is a representative sample of the target population at the time the survey is conducted. Therefore, these types of surveys *cannot* speak to changes *within* individual respondents over time. With different random samples from a large population, the probability that the same individual respondents would appear in successive surveys is rather small, making it impossible to track individual changes. Successive cross-sectional surveys do not necessarily reflect average individual change either, because population change is affected both by changes in individual population members and by changes in the composition of the population.

Panel Studies

More often than not, clinicians tend to be more interested in changes that occur *within* individual respondents over time. Only repeated interviews with the *same individual respondents* allow documentation of changes in individual respondents over time. Surveys that use repeated interviews with the same subjects are called **panel studies.** During the last decade, there has been a veritable explosion in the number of panel studies funded by the National Institutes of Health. Although the design and conduct of panel studies can be difficult and data analysis is almost always complex, the popularity of panel studies is easily explained in terms of their potential to address many questions of interest to health researchers.

As previously noted, however, mere interest in individual change over time would not necessarily require the use of panel studies. If people had perfect memories and could recall all events of interest to the researcher, there would be no need for panel studies because all of the necessary information could be collected retrospectively. For example, if patients with cancer could report not only their current symptoms, but also their past symptoms, with a high degree of accuracy, information from a single interview would allow us

to reconstruct the time path and changes in symptoms since diagnosis. Of course, patients usually cannot do this; thus, repeated measurements or interviews are required to record changes over time (Kurtz, Kurtz, Stommel, Given, & Given, 2002). In short, the fundamental rationale for panel surveys is that they yield data that allow us to examine changes occurring at the individual level (Korn & Graubard, 1999).

Timing of Interviews in Panel Studies. Panel studies are inherently prospective because the interviews can only be planned and conducted in the present and the future. However, it is important to recognize the fundamental distinction between the timing of the *events* of interest and the timing of the interviews during which the information is collected. *In fact, what should be considered the "proper" timing of the interviews in panel studies is one of the difficulties in designing such studies.* Ideally, one would like the interviews to occur at such times that the major changes in subjects are adequately captured. For instance, it is a well-known phenomenon that, after a myocardial infarction, many patients exhibit high levels of depressive symptoms. To capture these elevated levels of depression as well as their eventual decline, the survey interviews must be timed to reflect the changes occurring (Barber, Stommel, Kroll, Holmes-Rovner, & McIntosh, 2001). Similarly, the "best" timing of panel interviews that reflect major events in the course of a disease or its treatment requires either substantial prior information or trial and error (Given et al., 1999). To some degree, there is no adequate general solution to this problem of timing of panel interviews because disease and illness trajectories vary considerably from patient to patient. On the other hand, if the study target population is defined in terms of a signal event, such as the initial diagnosis of a disease, such event-*based samples* (Campbell, 1991) or *inception cohorts* (Given et al., 1999) offer greater chances of making sense of postevent developments or changes because all study participants start from a common baseline. Yet, even in the case of an inception cohort of newly diagnosed patients with cancer, fixed time intervals to the next follow-up interviews may find some panel respondents undergoing chemotherapy during a follow-up interview and others not, a situation that surely affects the responses to questions about physical and depressive symptoms (Kurtz et al., 2001). When panel studies involve heterogeneous samples with respect to the onset of a critical relationship or event, as would be the case in caregiver studies that enroll caregivers who differ in terms of the length of time that they have been involved in caregiving (short-term, medium-term, or long-term caregiver cohorts), patterns of change observed during the panel study may differ depending on cohort membership.

Panel Studies and Cohort Studies. Very little distinguishes a panel survey from a cohort study. Both are non-experimental, observational studies with repeated measures of the study participants. The differences are largely based on:

- The data collection method
- The selection of the study participants
- The focus of the research question

Panel surveys rely on interviews for data collection. In contrast, cohort studies often add available external records as additional sources of information, especially with outcomes such as death (vital records) or hospitalization (insurance records). However, *if such external data sources are not available and all information collected stems from a few repeated interviews, then cohort studies are indistinguishable from panel studies.*

However, although cohort studies that rely exclusively on interview data are panel studies, not all panel studies should be considered cohort studies. It is usually possible to tell the difference by considering the *selection process* by which study subjects are sampled. As discussed in chapter 9, study subjects in cohort studies are either initially selected based on their exposure to putative risk factors (special cohort study), or if exposure occurs after the first interview (general cohort study), subjects are later assigned or reclassified from "nonexposed" to "exposed" status. In both cases, the intent is to obtain evidence that sheds light on a causal relationship between risk factors and disease outcomes. Thus, the main focus of a cohort study is on the comparison of groups of subjects that differ with respect to their exposure status.

In contrast, in general panel studies, the goals of researchers tend to be broader. Rather than maintaining the narrow focus on disease outcomes or mortality rates, non-cohort panel studies are used as a means of examining developmental as well as growth and decline processes in individual respondents and groups of respondents. Thus, the emphasis is more on describing processes of change than on finding the causes for a few well-defined outcomes.

Age, Period, and Cohort Effects

Health researchers are often interested in understanding "age effects." However, the interpretation of statistically significant age effects can often be challenging, not only when based on cross-sectional data, but also when based on panel data. For example, consider a typical cross-sectional study. The subjects enrolled in such a study may be of varying ages, say, caregivers between 30 and 80 years old. Now suppose that the analysis shows that, even after controlling for many confounders, such as sex, education, income, relationship to the care recipients (spouse versus child caregivers), and so forth, there is a statistically significant positive relationship between age and scores on a standardized depression scale. Should such a finding be interpreted to mean that depression increases with age? Even if there are good reasons to believe that most or all relevant confounding variables were controlled for, there remains a fundamental problem with interpreting an age effect.

Essentially, when an age effect is inferred based on cross-sectional data, the *assumption* is made that, when the younger study subjects grow to be as old as the older study subjects, they will exhibit the same levels of depression as the older subjects do now. A similar issue arises with other time-related processes. Suppose that, in a cross-sectional study, a researcher compares patients whose cancer was diagnosed at different times in the past. Using a variable such as "months since diagnosis," the researcher would, in effect, make the assumption that patients with recent diagnoses will eventually "look like" patients with more distant diagnosis dates. In other words, it is assumed that the future states of recently diagnosed patients are adequately described by the current states of other patients who have survived the disease for longer periods. This may or may not be the case, however.

The key issue with "growth" or "change" interpretations based on cross-sectional data is that cross-sectional studies entail a complete confounding of **age, period,** and **cohort effects.** To see why, consider the data presented in Table 11-1. The rows in this table show five **birth cohorts,** or generations (groups of persons defined in terms of their year of birth, from 1940–1980). The columns indicate the years, or **periods,** of observations and the numbers show the birth cohorts' **age** at the time of observation. Suppose, in 2000, a researcher conducted a cross-sectional survey of persons 20 through 60 years of age to determine age-related changes in depression. A cross-sectional sample drawn in this year (period) would correspond to the shaded column labeled "2000."

It is clear that, by necessity, the age of the respondents and their birth cohorts are completely confounded. For instance, respondents who were 60 years old in 2000 were born during World War II, whereas those who were 30 years old in 2000 were born at the end of the Vietnam War. Thus, the two groups represent both differences in biologic age and two birth cohorts with substantially different historical experiences. These experiences include exposure to many health-relevant factors, such as nutrition, environmental pollution, medical knowledge and technology, immunization rates, access to health services, and so forth.

| Table 11.1 | | | Age, Period, and Cohort Effects* | | | | |

	Year (Period) of Observation						
Birth Year	**1950**	**1960**	**1970**	**1980**	**1990**	**2000**	**2010**
1940	10	20	30	40	50	60	70
1950		10	20	30	40	50	60
1960			10	20	30	40	50
1970				10	20	30	40
1980					10	20	30

*Numbers indicate ages of persons belonging to different birth cohorts in the year or period of observation.

Now, suppose that the researcher had obtained depression data from a panel study of a single birth cohort conducted over four decades. In Table 11-1, four cells of the first row are shaded, corresponding to a panel study that began with 30-year-old study participants in 1970 who were re-interviewed every 10 years. This time, the study design will allow us to generate data that reflect intraindividual changes in depression over time; however, these changes are completely confounded with the period effects. These may include general social changes that are independent of the aging effects. For instance, society may have changed with respect to the acceptability of reporting on mental health problems. If so, higher depression rates reported in later years may simply reflect social change rather than a true age effect. Finally, suppose that the available panel data include members of several birth cohorts. In Table 11-1, this situation is depicted with heavy lines shown around a rectangular array of entries. Thus, the panel study starts by enrolling 20-, 30-, and 40-year-old subjects in 1980 and follows them for three decades. The resulting data will, over time, produce information about subjects of the *same age*, but who are in *different birth cohorts*. This is shown in the diagonal entries. For instance, the 1980 interviews contain data from 40-year-old subjects who are part of the 1940 birth cohort, the 1990 data contain information from 40-year-old subjects who are part of the 1950 birth cohort, and so forth. With a complex design such as this, it will be possible to disentangle at least partially the age and cohort effects (Wolinsky, 1990). Although a detailed discussion of various panel–cohort designs is beyond the scope of this book, the purpose of this discussion is to provide a note of caution when interpreting study results in terms of age effects. As time passes and different age cohorts appear, with different historical experiences, age effects themselves are subject to change.

VALIDITY OF DATA OBTAINED FROM SURVEY STUDIES

It is always important to consider whether the questions asked of survey respondents have been answered truthfully. This is not a small matter when designing and evaluating surveys concerned with health and illness issues; yet, it is an issue that has received insufficient attention in the interpretation of results from survey studies. This section presents an overview of some survey validity issues.

The Use of Proxy Informants

The issue of what kinds of information can appropriately be asked of respondents arises in several situations. One issue goes back to the unit of analysis problem, which arises when the researcher seeks information about persons, organizations, or other entities that differ from the source of information. For example, suppose the respondent answering the questions (the informant) is asked to provide information about family matters. In such cases, the researcher needs to know *which* potential informant or survey respondent is likely to be the most knowledgeable about the subject area addressed in the survey questions. Choosing the wrong informants may result in data that are not useful in addressing the research questions. For instance, parents are not always knowledgeable informants about the risk-taking behaviors of their adolescent children. Spouses may or may not be aware of clinically significant depression in their partners. As these examples make clear, *identifying the best source of information for the questions in the survey is of fundamental importance to the successful execution of a survey.*

The use of informants (other than the patients themselves) is widespread in health care surveys, particularly in studies of older adults (Basset, Magaziner, & Hebel, 1990). The reasons are simple: older patients may have substantial cognitive impairment as a result of stroke or dementia, for example. Many other groups of interest to health researchers, such as the mentally ill, may also be unable to provide valid self-report data. This issue highlights the importance of understanding the limitations of using proxy informants. As a general principle, the informant must have access to the information in question, and this may well preclude the use of informants concerning most subjective experiences and preferences. More specifically, if a researcher wants to know about a person's attitudes, beliefs, or pain experiences (highly personal, subjective experiences or perceptions), the person must be asked directly. Friends and family members, even if they are close to the person about whom the information is sought, may not be reliable substitutes. Even in the case of observable *behaviors,* the use of informants can be problematic. Did the informant really have the opportunity to observe the behaviors in question? That depends on how "public" the behavior is and whether the informant is typically present when the behavior occurs. For instance, caregivers who live with their care recipients are likely to be better informed about the care recipients' limitations in activities of daily living, certainly compared with caregivers who live in different homes. On the other hand, the living arrangement of caregivers may not affect their knowledge of the care recipients' hospitalizations during the previous month.

Another example that is quite familiar to almost all nurses is inferences about the amount of pain experienced by patients who recently had surgery. There is now a substantial body of research showing that nurses have historically underestimated the amount of pain experienced by patients, based on the belief that the observed behavior of the patient is a reliable indicator of pain. For example, past studies have shown that many nurses believe that patients who are quiet, appear relaxed, are not spontaneously expressing pain (with sighs, groans, or other verbal indications), and are otherwise cooperative with care "can't be in much pain," and therefore should not need pain medica-

tion. Thus, the clinical care of patients has often been based on nurses' observations of the behaviors of patients, as opposed to asking patients directly about their levels of pain (Hollen, Hollen, & Stolte, 2000; Moore, 2001). Such studies have resulted in a reevaluation of pain assessment. In turn, new clinical care guidelines have been developed, including national initiatives for acute pain management, which incorporate measures of pain that rely more directly on patient self-reports, such as asking the patient to rate the severity of pain on a scale of 1 to 10, to guide clinical decisions about the type and dosage of pain medication used.

Despite these examples, which show the importance of respondents' self-reports with respect to many subjects, for some questions, informants other than the primary survey respondents may, in fact, be *better* sources of information. For example, in the age cohorts born before World War II, among couples in traditional marriages, it is not uncommon to find that only the husbands are knowledgeable enough to answer questions about the family's finances, whereas wives are the better informants about nutrition or the use of health services. *Overall, there are few general rules concerning the acceptability of proxy informants other than this: the behaviors and actions must be observable in principle, and the proxy informant must have been exposed to them* (Basset, Magaziner, & Hebel, 1992). Using informants to obtain information about third parties may also raise ethical concerns because the persons about whom information is gathered may not have consented to participate in the survey (Bersoff & Bersoff, 2000).[9]

Problems with Recall

Even if survey respondents are asked about their *own* attitudes, opinions, or behaviors, the problem of what can be reasonably asked of survey respondents remains an important one. Health care and nurse researchers are often interested in events, behaviors, or attitudes about which respondents may find it difficult to offer truthful information. Principally, there are two reasons for not obtaining the desired information from respondents: they may be *unable* to answer the questions or they may be *reluctant* or *unwilling* to answer them.

Health care and nurse researchers often want to obtain information about respondents' past behaviors or about past events that might explain current health outcomes. For example, a researcher might ask a sample of adult respondents to list all vaccinations received during childhood, to indicate how often they have been taking certain medicines

---

[9]A detailed discussion of confidentiality issues is presented in chapter 24.

over the last 3 months, and so forth. Even if the respondents are perfectly willing to answer such questions, they may have substantial recall or memory problems. Often, when past behaviors are not salient in the memory of a respondent, it may be difficult to obtain accurate information. This is particularly important in health-related research because subjects are very often identified *after* a signal health or illness event, such as a myocardial infarction or a diagnosis of breast cancer. Thus, patients' recall may be the only way to obtain information about causally important events that occurred *before* subject identification.

For instance, when studying depression among patients newly diagnosed with cancer, it is important to distinguish between depressive symptoms that occur as a temporary response to the initial diagnosis or treatment and long-standing depression that is independent of the cancer diagnosis (Stommel, Given, & Given, 2002). However, because cases are identified only after the diagnosis, the question arises as to how accurate such retrospectively obtained information might be. Research on recall basis and response shift (Kreulen et al., 2002) indicates that it may not be possible to obtain accurate information on past emotional states and attitudes in current survey interviews because they are heavily colored by the respondent's current experience. One approach to this issue is to have the patient or another informant provide "verification" of mood states via ratings of specific behaviors that are likely to be well-correlated with the emotional states or attitudes, such as functional status, days missed from work because of depression (depression disability days), and so forth. However, this approach to validation of psychological distress information does not fully address recall bias or response shift issues, especially when data about behaviors are gathered during the interview as opposed to being audited from archival measures obtained at the time in question. Sometimes attitudes and judgments, such as those about the severity of symptoms, may well be subject to a change in the frame of reference. This situation is technically known as a *response shift* (Kreulen et al., 2002). For example, when asked how burdensome a current physical limitation is or how "fit" the respondent feels, it is worth remembering that such questions are answered with a certain frame of reference in mind. *After* an automobile accident, for instance, a recovering surgical patient may consider the ability to climb stairs "excellent," even though it does not nearly reflect the patient's abilities before the accident.

Recall issues also come into play, when respondents are asked to give detailed information about frequently occurring behaviors and actions, such as nutritional patterns or

out-of-pocket expenditures for various medications or health care services. As a general rule, the less context-based, the less emotionally salient, and the more frequent and routine the actions of interest are, the more difficult it is for most respondents to give accurate information (Menon & Yorkston, 2000; Kihlstrom, Eich, Sandbrand, & Tobias, 2000). Finally, recall of past behavior is often subject to a *recency effect:* respondents' recent experiences with the behavior and actions in question tend to dominate questions about long-term patterns of such behaviors (Neath, 1993).

Other Sources of Response Bias in Health-related Survey Research

Memory problems, although certainly an important issue in survey studies, are not the only sources of bias in subject responses. Recent research has shown that a respondent's awareness of symptoms depends, to some extent, on the competition among cues (Pennebaker, 2000; Barsky, 2000). For instance, people who live alone tend to report more physical symptoms (Mahon, Yarcheski, & Yarcheski, 1993), as do respondents who are under stress (Goldman et al., 1996). Similarly, questions asked by health researchers sometimes provoke socially acceptable responses, as when patients who are asked about their adherence to medical regimens may be tempted to err on the side of the "expected" responses (Rand, 2000).

Finally, it is important to acknowledge that people sometimes have good reasons for refusing to participate in a survey, for refusing to answer some questions, or even for lying in response to specific questions. For instance, when claims are made about the proportion of men or women who engage in homosexual behavior, the proportion of women who are physically abused, or the number of people who use illegal drugs or possess firearms, then it is time to reflect on the limitations of surveys as sources of information or at least to recognize that the survey estimates may be biased, even when proper probability sampling was used. For an example, see Box 11-3.

It is important to keep in mind that there are many sensitive subject areas, other than sex, that may provoke respondents to be less than forthcoming. For example, the veracity of survey responses about income or urinary incontinence could be open to challenge as well as the responses to questions about some alternative medicines, given the highly sensitive nature of this kind of information in American society. The real problem with such questions is that researchers often lack an independent means of verification of self-reports: it is not always possible to

---

BOX 11.3   Sexual Practices and Behaviors in the United States

A few years ago, a renowned Harvard biologist published a strongly worded polemic directed at the authors of a study on sexual practices and behaviors in the United States (Lewontin, 1995). The authors' study was based on data from the *National Health and Social Life Survey* conducted by the National Opinion Research Center at the University of Chicago (Laumann et al., 1995). Among its many findings, the survey results showed that, *on average,* men report 75% *more* female sexual partners than women report male sexual partners.

Because it is a law of arithmetic that the *average* number of heterosexual partners in the population must be the same for men and women, it is necessary to conclude that either men "brag" or women "underreport." Of course, there are other logical possibilities, such as that American men have more sex abroad than American women, but these "explanations" lack credibility, given available information on travel abroad.

---

observe the underlying behaviors on which the survey responses are supposed to be based.

Despite these examples of validity problems in survey data, we hasten to add that none of this means that survey studies should be subject to generalized suspicion. It might be tempting to conclude that only "objective" measures, such as biophysiologic measures, are truly valid. However, these data collection methods often have their own sources of error that are no less problematic than those associated with survey data (see chapter 14). In addition, there are many areas in which survey results can be (and have been) compared with independent sources of information, such as medical records (Palmore, 1991). However, a user of survey data should ask the following questions of survey studies. These questions provide guidance about situations in which the survey results may not provide fully valid information:

- Are the questions that are being asked of survey respondents "answerable"? For example, do they overtax the ability of respondents to give correct answers because they require impossible memory feats?
- Are some of the questions that are being asked "socially sensitive"? For example, are there possible motives for respondents to be less than forthcoming about how they really think, feel, or behave?
- Should biases be expected because of the mental or emotional state of the respondents?
- Are there any independent sources of information that can corroborate the survey responses?

USE OF SURVEYS IN CLINICAL SETTINGS

It is not uncommon for APNs and other health professionals to conduct small-scale surveys in clinical settings.

Some of these surveys are conceived as research projects from the start, whereas others are conducted primarily to obtain data that serve as feedback to clinicians or administrators. Regardless of the primary purpose, survey studies should never be conducted without explicit statements of their objectives and explicit rules for eligibility, recruitment, and selection of survey respondents or without survey instruments whose contents are clearly related to the survey objectives. Furthermore, successful completion of a survey, like any other study, requires observation of the rights of human subjects, confidentiality in data handling, and special skills in data entry and data analysis procedures. Thus, before any survey is begun in a clinical practice setting, it should undergo a realistic assessment of the required resources and costs in terms of time, personnel, and equipment. Given the limited funding usually available, decisions must be made carefully, with expert consultation, about the scope of the survey project and the avoidance of sampling or measurement biases.

Although the discussion in this chapter has been concerned with design and validity issues involved in survey studies, we will list here some of the basic skills that are needed for the successful completion of a survey. Two key components of any survey are questionnaire design and sampling techniques, both of which will be discussed at greater length in later chapters. For other skills, we list several excellent references that describe the necessary steps involved in designing and implementing survey studies (Box 11-4).

►CLINICAL NURSING RESEARCH IN ACTION
Examples of Survey Studies

In this section, we briefly discuss two recently published survey studies. One is a cross-sectional study, and the other is a longitudinal panel study. The first study is a small-scale

> ## BOX 11.4 Steps and Skills for Conducting Surveys
>
> The conduct of any survey requires the following steps and skills. Depending on the scope of the survey and its sample size, a study may demand the cooperation of tens, if not hundreds, of people, some with highly specialized skills. On the other hand, a small-scale survey can sometimes be conducted "in-house" by a single person, perhaps with some clerical and technical support. Still, the same general issues and skills must be addressed:
>
> * Formulating survey goals includes identifying what information is needed and why and determining whether survey methods are the best way to obtain this information.
> * Covering important concepts and choosing measurement instruments involves evaluating existing measurement tools.
> * Designing the overall questionnaire requires skills in formulating and formatting questions.
> * Defining the target population and establishing eligibility criteria, recruitment procedures, and sampling plans involves skills in sampling techniques and determination of sample size.
> * Interviewing survey participants includes deciding on the best mode of survey administration.
> * Conducting interviews in a manner appropriate for the target population requires interviewing skills as well as graphic design skills for written questionnaires.
> * Devising procedures for collecting and recording data that minimize error and maximize confidentiality involves knowledge of available technologies, such as appropriate computer programs.
> * Assuring competence in data management and data cleaning procedures requires quality control procedures that are designed to ensure consistency, especially in long-term, ongoing data collection efforts.
> * Performing statistical analysis requires specific skills as well as familiarity with appropriate software.
> * Writing final reports and interpreting results.
>
> This list is not intended to discourage beginning researchers from conducting small-scale surveys in clinical settings. However, it is important to systematically consider each of these issues in advance. Many very useful tools are now available for the beginner (Fink, 2002), and with increased confidence and competence, beginning researchers will develop the skills needed to conduct more complex surveys.

(N = 31), cross-sectional survey of rural homeless women in Iowa (Craft-Rosenberg et al., 2000). Although the study reports only on homeless women affiliated with one particular rural shelter, it exemplifies the use of survey techniques to obtain a rich descriptive account of women's health problems and access to health resources. A major rationale for the study was that most of the literature on homelessness focuses on the urban homeless, so that even a report on a *specific* group of rural homeless women would make a contribution toward widening the debate about homelessness. Using the existing literature on urban homelessness as a foil, the researchers argued the need for descriptive information on these women's physical and mental status, dental status, and substance use, as well as the identification of previous adverse life events. They also explored the health status of the women's children as well as their resources and access to health care providers. For each of these areas of focus, the researchers either identified existing standardized instruments (such as Beck's Depression Inventory to gauge the prevalence of depression in this population as part of the mental health evaluation) or modified existing tools to address such issues as health history, family structure, and personal resources. The survey's respondents included all

of the women at a particular shelter (N = 31). Thus, the data may be considered a convenience sample from the much larger target population of rural homeless women in America, but it could also be seen as a population census, albeit from a very narrowly defined target population, consisting of the members of a particular shelter. The researchers obtained 100% cooperation from all women in the shelter, the likely effect of an incentive to combine the interview with a free physical and dental assessment at the shelter. The results are reported in terms of descriptive statistics (such as means and frequency distributions), which is appropriate in the absence of probability sampling and the lack of specific hypotheses to be tested. This study also highlights the sometimes problematic use of proxy informants: many women in the shelter were unable to report on their children's health, especially if the children were in foster care, had been adopted, or were cared for by others. The researchers reported inconsistencies even in the numbers of children reported by the women, pointing to the possibility that questions about their children were a very sensitive area for these women. All in all, this study provides a good example of the usefulness of descriptive surveys, even when done on a small scale. By reporting the descriptive results against the background of the wider (urban) homelessness literature, the researchers show how description can be enhanced with the use of a comparative context.

Armstrong-Stassen, Cameron, Mantler, & Horsburgh (2000) examined the effect of hospital mergers on nurses' job attitudes and morale. Specifically, the researchers examined panel data obtained on job satisfaction and organizational trust and commitment from nurses in (originally) four hospitals. Data were collected at three points in time: 2 years before the announcement of the hospital merger, at the beginning of the merger negotiations, and at the completion of the merger. The panel data were used to test specific hypotheses suggested in the literature: that employees in merged organizations are likely to experience a decline in job satisfaction as well as organizational trust and commitment and that employees in acquired organizations would show a bigger decline in these attitudes as well as in job satisfaction than employees in acquiring organizations. A total of 146 nurses (53 in acquired and 93 in acquiring hospitals) provided data at all three interviews and remained working at the same institution. Although the authors examined turnover *intentions,* indicated by the respondents in the interviews, they did not examine actual turnover among early interviewees who later dropped out of the study. The value of this study, however, derives from the fact that it examines attitude data obtained before, concurrent with, and immediately after ongoing merger events, thus allowing for direct comparisons before, during, and after the mergers. Data such as job satisfaction scores, organizational trust ratings, or intentions to quit could not have been obtained validly retrospectively. The study also provides an example of the use of panel data to test hypotheses as well as to provide more descriptive, exploratory evidence.

CONCLUSION

In this chapter, we introduced survey studies as one of the quantitative observational study designs. As with all other nonexperimental study designs, causal interpretation of relationships identified through survey data must be handled with caution because the lack of manipulation of a treatment variable and the lack of control over confounding variables can be alleviated only through the usual mechanism of statistical control. Thus, surveys should be considered primarily a tool to *describe* various target populations. However, their unique advantage lies in the fact that, when combined with probability or random sampling and the use of standardized instruments, they can produce highly accurate data representative of very large populations. As such, they have become an indispensable tool for describing the health and illness status as well as the health care needs of entire nations, state populations, or other specific populations, such as enrollees in specific health care plans. Furthermore, re-

peated cross-sectional surveys can be used to track changes in populations over time, and panel studies allow for monitoring changes over time in persons and groups of persons. Because survey studies, whether cross-sectional or longitudinal, rely on self-report data, their principal limitations derive from the inability or unwillingness of persons or certain groups of persons to participate and to provide accurate responses. Because health care researchers are often interested in vulnerable subpopulations, these limitations are occasionally substantial, but creative approaches to sampling and questioning can overcome many of them.

Suggested Activities

1. An APN would like to survey patients about their level of satisfaction with nurse coaching for a diabetes self-care program. The patient population includes about 70 patients with Type I diabetes who regularly attend primary care follow-up visits, including appointments with physicians and the APN.
   a. What sampling design (population census versus sample survey) would you recommend that the APN use? Justify your choice with respect to the likely advantages and disadvantages of each approach.
   b. What issues in terms of patient responses must be considered with regard to:
      i. Nonresponse or lack of response
      ii. Other validity issues with data and responses
   c. What are possible strategies for managing the issues identified in points i and ii above?
2. Read one or both of the Clinical Nursing Research in Action sections discussed in this chapter. Then critique the following:
   a. What are the possible or likely sources of biases in the survey sample that was used?
   b. To what extent were biases controlled for or explained by the researcher?
   c. Suggest feasible improvements for the limitations that you identified that could be implemented in a similar future study.

References

Aday, L. A. (1996). *Designing and conducting health surveys* (2nd ed.). San Francisco: Jossey-Bass.

Andersen, R., Kasper, J., Frankel, M. R. and Associates (1979). *Total survey error: Applications to improve health surveys.* San Francisco, CA: Jossey-Bass Publishers.

Armstrong-Stassen, M., Cameron, S. J., Mantler, J., & Horsburgh, M. E. (2000). The impact of hospital amalgamation on the job attitudes of nurses. *Canadian Journal of Administrative Sciences, 18,* 3, 149–162.

Barber, K., Stommel, M., Kroll, J., Holmes-Rovner, M., & McIntosh, B. (2001). Cardiac rehabilitation for community-based patients with myocardial infarction: factors predicting discharge recommendation and participation in such programs. *The Journal of Clinical Epidemiology, 54*, 10, 1025–1030.

Barsky, A. J. (2000). The validity of bodily symptoms in medical outpatients. In Stone, A. A., J. S. Turkkan, C. A. Bachrach, J. B. Jobe, H. S. Kurtzman, & V. S. Cain (Eds.), *The science of self-report: Implications for research and practice* (pp. 339–361). Mahwah, NJ: Lawrence Erlbaum.

Bassett, S. S., Magaziner, J. and Hebel, J. R. (1990). Reliability of proxy response on mental health indices for aged, community-dwelling women. *Psychology and Aging, 5, 1*, 127–132.

Bersoff, D. M., & Bersoff, D. N. (2000). Ethical issues in the collection of self-report data. In Stone, A.A., J. S. Turkkan, C. A. Bachrach, J. B. Jobe, H. S. Kurtzman, & V. S. Cain (Eds.), *The science of self-report: Implications for research and practice* (pp. 9–24). Mahwah, NJ: Lawrence Erlbaum.

Bradley, F., Smith, M., Long, J. and O'Dowd, T. (2002). Reported frequency of domestic violence: cross sectional survey of women attending general practice. *British Medical Journal, 324, 2*, 271–4.

Campbell, R. T. (1991). Longitudinal research. Pp.1146–58 in: E. F. Borgatta and M. L. Borgatta (Eds.), *Encyclopedia of Sociology, Vol. 3;* New York, NY: MacMillan.

Craft-Rosenberg, M., Powel, S. R., & Culp, K. (2000). Health status and resources of rural homeless women and children. *Western Journal of Nursing Research, 22, 8*, 863–878.

Fink, A. (2002). *The survey kit* (2nd ed.). Thousand Oaks, CA: Sage.

Fischbacher, C. M., Bhopal, R., Unwin, M., Walker, M., et al. (2001). Maternal transmission of type 2 diabetes varies by ethnic groups: cross-sectional survey of Europeans and South Asians. *Diabetes Care, 24, 9*, 1685–6.

Fowler, F. J. (2002). *Survey research methods* (3rd ed.). Thousand Oaks, CA: Sage.

Given, C. W., Given, B. A., Stommel, M., & Azzouz, F. (1999). The impact of new demands on caregiver depression: tests using an inception cohort. *The Gerontologist, 39*, 1, 76–85.

Goldman, S. L., Kraemer, D. T., & Salovey, P. (1996). Beliefs about mood moderate the relationship of stress to illness and symptom reporting. *Personality & Individual Differences, 41*, 115–28.

Hofferth, S. L., Reid, L. and Mott, F. L. (2001). The effects of early childbearing on schooling over time. *Family Planning Perspectives, 33, 6*, 259–67.

Hollen, C.J., Hollen, C.W., & Stolte, K. (2000). Hospice and hospital oncology unit nurses: a comparative survey of knowledge and attitudes about cancer pain. *Oncology Nursing Forum, 27*, 10, 1593–1599.

Kihlstrom, J. F., Eich, E., Sandbrand, S., & Tobias, B. A. Emotion and memory: implications for self-report. In Stone, A.A., J. S. Turkkan, C. A. Bachrach, J. B. Jobe, H. S. Kurtzman, & V. S. Cain (Eds.), *The science of self-report: Implications for research and practice* (pp. 81–100). Mahwah, NJ: Lawrence Erlbaum.

Korn, E. L., & Graubard, B. I. (1999). *Analysis of health surveys*. New York: John Wiley.

Kreulen, G. J., Stommel, M., Gutek, B. A., Burns, L. R. and Braden, C. J. (2002). The utility of retrospective pretest ratings of patient satisfaction with health status. *Research in Nursing & Health, 25, 3*, 233–41.

Kurtz, M. E., Kurtz, J. C., Stommel, M., Given, C. W. and Given, B. A. (2001). Physical functioning and depression among older persons with cancer. *Cancer Practice, 9, 1*, 11–18.

Kurtz, M. E., Kurtz, J. C., Stommel, M., Given, C. W., & Given, B. A. (2002). Predictors of depressive symptomatology of geriatric patients with lung cancer: a longitudinal analysis. *Psycho-Oncology, 11*, 12–22.

Laumann, E. O., Gagnon, J. H., Michael, R. T., & Michaels, S. (1995). *The social organization of sexuality: Sexual practices in the United States.* Chicago: University of Chicago Press.

Lewontin, R. C. (1995). Sex, lies, and social science. *The New York Review of Books, 37*, 7, 24–29.

Mahon, N. E., Yarcheski, A., & Yarcheski, T. J. (1993). Health consequences of loneliness in adolescence. *Research in Nursing & Health, 16*, 1, 23–31.

Menon, G., & Yorkston, E. A. (2000). The use of memory and contextual cues in the formation of behavioral frequency judgements. In Stone, A.A., J. S. Turkkan, C. A. Bachrach, J. B. Jobe, H. S. Kurtzman, & V. S. Cain (Eds.), *The science of self-report: Implications for research and practice* (pp. 63–80). Mahwah, NJ: Lawrence Erlbaum.

Moore, S.E. (2001). A growth of knowledge in pain management. *Pediatric Nursing, 27*, 3, 307.

Moser, D. K., Dracup, K., & Doering, L. V. (2000). Factors differentiating dropouts from completers in a longitudinal, multi-center clinical trial. *Nursing Research, 49*, 2, 109–116.

NCHS (2003). *National Center for Health Statistics: Surveys and Data Collection Systems.* http://www.cdc.gov/nchs/express.htm

Neath, I. (1993). Distinctiveness and serial position effects in recognition. *Memory & Cognition, 21, 5,* 689–98.

Neumark, D. E., Stommel, M., Given, C. W., & Given, B. A. (2001). Research design and subject characteristics predicting nonparticipation in a panel survey of older families with cancer. *Nursing Research, 50,* 6, 363–368.

Palmore, E. C. (1991). Medical records as sampling frames and data sources. In Lawton, M., & R. Herzog (Eds.), *Special research methods for gerontology* (pp. 127–135). Amityville, NY: Baywood.

Pennebaker, J. W. (2000). Psychological factors influencing the reporting of physical symptoms. In Stone, A.A., J. S. Turkkan, C. A. Bachrach, J. B. Jobe, H. S. Kurtzman, & V. S. Cain (Eds.), *The science of self-report: Implications for research and practice* (pp. 299–316). Mahwah, NJ: Lawrence Erlbaum.

Rand, C. (2000). 'I took the medicine like you told me, doctor': self-report of adherence with medical regimens. In Stone, A.A., J. S. Turkkan, C. A. Bachrach, J. B. Jobe, H. S. Kurtzman, & V. S. Cain (Eds.), *The science of self-report: Implications for research and practice* (pp. 257–276). Mahwah, NJ: Lawrence Erlbaum.

Rothert, M. L., Holmes-Rovner, M., Rovner, D., Kroll, J., Breer, L., Talarczyk, G., Schmitt, N., Padonu, G., & Wills, C. (1997). An educational intervention as decision support for menopausal women. *Research in Nursing & Health, 20,* 377–387.

Schwartz, L. M., Woloshin, S., Sax, H. C., Fischhoff, B., Welsh, H. G. (2000). U.S. women's attitudes to false-positive mammography results and detection of ductal carcinoma in situ: cross-sectional survey. *Western Journal of Medicine, 173, 5,* 307–12.

Scragg, R. K. R., Mitchell, E. A., Stewart, A. W., Ford R. P. K., Taylor B. J., et al. (1996). Infant room-sharing and prone infant position in sudden infant death syndrome. *The Lancet, 347, 1,* 7–12.

Stommel, M., Given, B. A., & Given, C. W. (2002). Depression and functional status as predictors of death among cancer patients. *Cancer, 94,* 10, 1–9.

Stone, A. A., Turkkan, J. S., Bachrach, C. A., Jobe, J. B., Kurtzman, H. S., & Cain, V. S. (Eds.), (2000). *The science of self-report: Implications for research and practice.* Mahwah, NJ: Lawrence Erlbaum.

Thompson, M. G., Heller, K., and Rody, C. A. (1994). Recruitment challenges in studying late-life depression: Do community samples adequately represent depressed older adults? *Psychology and Aging, 1,* 121–5.

Willinger, M., Hoffman, H. J., Wu, K. T., Hou, J. R., Kessler, R. C., et al. (1998). Factors associated with the transition to nonprone sleep positions of infants in the United States: The National Infant Sleep Position Study. *Journal of the American Medical Association, 280,* 329–335.

Wolinsky, F. D. (1990). *Health and Health Behavior among Elderly Americans: An Age-Stratification Perspective.* New York, NY: Springer Publications.

Special Resources for the Beginning Survey Researcher

Converse, J.M., & Presser, S. (1986). *Survey questions: Handcrafting the standardized questionnaire* [QASS No. 63]. Thousand Oaks, CA: Sage.

Fink, A. (2002). *The survey kit* (2nd ed.). Thousand Oaks, CA: Sage.

Fowler FJ. (2002). *Survey research methods* (3rd ed.). Thousand Oaks, CA: Sage.

Henry GT. (1990). *Practical sampling.* Thousand Oaks, CA: Sage.

CHAPTER 12 Qualitative Research Approaches

AN INTRODUCTION TO QUALITATIVE RESEARCH

Thus far in this book, we have focused almost exclusively on quantitative approaches to clinical research. In this chapter, as well as in chapters 18 and 21, we concentrate on some key conceptual and methodologic aspects of **qualitative research** to show how qualitative research is both distinctive and complementary to quantitative research. Our approach does not provide a comprehensive discussion of qualitative research methods and their associated philosophic underpinnings. Instead, we compare and contrast qualitative and quantitative research, including an emphasis on the usefulness of the two research approaches for addressing particular kinds of research problems. To get a sense of the kinds of issues and problems often addressed in qualitative research inquiry, consider the following research questions taken from six qualitative studies:

- Using a *phenomenologic research method* as a guide, a study uses in-depth, face-to-face interviews to explore the lived experience of 15 Taiwanese women with breast cancer (Chiu, 2000).
- Using *interpretive interactionism,* ten members of the Mt'kmaq, First Nation Community in New Brunswick, Canada, are interviewed in depth to gain an understanding of their hospitalization experiences from their perspectives in a culturally sensitive way (Baker & Daigle, 2000).
- Using participant observations, diaries, and field notes obtained in homes and at a day care center, 15 elderly Iranian immigrants to Sweden are studied *ethnographically* to explore the cultural appropriateness of a Swedish municipality's day care intervention program (Emami, Torres, Lipson, & Ekman, 2000).
- In-depth, cross-sectional interviews guided by a *feminist approach* are used to explore the meanings of menopause among 21 low-income Korean immigrant women, with a focus on how these meanings are constructed within their daily life experiences (Im & Meleis, 2000).
- *Grounded theory* is used to devise a theoretic framework that describes the problem of sexual violence by male intimates from the point of view of 23 women who have experienced such violence at some time in their lives (Draucker & Stern, 2000).
- *Heideggerian hermeneutic phenomenology* provides the framework and methods for a study of 24 U.S. Army nurses to explore the experiences of these nurses as they engage in advocating practices and to describe the shared practices and their common meaning (Foley, Minick, & Kee, 2000).

All of these studies are examples of using qualitative research approaches to provide "qualitative description," albeit with different "hues, tones, and textures" (Sandelowski, 2000a) that depend on the specific qualitative methods that are used. These studies focus on types of research questions that are generally more difficult to address with quantitative research approaches, such as *exploration of the meanings that study participants or patients give to events, decisions, or experiences.* This emphasis on *meaning* in qualitative research is often viewed as one of its most distinctive traits (Streubert & Carpenter, 1999).

Research Questions: Meaning Versus Causation

Qualitative approaches are sometimes used in combination with quantitative methods. For example, quantitative research is appropriate for studying the prevalence of AIDS or HIV infection in various population groups (Valleroy, MacKellar, Karon, & Rosen, 2000), the pressure-reducing properties of alternative cushion surfaces to provide relief from decubitus ulcers (DeFloor & Grypdonck, 2000), racial disparities in access to standard cancer therapy (Breen, Wesley, Merrill, & Johnson, 1999), or the (causal) effectiveness of various nursing interventions (Brown, 2002). These kinds of research questions require either large, representative samples of major population groups—using sample surveys, insurance files, or population registries—or controlled experiments or quasi-experiments that can isolate intervention effects from among a host of other (confounding) variables. As just mentioned, however, qualitative methods can be very useful in addressing certain questions in quantitative studies. For instance, the finding that among persons enrolled in Medicare, African Americans are less likely to be screened for breast cancer, less likely to receive beta-blockers after an acute myocardial infarction, or less likely to receive follow-up for mental illness after hospitalization (Schneider, Zaslavsky, & Epstein, 2002) invites further exploration and explanation. As part of this exploration, a qualitative study of interactions between providers and patients of different racial or ethnic groups may be useful in understanding the source of these health disparities.

Other examples of problems that are best studied with quantitative research methods include the physiologic benefits of exercise (Lee, Rexrode, Cook, Manson, & Buring, 2001) and the efficacy of mammography in saving lives (Olson & Gotzsche, 2001a; Olson & Gotzsche, 2001b). These study questions require quantitative research approaches for two reasons:

1. The efficacy of exercise or mammography can be assessed only on the basis of data from large study samples.
2. The *efficacy of many interventions is established without reference to human motives or intentions.*

The second point is essential. The various types of qualitative research emphasize the importance of the meanings that humans give to their actions and strive to *understand* human actions in terms of the meanings that the actors attach to them. Empathy and the ability to understand "where patients are coming from" or "what they are going through" are also important attributes for the successful clinician, and findings from qualitative studies can be particularly useful in providing clinicians with the knowledge needed to offer patients anticipatory guidance or successful coaching (Kearney, 2001). Yet, as the mammography example shows, there are many other important questions to be researched. For example, understanding why women participate or do not participate in mammography screening may also involve population-based evidence concerning the role of insurance status, household income, education, or residency patterns; evidence concerning attitudes toward risk-taking; or sociologic and ethnographic evidence concerning cultural barriers to participating in screening programs. Yet, the question of whether mammography programs are *effective* (i.e., whether the early discovery of a tumor actually improves life expectancy or reduces the morbidity rate among screened individuals) does not necessarily require information about human motives or understanding of human actions because it is a *causal* question.

Human Actions Versus Behavior: Implications for Choices of Research Methods

The question of *meaningful* (i.e., interpretable) actions can be looked at from a slightly different angle. We start by making a distinction between human action and human behavior. Human action is oriented toward an actor's "self-understanding," which provides the motives and rationales for actions. The basis for understanding such action is to see them in the context of the underlying intentionality (Searle, 1983; Fay & Moon, 1998). Human behavior, on the other hand, casts a wider net. At times, it may be *unconscious, unintentional,* or simply the expression of *chemical-physiologic processes.* To the extent to which behavior is the outcome of unconscious or unintentional behavior, qualitative approaches that rely on an assumption of constructed meanings to understand behavior will not be fully useful, or necessarily even appropriate. For example,

consider the experience of depression. There are a number of different theories about the causes of depression, including social and interpersonal as well as biochemical theories. To use only a quantitative research approach focusing only on the biochemistry of depression (e.g., neurotransmitter dysfunction) would not be sufficient to provide a complete understanding of the other types of factors influencing the development and course of depression. Likewise, to use only a qualitative research approach focusing on the "lived experience" of depression would not be sufficient to provide an understanding of the physiologic factors underlying the phenomenon of depression. Thus, a holistic, full explanation of depression draws on multiple types of theories, some of which are causal (e.g., What types of neurotransmitter dysfunctions cause depression?) and some of which concern meaning (e.g., What is the lived experience of depression as related to interactions with others?). Both kinds of questions and explanations are important in nursing and health care research.

MAIN FEATURES OF QUALITATIVE RESEARCH

In this section, we juxtapose the main features, or characteristics, of qualitative and quantitative approaches to research. Because we are primarily concerned with research design issues in this chapter, the juxtaposition is intended to clarify the different roles played by research *design* within the two research traditions. As with any classification system that is meant to differentiate complex sets of ideas, there is no claim that the list of contrasts is exhaustive or even mutually exclusive. For example, not all qualitative researchers eschew the use of numbers (Sandelowski, 2001); likewise, quantitative researchers do not deny the necessity of interpretation (Campbell, 1994). Yet, to orient the reader to the main differences, this *idealtypical* (Weber, 1949) portrayal of the two research traditions can be valuable.

Comparison of the descriptions of qualitative and quantitative research approaches shown in Box 12-1 shows that one important underlying distinction is that between *qualitative as exploratory* research and *quantitative as confirmatory* research. Although this distinction should not be overemphasized, a key contribution of qualitative research to nursing knowledge is its **heuristic value,** or its usefulness as a *tool for exploration* related to knowledge development. Qualitative research often informs clinical practice by raising questions and providing fertile ideas for additional research activities, specifically with regard to social or psychological phenomena, such as patient

---

BOX 12.1   Features and Comparative Characteristics of Qualitative and Quantitative Approaches to Research

Qualitative Research	Quantitative Research
Oriented toward theory discovery and the development of conceptual frameworks (inductive)	Oriented toward theory testing (deductive)
Attempts exploration in a "naturalist" way, under *uncontrolled* conditions	Attempts to control conditions and variables (experimental or statistical control)
Goal is to understand behavior or actions within their naturally occurring contexts	Goal is to isolate variables (lack of context)
Focus on behavioral or meaningfully understood action variables only	Focus on both biophysiologic and behavioral variables
Tendency to focus on smaller samples	Tendency to work with larger samples
Preferred sampling method: theoretical sampling	Preferred sampling method: probability sampling
Preference for open-ended, unstandardized, reactive data collection procedures	Preference for standardized measurement and data collection procedures
Oriented toward completeness of description	Oriented toward reproducibility of results
Open-ended inquiry (reactive to preliminary results)	Focus on predetermined variables
Emphasis on uniqueness of individuals or special population groups	Emphasis on predictable, repeatable aspects of human behavior
Preference for narrative summaries or descriptions	Preference for statistical and numerical summaries or description
Interpretative	Analytical
Explanation in terms of motivational theories ($\rightarrow$ understanding)	Explanation in terms of causal theories ($\rightarrow$ prediction)

---

behaviors, ideas, and values, about which relatively little is known.

Qualitative research approaches are often used as an initial step to understand the needs and perspectives of particular populations, to understand what questions should be asked in surveys, to develop new instruments to measure phenomena of interest (see chapter 18), and to tailor more generic interventions to meet the needs of specific populations (Hutchinson, 2001; Sandelowski, 2000b). These studies focus on description and on identifying and exploring the dimensions of a given phenomenon, often as a prerequisite to further research. These goals of qualitative research enable researchers to find appropriate labels for phenomena,[1] to develop new conceptual frameworks to better understand the nature of the phenomena, and to describe the scope and impact of the phenomena.

The emphasis on exploration means *deemphasizing the use of fixed or predetermined procedures*. It might, there-

---

[1]Phenomena may involve multiple interrelated concepts, but we use the terms "phenomenon" and "concept" somewhat interchangeably in this chapter because both are the focus of qualitative research. See chapter 2 for a discussion of the nature of concepts in relation to research.

---

fore, be considered misleading to talk of qualitative research *designs,* especially if we use the term "design" in the same sense as in our discussion of quantitative designs:

> "A research design is a plan . . . (it) suggests what observations to make, when to make them, and how to analyze the . . . variables" (chapter 2).

This notion of research design implies the exercise of control over the conditions under which data are collected as well as a focus on a predetermined set of variables, measured in a standardized way. Especially in the interest of generating *replicable* studies, such quantitative research is usually well planned and progresses in orderly steps. Because at least some unforeseeable events are likely to occur over time, most research of any complexity (whether quantitative *or* qualitative) involves moment-to-moment decisions and "fine-tuning" of research design and data collection activities to deal with contingencies. However, in general, quantitative researchers tend to stick to a "game plan" as outlined in the design statements, from which they do not deviate, unless there are justifiable reasons to do so. Qualitative research, on the other hand, is more *flexible* in its approach to data collection. The process of designing and refining a study as data collection unfolds, in part, in reaction to preliminary information, is referred to as an **emergent research design.**

Reliance on emergent design decisions does not imply haphazard or impulsive decisions. High-quality emergent design decisions require considerable thought, experience, and skill on the part of the researcher if rich and valid data are to be obtained. However, the hallmark of these decisions is that they are *reactive* (i.e., they incorporate observations and information about study subjects and contexts as they develop). Thus, qualitative research tends to be **less structured** than quantitative research[2] because less is assumed to be known about the concepts and subject matter being studied.[3]

Differences in Qualitative and Quantitative Philosophic Assumptions

The relative lack of structure is expressed in the open-endedness of the inquiry (i.e., an unwillingness to stick to a predetermined set of questions, hypotheses, or variables), which is an advantage during an exploratory phase of research. Some qualitative researchers do not view their work as exclusively exploratory or preparatory for later quantitative research, but may see it as a better alternative (e.g., see Streubert & Carpenter, 1999) when the goal is a fuller understanding of human motivation and action. Furthermore, some qualitative researchers believe that human actions can be understood only within a particular social context, and that any attempt to convert verbal utterances into standardized numerical scores would alter the meaning of the data unacceptably. This is a key source of disagreement among researchers who are exclusively devoted to *either qualitative or quantitative* research models (i.e., there are differences in viewpoints concerning the possibility of measurement expressed in numerical scores). As some qualitative researchers have stressed (Sandelowski, 2001), the difference of opinion is not (or at least should not be) about the use of numbers and numerical strategies because the operation of counting can always be performed with any classificatory (i.e., nominal) level of measurement.[4] The difference of opin-

ion concerns the possibility of measuring and understanding human attitudes, opinions, and emotions, regardless of context, on numerical rating scales.[5] Thus, to some degree, the labels of "qualitative" and "quantitative" research are misnomers. The principal difference is not that a qualitative researcher always eschews numerical analysis or that a quantitative researcher avoids interpretation of results in light of contextual knowledge. Rather, the principal difference lies in their attitudes toward standardized measurement.[6]

Another important difference can be observed with respect to the treatment of **context.** Most quantitative research tends to be analytical, which means that it attempts to *isolate* variables from their contexts (through either experimental or statistical control), whereas qualitative researchers attempt to understand human actions and decisions *within* their contexts. Rather than viewing contextual variables as nuisance factors that need to be controlled for, qualitative researchers see them as constituting and contributing to the very understanding of the observed human behavior. Again, this difference in viewpoint reflects the differences in research goals: the analytical tradition is primarily interested in causal analysis and prediction, which requires the *isolation* of factors and variables so that their *independent* contribution to an outcome of interest can be identified (Shadish, Cook, & Campbell, 2002). This type of analysis must, by necessity, go beyond a particular context, comparing, for instance, how asthma control is achieved in *different* social and ethnic groups (Butz, Malveaux, Eggleston, Thompson, Thompson, Huss, Kolodner, & Rand, 1995). In contrast, with its emphasis on interpretation and *understanding* of human action, qualitative research focuses on collecting information about, in principle, all contextual features that the subjects (i.e., human actors) consider relevant to their decisions. It is about reconstructing the "world view" or "lived experience" of the human actors involved.

THE RELEVANCE OF QUALITATIVE RESEARCH TO CLINICAL PROBLEMS

It is important to emphasize that obtaining information on patients' "world views" or "lived experience" requires either historical or current **narrative data.**[7] Narrative data

---

[2]Most quantitative researchers, even if they acknowledge the gain in flexibility, tend to emphasize the price to be paid for this flexibility, including greater difficulty in replicating studies and the greater trust or faith the reader must put in the individual researcher's ability to make the "right" decisions.

[3]As discussed in the chapters on measurement (chapters 13–17), successful quantitative studies require that the measurement tools are "valid" and "reliable" representations of the concepts. Thus, previous measurement studies and ubiquitous "pilot" studies are needed for a successful quantitative study.

[4]See chapter 13 for a more detailed discussion of levels of measurement.

[5]See chapter 18 for more discussion on qualitative "measurement."

[6]Again, measurement issues will be discussed in more detail in chapters 13 through 18.

[7]Qualitative researchers make use of all kinds of data, including direct observations. If the goal is to reconstruct the meaning that a human actor attributed to his or her action, reliance on verbal expressions by these actors must be a major component of this research. Inference of meanings from mere *observations* of behavior is always problematic.

can be obtained through open-ended, in-depth individual interviews, focus group interviews, or historical records that might even include novelistic descriptions of illness and care.[8] These data go well beyond quantifying the "level" and "nature" of pain on rating scales or measuring serum cortisol levels as an index of stress, as might be done in a strictly quantitative approach to pain measurement. Qualitative research approaches would strive to provide rich data about the experience and meaning of pain that could not be captured through standardized measurements of pain severity or stress associated with pain.

An important feature of qualitative clinical research is its potential to add to the current level of understanding by providing detailed information that would not necessarily be discovered on the basis of intuition or casual observation alone or through standardized measures that do not allow for the discovery of unanticipated responses.

For instance, enumeration of the different labels that small children use to describe pain and pain abatement through care (Woodgate & Kristjanson, 1996) can help pediatric clinicians to become more sensitized to the needs of hospitalized children.[9] Kearney (2001) has suggested four ways in which qualitative research can improve clinicians' judgments about what patients need. They include (1) insight and empathy, (2) assessment of status and progress, (3) anticipatory guidance, and (4) coaching. Each of these is discussed below in more detail.

1. With its emphasis on the variety of lived experiences, qualitative research helps to provide greater *insight and empathy* concerning variations in human behaviors, traditions, values, actions, and ideas. No clinician can do without knowledge of these differences, but a generalized sensitivity may be the best outcome of all. After all, we cannot expect to know intimately all of the different cultural preferences of every potential patient, but we can train ourselves to be ready to accept the idea that our assumptions may not apply in any given case, and to be aware of variations. Good qualitative research provides such a teaching tool.
2. Given its emphasis on description, qualitative research can provide clinicians with detailed information on illness trajectories and the attendant patient experiences,

thus offering an important contribution to the *assessment of a patient's status and progress*.
3. *Anticipatory guidance* is discussion of illness experiences with patients, including using the available evidence on illness trajectories to help patients to anticipate and cope with various stages in their illness or treatment.
4. Successful *coaching* of patients requires substantial knowledge of the fit between the teaching model and its content on one side and the patient's specific needs on the other. Thus, going beyond a generalized sensitivity to each patient's circumstances, the coach must be able to make (and negotiate) an accurate assessment of how the patient can integrate recommended treatment into his or her life.

The translation of research results into clinical practice always assumes that *patterns* discovered in research can be applied to new clinical situations. Thus, paradoxically, context-sensitive research ultimately must produce results that can be carried over to *new* contexts. Otherwise, the results have only historical interest.

In this context, it is also important to note that high-quality qualitative research does not focus on trivial, obvious understandings or on knowledge that would be expected to be validated as part of a standardized measurement procedure (e.g., pain hurts, pain is unpleasant, or, postsurgical patients have pain). Quantitative research can also produce trivial results. Research of any type (quantitative or qualitative) is ultimately justified in terms of the contributions it makes to new knowledge that is usable in clinical practice. For example, mere reiterations of the importance of social support in contributing to a patient's ability to cope are not new research findings.

For a practical example of how qualitative research can serve as a tool for exploration, consider the clinical issues described in Research Scenario 12-1.

This scenario shows a clinical situation in which qualitative research approaches are likely to be very useful. Note that little existing information is assumed to be available about either the nature of the study population or the phenomenon of interest as it occurs in the study population. Thus, basic information would be needed concerning the needs and perspectives of the population of interest, including what questions to ask. When researchers or clinicians begin an inquiry without even knowing what the relevant problems and issues are, they must, by necessity, begin with an informal exploration that relies on informants and members of the target population. The advance practice nurse (APN) needs this type of information to be able to develop relevant standardized measures of variables and to design, implement, and evaluate theoretically

---

[8]For an interesting description of a care relationship, see Doris Lessing's novel *Diary of Jane Somers*.

[9]There is an interesting paradox here: such research is useful only to the extent that it uncovers *general patterns* that do not apply only to the subjects under investigation, but can be generalized, or "carried over," to the reader's patients. Thus, generalizability is always a concern when judging the usefulness of research results. See chapter 21 for a more detailed discussion of generalizability in qualitative studies.

Example of a Research Study For a Limited-Information Context

An advance practice nurse (APN) who is interested in research would like to find out more about factors that affect primary care patients' interest in and ability to carry out health self-assessment activities, such as breast and testicular self-examinations, monitoring of skin for unusual lesions or changes to moles, monitoring for symptoms of sexually transmitted diseases, and asthma and diabetes self-monitoring. To inform her practice in this area, the APN has already done a thorough review of the literature on self-care and monitoring activities, and is knowledgeable about the general factors that contribute to interest level and follow-through with a variety of self-care activities. She regularly scans the literature for new developments in this area.

    Some of the patients the APN sees in her clinical practice seem to be different from the populations that have been studied and reported on in the research literature. For example, the APN works with a small population of indigent indigenous people who reside in a remote area of a northern state. These people appear to have substantially nonmainstream beliefs about self-care practices, at least on the basis of the APN's informal interactions with them at the primary care clinic. Although the APN believes that she has relatively good rapport with her patients, she also thinks about how many of them do not follow professional recommendations for their health monitoring and self-care practices. The population has clinically significant health disparities as manifested by relatively high rates of certain diseases that are detected later by health care providers in relation to other "mainstream" populations seen in the clinic. For example, women with suspicious breast lumps usually delay seeking help for 3 to 6 months. In comparison, other women often seek help within 1 month of noticing a lump. Overall, except for serious illness, this population of patients has little formal contact with the primary care clinic. The population is quite insular, having little contact with others outside the group, except for emergency situations.

    One morning at a weekly provider meeting, someone suggests that the APN could "do a study" to find out why this population of patients declines to follow professional recommendations. The APN is asked about how she would go about designing a study to address this question. The APN thinks about existing standardized survey measures that she might use in a quantitative approach to measuring the interest and ability of this population in regard to self-care activities. However, none of the measures the APN is aware of appears to have been validated (tested for reliability and validity) with this population. She is not certain that the use of surveys would be culturally appropriate for the population, and she has little information about their reading levels, beliefs, culture, or interest in participating in research.

    What recommendations would you make to this APN for designing her study?

based clinical interventions to improve the health of the population. Likewise, if the APN had already implemented an intervention to improve care-seeking behavior in the target population, qualitative research approaches could have a very important "explorative" role in the evaluation of existing clinical interventions and programs (Sandelowski, 1996). For further information, see the discussion of combining quantitative and qualitative research approaches that appears later in this chapter.

TYPES OF QUALITATIVE RESEARCH

Historical Background

Historically, many different social and behavioral science disciplines, such as anthropology, sociology, and social

psychology, have extensively debated and used qualitative approaches to social research. These debates have been fueled, in part, by philosophic arguments about the nature of knowledge and by evidence in the humanities and historical disciplines as opposed to the natural sciences. Specifically, German philosophic traditions as diverse as phenomenology, hermeneutics, and existentialism, and in a somewhat different way, even psychoanalysis, have emphasized the importance of "understanding" human behavior rather than identifying "laws of human behavior."[10] Because the social sciences deal with patterns and regularities in human behaviors as well as with human actions whose

---

[10]A classic text that is still worth reading because it embraces *both* the search for "empirical regularities" and "verstehen," or interpreting and understanding human actions in terms of culturally specific social norms, is Max Weber's (1949) *Methodology of the Social Sciences.*

intentionality can be understood with reference to group-specific social and cultural ideals, norms, and attitudes, it is not surprising that the debate over the proper goals of the social sciences has been going on for decades, if not more than a century.[11] By contrast, the history of nursing research and methodologic debate is much shorter.[12] However, by the mid 1980s, a lively debate about methods was underway in nursing, focusing on the relative merits of quantitative versus qualitative research.[13]

Before the mid to late 1980s, the quantitative approach was the main paradigm guiding nursing research that was published in nursing and other health-related journals. By the late 1980s, however, increasing interest in and use of qualitative research fostered the development of several new nursing and health-related research journals focusing on this research, such as *Nursing Science Quarterly* and *Qualitative Health Research.* Many other journals publishing nursing research, such as *Scholarly Inquiry for Nursing Practice,* the *Journal of Advanced Nursing,* the *Western Journal of Nursing Research,* and *Advances in Nursing Science,* also began to include qualitative research studies.[14]

More recently, top-ranked general nursing research journals, in particular *Research in Nursing & Health* and the *Western Journal of Nursing Research,* have devoted considerable space to qualitative research as well as to methodology corners or methods sections that include regular "spotlights" on qualitative approaches to research. Still, quantitative approaches to nursing research continue to predominate in publications, and certainly, funding opportunities for clinical research remain more oriented toward quantitative research (Hutchinson, 2001) and selected types of qualitative research. This tendency is consistent with the emphasis that many funding agencies place on the generation of *instrumental* knowledge, which includes causal analysis and prediction, a strong suit of the quantitative research tradition.

The history of the methods debate in nursing has sometimes been acrimonious,[15] but it is increasingly acknowledged by a majority of nurse researchers that many research problems can benefit from a blend of methods, depending on the particular nursing research questions posed in a clinical study. Extreme methodologic "camps" have become less common over time, as witnessed by such attempts to see the merits of both approaches to research (Sandelowski, 2000b). For the rest of this chapter, we will provide very brief introductions to the major qualitative research approaches, most of which were already mentioned in the introductory examples of qualitative research at the beginning of this chapter.

Specific "Schools" of Qualitative Research

Currently, nurse researchers use a wide variety of qualitative research approaches.[16] In this section, we provide an overview of some key approaches that have most often been used in conducting qualitative nursing research, starting with those that are more congruent with "pure" qualitative research paradigm assumptions and concluding with those that are relatively more consistent with the quantitative research paradigm. One problem with any classification system of qualitative approaches to research is that some approaches differ in terms of the philosophic assumptions that they make about "reality" rather than in terms of any unique approach to the research methods. Other distinctions among qualitative research approaches are more methods-oriented, concerning, in particular, approaches to data collection and interpretation. Although these approaches will be mentioned here, they are more properly treated in chapter 18, which deals more explicitly with qualitative approaches to data collection and interpretation.

The approaches described here have certain unifying dimensions, including a central focus on description and interpretation of the meaning of phenomena and concepts. In contrast, there is typically an absence of (causal) explanation and, in particular, of prediction of outcomes, which are usually the focus of quantitative research approaches. Our coverage of various types of qualitative research is necessarily less than comprehensive, focusing on the approaches that have been used most often in nursing re-

---

[11]Its first major manifestation was the "Methodenstreit" or "methods dispute" at the turn of the 20th century among the members of the German Association for Social Research. See the foreword in Max Weber's (1949) *Methodology of the Social Sciences.*

[12]Although there were some nurse researchers before World War II who made extraordinary contributions to nursing (e.g., Florence Nightingale), it was only in the early 1950s that enough nursing research was being done to foster the development of the first journal devoted fully to publishing nursing research (*Nursing Research,* in 1952). For an excellent review of key issues in American nursing that have affected nursing research as well as other aspects of nursing, see Baer, D'Antonio, Rinker, and Lynaugh (2001).

[13]See Hinshaw, Feetham, and Shaver (1999), chapters 1 through 4, for an excellent review of the evolution of research methods in nursing.

[14]A number of additional journals focus on qualitative research and publish qualitative nursing research studies. Our examples of journals are intended to be neither inclusive nor exclusive; the examples are provided only as illustrations.

[15]The same can be said about similar debates in other disciplines.

[16]In chapters 18 and 21, additional information will be provided about specific approaches to qualitative research data collection, quality issues, and sampling.

search. See the list of suggested readings for references that provide additional, in-depth discussions of the research approaches we review below. Each approach is considerably more complex than the brief overview of concepts we present in this chapter,[17] and any given approach would require additional study and skills before it could be used in a valid way in a research project.

Phenomenology

Phenomenologic inquiry and the related area of **hermeneutic inquiry (hermeneutics)** are modes of qualitative inquiry that are rooted in concepts from philosophic phenomenology and hermeneutics, although their use in qualitative health care research may deviate substantially from the original philosophic conceptions.[18] Phenomenologic inquiry has become a frequently used approach to qualitative nursing research. See Barnard, McCosker, and Gerber (1999) for a recent review of philosophic assumptions related to the use of phenomenology in health-related research. Phenomenologic research focuses on the "lived experiences" of individuals as a tool for understanding the broader sociopolitical, cultural, and historical contexts of living. A central focus of phenomenologic hermeneutics is the interpretation of "intentional acts" or meanings of lived experiences. Phenomenology is based on methods that are posited to allow the researcher to understand or view phenomena in their "pure essence," unobstructed by preexisting prejudices or preconceived biases. The procedure designed to put preconceived notions into abeyance is called **bracketing** one's existence. Researchers attempt to immerse themselves in the data in ways that allow the intended meanings to emerge. The ultimate criterion for the validity of one's interpretations, or the arrival at "pure essences," is the use of **intuition** and reflective thinking. Making sense of the data also relies on such criteria as **coherence** and **intelligibility.** There are no objective (interpersonal) criteria for the "correct" interpretation of data (i.e., because of the uniqueness of the lived and constructed experience, intuition is relied on to arrive at truth in interpretation of data).

Van Manen (1990) identified the following four areas of "lived experience" that constitute metaboundaries for phenomenologic research:

1. Space
2. Bodily experience
3. Human relationships
4. Time

Nursing research topics that are the subject of phenomenologic studies have focused predominantly on the bodily experience (such as the lived experience of pain) and human relationships aspects of lived experience.

▶CLINICAL RESEARCH IN ACTION
Living with a Urinary Catheter
For instance, Wilde (2002) performed a phenomenologic study of the experience of living with a urinary catheter. Wilde likened life with a catheter to "living with the forces of flowing water," a core concept that was meant to be a potentially useful metaphor for helping people to adjust to long-term use of a urinary catheter. Other phenomenologic studies include Bondas and Eriksson's (2001) study of women's lived experiences with pregnancy and McInnis and White's (2001) study of loneliness among older adults.

Ethnography

Ethnographic studies are rooted in the disciplinary traditions of anthropology. With its origin in the investigation of non-Western societies, the primary focus of ethnography is to understand and describe the cultural processes of particular population groups. These cultural processes include the experiences of the collective group, their beliefs and value systems, their symbols and cultural artifacts in the form of tools and other objects, and their behaviors and patterns of relating. The primary goal of the researcher is to understand a "society" or a distinct cultural subgroup, *as if he or she were a member of that group.* In ethnographic research, it is assumed that certain cultural processes are so entrenched within the society or culture that self-reports of group members *about* their experiences *must be augmented by substantial periods of immersion of the researcher within the culture or society.* In this immersion process, the researcher takes on the role of a **participant–observer,** meaning that the researcher actually lives with and interacts intensively on a daily basis with the group members to develop a deep level of understanding that is possible only through this level of immersion in the culture or society. However, most ethnographers acknowledge the impossibility of becoming a complete insider ("going native" or acquiring the "emic" view), which, in the language of phenomenology, amounts to "bracketing one's prior life." Instead, they strive to interpret and describe life in a cultural group in theoretic terms that go beyond the

---

[17]Additional details about qualitative research approaches are presented in chapter 18, which discusses data collection and interpretation, and chapter 21, which discusses sampling issues in qualitative research.

[18]For a lively exposition of philosophic phenomenology, see the article on "Phenomenology" in the *Encyclopedia of Philosophy* by Richard Schmitt.

language of the native group. This description also implies at least partial adoption of the "etic" view (i.e., an outsider's view of the culture).[19]

The primary mode of data collection in ethnographic studies is the performance of **fieldwork** as a participant–observer.[20] Fieldwork may include unstructured interviews, but relies heavily on observations as captured in field notes. Other sources of information may include artifacts, written documents, and so forth. Ethnography shares with other qualitative approaches to research the *rejection of a fixed, preplanned research design*. This is a necessary component of fieldwork as performed by a participant–observer because the question of which events to observe and participate in is often determined by decisions made by other group members: a participant–observer must, at least to some degree, go with the flow.

One of the most famous programs of ethnographic research, familiar to many people, involved the study not of human beings, but of chimpanzees. Jane Goodall, a world-famous ethnographic researcher of chimpanzee behavior and culture, spent decades living in remote geographic regions populated by civilizations of chimpanzees. During this time, she lived with and befriended many members of the chimpanzee group.[21]

▶CLINICAL RESEARCH IN ACTION
Recent Ethnographic Nursing Studies

Estroff (1981) published a seminal book on the experiences of mentally ill people living in a Midwestern community. In this study, the primary method of data collection involved participant observation. Ethnographic methods have been used in a limited, but growing, number of nursing research studies. For example, Denham (1999) reported on several studies of family health among Appalachian families. The goal was to describe how families "defined and practiced" family health within their households. Lobar and Phillips (1996) reported an ethnographic analysis of parents adopting infants. Mahoney (2001) reported the results of a study to understand the illness experiences of patients with congestive heart failure and their families. Finally, Emami et al. (2000) focused on the experience of elderly Iranian women who immigrated to Sweden.

Although the origin of ethnographic studies is rooted in the anthropologic concern for understanding whole cultures, the interpretive *practice* of ethnographic studies in nursing and other health-related disciplines may not always be clearly distinguishable from that of other qualitative approaches, except for the greater emphasis on observational data as opposed to exclusive reliance on narrative text obtained through open-ended interviews.

Grounded Theory

Grounded theory is another qualitative research approach. It originally developed within the discipline of sociology, in particular through the work of Glaser and Strauss (1967).[22] The focus of grounded theory studies is on social and psychological processes in general, but with the more specific aim of *discovering* theoretic concepts. Like phenomenology and ethnography, the grounded theory approach is primarily *inductive* (i.e., it starts with some form of "data," such as observations or transcripts of in-depth interviews), and it attempts to generate concepts and theories that encapsulate the data in theoretically meaningful terms. Grounded theory approaches rely on a process of **constant comparative analysis,** in which data obtained through time are continuously and explicitly compared to detect themes and emerging meanings.

As is common in other qualitative approaches, researchers adopting the grounded theory approach do not wish to begin the research process with tightly focused research questions or hypotheses, which could have been developed only through previous research and reliance on literature. Instead, the data are supposed to "yield," in a series of increasingly abstract **coding** steps, the emerging concepts and theories. The first level of coding, **open coding,** is an attempt to apply codes, line by line, to the narrative text that is being examined. These codes may consist of concepts used, or at least implied, by the study participants. In the second level of coding, the method of constant comparison comes into play as first-level codes, abstracted from different data, are compared and grouped into categories, which are often newly created **substantive codes** or concepts. These emergent categories are then compared for their distinctness and mutual exclusiveness. An attempt is made to reduce the number of codes and concepts by combining similar codes into broader concepts. Finally, the researcher undertakes **theoretic coding,** which is designed to move beyond a descriptive to a theoretic analysis that integrates the concepts into an explanatory theory.

---

[19]A classic anthropologic study by Malinowski (Young, 1976) of the Trobriand Islanders uses a modified psychoanalytical framework to understand and explain the culture of that society.

[20]In chapters 16 and 18, we will discuss general issues associated with observations.

[21]Generations of young people have been fascinated by Goodall's work (including photographs of interactions with chimpanzees) that has been published in *National Geographic Magazine*.

[22]For several references, see the suggested readings list.

►CLINICAL RESEARCH IN ACTION
Grounded Theory Approaches to Nursing Research

There are many examples of qualitative nursing studies that use grounded theory approaches, and many qualitative nursing studies cite grounded theory foundations as the later basis for middle-range theory testing. For example, Crooks (2001) studied older women with breast cancer and used a grounded theory approach for data collection and analysis. Kearney (1998) described the development of a formal grounded theory of women's addiction recovery based on a derived concept of "truthful self-nurturing."

Like other qualitative research approaches, the grounded theory approach is intended to be **inductive.** The great merit of inductive approaches is that they can be very helpful as *exploratory devices* to generate new hypotheses or theories. They carry the very useful exhortation not to close our minds before we have explored a subject, and they offer avenues toward theory generation, a topic about which traditional quantitative approaches have little to say.[23] However, there remains a difference between "avenues toward theory generation" and an inductive *method* of arriving at true theories. Whether induction of the latter kind is possible remains doubtful. When a researcher "codes" a text, or looks for similarities and differences, he or she inevitably *imposes* a category system. This also applies to "emergent" categories, which are *picked* by the researchers. Furthermore, any decision about "sameness" or "difference"—an argument, for instance, that two different actions described in a text are examples of "fear" or "joy"—is an interpretative and conceptual leap made by the researcher, however defensible or justified it may seem. Thus, coding (i.e., interpretation and categorization) is an act of imagination and creativity that the researcher *brings to* the task. No person approaches research with an *empty mind,* because an empty mind is without categories and, in fact, without any language!

Historical Research

Although we continue the practice of including **historical research** among the qualitative research approaches, it is worth emphasizing that historical research by no means excludes quantitative data or even quantitative data analysis.[24]

Historical research encompasses a variety of methods for analyzing archival records, with the goals of description and interpretation of the historical record in relation to contemporary life. Because historical research involves interpreting past records and uncovering previously unknown "facts" and relationships about the past, it generates *new* knowledge, and this characteristic differentiates it from a standard summary of literature. Historical research is usually substantially *integrative* in compiling and analyzing information from multiple sources, ranging from written records to diverse archival material, which may include audio and video records for more recent historical periods.

Historians usually distinguish carefully between **primary** and **secondary** source materials. A primary source is an "original" record in the sense that it is closely linked in time, space, and access to the event under study. For example, a historical researcher who wanted to interpret the works of Florence Nightingale would be substantially interested in obtaining the original writings of Florence Nightingale for analysis as opposed to what others may have reported about Nightingale's writings, perhaps decades later. Secondary sources are distinguished in terms of "how far away" they are in relation to actual historical events. For example, public health records, newspaper clippings, and actual excerpts from people's diaries from 1919 reporting on the worst influenza pandemic of the 20th century would be considered primary source material, whereas an analysis of the pandemic based on interviews with flu survivors reported in a journal in 1947 would be considered a secondary source.

Historical research in nursing and other health-related disciplines rarely deals directly with clinical problems. The bulk of historical research in nursing has focused on the nursing *profession* itself. Historical analyses usually go beyond "simple" description and provide an interpretation of the larger context and meaning of the sequence of events under investigation. For example, Baer, D'Antonio, Rinker, and Lynaugh (2001) published an anthology of nursing history articles, with the goal of showing how certain issues in nursing are "enduring," providing the reader with a perspective on and explanation of the current status of the nursing profession. Likewise, Reverby (1987) published a history of U.S. nursing from 1850 to 1945, with a goal of critically reviewing legal and social constraints on nursing practice. Currently, few programs of nursing research in the United States focus on historical research, and funding for historical research in nursing has often been limited to that provided by professional organizations or foundations.

---

[23]Being deductively oriented, quantitative research approaches *assume* that the researcher starts with research questions, theories, and hypotheses that were generated based on previous research or reading the existing literature.

[24]The branch of historical research that is primarily concerned with the quantitative analysis of historical records is called *cliometrics.*

Case Study Research

Case study research is another research approach that is often, but not always, qualitative in its orientation. It is being practiced in a variety of ways, most notably in medicine and nursing through descriptive **case histories.** An example that is probably familiar to most readers is the "unusual disease" case report feature that appears in a number of clinically oriented medical journals. Such case reports include an in-depth description and analysis of a particular occurrence of illness, including its putative etiology, defining features, and illness trajectory. These reports are often based on the history of a single patient. Such case histories are not confined to qualitative data, such as patient self-reports or clinical observations, but include quantitative test results and standardized physiologic measures.

▶CLINICAL RESEARCH IN ACTION
Case Studies

In nursing research, case studies usually have been qualitatively oriented. They have been used to gain an in-depth understanding of illness experiences and patient perceptions about other events. For example, Lewis (1995) reported a case study analysis of a year in the life of a woman who was experiencing premenstrual syndrome. Perry and Olshansky (1996) used case study methods to examine how a family adjusted to Alzheimer's disease in a family member. In these and other studies, the goal is to understand the meaning that the study participants attached to various events.

A key strength of case studies is their emphasis on detailed observation[25] with the concomitant ability to gather *rich* data that are often suggestive of new connections and hypotheses. However, the obvious limitation of case studies lies in their limited generalizability and the impossibility of disentangling causal relationships when dealing with many pieces of information (variables) and a single case.

Case study research is not confined to case histories of individual patients. The "case" in question may be an agency, hospital, or other organization. In addition, case study research may not be confined to a single case, but may incorporate an explicit comparative perspective in **multiple-case designs** (Yin, 1994). These multiple-case designs are often used in **program evaluation** (King, Morris, & Fitz-Gibbon, 1987). For instance, a comparison of a

nurse-managed clinic with a physician-managed clinic might focus on differences in internal organization and hierarchies, referral patterns and external networks, patient outcomes and costs, and so forth. These case studies may involve the collection of qualitative and quantitative data from computerized records, direct observations of provider–patient contacts, interviews with key informants, or written organizational charts.

COMBINING QUALITATIVE AND QUANTITATIVE RESEARCH APPROACHES

In this chapter, we have already referred to multiple ways in which qualitative and quantitative research approaches can be complementary. In addition, some research approaches, such as historical research and case studies, explicitly combine qualitative and quantitative data. As we have emphasized in this chapter, qualitative research approaches are particularly valuable for the earlier phases of research, when the focus is on identifying, describing, and exploring key phenomena or concepts. The results of such explorations may lay the foundation for theoretically based quantitative research that focuses on testing theories, explaining cause and effect relationships, and testing the effectiveness of selected interventions through their manipulation under controlled conditions.

Qualitative approaches to research can also play a very important role in the evaluation of existing clinical interventions and programs that occur as part of clinical practice or research studies (Sandelowski, 1996). In addition to obtaining information about whether an intervention works, clinicians need information on the context in which interventions are particularly effective so that they can "fine-tune" interventions for different age groups, sociocultural contexts, and so forth. Specifically, process evaluations of clinical interventions and programs often use qualitative methods that help us to understand the specific circumstances under which interventions are effective as well as other social and psychological factors that are of interest to researchers and clinicians. A **process evaluation** focuses on the process or activities of implementing an intervention or program, whereas an **outcomes evaluation** is concerned with the overall effects of an intervention or program. For instance, a nurse researcher might use a process evaluation based on qualitative methods (e.g., focus group interviews; see Part V) to understand how study participants view a clinical intervention or to gain specific information about needed adjustments to the intervention.

---

[25]The case study as an *observational* study approach is distinct from a single-subject *experiment,* in which the researcher implements an intervention for a single individual and observes the effects.

These kinds of qualitative approaches to research are especially useful when the clinical intervention or program is new or is tested on a new population group or under a novel set of circumstances. In summary, the use of qualitative approaches can substantially add to our understanding of the circumstances under which an intervention is well received and, therefore, is likely to be effective with a target population.

Some specific approaches to combining quantitative and qualitative methods have become more common in nursing research over the last decade. In one area, quantitative scale development based on questionnaire items, it is common practice to start with qualitative approaches to *generating* such questions.[26] Beyond scale development, combining or blending qualitative and quantitative methods is now considered conventional and even desirable, particularly when the research program is concerned with psychosocial problems that involve little-studied phenomena or concepts or when the concern is with the development of middle-range theories with relevance for nursing theory, practice, and research. Combining different methods is also referred to as **multi-method, mixed-method,** or **triangulation** research (Murdaugh, 1999; Sandelowski, 2000b). There is still substantial controversy concerning the ways in which methods can be combined.[27] If a single study uses multiple methods to collect data, it is a case of **across-methods triangulation** (Murdaugh, 1999). It is this definition of triangulation that we will use for our discussion of combining qualitative and quantitative approaches within a single study.

Although many researchers are now moving to across-methods triangulation approaches, a substantial amount of methodologic research and consensus building must be done regarding "best practices" for methods triangulation. In brief, key issues in across-methods triangulation (Murdaugh, 1999) concern:

- How to combine numerical and narrative data
- Data weighting methods
- Interpretation of discrepant results between methods
- How to reconcile differences in definitions of the same concept between methods[28]
- Sampling issues

Recently, some researchers (Morgan, 1998; Sandelowski, 2000b) proposed strategies for combining qualitative and quantitative approaches in health-related research to address the issues raised by Murdaugh (1999). Morgan (1998) discussed the idea of "assigning priority" to one approach over the other and making a decision about the "sequence" of carrying out the methods, whether the complementary method precedes or follows the principal method.[29] Morgan (1998) provided as a rationale for this suggestion the idea that the two methods probably cannot have equal priority within a given study because of the problem that is created in analyzing data, particularly if apparently discrepant results are obtained between methods. In addition, Morgan (1998) indicated that sequencing of qualitative and quantitative methods would be needed so that the complementary method would be helpful or able to "effectively assist" the primary method. Morgan (1998) envisioned a "priority-sequence model," in which both priority and sequencing decisions are made based on the primary study goals. For instance, poorly understood quantitative survey results may need to be followed up with in-depth interviews for better interpretation, or promising qualitative case study results may need to be followed up with larger-scale samples that are representative of the intended target population.

Sandelowski (2000b) provided an integrative critique of several key issues in methods triangulation, classifying controversies, and uncertainties in terms of philosophic assumptions, methods, and specific techniques. Drawing on the work of Morgan (1998) and others, Sandelowski (2000b) presented seven possible hybrid, combination, or mixed-method research design "templates," reflecting combinations of priority, temporality, and the research goals associated with each method. Sandelowski's proposal allows for the possibility that quantitative and qualitative research methods could be of either different or equal priority or time sequence and also allows for going back and forth between methods.

In summary, for psychosocial research, there can be substantial advantages to across-methods triangulation, or the combination, of quantitative and qualitative research approaches. There are ongoing debates about the extent to which methods can be combined and in what manner the combination can occur. More research is needed concerning "best practices" in methods triangulation.

---

[26]One common approach is the use of focus groups that include members of the target population. Because the use of focus groups is primarily an approach to data collection, it will be addressed in chapter 18, which discusses measurement and data collection issues in qualitative research.

[27]Some researchers believe that it is not possible to combine methods that have fundamentally different philosophic assumptions. See Leininger (1992) and Phillips (1988).

[28]See Masse (2000) for a recent example.

[29]Note that quantitative scale development involves a definite sequence of qualitative followed by quantitative approaches.

CONCLUSION

As this chapter has shown, qualitative research approaches are intended to provide a researcher and others with an in-depth understanding of a phenomenon of interest, in terms of the meanings that study participants ascribe to their experiences. Qualitative research approaches are quite diverse, but share the methodology of collecting and analyzing self-report data from human subjects. Qualitative and quantitative approaches are largely complementary and are often used in combination to provide a more holistic view of phenomena. More recently, conceptual work has focused on understanding how to best integrate quantitative and qualitative methods, including the specific ways to "triangulate" methods, and the boundary conditions under which specific triangulation approaches are appropriate. In chapters 18 and 21, qualitative research methods and sampling are addressed in greater detail.

Suggested Activities

1. After reviewing the scenario in Research Scenario 12-1, propose specific recommendations with rationales for the APN researcher. Include a discussion of specific qualitative research approaches that may be most appropriate for this situation, and justify your recommendations.

2. Based on what you know about quantitative and qualitative research paradigms thus far, do you view yourself as more interested in one research paradigm versus the other? If you feel more interested in one versus the other, discuss your rationale with an interested colleague. Include possible implications for specific research ideas and studies and considerations of methods triangulation issues.

3. Read several of the research references in the suggested readings list that reflect different types of qualitative research approaches.
   a. Do the study findings have implications for clinical practice or research?
   b. As applicable, identify some specific implications, and critique the strength of the evidence in support of the study findings.
   c. If you wanted to do similar studies, what changes, if any, might you recommend to the designs and data collection approaches used? Provide a rationale for any changes you recommend.

Suggested Readings

Atkinson, P., Coffey, A., Delamont, S., Lofland, J., & Lofland, L. (Eds.). (2001). *Handbook of ethnography.* Thousand Oaks, CA: Sage.

Baer, E. D., D'Antonio, P., Rinker, S., & Lynaugh, J.E. (Eds). (2001). *Enduring issues in American nursing.* NY: Springer.

Barnard, A., McCosker, H., & Gerber, R. (1999). Phenomenography: A qualitative research approach for exploring understanding in health care. *Qualitative Health Research, 9,* 212–226.

Beck, L. W. (Ed.). (1949). *Critique of practical reason and other writings in moral philosophy* (translated from by I. Kant's *Werke,* edited by B. Cassirer, 1922–23). Chicago: University of Chicago Press.

Beyea, S. C., & Nicoll, L. H. (2000). Learn more from using focus groups. *AORN Journal, 71,* 897, 899–900.

Bondas, T., & Eriksson, K. (2001). Women's lived experiences of pregnancy: A tapestry of joy and suffering. *Qualitative Health Research, 11,* 824–840.

Brooks, E. L., Fletcher, K., & Wahlstedt, P. A. (1998). Focus group interviews: Assessment of continuing education needs for the advanced practice nurse. *Journal of Continuing Education in Nursing, 29,* 27–31, 46–47.

Butz, A. M., Malveaux, F. J., Eggleston, P., Thompson, L., Huss, K., Kolodner, K., & Rand, C. S. (1995). Social factors associated with behavioral problems in children with asthma. *Clinical Pediatrics,* 581–590.

Cohen, M. Z., Kahn, D. L., & Steeves, R. H. (2000). *Hermeneutic phenomenological research: A practice guide for nurse researchers.* Thousand Oaks, CA: Sage.

Cote-Arsenault, D., & Morrison-Beedy, D. (1999). Practical advice for planning and conducting focus groups. *Nursing Research, 48,* 280–283.

Cowling, W. R. (1998). Unitary case inquiry. *Nursing Science Quarterly, 11,* 139–141.

Crabtree, B. F., & Miller, W. L. (1999). *Doing qualitative research.* Thousand Oaks, CA: Sage.

Creswell, J. W. (2002). *Research design: Qualitative and quantitative approaches* (2nd ed.). Thousand Oaks, CA: Sage.

Crooks, D. L. (2001). Older women with breast cancer: New understanding through grounded theory research. *Health Care for Women International, 22,* 99–114.

Denham, S. A. (1999). Introduction to three ethnographic studies on family health with Appalachian families. *Journal of Family Nursing, 5,* 130–132.

Denzin, N. K., & Lincoln, Y. S. (2002). *The qualitative inquiry reader.* Thousand Oaks, CA: Sage.

Denzin, N. K., & Lincoln, Y. S. (2000). *Handbook of qualitative research* (2nd ed.). Thousand Oaks, CA: Sage.

Eldridge, J. E. T. (Ed.). (1975). *Max Weber: The interpretation of social reality.* New York: Scribner.

Fetterman, D. M. (1998). *Ethnography: Step-by-step* (2nd ed.). Thousand Oaks, CA: Sage.

Flick, U. (2002). *An introduction to qualitative research* (2nd ed.). Thousand Oaks, CA: Sage.

Glaser, B. G. (1992). *Basics of grounded theory analysis: Emergence vs. forcing.* Mill Valley, CA: Sociology Press.

Glaser, B. G. (1995). *Grounded theory, 1984–1994* (Vols. 1–2). Mill Valley, CA: Sociology Press.

Glaser, B. G. (1998). *Doing grounded theory: Issues and discussions.* Mill Valley, CA: Sociology Press.

Glaser, B. G. (1999). The future of grounded theory. *Qualitative Health Research, 9,* 836–845.

Glaser, B. G., & Strauss, A. L. (1967). *The discovery of grounded theory: Strategies for qualitative research.* Chicago: Aldine.

Gomm, R., Hammersley, M., & Foster, P. (Eds.). (2001). *Case study method: Key issues, key texts.* Thousand Oaks, CA: Sage.

Hall, W. A., & Callery, P. (2001). Enhancing the rigor of grounded theory: Incorporating reflexivity and relationality. *Qualitative Health Research, 11,* 257–272.

Hammersley, M., & Atkinson, P. (1995). *Ethnography: Principles in practice* (2nd ed.). New York: Routledge.

Holliday, A. (2002). *Doing and writing qualitative research.* Thousand Oaks, CA: Sage.

Huberman, A. M., & Miles, M. B. (2002). *The qualitative researcher's companion.* Thousand Oaks, CA: Sage.

Hutchinson, S. A. (2001). The development of qualitative research: Taking stock. *Qualitative Health Research, 11,* 505–521.

Kearney, M. H. (1998). Truthful self-nurturing: A grounded formal theory of women's addiction recovery. *Qualitative Health Research, 8,* 495–512.

Kennedy, C., Kools, S., & Krueger, R. (2001). Methodological considerations in children's focus groups. *Nursing Research, 50,* 184–187.

Krueger, R. A., & Casey, M. A. (2000). *Focus groups: A practical guide for applied research* (3rd ed.). Thousand Oaks, CA: Sage.

Lewis, L. L. (1995). One year in the life of a woman with premenstrual syndrome: A case study. *Nursing Research, 44,* 111–116.

Mahoney, J. S. (2001). An ethnographic approach to understanding the illness experiences of patients with congestive heart failure and their family members. *Heart and Lung, 30,* 429–436.

Masse, R. (2000). Qualitative and quantitative analyses of psychological distress: Methodological complementarity and ontological incommensurability. *Qualitative Health Research, 10,* 411–423.

McDougall, G. J., Blixen, C. E., & Suen, L. J. (1997). The process and outcome of life review psychotherapy with depressed homebound older adults. *Nursing Research, 46,* 277–283.

McInnis, G. J., & White, J. H. (2001). A phenomenological exploration of loneliness in the older adult. *Archives of Psychiatric Nursing, 15,* 128–139.

May, T. (2002). *Qualitative research in action.* Thousand Oaks, CA: Sage.

Miller, S. I., & Fredericks, M. (1999). How does grounded theory explain? *Qualitative Health Research, 9,* 538–551.

Morrison, R. S., & Peoples, L. (1999). Using focus group methodology in nursing. *Journal of Continuing Education in Nursing, 30,* 62–65, 94–95.

Morse, J. M., & Richards, L. (2002). *Read me first for a qualitative user's guide to qualitative methods.* Thousand Oaks, CA: Sage.

Morse, J. M., Swanson, J., & Kuzel, A. J. (2001). *The nature of qualitative evidence.* Thousand Oaks, CA: Sage.

Moutsakas, C. (1994). *Phenomenological research methods.* Thousand Oaks, CA: Sage.

O'Rourke, M. E., & Germino, B. B. (1998). Prostate cancer treatment decisions: A focus group exploration. *Oncology Nursing Forum, 25,* 97–104.

Paley, J. (2001). Positivism and qualitative nursing research. *Scholarly Inquiry for Nursing Practice, 15,* 371–387.

Pasacreta, J. V. (1999). Psychosocial issues associated with increased breast cancer and ovarian cancer risk: Findings from focus groups. *Archives of Psychiatric Nursing, 13,* 127–136.

Patton, M. Q. (2002). *Qualitative research and evaluation methods* (3rd ed.). Thousand Oaks, CA: Sage.

Perry, J., & Olshansky, E. F. (1996). A family's coming to terms with Alzheimer's disease. *Western Journal of Nursing Research, 18,* 12–28.

Rees, C. E., & Bath, P. A. (2001). The use of between-methods triangulation in cancer nursing research: A case study examining information sources for partners of women with breast cancer. *Cancer Nursing, 24,* 104–111.

Roper, J. M., & Shapira, J. (1999). *Ethnography in nursing research.* Thousand Oaks, CA: Sage.

Sandelowski, M. (1996). Focus on qualitative methods: One is the liveliest number. The case orientation of qualitative research. *Research in Nursing & Health, 19,* 525–529.

Scholz, R. W., & Tietje, O. (2002). *Embedded case study methods: Integrating quantitative and qualitative knowledge.* Thousand Oaks, CA: Sage.

Sharts-Hopko, N. C. (2001). Focus group methodology: When and why? *Journal of the Association of Nurses in AIDS Care, 12,* 89–91.

Stebbins, R. A. (2001). *Exploratory research in the social sciences.* Thousand Oaks, CA: Sage.

Stewart, D. W., & Shamdasani, P. N. (1990). *Focus groups: Theory and practice.* Thousand Oaks, CA: Sage.

Streubert, H. J., & Carpenter, D. R. (1999). *Qualitative research in nursing: Advancing the humanistic imperative* (2nd ed.). Philadelphia: Lippincott.

Struthers, R. (2000). The lived experience of Ojibwa and Cree women healers. *Journal of Holistic Nursing, 18,* 261–279.

Tashakkori, A., & Teddlie, C. (2002). *Handbook of mixed methods in the social and behavioral sciences.* Thousand Oaks, CA: Sage.

Walcott, H. F. (2001). *Writing up qualitative research* (2nd ed.). Thousand Oaks, CA: Sage.

Wills, C. E. (1997). Young adult medication decision making: Similarities and differences among mental versus physical health treatment contexts. *The Journal of Nursing Science, 2,* 59–72.

References

Baer, E. D., D'Antonio, P., Rinker, S., & Lynaugh, J. E. (Eds.). (2001). *Enduring issues in American Nursing.* New York: Springer.

Baker, C., & Daigle, M. C. (2000). Cross-cultural hospital care as experienced by Mi'kmaq clients. *Western Journal of Nursing Research, 22,* 1, 8–28.

Barnard, A., McCosker, H., & Gerber, R. (1999). Phenomenography: A qualitative research approach for exploring understanding in health care. *Qualitative Health Research, 9,* 212–226.

Bondas, T., & Eriksson, K. (2001). Women's lived experiences of pregnancy: A tapestry of joy and suffering. *Qualitative Health Research, 11,* 824–840.

Breen, N., Wesley, M. N., Merrill, R. M., & Johnson, K. (1999). The relationship of socio-economic status and access to minimum expected therapy among female breast cancer patients in the National Cancer Institute Black-White Cancer Survival Study. *Ethnicity & Disease, 9,* 1, 111–125.

Brown, S. J. (2002). Nursing intervention studies: A descriptive analysis of issues important to clinicians. *Research in Nursing & Health, 25,* 4, 317–327.

Butz, A. M., Malveaux, F. J., Eggleston, P., Thompson, L., Huss, K., Kolodner, K., & Rand, C. S. (1995). Social factors associated with behavioral problems in children with asthma. *Clinical Pediatrics, 34,* 11, 581–590.

Campbell, D. T. (1994). Foreword. In Yin, R.K. (1994). *Case study research: Design and methods.* Thousand Oaks, CA: Sage.

Chiu, L. (2000). Lived experience of spirituality in Taiwanese women with breast cancer. *Western Journal of Nursing Research, 22,* 1, 29–53.

Crooks, D. L. (2001). Older women with breast cancer: New understanding through grounded theory research. *Health Care for Women International, 22,* 99–114.

DeFloor, T., & Grypdonck, M. H. F. (2000). Do pressure relief cushions really relieve pressure? *Western Journal of Nursing Research, 22,* 3, 335–350.

Denham, S. A. (1999). Introduction to three ethnographic studies on family health with Appalachian families. *Journal of Family Nursing, 5,* 130–132.

Draucker, C. B., & Stern, P. N. (2000). Women's responses to sexual violence by male intimates. *Western Journal of Nursing Research, 22,* 4, 385–406.

Emami, A., Torres, S., Lipson, J. G., & Ekman, S.-L. (2000). An ethnographic study of a daycare center for Iranian immigrant seniors. *Western Journal of Nursing Research, 22,* 2, 169–188.

Estroff, S. E. (1981). *Making it crazy: An ethnography of psychiatric clients in an American community.* Berkeley, CA: UCLA Press.

Fay, B., & Moon, J. D. (1998). What would an adequate philosophy of social science look like? In Klemke, E. D., R. Hollinger, & D. W. Rudge (Eds.), *Introductory readings in the philosophy of science* (pp. 171–189). Amherst, NY: Prometheus Books.

Foley, B. J., Minick, P., & Kee, C. (2000). Nursing advocacy during a military operation. *Western Journal of Nursing Research, 22,* 4, 492–507.

Glaser, B. G., & Strauss, A. L. (1967). *The discovery of grounded theory: Strategies for qualitative research.* Chicago: Aldine.

Hinshaw, A. S., Feetham, S. L., Shaver, J. L. F. (Eds.). (1999). *Handbook of clinical nursing research.* Thousand Oaks, CA: Sage.

Hutchinson, S. A. (2001). The development of qualitative research: Taking stock. *Qualitative Health Research, 11,* 505–521.

Im, E.-O., & Meleis, A. I. (2000). Meanings of menopause to Korean immigrant women. *Western Journal of Nursing Research, 22,* 1, 84–102.

Kearney, M. H. (1998). Truthful self-nurturing: A grounded formal theory of women's addiction recovery. *Qualitative Health Research, 8,* 495–512.

Kearney, M. H. (2001). Levels and applications of qualitative research evidence. *Research in Nursing & Health, 24,* 2, 145–153.

King, J. A., Morris, L. L., & Fitz-Gibbon, C. T. (1987). *How to assess program implementation.* Newbury Park, CA: Sage Publications.

Lee, I.-M., Rexrode, K. M., Cook, N. R., Manson, J. A., & Buring, J. E. (2001). Physical activity and coronary heart disease in women: Is 'pain, no gain' passé? *Journal of the American Medical Association, 285,* 21, 1447–1454.

Leininger, M. (1992). Current issues, problems, and trends to advance qualitative paradigmatic research methods for the future. *Qualitative Health Research, 2,* 392–415.

Lewis, L. L. (1995). One year in the life of a woman with premenstrual syndrome: A case study. *Nursing Research, 44,* 111–116.

Lobar, S. L., & Phillips, S. (1996). Parents who utilize private infant adoption: An ethnographic analysis. *Issues in Comprehensive Pediatric Nursing, 19,* 65–76.

Mahoney, J. S. (2001). An ethnographic approach to understanding the illness experiences of patients with congestive heart failure and their families. *Heart and Lung, 30,* 429–436.

Masse, R. (2000). Qualitative and quantitative analyses of psychological distress: Methodological complementarity and ontological incommensurability. *Qualitative Health Research, 10,* 411–423.

McInnis, G. J., & White, J. H. (2001). A phenomenological exploration of loneliness in the older adult. *Archives of Psychiatric Nursing, 15,* 128–139.

Morgan, D. L. (1998). Practical strategies for combining qualitative and quantitative methods: Applications to health research. *Qualitative Health Research, 8,* 362–376.

Murdaugh, C. L. (1999). Relationship of research perspectives to methodology. In Hinshaw, A. S., S. L. Feetham, & J. L. F. Shaver (Eds.), *Handbook of clinical nursing research* (pp. 61–70). Thousand Oaks, CA: Sage.

Olsen, O., & Gotzsche, P. C. (2001a). Cochrane review on screening for breast cancer with mammography. *The Lancet, 358,* 9290, 1340–1342.

Olsen, O., & Gotzsche, P. C. (2001b). *Systematic review of screening for breast cancer with mammography.* Copenhagen: The Nordic Cochrane Center.

Perry, J., & Olshansky, E. F. (1996). A family's coming to terms with Alzheimer's disease. *Western Journal of Nursing Research, 18,* 12–28.

Phillips, J. R. (1988). Research blenders. *Nursing Science Quarterly, 1,* 4–5.

Reverby, S. M. (1987). *Ordered to care: The dilemma of American nursing, 1985–1945.* New York: Cambridge & University Press.

Sandelowski, M. (1996). Focus on qualitative methods: Using qualitative methods in intervention studies. *Research in Nursing & Health, 19,* 359–364.

Sandelowski, M. (2000a). Whatever happened to qualitative description? *Research in Nursing & Health, 23,* 334–340.

Sandelowski, M. (2000b). Combining qualitative and quantitative sampling, data collection, and analysis techniques in mixed-method studies. *Research in Nursing & Health, 23,* 246–255.

Sandelowski, M. (2001). Real qualitative researchers do not count: The use of numbers in qualitative research. *Research in Nursing & Health, 24,* 230–240.

Schmitt, R. (1967). Phemomenology. *The Encyclopedia of Philosophy, Vol. 6.* New York, NY: MacMillan Publishing Company & The Free Press.

Schneider, E. C., Zaslavsky, A. M., & Epstein, A. M. (2002). Racial disparities in the quality of care for enrollees in Medicare managed care. *Journal of the American Medical Association, 287,* 10, 1288–1294.

Searle, J. R. (1983). *Intentionality: An essay in the philosophy of mind.* New York: Press Syndicate of the University of Cambridge, UK.

Shadish, W. R., Cook, T. D. and Campbell, D. T. *Experimental and Quasi-Experimental Designs for generalized causal Inference.* Boston, MA: Houghton Mifflin Company; 2002.

Streubert, H. J., & Carpenter, D. R. (1999). *Qualitative Research in Nursing: Advancing the Humanistic Imperative* (2nd ed.). Philadelphia: Lippincott.

Valleroy, L. A., MacKellar, D. A., Karon, J. M., & Rosen, D. H. (2000). HIV prevalence and associated risks in young men who have sex with men. *Journal of the American Medical Association, 284,* 2, 198–204.

Van Manen, M. (1990). *Researching lived experience: Human science for an action sensitive pedagogy.* London, Ontario: Althouse.

Weber, M. (1949). *Max Weber on the methodology of the social sciences* (translated and edited by Shils E. A., & H. A. Finch). Glencoe, IL: Free Press.

Wilde, M. H. (2002). Urine flowing: A phenomenological study of living with a urinary catheter. *Research in Nursing & Health, 25,* 14–24.

Woodgate, R. and Kristjanson, L. J. (1996). "Getting Better from my hurts": Toward a model of the young child's pain experience. *Journal of Pediatric Nursing, 11,* 4, 233–242.

Yin, R. K. (1994). *Case study research: Design and methods.* Thousand Oaks, CA: Sage.

Young, M. W. (Ed.). (1979). *The ethnography of Malinowski: The Trobriand Islands 1915–18.* London: Routledge & Kegan.

THE CONCEPT OF MEASUREMENT

It is no exaggeration to say that measurement is the most fundamental of all problems in science (Campbell, 1952; Nagel, 1961). If we cannot be reasonably sure that we are actually measuring the variables we intend to measure, then basing our decisions on "empirical evidence" loses all meaning. The same holds for clinical practice: without measurement procedures that empirically "capture" an outcome, such as urinary incontinence, we would not be in a position to decide whether a behavioral intervention, such as to control incontinence, is effective (Dougherty, Dwyer, Pendergast, Boyington, Tomlinson, Coward, Duncan, Vogel, & Rooks, 2002). In general, test results and observations used in clinical practice or research must "reflect" reality to a sufficient degree that they can be useful tools in decision-making.

In a classic article, Stevens (1946) introduced a definition of measurement that is still widely used today: "Measurement is the assignment of numerals to objects or events according to rules." Even more succinctly, Campbell (1952) defined measurement as the "assignment of numbers to properties." This second definition has the advantage of turning our attention to the fact that we do not measure objects *per se;* instead, we measure certain characteristics, features, or *attributes* of objects. For instance, we do not measure "people," but we do measure their height, weight, blood pressure, anxiety level, and so forth, to characterize them with regard to these attributes. Thus, measurement requires *abstraction* (e.g., objects or persons are usually compared based on how they rate on a single conceptual dimension or unitary attribute). Ideally, instruments that are used to obtain measurements, whether they are blood pressure cuffs or survey instruments to assess attitudes, should be **unidimensional** in this sense. For example, when weighing a person on a scale during a routine primary care visit, the goal is to get an accurate or "true" measure of body weight, not of shoes, clothes, or a recent meal. Likewise, measures of depression that are derived from interview responses often include somatic symptoms, such as sleeplessness or loss of appetite, among the indicators.[1] However,

if sleeplessness or loss of appetite were the result of an extraneous factor, such as the adverse side effects of a medication, then the final depression score would no longer be an "uncontaminated" reflection of "true" symptoms of depression. For various reasons (such as these examples illustrate), uncontaminated measures that measure only the attribute of interest are sometimes difficult to come by.

MEASUREMENT RULES AND STANDARDIZATION

The definition of measurement given by Stevens emphasizes that the assignment of numbers in the measurement process occurs according to some *rule system*. The rule may appear simple or "obvious," as in the example of using a ruler to measure the length of a sheet of paper. However, the rules are often more complex and not as intuitively obvious. Consider the use of a thermometer to measure temperature. On the face of it, this also seems to be a simple measurement procedure: whenever temperature rises by 1°F, the column of mercury in a particular thermometer may rise by 2 mm. However, for this measurement procedure to make sense, one must accept as true the physical theories about the behavior of matter under different temperatures (e.g., the volume of mercury expands as temperature rises). Can it be confidently assumed that there are no other factors that might influence the changing volume of mercury? Because many psychological concepts of interest to nurses and health care researchers are only indirectly observable—think of such concepts as depression, hardiness, anxiety, or coping abilities (Pollock, 1989; Radloff, 1977; Spielberger & Vagg, 1984; Folkman & Lazarus, 1983)—it is vital to have rule systems that spell out clearly how to measure the presence and intensity of the observable manifestations of a concept. These measurement rules not only spell out how a concept is operationalized, but also accomplish the **standardization** of the measurement procedures (i.e., the use of the same measurement criteria across different occasions and objects).

Advantages of Standardized Measurement Procedures

The use of standardized measures offers several advantages. In fact, the word "advantage" may be too weak a term to capture the essential point. Progress in science would be extremely difficult (if not sometimes impossible) without standardized measurements. Consider briefly the

---

[1]Depression scales that are often used for research purposes include the CES-D (Radloff, 1977; Devins & Orme, 1983), the Beck Depression Inventory (Beck et al., 1961), the Hamilton Depression Rating Scale (Hamilton, 1960), and the Zung Depression Scale. These measures, especially the CES-D, are still sometimes used in primary care settings to screen for depression. In recent years, other screening measures for mood, anxiety, and substance abuse disorders have been developed for their ease of use in primary care settings. These measures include the PRIME-MD and the Patient Health Questionnaire (Spitzer, Williams, et al., 1994; Spitzer, Williams, and PHQ Primary Care Study Group, 1999).

BOX 13.1   Measuring Body Temperature

Suppose that the only way to measure a person's body temperature is through an assessment based on physical touch. Instead of referring to a "body temperature of 102° Fahrenheit," we would be talking about a "high temperature," or a "feverish state." Although procedures such as assessing body temperature by touch are often perfectly acceptable and valuable for a first "rough estimate" of the state of the patient, it would be difficult to determine whether an elevation in body temperature has reached a critical threshold so that decisions could be made about what should be done, such as cold compresses or a cooling bath. In fact, the very notion of a threshold, which is implicit in the critical values of all screening tests, would be quite meaningless, because "measurement" would be reduced to subjective appraisals involving situation-specific judgments.

hypothetical situation described in Box 13-1, which was not an uncommon everyday situation approximately 200 years ago.

In contrast, the availability of standardized measures for body temperature or any other variable of interest reduces the need for situation-specific judgments that depend largely on the skills of the appraiser. As a result, at least five major benefits are associated with standardized measurement procedures:

1. Objectivity
2. Precision
3. Replicability
4. Comparison
5. Development of population norms

Objectivity

Both clinicians and researchers need to come to reasonable agreement about observations of empirical events. For example, imagine a situation in which several clinicians are interpreting a radiograph and cannot agree about what the radiograph shows. If there are no agreed-on procedures for confirming observations, discourse may break down. In this situation, it could be difficult for the clinicians to come to agreement. Such lack of agreement has important implications for patient care because it is unclear what course of action should be recommended in the absence of agreement among the clinicians.

It is important to note that we are talking about agreements with respect to *observations,* not theories or hypotheses. For instance, two psychologists may have competing theories about how the experience of child abuse leads to aggressive and destructive behavior among adolescents. As long as both agree on how to measure "child abuse" and "aggressive and destructive behavior," it is possible to put the theories to an empirical test to decide be-

tween them. Of course, scientists debate all the time about the appropriateness of their measurement procedures. However, the key to objectivity is the *separation* of disputes over measurement issues from disputes over theories. In other words, it is possible for researchers to come to an agreement on measurement, or what constitutes an appropriate empirical test, even if they strongly disagree on theory.

Precision

Standardized measurement tools yield numerical scores that allow for the expression of finer detail in the observations. For instance, we may use a precise definition of hypertension as a condition that entails a systolic blood pressure reading of at least 140 mm Hg and a diastolic reading of at least 90 mm Hg. Such precision facilitates decisions by clinicians and researchers alike because it allows for the establishment of objective criteria that are independent of the specific situations in which observations take place.[2] Precision in measurement and numerical scoring also allows for *modeling the shape of a relationship* between two or more variables. Rather than simply asserting that "two variables are related" or that "the values of one variable increase with those of another," precision in measurement and numerical scoring allows us to describe the relationships in terms of specific mathematical functions and substantially improves our ability to predict specific outcomes.

Replicability

We have repeatedly emphasized in the study design chapters that truly convincing evidence requires more than the

---

[2]Precision in measurement can be taken too far. Contrary to popular media portrayals of the "mad scientist," precision in measurement is not an end in itself. The usefulness of measurement precision depends on the purpose of measurement. For example, there is no point in trying to measure the distance between two cities in inches!

results of a single study. Yet, to replicate any study, one must be able to describe its conditions and circumstances with the desired level of accuracy. For example, an intervention study to improve pulmonary functioning may use as one of its eligibility criteria for subject recruitment a pulse oximetry reading of 90% or lower, rather than "low oxygen saturation." Likewise, an experimental subject in a drug trial may receive x mg of a particular drug, not just a "spoonful." Without standardized measures, we would lack the essential communication tools to replicate any study at a different time or in a different place.

Comparison

When we compare patients and study subjects, we usually compare them with respect to a measurable attribute. To say that some persons are "heavy" means that we score them higher on some weight scale than most other persons. To say that hypertension in some patients "has been controlled" is to say that blood pressure readings show a decline over time. These comparisons, whether they involve measures obtained from different subjects at a single moment in time or several measures obtained from the same subjects at different times, presuppose that the measurement tool itself remains invariant (i.e., it does not change between the measurement occasions [Stommel, Wang, Given, & Given, 1992]). If we were to compare the length of two tables with a soft ruler that easily expands or contracts at the slightest temperature change, we would have little confidence in the comparison because observed differences may reflect both differences in the attribute measured and variations in the measurement tool used. Only through standardization of the measurement procedures can we minimize this problem. That is, of course, the reason for the calibration of measurement instruments used in clinical practice, including blood glucose measurement machines, magnetic resonance imaging scanners, and so forth.

Development of Population Norms

Many measures acquire meaning only with reference to population norms. Achievement tests, such as the Scholastic Aptitude Test (SAT) that many high school students take as part of the admission requirements for college, are explicitly constructed with reference to a population average. Knowing what a "typical score" is on a measure (such as the SAT) for the entire U.S. population provides a researcher or clinician with a benchmark against which to judge the severity of a phenomenon in a particular patient population or individual. For instance, one study has shown mean Center for Epidemiologic Studies Depression Scale (CES-D) scores of more than 20 in a specific group of caregivers (Robinson & Austin, 1998). Mean CES-D

scores in the general adult U.S. population are approximately 7 to 9, with a standard deviation of 6 to 8 (Devins & Orme, 1985). This information provides the context for the inference that depression scores tend to be elevated among the caregivers. Yet, population norms can be constructed only if measurement procedures are standardized so that scores across individuals are comparable. Paradoxically, it is the availability of population norms that highlights the uniqueness of individuals: the detection of individual differences and, in particular, of individuals with "extreme" values presupposes the existence of measurement scales that are applicable to the entire target population.

Levels of Measurement

In chapter 2, we introduced levels of measurement as one of the important characteristics that distinguish different types of variables.

When we operationalize a variable (i.e., translate a concept into measurable scores), we apply a rule system that specifies how we get from observations to scores. Thus, measurement can be understood to involve the *mapping* of elements of a set of real attributes onto a set of symbolic objects (usually numbers). The rule system that underlies the mapping operation determines what kinds of symbolic operations (i.e., mathematical procedures) are defensible or appropriate. To lend substance to this rather abstract formulation, consider the rule systems that distinguish the four levels of measurements that are commonly encountered in health care research and clinical practice.

Nominal or Categorical Variables

The first step in the process of measurement is classification.[3] The construction of **nominal categories** entails grouping objects with respect to a common attribute of interest (e.g., grouping respondents by sex or religious preference as indicated by their survey responses). The numerical labels applied to a group are, in a sense, arbitrary, because they only serve the purpose of distinguishing among the groups. Whether we code female as "1" or "5" and male as "0" or "9" is unimportant, except that the same label cannot be used for two different categories. Likewise, objects that are classified on the basis of a categorical variable must belong to one, and only one, category. In other words, the categories of such a variable must be **mutually exclusive.** This does not mean that the actual decision to classify an object or individual as belonging to a particular category is error-free, or even simple. For instance, with self-report data ob-

---

[3]Not everyone considers "mere" classification an example of measurement, although it is a necessary ingredient (Jones, 1971).

tained in surveys, researchers provide the categories, but it is the respondents who choose the most appropriate category. As shown by the recent change in the race and ethnicity categories used by the U.S. Census Bureau and the National Center of Health Statistics, such classifications and reclassifications can be quite problematic (Box 13-2). Yet, in the end, any classification scheme must be constructed so that subjects belong to mutually exclusive

---

BOX 13.2   Classification of Race and Ethinicity in Federal Surveys

In October 1997, the Office of Management and Budget issued a new standard for the classification of race and ethnicity information in federal surveys. This new standard was implemented in the 2000 Census and has also become the standard in the surveys conducted by the National Center for Health Statistics (NCHS). The former (pre-1997) standard included one "race" variable with four categories: "White," "Black," "American Indian," or "Alaskan Native," "Asian or Pacific Islander"; and a separate "ethnicity" variable with two categories: "Hispanic origin" and "not of Hispanic origin." Under this system, each survey respondent must make two choices: he or she can choose one of the four race categories and one of the two ethnicity categories, allowing, for instance, for such combinations as "Hispanic Black" and "non-Hispanic White."

In recent decades, the U.S. population has experienced a substantial increase in interracial and interethnic marriage as well as accelerated immigration. To accommodate persons who claim a heritage that includes multiple races or ethnic groups, the race variable was substantially revised and now allows for multiple choices. The new format used by Census and NCHS interviewers looks like this:

Is this person Spanish/Hispanic/Latino?

(1)_____ No, not Spanish/Hispanic/Latino
(2)_____ Yes, Mexican, Mexican American, Chicano
(3)_____ Yes, Puerto Rican
(4)_____ Yes, Cuban
(5)_____ Yes, other Spanish/Hispanic/Latino—Print group _____

What is this person's race?
(Mark *one or more* races to indicate what this person considers himself/herself to be)

(1)_____ White
(2)_____ Black, African American, or Negro
(3)_____ American Indian or Alaska Native
(4)_____ Asian Indian
(5)_____ Chinese
(6)_____ Filipino
(7)_____ Japanese
(8)_____ Korean
(9)_____ Vietnamese
(10)_____ Other Asian—Print race _____
(11)_____ Native Hawaiian
(12)_____ Guamanian or Chamorro
(13)_____ Samoan
(14)_____ Other Pacific Islander—Print race _____
(15)_____ Some other race—Print race _____

Even if categories 4 to 10 are collapsed into "Asian" and categories 11 to 14 into "Pacific Islander," there remain six "race" categories (White, Black/African American, American Indian, Asian, Pacific Islander, other race) that can form up to 720 combinations, with 57 combinations actually reported in the 2000 Census. In that year, almost 7 million U.S. residents chose two or more race categories, including 823 persons who chose all six major categories. Cross-classification of the race and ethnicity categories reveals some confusion about these terms, especially among Hispanics/Latinos: Some 48% of all Hispanics reported their race as "White," 42% indicated some other race," and 6% chose multiple race categories (U.S. Census Bureau, 2001).

BOX 13.3   Grading and Ranking Term Papers

For example, when instructors grade term papers, they rank-order them according to a perceived quality gradient. The resulting piles of term papers labeled "A—4.0," "B—3.0," "C—2.0," "D—1.0," and "F—0.0" not only contain distinct papers, but are also thought to possess distinguishable quality attributes, such that A > B > C > D > F. In other words, any paper in A is expected to be better than any paper in B, and so forth. In addition, this property is transitive, meaning that it carries through to nonadjacent piles. In other words, any paper in B is better than any paper in D. In more general terms, ordinal measurement requires that if A > B (objects in A are ranked higher than objects in B) and B > C (objects in B are ranked higher than objects in C), then A > C (objects in A are always ranked higher than objects in C). Note, however, that rank-orders do not require measurement of distance or intervals. For instance, the perceived difference in quality between the "worst" B paper and the "best" C paper may be quite small (boundaries have to be drawn somewhere!); in fact, this difference may be smaller than the perceived difference in quality between two papers that are assigned the same grade.

groups. Similarly, medical and nursing diagnoses may involve multiple, complex steps that draw on test results, individual observations, and judgments. The outcome of diagnosis is a case classified as either having or not having strep throat or mononucleosis, for instance.

The "common" characteristic that defines membership in a group or category depends on the researcher's or clinician's purposes, and its scope may be broad or narrow. For example, for some purposes, it may suffice to divide a clinical population into hypertensive and normotensive patients, without paying much attention to finer individual variations in blood pressure *within* such groups. As always in such situations, the usefulness of a category system ultimately depends on what it shows in terms of its relationship to other variables of interest.

Given the mapping rules just outlined, we cannot rank-order the categories, nor can we assign meaningful distances to them, but we can count the cases that fall into the various categories. Although this limitation restricts the kinds of statistical analyses that legitimately can be used,[4] during the last two decades, powerful multivariate statistical models have been developed to analyze such count data, including Logit, Probit, and Poisson regression models (Agresti, 1990; Agresti, 1996). These models are now widely available in major statistical analysis software packages.

Ordinal Variables

Ordinal-level measurement goes beyond classification and involves *ranking* the categories according to an attribute of interest (Box 13-3).

From this example, it follows that the numbers associated with the ranks cannot be assumed to indicate precise magnitudes of the measured attribute. Thus, 4 minus 2 is not necessarily equal to 3 minus 1. Because the numbers do not indicate magnitude, their assignment as indicators of rank is arbitrary *within limits:* a higher (lower) rank must always be indicated by a higher (lower) number, but sequences such as 1, 2, 3; 2, 6, 11; and 1.5, 2.8, 4.5 are all equivalent ways of assigning ranks to just three objects from lowest to highest. Thus, in addition to counting procedures, the median and percentiles can be used to indicate central tendency and the relative position of cases within a distribution. A variety of more complex statistical analysis tools are also available, including rank-order correlation coefficients (e.g., Spearman's rho, Kendall's tau), rank-order analysis of variance models (e.g., Wilcoxon-Mann-Whitney test, Kruskal-Wallis one-way ANOVA), and sophisticated multivariate statistical models (e.g., ordered Logit and ordered Probit models).[5]

Rank-order information is quite common in clinical practice because the clinician is often called on to rate the strength or weakness of an attribute or the relative "healthiness" of a subject. A classic example of a routinely used clinical rating scale is the Apgar score, which requires the clinician to score a newborn baby on five dimensions: muscle tone, pulse, reflex irritability, skin color and appearance, and respiratory capacity. Within each of the five dimensions, 0 to 2 points are assigned. For example, the rating scale for the newborn's muscle tone includes these category definitions: absent (0), arms and legs flexed (1), active

---

[4]Traditional analysis of variance and linear regression models assume, among other things, that the dependent or outcome variables are continuous and are measured at the interval or ratio level. Such models are not appropriate for categorical outcome measures.

[5]For detailed information on basic ordinal statistics, see Siegel and Castellan (1988); for advanced multivariate ordinal statistical models, see Agresti (1990) and Long (1997).

movement (2). Assignment of babies to these categories clearly requires the observer to make rank-order judgments. In the case of Apgar rankings, such judgments tend to be highly reliable, and the total score is a good predictor of neonatal outcome (Casey, McIntire, & Leveno, 2001).[6]

Ordinal ratings are also common in survey data. The categories of the widely used Likert response scales, such as "strongly disagree" (1), "disagree" (2), "indifferent" (3), "agree" (4), and "strongly agree" (5) are ordinal ratings that only imply greater or lesser degrees of agreement, without necessarily fixing the *amount* of agreement.

Interval Variables

Interval-level variables possess all of the characteristics of nominal and ordinal measures (i.e., mutually exclusive categories that can be rank-ordered), but have the additional feature of a defined distance between the categories. With interval-level measures, numerical distances of a given magnitude correspond to "real distances" of the same magnitude in the attribute being measured. To some degree, this is a word game. Take the classic example of a temperature scale. This type of scale *defines* a degree of temperature, whether expressed in Fahrenheit or Celsius,[7] as corresponding to a given amount of expansion or contraction in the volume of mercury as temperature rises or falls. Once defined, the distance, or interval, between 30° and 40° is equal to the distance, or interval, between 50° and 60°, as long as degrees are measured consistently using the same scale. The importance of this property of *defined intervals* lies in the fact that it is possible to add and subtract scores and to compute means, variances, and standard deviations, all of which are the basic building blocks of parametric statistics, such as regression analysis, analysis of variance, and factor analysis.[8]

One of the enduring controversies in measurement theory is the interval-level properties of many composite scale scores used in health care research. For example, health care and nursing researchers routinely use statistical analysis tools (such linear regression or ANOVA) on depression and quality-of-life scales that are often based on averaged, or summated, scores of questionnaire items with Likert-type

response scales. This is done even though the statistical tools require, strictly speaking, interval-level measurements. More will be said about this controversy in chapter 14.

Ratio Variables

Interval scales lack one property that is necessary for being able to apply all four arithmetic operations (addition, subtraction, multiplication, division) to variable scores: they do not have an absolute zero point. Consider the Fahrenheit scale again: *100°F is not twice as hot as 50°F,* simply because 0°F is an arbitrary number. One way to see this is to convert Fahrenheit degrees into Celsius:

$$°C = 5/9 \ (°F - 32)$$

Thus, 100°F = 37.8°C and 50°F = 10°C

Whereas 100°F/50°F = 2, 37.8°C/10°C = 3.8

In other words, the ratio of two temperatures does not remain invariant after the conversion of scores from one scale to another. Similarly, many psychological instruments that measure concepts such as depression, anxiety, aggression, or hardiness (Bowers, 1999; Devins & Orme, 1985; Pollock, 1989; Spielberger & Vagg, 1984) may attain interval levels of measurement, but surely not ratio levels.[9] There is little sense in speaking of the complete absence of aggression or depression, or of some person having literally "no" (i.e., zero) intelligence. On the other hand, many variables that are used in health care research do meet the ratio test. Among them are biophysiologic measures, such as forced expiratory volume (FEV) or blood pressure, as well as costs (measured in dollars) or time.[10] In sum, ratio-level variables possess all of the qualities associated with lower levels of measurement (e.g., mutually exclusive categories, ranks, defined intervals), with the addition of an absolute zero point. Because most statistical models do not require ratio-level measurements, interval-level and ratio-level measures are usually lumped together as variables that can be analyzed with "parametric" statistics. Occasionally, other scales are seen in the literature, such as logarithmic interval scales to measure pain, for example. Such magnitude estimation scales are constructed so that equally distant intervals on the scale represent *proportionate* increases (or decreases) in the attribute being measured. For example, a/b = c/d or ln(a) −

---

[6]The full meaning of the term "reliability" will be explored in the next chapter.

[7]Degrees Celsius can easily be converted into degrees Fahrenheit and vice versa: F = 9/5 C + 32.

[8]Consider the definition of the arithmetic mean: $\Sigma X_i/n$ (i.e., the sum of the observation values divided by the number of observations). For instance, the mean of three diastolic blood pressure readings of 80, 85, 90 = (80 + 85 + 90)/3 = 85, whereas the mean of 80, 85, 96 = 87. These computations make sense only if we can assume that the distance between 85 and 96 is greater than the distance between 85 and 90 or, in other words, if the distances are defined.

---

[9]See Wills and Moore (1994) for a critique of the debate about magnitude estimation versus category rating scales in nursing.

[10]Time in general may have no meaningfully defined zero point or origin, but starting points can nonetheless be defined in practice, as when measuring days until rehospitalization (with a given hospital discharge date as the starting point for counting).

ln(b) = ln(c) − ln(d). Readers who are interested in further detail about such scales are referred to the measurement literature (Nunnally & Bernstein, 1994; Waltz, Strickland, & Lenz, 1991).

MEASUREMENT ERROR IN CLINICAL PRACTICE AND RESEARCH

When clinicians make decisions based on the results of clinical tests, they implicitly assume or hope that the tests can be trusted to provide a sufficiently accurate picture of the underlying reality. Yet, any experienced clinician knows that measurement of even the most mundane variables, such as body weight, is prone to errors. The three clinical examples described in Box 13-4 illustrate this point.

Example 1 highlights a common problem. Anyone who is familiar with primary care practices knows that the practice of weighing patients at the beginning of a routine visit is imprecise. A patient may be weighed with or without shoes, with or without an overcoat, with or without any instruction as to posture, before or after a heavy meal, and so forth. As a result, even for a person who maintains a very steady body weight, readings from different visits may fluctuate within a range of ± 5 lb. To the extent that such readings differ from the "true" weight at the time of measurement, they may be said to contain measurement error.

Examples 2a and 2b show a similar issue. As a clinician, you are familiar with the fact that successive blood pressure readings taken on the same patient vary from one occasion to the next. The problem is that you must draw inferences about a patient's "true" blood pressure based on fallible readings. The problem is even more complicated. The very notion of a "true," or "normal," blood pressure is elusive because physiologic variables, such as blood pressure or weight, tend to fluctuate naturally. Thus, the observed fluctuation in blood pressure readings represents *both* physiologic changes *and* measurement error. Furthermore, some degree of actual fluctuation in blood pressure, if it remains within a "normal" range, may have no pathologic significance. Under these conditions, how can we make sense of the blood pressure readings obtained? The most general answer is that we need a context that allows us to make judgments about test results.

In Examples 2a and 2b, most of us would be inclined to "write off" the third reading from the first patient as a possible error, but would not conclude that the fourth reading from the second patient constitutes an error, *even though*

BOX 13.4   Clinical Examples of Measurement Error

Example 1
One of the authors of this book recently had a routine medical checkup, during which the nurse asked him to stand on a scale to measure his weight. The resulting number was an astounding 21 lb higher than his normal weight, which he knew from experience did not fluctuate that widely. He disputed the accuracy of the reading. A second reading was taken, with a similar result. After that, he could not persuade the nurse that there might be something wrong with the scale. This story has an ending that resulted in at least some justice. A week later, the nurse called the patient at home and remarked that two other patients had also disputed the accuracy of the weight readings. Service personnel were called and found a mechanical problem with the scale. The moral of this story is that clinicians and researchers should be prepared for the possibility of measurement errors.

Example 2A
You obtain the following blood pressure measurements on a new primary care patient who is 52 years old: 143/95 mm Hg. At the end of the visit, you suggest some dietary changes, such as reduced salt intake, and recommend moderate exercise, such as a walking program during lunch break. You provide the patient with written information about the likely consequences of prolonged hypertension and ask him to come back once every 2 months for a checkup. After three additional visits, each about 2 months apart, you record the following blood pressure readings for this patient: 143/95 mm Hg (visit 1), 140/93 mm Hg (visit 2), 132/85 mm Hg (visit 3), and 141/94 mm Hg (visit 4).

Example 2B
A second patient has blood pressure readings taken at the same time. He receives the same recommendations for dietary changes and exercises and his four readings taken at 2-month intervals: 143/95 mm Hg (visit 1), 141/94 mm Hg (visit 2), 140/93 mm Hg (visit 3), and 132/85 mm Hg (visit 4). How would you interpret these results?

both sequences contain the same readings and thus the same magnitudes of departure from the first reading. However, the successive blood pressure readings of the second patient represent a *trend* for which we have a ready explanation: namely, that we see the effects of the patient following the dietary and exercise recommendations. In contrast, the third reading for the first patient is both unusually low and out of sequence. Thus, it is not unreasonable to assume that an error occurred. Before making a final judgment, we would at least require "more data" or "more evidence." Clinicians sometimes offer patients several explanations as to why one of their blood pressure readings might be "unusually" high or low at a given office visit. A reading might be erroneous because of a problem with the equipment, the technique used, interference of the patient's clothing, an unusually high room temperature because of failing air conditioning, and so forth. This type of explanation clearly would not be a convincing argument for the blood pressure readings observed in the second patient (Example 2b), even though a good clinician would want to see at least one more follow-up reading to be sure that the numbers really have come down. What emerges from this is that the "true" state of the patient's hypertensive status will be known only through *repeated* blood pressure assessments over time. Only a repeated and repeatable pattern of blood pressure readings allows us to classify patients with reasonable certainty as being hypotensive, normotensive, or hypertensive.

Consider Example 1 again. It is a case of a *systematic* measurement error. The scale was miscalibrated, overestimating every patient's weight. The only way that such an error can be discovered is if patients use an external standard, such as their weighing experiences outside the primary care practice, as a reference point. Likewise, the nurse's reaction to the challenge that the scale might produce false readings is a correct one: "file away" in working memory a single challenge as an "unexplained aberration," but investigate further when the challenges continue. This is very much the basis of the scientific, or statistical, approach to measurement: *try to distinguish between unexplained, and perhaps unexplainable, random fluctuations and systematic variation in measurement.*

STATISTICAL MODELS TO EVALUATE MEASUREMENT ERROR

Types of Measurement Errors

In the example of the two series of blood pressure readings, we interpreted fluctuations in blood pressure readings in two ways:

1. There may have been *true* changes in blood pressure.
2. *Measurement errors* may have produced variations in readings from one occasion to the next.

In "real-life" clinical practice and research, both of these explanations are likely to apply. Consider some of the many possible reasons for fluctuations in real blood pressure: the patient may have had a vigorous physical workout an hour before the blood pressure measure was taken (resulting in a lower than usual reading) or the patient may be angry about a traffic incident that took place just before the primary care visit (raising the blood pressure reading). Likewise, some of the possible sources of measurement error include:

- Use of a different arm compared with previous measurements
- Inflation of pressure cuffs to different air pressures
- Application of the pressure cuff to different locations on the same arm
- Variations in room temperature when blood pressure is measured
- Variations in the nurse's auditory or visual capacity as a result of a cold or allergies
- Different nurses measuring blood pressure
- Assessment of blood pressure in a noisy location
- Patient activity, such as talking, during blood pressure assessment

These examples show that there are many possibilities for measurement error; further, multiple sources of error could be occurring simultaneously.

Now, consider some of the typical sources of measurement error in a survey. Any particular question on a survey may be misread by the interviewer or misunderstood by the respondent for a variety of reasons, such as hearing loss or trouble with reading comprehension. A response may be incorrectly recorded, or there may be errors in coding, transcribing, or programming. Again, the list of potential sources of error is large. Even if standardized measures are used, their application or use at different occasions by different people inevitably varies at least somewhat from one occasion to the next. Although researchers often go to great lengths to minimize such errors (e.g., extensive training of interviewers and observers, duplication of data entry to discover inconsistencies), complete elimination of measurement error is impossible. In fact, it is not too strong a statement to say that *where there is measurement, there is bound to be at least some measurement error.*

If measurement error is unavoidable, how do researchers deal with it? How can they be reasonably sure that their findings reflect reality and do not represent erroneous inference based on inaccurate measurement results? To make headway with this problem, one must be able to estimate the *magnitude* of measurement errors present in a particular data set or a particular variable. Furthermore, one must be able to distinguish between two kinds of measurement errors: **systematic error,** also known as "measurement bias," and **random error.**

If we could measure a variable without any measurement error, its observed measurement outcome would be identical to the true state of affairs. When measurement error is present, the observed measurement score deviates from a true score. There are two kinds of such deviations:

1. Measurement results may deviate from the true scores in a *predictable* (or *systematic*) way.
2. They may fluctuate in a more or less *random* fashion, sometimes overestimating and sometimes underestimating the true score.

Systematic Measurement Error

Consider the example of a weight scale that is based on a spring mechanism. The spring inside the scale gradually suffers from metal fatigue. As a result, the scale will eventually produce systematic overestimates of weight (i.e., each patient weighed on the scale is likely to show a weight higher than his or her true weight). If the magnitude of this systematic error is known, and if the error is reasonably stable over the short run,[11] it is possible to use the scale and subtract the systematic measurement bias from the obtained readings. Of course, the problem is often that one does not know exactly how much systematic measurement error occurs unless one has an *external* device to recalibrate the scale.

In clinical practice, systematic measurement error is often disregarded, usually because it is not considered large enough to be clinically meaningful. Some clinicians may simply attempt to compensate for systematic measurement error, as when patients are not requested to remove their shoes or coats before standing on a scale, but are asked for a "best guess" about how much their clothing weighs. Although some clinicians may subtract a patient's estimate of the weight of clothing from the obtained weight, others may not. Without a policy, or standardization, of how to proceed, weights obtained at successive visits may fluctuate depending on the inclusion or exclusion of the weight of major articles of clothing. Thus, what initially may be considered a systematic error becomes a *random error* in the long run.

Random Measurement Error

Random measurement errors produce *unpredictable variation* in measurement results *from one instance to the next*. At first glance, this seems to be an even more difficult problem, but on reflection, it is more manageable than systematic measurement error. To the extent that measurement errors are unpredictable, or random, at given instances of measurement, they do not produce predictable patterns of *change* in the long run. That is, they fluctuate around the underlying true scores. Because a random error is just as likely to yield an overestimate as an underestimate of the true score, we can assume that the long-run *average* of many obtained measurements approaches the true score.[12] As the example in Box 13-5 shows, we can think of every observed measurement score as consisting of two components: a true score and measurement error.[13] Thus, $O_i = T + e_i$ or, for example, $82 = 80 + 2$ or $79 = 80 − 1$. The example in Box 13-5 also shows that the sum of all error terms equals zero, or $\Sigma e_i = 0$. Although that is true "in the long run," if the measurement error is truly random, it may be only approximately true after just ten measurements are taken.[14] Nevertheless, if measurement errors cancel each other out "in the long run," *as more measurements are taken, the mean of many scores must come closer and closer to the true score.* Thus, after repeated measurements of a given attribute of the same subject, we can obtain at least an estimate of the true score and, therefore, also an estimate of measurement error. The variance of these error terms gives an indication of how large the average (squared) measurement error is. It plays a central role in the notion of measurement **reliability,** as we will see shortly.

Suppose that diastolic blood pressure readings are obtained from a sample of 200 patients. We can think of each of these scores as being composed of the true underlying blood pressure of that individual plus or minus some unavoidable measurement error. To the extent that measurement error is random, it is not correlated with the true score.[15] Because the variance of the sum of two uncorrelated variables equals the sum of their variances (Nunnally & Bernstein, 1994), we can think of the variance of the ob-

---

[12]We assume here that the "real" attribute does not change for the duration of the repeated measurements.

[13]This model does not incorporate systematic error. This kind of error does not fluctuate from one measurement occasion to the next and can be detected only through comparisons with external standards.

[14]The principle here is the same as in games of chance. With a completely unbiased die, each of the six sides (numbers) has the same probability of coming up on top, but one would not expect that, after only 12 throws, all six possible outcomes occurred exactly twice.

[15]Recall that "randomness" means unpredictability; however, if two variables are correlated, one can predict the scores of one from the other.

---

[11]Of course, as metal fatigue continues to occur, overestimates will become larger with time.

BOX 13.5   Example of Measurement Error: 10 Diastolic Blood Pressure Readings Obtained From a Single Patient within 10 Minutes

		Measurement error	
Observed diastolic blood pressure readings O_i	Assumed "true" and stable diastolic blood pressure: T	Deviation from true score: e_i	Squared deviation: e_i^2
78	80	−2	4
81	80	+1	2
79	80	−1	2
76	80	−4	16
82	80	+2	4
83	80	+3	9
80	80	±0	0
78	80	−2	2
79	80	−1	1
84	80	+4	16
$\mu_O = t = \Sigma o_i/n = 80$	t = 80	$\Sigma e_i = 0$	$\Sigma e_i^2 = 56$

Error variance $= V_e = \Sigma e_i^2/(n-1) = 56/9 = 6.2$

served scores (V_o), as comprising the variance of the true scores (V_t) between the individuals and the variance of the measurement errors (V_e):

$$V_o = V_t + V_e$$

Although we can never actually observe the true scores and their variance, this equation suggests that if we can obtain an estimate of the error variance, we will also get an estimate of the true variance:

$$V_t = V_o - V_e$$

Furthermore, if we divide both sides of this equation by the variance of the observed score (V_o), we get an expression for reliability in measurement:

$$R = V_t/V_o = 1 - V_e/V_o$$

On the right-hand side of the first equal sign, we have *the ratio of true score variance divided by observed variance* (V_t/V_o). That is the formal definition of measurement reliability. Assume for a moment that we are in possession of an error-free measurement procedure. Then error variance would be zero ($V_e = 0$), and consequently, observed variance would equal true variance.[16] However, if $V_t = V_o$, the ratio of V_t/V_o must be equal to one (i.e., the measurement is perfectly reliable). Now, assume that the measured

individuals do not differ from each other at all (i.e., true variance would equal zero, all observed variance would be due to measurement error, and the reliability coefficient would equal zero).

In general, if V_e/V_o, the proportion of the variance of observed scores accounted for by measurement error declines, then V_t/V_o, the proportion of observed variance accounted for by the true scores, must increase. Thus, a measurement procedure is reliable to the extent that it produces relatively few random measurement errors. Although this definition of reliability in measurement is straightforward, we do not yet have a practical way of *assessing* or *estimating* reliability in measurement. This discussion will be taken up in chapter 14.

MEASUREMENT AS A SAMPLING PROCESS

Many of the examples of measurement error given so far have involved repeated measurements. Consider again the examples in Box 13-1 of taking several blood pressure measurements of the same patient in short succession. We can think of these obtained measures as a *sample* of all possible measures that we could have taken. Because measurement is fallible, this sampling process is subject to sampling error (i.e., the obtained measures will not always

---

[16]Since $V_o = V_t + V_e$, $V_e = 0$ implies that $V_o = V_t$.

result in identical estimates of the true underlying attribute, and a different collection, or sample, of measures would likely return slightly different results).[17]

Knowledge and attitude tests can also be thought of in this way. For example, consider the NCLEX-RN examination, taken for licensure as a registered nurse in the United States. In any given year, graduating nursing students are tested on their nursing knowledge with a different examination. Each examination represents a sample of all possible knowledge questions that could be asked of nursing students prepared to take the test. Suppose the test consists of only 10 randomly chosen questions out of a pool of 10,000 such questions, and suppose further that a particular student gets 9 of the 10 answers right, for a score of 0.9. Almost everyone would agree that such a test would be too short to cover the relevant domain of knowledge. A student's overall test score (the proportion of correct answers) would depend a fair amount on the luck of the draw (i.e., whether the student happens to know the 10 randomly drawn questions). Now, suppose that we draw 100 questions from the same question pool, which constitutes our "knowledge universe." If the student also scores 0.9 on this expanded test, we would have much greater confidence that the expanded test reflects the student's "true" knowledge of nursing. The reason is simple: the probability that a student who *really* knows the answers to only 70% of the 10,000 questions covering the relevant knowledge domain for nursing will get at least 90 of 100 randomly chosen questions right is quite small ($P < .0000015$), whereas the probability that this student will get at least 9 of 10 questions right is nonnegligible ($P = .1493$).[18]

This result is consistent with our intuitive understanding: longer tests are harder to "fake." It also means that *longer tests are more reliable and accurate.* For instance, among students who know 90% of the potential test material, we can expect that only 58.8% will obtain a test score of .88 to .92 on the 100-item test, but 81.6% will obtain a test score in this range on a 400-item test.[19] This is precisely the reason why we repeat tests when we suspect that they may be unreliable: the average of several obtained measures is likely to provide a better estimate of the true score than a few measures or a single observation or test result. To avoid any confusion about the meaning of the sampling process involved in measurement, *it is not a question of sampling more study subjects, but of sampling more measurements or observations!*

CONCLUSION

In this chapter, we have introduced the concept of measurement as the assignment of numbers to attributes of objects according to a rule system. Two aspects of the rule system are of paramount importance. First, the rules used to assign numbers to attributes implicitly define the levels of measurement (nominal or categorical, ordinal, interval, or ratio) and thus determine the kinds of mathematical operations and manipulations that are permissible when analyzing variables generated at the various measurement levels. Second, rule systems impose, to the degree that it is possible, a standardization of measurement procedures. That is, they are the only guarantors we have to produce reliable (i.e., dependable and consistent) measurement results across different locations and times. However, even the most dependable measurement procedures produce unexplained and unpredictable fluctuations in measurement scores; thus, measurement error is endemic in the measurement process.

The distinction between systematic and random variation in observed scores underlies all efforts to estimate the magnitude of (random) measurement errors; however, acceptance of the idea of randomness in measurement does not imply a particular worldview or set of philosophic assumptions about the sources of randomness in measurement. If one talks at length with different researchers, especially from widely different fields of study, one would notice that they make different philosophic assumptions about how to view "error." For example, many researchers believe that there is inherent randomness in almost all processes of the known world. That would certainly be true of such physiologic processes as blood pressure, and it applies to just about any characteristic or attribute of living organisms. Further, it also applies to inanimate objects. For instance, an apparently stable metal rod contracts and expands ever so slightly when external temperature changes. Thus, one view is to say that no phenomenon in our world can really be considered "stable," and if sufficiently precise measurements were available, we would discover that "everything is in flux," even the measurement tool itself. Yet, the acceptance of apparently "random" fluctuations from one moment to the next does not, in itself, preclude a completely deterministic view of the world. In principle, one could conceive of all variations in measured outcomes as caused by some systematic, if unknown, factor. For instance, when you attempt to list all of the causative factors

---

[17]For a more detailed discussion of these ideas, see chapters 19 and 20.

[18]These calculations are based on the binomial distribution (Snedecor & Cochran, 1989; Siegel & Castellan, 1998).

[19]παντα ρει <greek letters pi alpha nu tau alpha rho epsilon iota> or "everything is in flux" was the first philosophic principle of the ancient Greek philosopher Heraklit (Jaeger, 1965).

that might account for variations in blood pressure readings (e.g., slight variations in the concentration level of the nurse measuring the blood pressure, differences in room temperature, fluctuations in lighting that affect the ability to read the number on the sphygmomanometer), it is easy to see that there is no end to the differences between any two measurement occasions. In other words, no two moments are exactly alike, so *the conditions under which measurement takes place are always changing somewhat* and, with them, the outcomes, scores, or readings that are obtained. In practice, neither researchers nor clinicians need to obsess about the minutiae of measurement fluctuations. What they need are ways to disentangle random fluctuations from true variations in the measured phenomenon. So far, we have simply posited that observed scores are composed of "true" scores and a random measurement component. In chapter 14, we will see how observed scores, together with some assumptions about the behavior of random errors, can be used to estimate the reliability of measurement instruments, and thus, true score variation.

Suggested Activities

1. Take your own pulse (count for 30 seconds) five times in a row within a span of 5 minutes, and write down the results. Repeat this process at least once a day for 4 days, and record the results.
   a. Based on the 20 pulse measures, estimate your overall mean ("true") pulse rate.
   b. Based on each of the five daily measures, estimate your *daily* mean pulse rate.
   c. If your daily mean pulse rates differ from your overall mean pulse rates, how do you interpret that finding?
   d. If individual pulse readings differ from the daily mean readings, how do you interpret that finding?
   e. Provide an estimate of the average random measurement error.
   f. Do you consider differences in mean daily pulse rates measurement error? Provide a rationale for your position.

2. Provide examples of measurement errors that you have encountered in your clinical practice.
   a. What strategies did you or your team members pursue to improve the reliability of the measurement results in question?
   b. Have you ever obtained readings from an instrument in clinical practice that you thought were "wrong?" If so, what information did you base that judgment on?
   c. Should clinicians disregard test results that they consider mistaken? Discuss the pros and cons of doing so, with reference to the content of this chapter.

References

Agresti, A. (1990). *Categorical data analysis*. New York: John Wiley & Sons.

Agresti, A. (1996). *An Introduction to Categorical Analysis*. New York, NY. John Wiley & Sons.

Beck, A. T., Ward, C. H., et al. (1961). An inventory for measuring depression. *Archives of General Psychiatry, 4,* 561–571.

Bowers, L. (1999). A critical appraisal of violent incident measures. *Journal of Mental Health, 8,* 4, 339–349.

Campbell, N. R. (1952). *What is science?* New York: Dover.

Casey, B. M., McIntire, D. D., & Leveno, K. J. (2001). The continuing value of the APGAR score for the assessment of newborn infants. *New England Journal of Medicine, 344,* 7, 467–471.

Devins, G. M., & Orme, C. M. (1985). Center for Epidemiological Studies depression scale. In Keyser, D. J., & R. C. Sweetland (Eds.), *Test critiques* (pp. 144–160). Kansas City, MO: Test Corporation of America.

Dougherty, M. C., Dwyer, J. W., Pendergast, J. F., Boyington, A. R., Tomlinson, B. U., Coward, R. T., Duncan, R. P., Vogel, G., & Rooks, L. G. (2002). A randomized trial of behavioral management for continence with older rural women. *Research in Nursing & Health, 2002, 25,* 3–13.

Folkman, S., & Lazarus, R. S. (1983). *Ways of coping questionnaire (WCQ)*. Redwood City, CA: Mind Garden.

Hamilton, M. (1960). A rating scale for depression. *Journal of Neurology, Neurosurgery and Psychiatry, 23,* 56–62.

Jaeger, W. (1965). *Paidaia: The ideals of Greek culture*. New York: Oxford University Press.

Long, J. C. (1997). *Regression models for categorical and limited dependent variables*. Thousand Oaks, CA: Sage.

Nagel, E. (1961). *The structure of science: Problems in the logic of scientific explanations*. New York: Harcourt, Brace.

Nunnally, J. C., & Bernstein, I. H. (1994). *Psychometric theory* (3rd ed.). New York: McGraw-Hill.

Pollock, S. E. (1989). The hardiness characteristic: A motivating factor in adaptation. *Advances in Nursing Science, 11,* 2, 53–62.

Radloff, L. S. (1977). The CES-D scale: A self-report depression scale for research in the general population. *Applied Psychological Measurement, 1,* 385–401.

Robinson, K., & Austin, J. K. (1998). Wife caregivers' and supportive others' perceptions of the caregivers' health and social support. *Research in Nursing & Health, 21,* 1, 51–57.

Siegel, S., & Castellan, N. J. (1988). *Non-parametric statistics* (2nd ed.). Boston: McGraw-Hill.

Snedecor, G. W., & Cochran, W. G. (1989). *Statistical methods* (8th ed.). Ames, IA: Iowa State University Press.

Spielberger, C. D., & Vagg, P. R. (1984) Psychometric properties of the State-Trait Anxiety Inventory: A reply. *Journal of Personality Assessment, 48,*1, 95–97.

Spitzer, R., Williams, J. B., Kroenke, K., Linzer, M., deGruy, F. V., et al. (1994). Utility of a new procedure for diagnosing mental disorders in primary care: The PRIME-MD 1000 study. *Journal of the American Medical Association, 272,* 1749–1756.

Spitzer, R. L., Kroenke, K., Williams, J. B. and the PHQ Primary Care Study Group. (1999). Validation and utility of a self-report version of PRIME-MD: The PHQ primary care study. *Journal of the American Medical Association, 282,* 1752–1759.

Stevens, S. S. (1964). On the theory of scales of measurement. *Science,* 103, 677–680.

Stommel, M., Wang, S., Given, C. W., & Given, B. A. (1992). Confirmatory factor analysis (CFA) as a method to assess measurement equivalence. *Research in Nursing & Health, 15,* 5, 352–360.

U.S. Census Bureau. (2001). *Overview of race and Hispanic origin: Census 2000 brief.* Washington, DC: U.S. Department of Commerce. C2KBR/01-1 (March 2001).

Waltz C. F., Strickland, O. L., & Lenz, E. R. (Eds.) (1991). *Measurement in nursing research* (2nd ed.). Philadelphia: F. A. Davis.

Wills, C. E., & Moore, C. F. (1994). A controversy in scaling of subjective states: Magnitude estimation versus category rating methods. *Research in Nursing & Health, 17,* 231–237.

CHAPTER 14 Judging the Quality of Measurement

OVERALL PRINCIPLES OF EVALUATION OF MEASUREMENT INSTRUMENTS

In the last chapter, we introduced a basic definition of measurement and the concepts of **levels of measurement** and **measurement error.** In this chapter, we build on these concepts to provide tools for the evaluation of measurement instruments and procedures. Historically, one of the challenges in interpreting measurement issues in the health care research literature has been that the vocabulary to describe measurement issues and problems is derived from two separate traditions: (1) the psychometric tradition and (2) the medical and public health tradition.

Psychometric Tradition: Reliability and Validity

The *psychometric tradition* has primarily been concerned with constructing more or less continuous measurement scales based on self-report measures. The basic building blocks of such measures are the patients' or study subjects' responses to multiple question items, with standardized response categories that are combined in some fashion to form a single, continuous scale measure (Box 14-1). This type of measurement tradition has produced a very rich and extensive body of literature (Hambleton & Swaminathan, 1994; Nunnally & Bernstein, 1994; Shavelson, 1991; Traub, 1994; Camilli & Shepard, 1994) concerned with the **validity** and **reliability** of such measurement instruments. The focus on creating continuous scales has meant that individuals are viewed as having finely graduated perceptions and attitudes, attributes, and experiences that may vary over a wide range. For example, the SF-36 and its subscales are scaled from 0 to 100, and fractional (between whole numbers) scores are possible (see box 16–1). Similarly, the Center for Epidemiologic Studies Depression (CES-D) scale, which has been discussed in previous chapters of this book, combines the responses to 20 items into a scale score with a potential range of 0 to 60.

Medical and Public Health Tradition: True Positives, True Negatives, False Positives, and False Negatives

In contrast to the psychometric tradition, the focus of the *medical and public health tradition* has been on biophysiologic tests. Such tests have been used primarily to *divide patients into a few diagnostic categories.* This makes sense in light of the major emphasis to medical practice on the causes, diagnosis, and cure of diseases. Although the medical and public health literature is also concerned with measurement error (see the discussion of **false positives** and **false negatives**), the interest in measurement error is in relation to the correct or accurate classification of patients into a limited number of diagnostic categories (Kraemer, 1992). However, the use of categories for diagnosis does not mean that the underlying *measurement procedure* is necessarily categorical. Actually, many biophysiologic tests produce measurement outcomes that approximate continuous scales, as we discussed in chapter 14, with the example of blood pressure and pulse oximetry testing. However, ultimately, for reasons of practicality and clinical decision-making, clinicians are often interested in finding cutoff points on such continuous tests to obtain the "best" possible classification of patients (for given diagnostic and treatment purposes) into *cases* and *non-cases.*

Merging Discrete Measurement Traditions

Both measurement approaches (psychometric and medical and public health) have their value in health care research, and a gradual merging of these traditions is taking place. However, clinicians and researchers alike tend to be familiar with the techniques and terminology of only one of these traditions. Although behavioral researchers who are not clinicians tend to be more familiar with measurement concepts derived from the psychometric tradition, clinicians who are not necessarily researchers tend to be more familiar with measurement concepts derived from the medical and public health tradition. In this chapter, we attempt to bridge this gap by emphasizing the common issues and similarities underlying the two approaches. A key advantage to understanding and comparing the ideas from both measurement traditions is that clinicians and researchers

---

BOX 14.1   SF-36: A Quality-of-Life Measure

For example, the SF-36, which was originally developed for a landmark research project called the Medical Outcomes Study (Ware & Sherbourne, 1992; McHorney, Ware, & Raczek, 1993, 1993b) is a measure of health status that is often interpreted as a quality of life measure. It assess overall health, functional status, emotional health, vitality, and so forth, by providing respondents with fixed response scales to 36 specific questions (indicator items) designed to cover these conceptual domains.

alike will have a richer understanding of quality-of-measurement issues.

RELIABILITY IN MEASUREMENT

In the last chapter, we defined **measurement reliability** *as the relative absence of unsystematic, random measurement error*. Although measurement error cannot be completely eliminated, both researchers and clinicians have a strong interest in measurement instruments and procedures that minimize this type of error. Thus, if the attribute that is being measured does not change, a reliable measurement instrument or procedure should produce *stable observations and scores*. The desirability of stable measurement results should be considered in the following contexts:

- *Measurement results should be independent of the person performing the measurement.* Ideally, it should not matter who among several trained clinicians performs a pulse oximetry test, nor should the final scores on a standardized instrument, such as the SF-36, vary systematically depending on who collected data from the SF-36 respondents.

- *Measurement results should be independent of the occasions on which they are performed.* "Occasion" is the timing of the act of measurement. If the measured attributes are relatively stable, such as the height and weight of an adult or traits such as generalized ("G factor") intelligence,[1] the obtained ratings should be similar, whether taken on Tuesdays or Thursdays, in the morning or the evening. Of course, as was emphasized in the last chapter, in reality, no two occasions are ever exactly alike. Room temperature, lighting, and a host of other factors will be slightly different from one occasion to the next. Yet, as long as no *systematic* changes in conditions affect all subsequent measurements, differences among occasions usually result in small random fluctuations. For example, an adult should not be 5 feet tall one day and 6 feet tall the next. Any measurement procedure that gave us such results would be considered completely untrustworthy.

- *Measurement results should be independent of the locations at which they are performed.* The classic example is the measurement of body temperature at different body locations (sublingual, armpit, rectal, tympanic, forehead), all of which, in theory, should return similar readings, if the "core" body temperature is being accurately assessed. Similarly, the location of an interview, such as in the hospital or postdischarge at home, should not systematically affect the answers given.

- *Measurement results should be independent of the particular measurement instruments being used.* The scale that is used in a primary care clinic and the scale used in a hospital emergency department should return similar weight readings for the same person. Likewise, whether we use the Beck Depression Inventory, the CES-D scale, or the Hamilton Depression Rating Scale, all of which are widely used, standardized instruments to assess current depressive symptoms, each scale should be similar in its ability to identify "depressed" versus "nondepressed" individuals.[2] Similarly, whether blood pressure is measured with a sphygmomanometer or an electronic gauge, such as DINAMAP (Ornstein, Markert, Litchfield, & Zemp, 1988), should not matter much in terms of the obtained results, particularly in the final categorization of people as "hypertensive" or "normotensive."

In sum, reliability is the consistency of measurement results across **persons, occasions, locations,** and **instruments.** Consistency can be detected only *if there are at least two measures to compare, and preferably more than two.* This means that the reliability (or lack of reliability) of a measurement tool or procedure can be established only if we have *multiple observations to compare.* A single measurement may or may not be accurate, but its reliability cannot be known.

Suppose, for example, that you want to determine the sex of a participant in a survey study. Most questionnaires contain only a single question about a respondent's sex (i.e., respondents check a box to indicate "male" or "female"). This makes sense in principle because respondents rarely make mistakes in response to this question, and errors can often be picked up when they do occur; for example, a respondent whose first name is "David" is unlikely to be female. Nonetheless, even this variable is not com-

---

[1]What constitutes a "stable" trait can be controversial in both research and clinical practice. For example, researchers and clinicians have debated over the extent to which personality "traits" remain stable or are amenable to change over time and circumstances. See McCrae and Costa (1990) for an example of research on personality change.

[2]Clinicians and researchers alike often debate the conceptual and practical merits of using one scale over another for a given purpose. For the example we cited, the Beck Depression Inventory is particularly useful for picking up the cognitive manifestations of depression; the CES-D is useful for detecting current generalized, multidimensional distress that is consistent with (but not exclusive to) major depression; and the Hamilton Depression Rating Scale is useful for measuring the severity of clinically significant depressive symptoms. Also, as we will address in chapter 15, factors such as feasibility considerations and cultural, developmental, and other differences among target populations must be carefully considered in selecting a specific measure.

pletely error-free. If nothing else, an occasional coding error leads to a mistaken sex code. How would you discover the mistake? As we have just illustrated in the example of "David" being unlikely to be female, errors can be picked up only through comparisons with other sources of information, for example, interview data and medical records, or through comparisons with other items on the same questionnaire.[3] This is the general principle when we *estimate* the reliability of a measurement tool or procedure.

As we mentioned in chapter 13, reliability is defined as *the ratio of true score variance divided by observed variance*. Yet, we can never directly compare an observed score with a true score because the only way to know the true score is to obtain *observations* about the attribute. In other words, observed scores are "all there is to go on."

The best we can do is to compare multiple fallible observations and use them to estimate the underlying true measurement score. In the next section, we look at three closely related concepts (types of reliability), all of which have found widespread application in the health-related research literature: internal consistency, test-retest reliability, and interrater reliability.

Reliability of Interview Data: Internal Consistency

A very common issue in health care research is the determination of the reliability of a composite scale based on a cross-sectional,[4] multi-item questionnaire instrument that has fixed response categories. Examples of composite scales include the SF-36 quality-of-life measure, the Coping Resources Inventory (Hammer, 1988), the Profile of Mood States scale (McNair, Lorr, & Droppleman, 1992) the Social Support Questionnaire (Norbeck, 1995), and the CES-D scale (Radloff, 1977; Devins & Orme, 1985). Given the complexity of concepts such as quality of life, social support, and depression, it is not surprising that these instruments are subdivided into several dimensions (subscales) that probe specific aspects of the overall, more complex concept. For instance, we already mentioned that the SF-36 contains 36 questions that form eight subscales, "tapping into" (assessing) concepts such as physical func-

tioning, social functioning, mental health, and vitality. Each of these concepts is explored with multiple questions. The physical functioning subscale, for example, includes 10 items, all of which are designed to measure the respondents' ability to perform various physical tasks. To the extent that these 10 items are indicators of a respondent's ability to perform basic physical tasks, they should generate similar or consistent responses in a given subject.

The most widely used measure to estimate the **internal consistency reliability** of a multi-item instrument administered in a single interview is Cronbach's alpha (Cronbach, 1951; Traub, 1994). Because of the widespread use (and occasional misuse) of this statistic in the literature, it is important for the reader to understand its meaning and purpose. We use data from the first wave of a panel study of patients with cancer (Given & Given, 1993) to demonstrate the estimation of the reliability of one of the subscales of the CES-D.

Cronbach's Alpha: A Measure of Internal Consistency and Reliability of Multi-item Scales

The CES-D (Radloff, 1977; Radloff & Locke, 1986; Devins & Orme, 1985; Stommel et al., 1993) is a 20-item measure of depressive symptoms that can be subdivided into four subscales, customarily thought to measure depressed mood or affect (7 items), somatic and retarded activity (7 items), absence of a sense of well-being (4 items), and interpersonal relations (2 items). Table 14-1 shows a list of all seven "depressed mood" items and their associated response categories. The table also shows the mean sample responses (and their standard deviations) for N = 787 patients newly diagnosed with cancer.

Because all means in Table 14-1 are less than 1, most of the patients must have responded "rarely or none of the time" to these questions.[5] However, for our purposes, we focus only on the *internal consistency* of the responses. Assuming that all seven items measure the underlying concept of "depressed mood," we would expect them to generate very similar responses because the respondents' underlying mood gives rise to the responses to individual questions. For example, an individual who indicated that he or she felt depressed only a little or none of the time in the last week would also be expected to indicate that he or she rarely felt sad during the same period. Of course, it is unlikely that all respondents would consistently choose a single response category across all seven items, such as

---

[3]For instance, surveys of caregivers usually ask about the "relationship" of the caregiver to the care recipient. If the answer to this question is "daughter" or 'niece," but the care recipient's sex is described as "male," the researcher would know that there is a problem. Additional information about how such errors can be prevented, such as "data cleaning" procedures, is given in chapter 23.

[4]That is to say, all questions are asked at more or less the "same" time.

---

[5]The total mean CES-D score for this sample is 11.0, indicating only minimally elevated scores over those of the general population, which generally have mean scores ranging from 8 to 10 (Stommel et al., 1993).

TABLE 14.1	Depressive Mood or Affect Subscale of the Center for Epidemiologic Studies Depression Scale (CES-D)

Question stem: During the past 2 weeks, how often have you felt this way
CES-D3:   . . . I felt that I could not shake the blues, even with the help of family and friends
CES-D6:   . . . I felt depressed
CES-D9:   . . . I thought my life had been a failure
CES-D10: . . . I felt fearful
CES-D14: . . . I felt lonely
CES-D17: . . . I had crying spells
CES-D18: . . . I felt sad

Answer categories and associated codes: 0 = rarely or none of the time; 1 = some or a little of the time; 2 = occasionally or a moderate amount of the time; 3 = most or all of the time.

Descriptive Statistics for Responses to CES-D Mood Items by Newly Diagnosed Cancer Patients (N = 787)

Questionnaire Item	Mean Response	Standard Deviation
CES-D3	0.35	0.65
CES-D6	0.49	0.65
CES-D9	0.15	0.43
CES-D10	0.43	0.63
CES-D14	0.38	0.63
CES-D17	0.21	0.47
CES-D18	0.44	0.59

(With permission from Given, B. A., & Given, C. W. (1993). Family home care for cancer: A community-based model. Grant RO1 N01915. Funded by the National Institute for Nursing Research and the National Cancer Institute.)

"some of the time."[6] In part, this is because no two questions are ever exactly alike in their ability to "tap into" an underlying psychological concept, but there are also other sources of measurement error associated with every question. These sources of error include differences in the language skills of respondents; the varying emotional significance of certain words, such as "sad" or "depressed," for different respondents; or simply the poor eyesight of a respondent who marks his or her answers on the printed page.

As long as we can reasonably assume that errors in measurement are unrelated to each other, we can use the correlations among the seven indicator variables (responses to items) to estimate internal consistency. Recall that each response to a specific indicator item is thought of as consisting of two components:

1. One reflecting the true magnitude of "depressed mood"
2. The other reflecting the random measurement error

In this situation, the only feature that two different CES-D subscale items share is that they are both indicators of depressed mood. To the extent that two items are tapping into the same characteristic (in this case, the absence or presence of depressed mood), observed responses to the items will correlate. In contrast, *the random measurement error will not contribute to the correlation among observed scores.*[7] To examine the data in Table 14-2, first look at the correlation matrix. It shows the Pearson correlations among the seven indicators of depressed mood, with the diagonal showing the correlation of a variable with itself, which is a perfect 1.00. In the lower triangle, you can find all possible 21 pairwise correlations among these indicator variables. As expected, they are all positive, yet they are far from perfect. The smallest correlation is 0.23 and the largest is 0.62, with a mean inter-item correlation ($\bar{r}$ = mean value of the 21 correlations in the table) of $\bar{r}$ = 0.43. Thus, we know from these bivariate correlations that each of the individual items in the depressive mood scale reflects the underlying mood imperfectly, and this is why the correlations are only moderately large, instead of a perfect 1.00.

---

[6]In the current sample, 37.5% of the respondents exhibit perfect consistency.

[7]If one takes two series of randomly generated numbers and correlates them, the observed correlation will be close to zero. Why? *Correlation* implies *systematic co-variation* between two variables, whereas *randomness* implies the *absence* of any systematic pattern. Thus, random error will not contribute anything to the correlation among observed scores.

| TABLE 14.2 | Correlation matrix for Seven CES-D-Mood Items (N = 787) |

	Bivariate Correlations							Item-Total Correlations
	CES-D3	CES-D6	CES-D9	CES-D10	CES-D14	CES-D17	CES-D18	
CES-D3	1.00							0.64
CES-D6	0.56	1.00						0.68
CES-D9	0.33	0.33	1.00					0.42
CES-D10	0.47	0.49	0.33	1.00				0.60
CES-D14	0.44	0.49	0.34	0.42	1.00			0.59
CES-D17	0.45	0.41	0.23	0.32	0.34	1.00		0.51
CES-D18	0.53	0.62	0.34	0.58	0.54	0.51	1.00	0.74

Mean interitem correlation: 0.43

Cronbach's alpha: A = 0.85

Next, look at the item-total correlations shown in the last column of Table 14-2. An **item-total correlation** is the correlation between a particular indicator item and the sum of all other indicator items that are part of the same subscale. For example, correlating the responses to CES-D10 with those to CES-D3 + CES-D6 + CES-D9 + CES-D14 + CES-D17 + CES-D18 yields a correlation value of 0.60. Such item-total correlations can be considered an index of how well the responses to any particular indicator item vary with the responses to the other subscale items. An item with very low item-total correlations does not produce responses that are consistent with the other items, and is thus an unreliable indicator of the underlying concept.[8] Finally, we consider the internal consistency reliability coefficient itself, **Cronbach's alpha:**

$$A = \frac{k}{k-1}\left(1 - \frac{k}{k + k(k-1)\bar{r}}\right).$$

Although this formula may appear relatively complicated, it actually contains just two variables. The k stands for the number of indicators, or items, used in the measurement instrument, and the r with the bar over it ($\bar{r}$) stands for the average correlation among the items. Applying the results from Table 14-1, with seven indicator items for "depressed mood" ($k = 7$) and an average inter-item correlation ($\bar{r} = 0.43$), we get an alpha value of:

$$A = \frac{7}{7-1}\left(1 - \frac{7}{7 + 7(7-1)0.43}\right) = 0.85.$$

This result is remarkable: it says that if we create a scale score that either sums or averages the scores across all seven items, this depressed mood scale will have an *impressive reliability* (alpha = 0.85), or 85% true score variance. Why should that be so? Remember that we assumed that the responses to each individual mood item are: (1) influenced by the "true" mood of the respondent and (2) influenced by all sorts of extraneous, unrelated factors, which we have collectively called "error." Because of the error component, the following statements are true:

• Some items tend to *overestimate* true depressed mood.
• Other items tend to *underestimate* true depressed mood.
• Taking an *average across several items* will "smooth out" the error component.
• The combined scale score will be closer to the true overall mood score than will the score of any single item.

It is clear that if we had more indicator items, that is, if we generated additional questions similar to the existing questions about depressed mood, they would also reflect both the true depressed mood of the subjects and some error component. However, the more items we have, the more likely it is that the combined random errors cancel each other out. As a result, additional items will improve scale reliability, even if they do not increase the average correlation among all items. Cronbach's alpha reflects that fact. For example, assume we had 10 question items that probe depressed mood. Even with the same mean inter-item correlation, the overall scale reliability would increase to 0.88.[9]

---

[8]A minimum item-total correlation of at least 30 is desirable. Items that have lower item-total correlations are usually excluded from the scale (Spector, 1990).

[9]You may want to try different values for k to see how it affects the alpha value.

	TABLE 14.3	Examples of Tradeoffs between the Numbers of Indicators and the Average Inter-item Correlations Holding Scale Reliability Constant at Alpha — 0.80

Cronbach's alpha	Number of items (k)	Mean Interitem correlation ($\bar{r}$)
0.80	5	0.44
0.80	10	0.29
0.80	20	0.17
0.80	40	0.09

$$A = \frac{10}{10 - 1} \left(1 - \frac{10}{10 + 10(10 - 1)0.43}\right) = 0.88$$

Although this change is not very large, it illustrates the principle that the larger the sample of items used to measure the same concept, the more reliable the combined measure. Again, this is intuitively obvious; as we saw in the example of the NCLEX examination (chapter 13), a longer test will provide a more accurate and reliable estimate of a student's nursing knowledge than a short one.

Now, we will look at Cronbach's alpha from a different angle. We hold k (the number of indicator items) constant, but vary $\bar{r}$ (the average correlation among the items). Suppose the average correlation among all question items is zero. Substituting zero for $\bar{r}$ in the formula for alpha yields an alpha that is also equal to zero. That is what we should expect: when responses to question items do not correlate at all, the items do not capture any common "true" score. With nothing but "error" variance, scale scores are completely unreliable. On the other hand, very high average correlations among indicator items of a scale indicate substantial communality: they measure the underlying concept consistently, with little measurement error. In the theoretic extreme, where each individual indicator item is a perfect measure of the underlying concept, all bivariate correlations should be equal to 1 because all items would produce perfectly consistent responses.[10] Yet, if the constituent items of a measurement scale are perfect measures of the concept, so is the scale itself, and its reliability is equal to 1.

Now, we have arrived at a key issue in the construction of multi-item or multi-indicator scales. *We can always*

strengthen the reliability of such scales by increasing the number of indicators or improving the quality of a given number of items. Items that produce relatively error-free responses have greater communality, which raises the average correlation among them. On the other hand, items that have a great deal of measurement error reduce the average correlation among the indicators. Thus, we can engage in a tradeoff between the number of indicators and their quality. For instance, Table 14-3 shows four different item combinations, all of which would achieve a scale reliability of .80. Several lessons can be drawn from this:

- It is *always* possible to achieve a high alpha value if one uses many indicator items, say, more than 20. As Table 14-3 shows, with more than 40 items, even an average inter-item correlation of less than .1 results in an "impressive" overall reliability of .80. However, low average correlations among a multitude of indicator items may not simply indicate the presence of a great deal of measurement error, but may conceal the fact that the items measure multiple concepts that are only weakly related.
- The key to a good *unidimensional* scale is to find relatively few items (say, 5–10) that nonetheless achieve high reliability. This is only possible if inter-item correlations are at least moderately strong ($r \geq .30$).[11] In practice, it is not easy to come up with a relatively few "best" items that both measure the desired concept and produce consistent results in different subpopulations.
- Implicit in this discussion is the idea that a reliable measurement instrument is one that maximizes variation among subjects, but minimizes variation among items, or alternative indicators.[12]

Substitute 1 for $\bar{r}$ in the formula for Cronbach's alpha:

$$A = \frac{k}{k - 1}\left(\frac{1 - k}{k + k(k - 1)\bar{r}}\right) = \frac{k}{k - 1}\left(\frac{k + k(k -) - k}{k + k(k - 1)}\right) =$$

$$\frac{k}{k - 1}\left(\frac{k(k - 1)}{k + k(k - 1)}\right) = \frac{k}{1}\left(\frac{k}{k + k(k - 1)}\right) = \frac{1}{1}\left(\frac{k}{1 + 1(k - 1)}\right) =$$

$$\frac{k}{1 + k - 1} = \frac{k}{k} = 1.$$

[10]Note the reference to *unidimensional* scales. Complex multidimensional scales (such as CES-D and SF-36), which have several (*unidimensional*) subscales, may have larger numbers of indicator items.

[11]The interest in determining different sources of measurement error has led to a generalized analysis of variance approach to measurement, known as generalizability theory. See Shavelson and Webb (1994).

[12]See Munro (2001).

- The reader of a research report should not be unduly impressed with high reliability values if the measurement instrument or scale has many ($k > 20$) items. This is particularly so when internal consistency reliability is the only index of reliability reported in an article. Often, the authors of research articles report the internal consistency reliability of the scales used, but do not provide any validity information. As we will see later, criteria such as validity considerations are at least as important in judging the quality of a multi-item measurement instrument.

Test–Retest, or Repeated-Measures, Reliability

The measurement instruments for many clinical variables do not produce multiple indicator scores designed to measure a single variable, but instead produce only a single observed score. To estimate the reliability of such a measurement tool or procedure, one can repeat the measurement a second time, or even more frequently, and examine the consistency of the results. *As long as there is no real change in the attribute being measured,* repeated measurement should produce stable results.

[13]For example, suppose you are interested in evaluating the magnitude of measurement error in blood pressure readings taken within a short time span on the same patients. One way to do this is to perform two successive blood pressure tests on a sample of 50 patients or so, with the tests taken within 15 minutes of each other. After recording and collecting the data, you would have information on four variables: two diastolic and two systolic readings for each of the 50 patients. Suppose that correlating each of the two successive readings yields a Pearson's $r = .94$ for the diastolic blood pressure and $r = .90$ for the systolic blood pressure. Because the squared Pearson's r can be interpreted as the proportion (or percentage) of shared variance between two variables, the diastolic readings have 88% shared variance ($R^2 = .88$) and the systolic readings have 81% shared variance ($R^2 = .81$).

What can be concluded from these data? Under the assumption that the patients' blood pressures remain stable over the 15-minute period, *the measurement procedure can be assumed to have yielded 88% true score variance, coupled with 12% measurement error, for the diastolic blood pressure and 81% true score variance, coupled with 19% error, in measuring systolic blood pressure.* The basis for this conclusion hinges on the behavior of the meas-

urement error. As discussed in the previous section, as long as it is random, measurement error does not contribute anything to the observed correlation. In other words, the correlations between observed scores reflect only the systematic co-variation as a result of true score variance. Should there ever be a measurement procedure without any error coupled with no change in the underlying "real" condition, we would expect a perfect correlation ($r = 1$) between the two sets of blood pressure readings. Thus, when interpreting the correlations, we are treating the departure from perfect correlation as the "error component" in measurement.

The 88% and 81% reliability estimates can actually be considered the *lower limits of the true test–retest reliability.* Recall that we assumed that the *only* reason why the two sets of blood pressure readings will not correlate perfectly is that there is error associated with measuring blood pressure. Yet, it is more realistic to assume that the "true" blood pressure would not remain completely stable over the two successive measurement occasions. Systolic blood pressure in particular is more susceptible to change over relatively brief periods. Because we did not, or could not, distinguish between real change and measurement error, we likely overestimated the amount of error in measurement, thus underestimating the true reliability of the blood pressure measurement. Our most appropriate interpretation in this situation would be to view the obtained reliability estimates as "conservative."

There are two important caveats when interpreting test–retest reliability estimates:

1. When the correlation between two successive applications of a particular measurement procedure is relatively "low," say, less than .7, it does not *necessarily* follow that the measurement procedure is unreliable. That is, if the measured characteristic itself changes within the measurement interval, then even a reliable measurement procedure will yield low correlations. It follows that it would be harder to establish test–retest, or repeated-measures, reliability of a measurement procedure if it is aimed at a phenomenon that fluctuates naturally, as many physiologic variables do. In such situations, shorter time intervals between the measurement points should increase the consistency of the results.

2. In some situations, estimates of test–retest reliability are biased *upward.* This occurs particularly with knowledge tests and other tests that involve human memory. When subjects take a test or answer questions a second time, they may remember their previous responses and repeat them. Obviously, in this case, the bias in favor of *overestimating* reliability would be greater, the shorter the interval between the test occasions.

---

[13]For a detailed discussion, see Siegel and Castellan (1988).

In sum, the assessment of test–retest reliability is not always straightforward. A researcher should have sound, conceptually based reasons for the assessment, including a good understanding of how variable the measured phenomena are over the period contemplated for subsequent measurement.

Reliability of Observational Data: Interrater Reliability

It is sometimes necessary to use either behavioral observations or proxy judgments of a patient's true state. For example, because of the "high stakes" involved in getting it right, a judge may ask two or three mental health experts to independently evaluate a person who appears to be experiencing marked symptoms of psychosis, to determine whether the person is legally competent to stand trial for a criminal charge. The evaluation would include clinical judgments by the mental health experts about the state of the patient, but would be based on specific information, such as observations of the person's behavior, medical records, and reports from family members and significant others. Behavioral or proxy measures may also be used when patients cannot answer self-report questions (e.g., patients with severe dementia, very young children or infants).

In an effort to standardize ratings involving observations, researchers often use two or more trained observers who are asked to rate the same observed behaviors *independently*. For example, during a change of dressings, two nurses may independently rate the pain experienced by patients in a burn unit who cannot reliably verbalize or record their pain ratings because of tracheal intubation, fluctuating delirium, and severe hand burns. The rating scale may consist of ordinal categories, such as:

Categories	Rating Scale
No apparent pain	0
Mild pain	1
Moderate pain	2
Substantial pain	3
Severe pain	4
Excruciating pain	5

Given these ordinal rankings, a simple way to assess the amount of agreement in the parallel observations would be to have the two nurse observers rate patient pain during three or more dressing changes and then to use a rank-order correlation coefficient, such as Spearman's r,[14] to estimate the correlation. Correlation values close to 1 would indicate near-perfect agreement between the observers, whereas a value of zero indicates no consistency between the ratings. If more than two raters are used, Kendall's W coefficient of concordance may be used to estimate the amount of agreement among the multiple raters.[15]

Cohen's Kappa

As mentioned earlier in the chapter, in many clinical situations, the main aim of making observations is to classify patients in some way. Essentially, all diagnostic activity amounts to assigning patients to preexisting diagnostic groups, a process that may be far from easy if the criteria are complex and the available evidence is ambiguous. For example, consider two radiologists who examine radiographs for the same set of 300 breast nodes to determine whether the visible nodes should be classified as "benign," "suspicious," or "cancerous." Table 14-4 presents hypothetical data comparing the classification ratings of the two radiologists.

At first, one might think that the percentage of agreements among all classifications could be used as a simple measure of the reliability in the diagnostic classifications. Table 14-4 shows this observed percentage (or proportion: p_o) as 67%. However, this simple tally does not take into account *how much agreement between two raters should be expected simply as a result of chance.*[16] Suppose the two radiologists use completely independent methods of node classification that share nothing in common. Under that assumption, each classification made by radiologist A is independent of each classification made by radiologist B. Because radiologist A classifies 180 (60%) of the nodes as benign and radiologist B classifies 150 (50%) of the nodes as benign, independent classifications would result in 90 ($180 \times 150/300$) or 30% of all nodes classified as benign by both radiologists. Likewise, 7 (2%) nodes could be expected to receive a classification of "suspicious" by both radiologists and 27 (9%) could be expected to be classified as "cancerous," resulting in total agreement on 41% of all nodes, *even though the hypothetical classification schemes used by the two radiologists do not share any criteria.*

---

[14]See Siegel and Castellan (1988).

[15]Although we did not discuss this in detail, the earlier method of comparing ordinal rankings through correlation coefficients also allows for random levels of agreement in rankings: a Spearman's r or Kendall's W value of zero does *not* imply complete disagreement about the rankings, only the unpredictability of one set of rankings on the basis of another.

[16]This cannot happen with the different marginal distributions shown in Table 14-4. "Perfect agreement" also implies that both raters classify the same number of persons into the various categories.

TABLE 14.4	Cohen's Kappa as a Measure of Interrater Reliability for Classifications of Nominal Groupings: Comparisons of Two Hypothetical Classifications of 300 Breast Nodes Based on Radiographs

		Classifications of Radiologist A			
		Benign	Suspicious	Cancerous	Total
Classifications	Benign	130	10	10	150
	Suspicious	30	10	10	50
of radiologist B	Cancerous	20	20	60	100
	Total	180	40	80	300

Observed agreement in classifications (p_o)

$(130 + 10 + 60)/300 = 200/300 = .67$ or 67%

Expected agreement (p_e) under null hypothesis of completely independent classifications

Benign—Benign: $(180 \times 150)/300 = 90$,
Suspicious—Suspicious: $(40 \times 50)/300 = 7$,
Cancerous—Cancerous: $(80 \times 100)/300 = 27$;
$\Rightarrow (90 + 7 + 27)/300 = 124/300 = .41$ or 41%

Interrater agreement as measured by Cohen's kappa

$K = (p_o - p_e) = (0.67 - 0.41)/(1 - 0.41) = 0.44$

As this example shows, under these circumstances, it would be more meaningful to ask whether the two radiologists can produce levels of agreement that are substantially better than those expected by chance alone. Perfect agreement would mean that all classifications in Table 14-4 end up on the diagonal, producing an agreed-on proportion of 1 (300/300).[17] Thus, the relevant range against which to judge the amount of actual agreement equals $1 - .41$ because we expect the radiologists to do better than chance. Cohen's kappa (Cohen, 1960) expresses the amount of agreement between two classifiers as a ratio of two differences: (1) the difference between the observed proportion of agreements and the expected proportion based on mere chance (in the numerator) and (2) the difference between perfect agreement and the expected proportion of agreements based on mere chance (in the denominator). If the proportion of observed agreements exceeds the expected

agreement, kappa must be larger than zero, and it will reach 1 if the proportion of observed agreements reaches unity.[18] According to Landis and Koch (1977), kappa values of .41 to .60 can be considered "moderate," values of .61 to .80 can be considered "substantial," and values of .80 to 1.00 are "almost perfect." Any classification procedure that results in a kappa value of .81 or higher is usually considered to have high *interrater reliability*.[19]

Reliability and Validity of Biophysiologic Measures: Sensitivity and Specificity

So far, we have discussed three ways to estimate reliability in measurement using terminology that was essentially

[17]Estimators of standard errors for Cohen's kappa are available for use in constructing confidence limits and significance testing. An extension to the case of multiple raters is also available (Landis & Koch, 1977). A good introduction can be found in Altman (1991).

[18]The cutoff points for kappa in determining the adequacy of agreement above chance are somewhat arbitrary and subject to debate, although it is agreed that higher or lower kappa values indicate higher or lower levels of agreement, respectively. For a review and critique of this debate, see Knapp & Brown, 1995.

[19]In the medical literature, the term *reproducibility* is more commonly used than *reliability* for this aspect of testing and measuring. For instance, the question might be whether different clinicians who use the testing instruments could reproduce the test results.

borrowed from the psychometrics tradition that we mentioned earlier. All three concepts of reliability share the fundamental characteristic that information is gathered from *multiple sources*. Test–retest reliability is assessed by collecting data at multiple time points (occasions). Internal consistency reliability is assessed by analyzing simultaneous responses to multiple indicator items. Interrater reliability involves the comparison of ratings from two or more observers. *The overall commonality among the various approaches to assessing reliability is to examine the consistency of multiple measurement results.*

The assessment of biophysiologic test results is rooted in a very different body of literature (what we referred to earlier as the "medical and public health tradition") using the somewhat different terminology of medical testing (Kraemer, 1992; Altman, 1991). Medical tests are performed to diagnose a disease, screen for the presence of disease markers, or evaluate the progress of treatment. In the end, clinicians typically use the information obtained from such tests to classify a patient as having a particular condition or disease ("positive" outcome, or patient identified as a "case"), or not having it ("negative" outcome, or patient identified as a "non-case"). Even though a particular test may produce finely graded continuous numbers, such as the percentage scores of oxygen saturation produced by oximeters, the test results are typically used for classification purposes. Clinicians then determine, for instance, whether certain clinical action must be taken based on their findings. In the instance of a pulse oximetry reading, a value lower than a certain percentage would indicate the need for supplemental oxygen, and the range into which a particular reading falls would determine the amount of oxygen provided; for example, 1, 2, or 3 L O_2 per nasal cannula, and so forth. As with all tests used for classification purposes, their value hinges primarily on the **accuracy** of their prediction.

The term *accuracy* refers not only to the *reliability* of a test,[20] but also encompasses aspects of **validity.** A measurement procedure is said to be valid to the extent that it accomplishes its stated goal, which, in the current context, means that it correctly classifies patients as having or not having a certain condition. But how does one know whether a test gives "correct" results? The answer is that we evaluate the accuracy of a medical or biophysiologic test by comparing test outcomes with a putative **gold stan-**

dard. Of course, that begs the question of how we assess the accuracy of the gold standard.

Earlier in this chapter, we mentioned that, in the assessment of the reliability of a new measurement procedure, we cannot actually compare the obtained measurement scores with the "true scores"; we can only compare multiple observed scores. That implies that, in the final analysis, *the gold standard for any test is itself a potentially fallible measure of the underlying reality.* Thus, when we use a **gold standard,** we have already accepted as fact that one existing measurement procedure or test is unquestionably superior to others that might be available. There may be good reasons for taking this approach. Historically, medical testing has often involved the choice of discrete outcomes as gold standards that could easily be observed, such as death or myocardial infarction. For the earlier example of radiographic evidence of breast tumors, the gold standard would be provided by the biopsy results. Yet, even biopsy results are not 100% error-free (Wong, Edwards, & Tuttle, 2001). Still, for many disease outcomes, an accurate determination eventually can be made, even if it involves a postmortem autopsy. Although gold standards may sometimes be more easily available in health research than in psychological testing, the principle remains that *all* outcome measures are potentially fallible.

Sensitivity and Specificity as Indicators of the Quality of a Test

Nurses who are active in clinical practice are familiar with many diagnostic tests that are commonly performed in clinical settings (e.g., electrocardiograms, radiographs, blood and urine tests). In addition, tests done for screening and prevention purposes are also commonplace, such as Pap smears, mammography, fecal occult blood testing, and lipid profiles. For any of these tests, the guiding premise is that some characteristic of the patient is being measured in the hope that it will yield accurate information about the presence or absence of a disease or disorder. In addition, a number of tests can also provide information about the level or severity of a disease process.

As with all measurements, it is unlikely that the results of screening and diagnostic tests are completely error-free. Thus, before the test results are used as a basis for clinical decision-making, it is of critical importance to know "how good" these tests actually are. In the previous section, we discussed the example of two radiologists independently rating radiographic images of women's breasts for evidence of tumors. In that example, there is no gold standard, just two independent judges with equal claims on the veracity of their judgments. Now suppose the radiographs

---

[20]This would be unusual because women whose nodes were rated "benign" by both radiologists most likely would not have undergone biopsy.

| TABLE 14.5 | Comparison of Test Predictions with Gold Standard Outcomes | | |

Test predictions (based on radiographic evidence)	True State of Affairs (based on surgery/biopsy results)		Predicted totals
	Patient has a malignant tumor	Patient does not have a malignant tumor	
Patient is predicted to have a malignant tumor	True-positive results N = 80	False-positive results N = 20	N = 100
Patient is predicted not to have a malignant tumor	False-negative results N = 40	True-negative results N = 160	N = 200
True totals	N = 120	N = 180	N = 300

Sensitivity (80/120) × 100 = 66.7%

Specificity (160/180) × 100 = 88.9%

Positive predicted value (80/100) × 100 = 80%

Negative predicted value (160/200) × 100 = 80%

come from patients who either underwent recent surgery or had a diagnostic biopsy.[21] In that case, we can compare a radiologist's predictions or classifications with the gold standard of postsurgery results, which presumably are an accurate reflection of the "true state of affairs." To simplify, we can ask a radiologist to classify patients on the preponderance of evidence into two groups: those who are likely to have a malignant tumor and those who do not have one. When we compare the radiologist's predictions with the actual state of affairs, there are four possible outcomes:

1. Some patients are correctly identified as having a malignant tumor (**true-positive** result).
2. Some patients are correctly identified as *not* having a malignant tumor (**true-negative** result).
3. Some patients are identified as having a malignant tumor, even though they do *not,* in fact, have one (**false-positive** result).
4. Some patients are *not* identified as having a malignant tumor, even though they do have one (**false-negative** result).

Sensitivity and Specificity of a Test

It is obvious that one would wish for any test or diagnostic procedure to *minimize* the occurrence of *false positives* and *false negatives.* At the same time, ideally, a test should identify all those who do have the disease or condition un-

[21]Any increase in the number of true-positive results necessarily means fewer false-negative results because their sum equals the fixed quantity of patients who actually have the disease. In Table 14-5, 80 + 40 = 120; with the total of 120 fixed, an increase in the 80 true positives comes at the expense of the 40 false negatives.

der consideration. If a test yields a high proportion of true positives, it is **highly sensitive.** A test should also be able to rule out cases correctly if those patients do not have the disease or condition in question. A test that yields a high proportion of true negatives is **highly specific.**

Table 14-5 provides a specific example. This time, we assume that we have data on 300 women who have undergone breast surgery or biopsy. According to this gold standard, 120 (40%) of the women have a malignant tumor and 180 (60%) are tumor-free (see row for "true totals"). Overall, examination of the radiographs led to the identification of 100 (33%) women with a tumor and 200 (67%) women without a tumor (see column of "predicted totals"). More interesting for our purposes is the distribution of cases. If we divide the number of cases identified as true positive by the number of cases with a tumor and multiply this proportion by 100, we obtain the **sensitivity** of the test or radiograph ratings. The sensitivity tells us what percentage of patients who do have the disease or disorder are positively identified by the test as having the disease or disorder. The **specificity** of a test refers to the percentage of patients who do *not* have the disease or disorder and are correctly *ruled out* by the test.

In the example in Table 14-5, we find that 80 of the 120 patients with a tumor were correctly identified (sensitivity of 66.7%) and 160 of 180 women without a tumor were correctly identified (specificity of 80%). It appears that this particular radiographic test is better at ruling out cases than at positively identifying them. This example also shows something else: *the greater the sensitivity of a test, the*

TABLE 14.6	Comparison of Test Predictions with Gold Standard Outcomes after a Change in the Prevalence of Malignant Tumors		
	True State of Affairs (based on surgery/biopsy results)		
Test predictions (based on radiographic evidence)	**Patient has a malignant tumor**	**Patient does not have a malignant tumor**	**Predicted totals**
Patient is predicted to have a malignant tumor	True-positive results N = 40	False-positive results N = 40	N = 80
Patient is predicted not to have a malignant tumor	False-negative results N = 20	True-negative results N = 320	N = 340
True totals	N = 60	N = 360	N = 420

Sensitivity (40/60) × 100 = 66.7%
Specificity (320/360) × 100 = 88.9%
Positive predicted value (40/80) × 100 = 50%
Negative predicted value (320/340) × 100 = 94%

smaller the proportion of false-negative results.[22] By the same argument, *greater specificity of a test implies fewer false-positive results.*[23]

Predictive Values of a Test

In our discussion of the sensitivity and specificity of a diagnostic test, we have approached the problem of the accuracy of such a test with this question: *What proportion of the patients who have or do not have the disease in question will be classified correctly by the test?* In a diagnostic situation, however, a clinician is usually interested in a slightly different (but related) question: *How well does the test predict the presence of the disorder?* In other words, a clinician usually wants to know: Given the test results, what is the probability that the patient has the disease in question?

The answer to this question is given in terms of a test's predictive values. Consider again the radiograph example in Table 14-5. This time, we ask: What proportion of patients with a positive radiograph actually has a tumor? This

is the *positive predictive value* (PPV) of the test. In Table 14-5, 100 patients were predicted to have a tumor (number of patients with a positive radiograph), and 80 of these actually have a tumor. Thus, the PPV = 80%, or the probability that a positively identified patient will actually have a tumor is .8. For the *negative predicted value* (NPV), we ask: What proportion of the patients with a negative radiograph actually is tumor-free? Based on the data in Table 14-5, the NPV = 80% also. Different from sensitivity and specificity, positive and negative values should *not* be used to evaluate the quality and accuracy of a test because these statistics also vary depending on the prevalence of the condition. To see this, look at the changed data in Table 14-6. The prevalence of true tumor cases has been changed from 40% (120/300) in Table 14-4 to 14% (60/420). At the same time, the sensitivity and specificity have been left unchanged. However, the PPV has decreased to 50% and the NPV has increased to 94%. The reason is simple: for a given error rate, the absolute numbers of true-positive and false-negative results decline, whereas the numbers of false-positive and true-negative results increase. Thus, the PPV (true positives)/(true positives + false positives) declines and the NPV (true negatives)/(true negatives + false negatives) increases.[24]

---

[22]Using the arrangement in Table 14-5, we recommend making up some numbers for true positives, true negatives, false positives, and false negatives. Then change the numbers and examine for yourself the effect of the changes on sensitivity, specificity, and the numbers of false negatives and false positives.

[23]The implications of these facts for the application of screening tests are explored in chapter 15.

[24]The implications of these these facts for the application of screening tests are explored in chapter 15.

| TABLE 14.7 | Blood Glucose Levels and Distribution of Patients with Diabetes Mellitus Diagnosis |

Grouped Blood Glucose Levels (mg/ 100 mL):	Patients with Diabetes Mellitus	Patients without Diabetes Mellitus
41–60	0	99
61–80	0	207
81–100	5	270
101–120	11	241
121–140	15	56
141–160	16	18
161–180	14	7
181–200	15	2
201+	24	0
Total N	100	900

Sensitivity and Specificity for Tests with Continuous Scores

The example of examining radiographs to predict malignant tumors is a case of comparing a *dichotomous prediction* (presence or absence of the tumor) with a *dichotomous true outcome*. However, most biophysiologic diagnostic and screening tests yield more than two values. For example, serum cholesterol and blood glucose tests result in continuous measures of milligrams per 100 milliliters. These tests yield widely varying scores, on the basis of which the clinician must decide whether they are indicative of the presence or absence of the disorder, and what specific action to take.[25]

Now, consider an example of a hypothetical distribution of blood glucose levels among a sample of 1000 persons, 100 of whom have been diagnosed with diabetes mellitus (see Table 14-7). It is easy to see that, with rising levels of blood sugar levels, more individuals are diagnosed with diabetes mellitus. However, the *distributions overlap*, as is often the case with diagnostic tests. Suppose the test results for a particular patient show a glucose level of 202 mg/100 mL. If glucose levels among patients with diabetes and those without diabetes in the general population are distributed as in the sample data shown in Table 14-7, we would conclude that this patient must have diabetes because *none* of the patients without diabetes has a glucose level above 200 mg/100 mL.[26] Consequently, we might adopt the following decision rule: whenever a test result shows a glucose level above the cutoff point of 200 mg/100 mL, the patient is classified as having diabetes; when the glucose level is below 200 mg/100 mL, the patient is classified as not having diabetes.

Is this a good decision rule? One way to find out is to calculate both the sensitivity and the specificity after collapsing the data into a 2 × 2 table constructed on the basis of the cutoff point of 200 mg/100 mL (Table 14-8). The advantage of this decision rule is that it has a specificity of 100%. In other words, all 900 patients without diabetes are correctly classified. On the other hand, the decision rule leads to a low sensitivity of only 24%, with 76% of the patients with diabetes unidentified (false negatives). Given the seriousness of unidentified diabetes mellitus, most clinicians would not be satisfied with a screening test that identifies only 24% of persons with the disease.[27] Therefore, we might choose a different cutoff point. Under the new rule, any patient who has a glucose level higher than 120 mg/100 mL is classified as having diabetes. This cutoff point results in a sensitivity of 84% and a specificity of 91% (Table 14-9). That means that 84% of all patients with diabetes will be identified while the test retains a respectable specificity of 91%. Still, under the new rule, the test will produce 83 false-positive results.

[25]In real-life clinical situations, such decisions would rarely be made on the basis of one test result because one result provides only one piece of information among many others. It is the consistency of the multiple indicators that offers convincing evidence for or against a particular diagnosis. In addition, the ranges of test values provide more guidance about what specific clinical actions should be taken. For example, a blood glucose value of 300 mg/100 mL will result in a different treatment decision than a blood glucose level of 150 mg/100 mL.

[26]To make the table manageable in size, the blood glucose levels were collapsed into nine categories, but normally, there is no need for such grouping.

[27]Given the natural fluctuation in blood glucose levels, it would also be advisable to repeat the test to guard against isolated elevated or depressed readings that might produce false positives or false negatives.

TABLE 14.8	Sensitivity and Specificity of Blood Glucose Measurements with Cutoff Point at 200 mg/100 mL	
Grouped Blood Glucose Levels (mg/100 mL)	Patients with Diabetes Mellitus (DM)	Patients without DM
≤ 200: Patient is predicted not to have DM	76	900
201+: Patient is predicted to have DM	24	0
Total N	100	900

Sensitivity (24/100) × 100 = 24%
Specificity (900/900) × 100 = 100%

TABLE 14.9	Sensitivity and Specificity of Blood Glucose Measurements with Cutoff Point at 120 mg/100 mL	
Grouped Blood Glucose Levels (mg/100 mL)	Patients with Diabetes Mellitus (DM)	Patients without DM
≤ 120: Patient is predicted not to have DM	16	817
121+: Patient is predicted to have DM	84	83
Total N	100	900

Sensitivity (84/100) × 100 = 84%
Specificity (817/900) × 100 = 91%

The most important point that emerges from this example is the inevitable tradeoff between the sensitivity and the specificity of a test. This can easily be seen in Table 14-10, which shows how sensitivity and specificity values change at the nine cutoff points in the original frequency distribution. Given this information, how can we choose between more and less accurate tests? One way to do so is to plot a receiver-operating characteristic (ROC) curve based on the available information about sensitivity and specificity at each cutoff point (Figure 14-1).[28] The ROC curve plots sensitivity, or the proportion of true positives, on the vertical axis against the proportion of false positives (1−specificity). A test for which some of the proportions of true positives and false positives is always equal to one is worthless because any

[28]ROC curves are often reported and illustrated in medical and public health research literature that is of relevance to advance practice nurses.

TABLE 14.10	Variation in Sensitivity and Specificity Depending on Cutoff Points for Blood Glucose Measurements	
Blood Glucose Level Cutoff	Sensitivity	Specificity
60	100%	11%
80	100%	34%
100	95%	64%
120	84%	91%
140	69%	97%
160	53%	99%
180	39%	99%
200	24%	100%

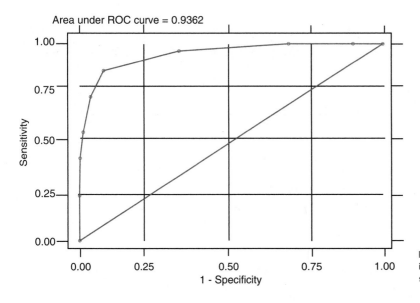

Area under ROC curve = 0.9362

FIGURE 14.1 Receiver operating curve incorporating trade-offs between sensitivity and specificity

increase in sensitivity is offset by an equal decrease in specificity. Such tests are graphically presented as moving along the straight diagonal line shown in Figure 14-1. On the other hand, if a test has both high sensitivity and high specificity, the ROC curve tends toward the upper left-hand corner because high rates of true positives are associated with low rates of false positives (1−specificity). In that case, the area under the ROC curve tends toward encompassing the whole square. As you can see, for the data in Table 14-10, the associated area under the ROC curve in Figure 14-1 encompasses 93.62% of the area of the square. One way to compare two diagnostic tests is to test whether the areas under their respective ROC curves are significantly different from each other (DeLong, DeLong, & Clark-Pearson, 1988). Tests with larger areas can have *both* greater sensitivity *and* greater specificity. Such tests have more discriminatory power (i.e., they result in *both* fewer false positives *and* fewer false negatives).

VALIDITY IN MEASUREMENT

In the previous section, we briefly mentioned that determining the *accuracy* of a biophysiologic or medical test includes both *reliability* and *validity*. Generally, a measurement procedure is considered valid if it measures the characteristics or attributes that it is intended to measure. Although this definition seems clear, the actual determination of the validity of a measurement tool, test, or proce-

dure is not that easy and may be quite involved. The approach taken with many medical tests is to compare the test results with a putative gold standard, which, of course, leads to the question of how one validates the gold standard. There is a certain circularity in this argument. As we have emphasized before, one can never compare one's measurement results with the "true state of affairs," only with other fallible measures. These other measures contain a certain amount of random measurement error and are, therefore, limited in their reliability; they are also subject to the same questions about their validity: Do they in fact measure what they are intended to measure?

Traditionally, in the psychometric literature, the establishment of measurement validity has been approached in three ways (Nunnally & Bernstein, 1994). We distinguish between content, criterion, and construct validity.

Content Validity

Content validity is probably the most common approach to establishing the validity of a measurement scale, in particular, a scale that is based on standardized responses to self-report questions. The main concern with content validity is that the question items selected as scale indicators all tap into this conceptual domain. For example, we might go back to the seven items that make up the depressed mood subscale of the CES-D (Table 14-1). Item CES-D9 asks the respondent, "How often have you thought your life has been a failure?" One could argue that, of the items contained in the depressed mood subscale, this is the only one that asks the respondent to contemplate his or her whole life history, not just recent moods. As such, it appears to differ somewhat from the conceptual core of the other mood items, a possible reason for the frequent empirical finding that shows this item to have the lowest item-total correlation among all seven subscale items.

The semantic distinction just made is an example of weighing the content validity of a particular indicator item. Ultimately, one would use "experts" in a given field to make judgments about the content validity of particular questions, or one would ask them to develop the questions. The experts in a given field may very well be members of the target population that the researcher intends to study. In that case, a more formal approach to developing question items with relevant content may be the use of focus groups (see chapter 18). Because the meanings of words and phrases often vary among different users and subgroups, there is probably no way to establish content validity "once and for all." Both the reliability and the validity of a measure can vary considerably as a function of the target population and other variables in the research context. Nonetheless, a consensus about the meaning of questions among experts of a particular subject area often can go a long way toward establishing content validity.

Criterion Validity

The establishment of **criterion validity** is concerned with using *external* criteria to validate a given measurement instrument. If the external criterion occurs some time in the future, this type of criterion validity is often referred to as **predictive validity.** To establish it, one uses the scores obtained through the new measurement tool to predict an external outcome or criterion. For instance, an in-house capstone test for nursing students that is administered shortly before graduation from a bachelor's degree program could be validated by comparing the scores with scores on the actual NCLEX-RN examination taken for licensure as a registered nurse in the United States. Suppose, however, that the external criterion is conceptually distinct from the measure in question, as when predicting "job success" within 5 years after graduation from nursing school on the basis of NCLEX scores. Although job success, however defined, could conceivably be considered a possible external criterion for the NCLEX, using it as a validation criterion for a knowledge test would require a validated theory that relates knowledge to job success. At this point, establishing criterion validity involves substantive research that examines the relationship between two conceptually distinct variables (Knapp, 1985).

If the external criterion used to establish validity occurs, more or less, at the same time at which the measurement scores were obtained, the validity is referred to as **concurrent validity.** The use of gold standards to validate medical tests is an example of concurrent validity. Note, however, that the boundaries between "predictive" and "concurrent" validity may be small or even arbitrary. When we use a gold standard to validate a diagnostic tool, or more generally, when we use an external criterion to validate any measurement tool, we usually assume that both measures are obtained "close enough" together so that they reflect the same underlying reality. To give an extreme counter-example, we would not try to validate interpretations or ratings based on radiographs using the results of biopsies that were performed 1 year later. What is considered an "acceptable" interval between the measurement of test scores and the determination of the criterion or gold standard outcomes depends on the phenomenon under investigation. *The faster it can change, the shorter the acceptable period for measurement validation.* Sometimes the criterion measure may refer to events *in the recent past,* as when researchers try to validate attitude scales, the scores of which are compared with information about actual recent behaviors. An example can be found in Collins, Stommel, and King (1991), in which the authors validated a scale for determining attitudes toward community services by correlating its scores with variables that measured recent actual use. The validity of this procedure hinges on, among other factors, the assumption that attitudes have not changed very much since the period to which the behavioral measures refer. Thus, temporal considerations should always be part of the evaluation of external validity criteria.

As previously discussed, with reference to gold standards, the establishment of criterion validity is dependent on the prior acceptance of the criterion as a valid reference point for the concept or variable. For instance, because attitudes do not necessarily translate into behaviors, behavioral measures may not be useful criteria to establish the validity of an attitude measure. Ultimately, we are forced to consider the question: How do we validate the criterion itself? That leads inevitably into theoretic considerations and justifications. If the **validity coefficient** (i.e., the correlation coefficient between the new measure and the criterion measure) is low, we have, in principle, two choices: (1) we can reject the validity of the new measure, or (2) we can question the validity of the gold standard or criterion as a measure of the concept.

Construct Validity

As stressed in the previous section, considerations of measurement validity ultimately are not just empirical, but also theoretic. For a measurement instrument to be valid, it must first and foremost "capture" the meaning of the concept that it is supposed to measure. It is often much more difficult to establish validity for psychosocial concepts, such as "coping behavior," "aggression," or "depression," than for biophysiologic variables.

In chapter 2, we made a distinction between **observational concepts** (i.e., those that are concrete in the sense that they almost suggest the measurement procedure), **indirectly observable concepts** (i.e., concepts that must be inferred from indicators), and **theoretic concepts or constructs.**

Many biophysiologic concepts are either "observational" or "indirectly observable." They also tend to be conceptually "simple" or *unidimensional* concepts, such as blood pressure or blood oxygenation. Although there may be multiple methods used to measure these concepts and evidence may be indirect, as in the case of pulse oximetry, the relationship between the concept and the measurement procedure tends to be one of simple "correspondence." Often, it is the measurement procedure that defines the concept.[29] On the other hand, up until now, psychosocial constructs have almost never been measured directly,[30] and are often *complex* and *multidimensional,* which makes it harder to validate their operationalization or measurement procedure.

Take, for instance, a psychosocial concept, such as "major depression." According to the *Diagnostic and Statistical Manual of Mental Disorders* (DSM-IV) criteria (American Psychological Association, 1994), "major depressive disorder" is present if a person experiences five or more of the following symptoms most of the day and nearly daily for at least 2 weeks:

1. Markedly diminished interest or pleasure in almost all activities
2. Depressed mood
3. Significant weight loss or gain
4. Insomnia or hypersomnia
5. Psychomotor retardation or agitation

6. Fatigue (loss of energy)
7. Feelings of worthlessness (guilt)
8. Impaired concentration (indecisiveness)
9. Recurrent thoughts of death or suicide

Because these symptoms encompass affective, cognitive, interpersonal, and somatic manifestations, it is clear that any measurement instrument that is designed to capture the concept of depression must also be multidimensional. A review of some major standardized self-report depression scales (BDI, CES-D, HDRS, GDS)[31] would show that they all use multiple questions that can be separated into distinct item groupings (subscales) that are designed to measure the various conceptual dimensions of depressive symptoms.[32] One way to explore and *empirically* test the construct validity of such multidimensional measurement instruments is to use factor analysis.

Use of Factor Analysis to Establish Construct Validity

At its most basic, **factor analysis** is a set of statistical techniques that can be used to find item groupings (exploratory factor analysis) or to test for the existence of predetermined groupings (confirmatory factor analysis).[33] Exploratory factor analysis is an indispensable tool for finding out if the question items that were developed result in uniform or multidimensional response patterns.[34] Table 14-11 shows an example of a correlation pattern that is consistent with a two-dimensional factor structure. For simplicity, we have chosen six CES-D items, three from the depressed mood subscale and three from the absence of well-being subscale.[35] On the assumption that all six items are indicators of overall depressive symptoms, the responses to these questions should, and do, correlate positively, because it is the underlying depression that gives rise to the joint occur-

---

[29]The philosophic position that the meaning of a concept is derived from its measurement is called "operationism."

[30]There is a quest to develop valid, reliable biophysiologic measures to diagnose mental disorders, particularly subtypes of disorders that vary in responsiveness to particular treatment approaches. The development of such measures also informs the development of more specific and effective treatments.

[31]BDI: Beck Depression Inventory; CES-D: Center for Epidemiologic Studies Depression Scale; GDS: Geriatric Depression Scale (Yesavage, Brink, Rose, Lum, Huang, Adey, & Lierer, 1983); HDRS: Hamilton Depression Rating Scale (Hamilton, 1960).

[32]These scales differ in the specific "flavor" of depression that is assessed most effectively (e.g., cognitive symptoms, severity).

[33]We do not intend to provide an introduction to factor analysis here. There is a huge body of literature on the various types of factor analytic procedures, and the serious study of factor analysis requires familiarity with matrix algebra. Nunnally and Bernstein (1994) provide an excellent, conceptually based introduction to factor analysis. The purpose of the current discussion is to show how empirical exploration of the multidimensionality of a measurement instrument can contribute to the establishment of measurement validity.

[34]Exploratory factor analysis is usually one step in the complicated, multistep process of developing a new measurement scale.

[35]The analysis is based on the data of Given and Given (1993).

TABLE 14.11	Example of a Correlation Pattern Consistent with Subscale Structure of a Two-Dimensional Scale: CES-D Items Divided into Two Subscales

Question stem: During the past 2 weeks, how often have you felt this way?

Mood items

CES-D3:   . . . I felt that I could not shake the blues, even with the help of family and friends?
CES-D6:   . . . I felt depressed?
CES-D18:   . . . I felt sad?

(Absence of) Well-Being items

RCES-D8:   . . . I felt hopeful about the future?
RCES-D12: . . . I was happy?
RCES-D16: . . . I enjoyed life?

*Answer categories for absence of well-being items are reverse (R) coded: 3 = rarely or none of the time; 2 = some or a little of the time; 1 = occasionally or a moderate amount of the time; 0 = most or all of the time.

Based on a sample of newly diagnosed cancer patients (N = 787)

Correlation Matrix

	CES-D3	CES-D6	CES-D18	RCES-D8	RCES-D12	RCES-D16
CES-D3	1.00					
CES-D6	0.56	1.00				
CES-D18	0.53	0.62	1.00			
RCES-D8	0.24	0.31	0.28	1.00		
RCES-D12	0.34	0.37	0.39	0.51	1.00	
RCES-D16	0.23	0.27	0.29	0.43	0.59	1.00

Mood subscale: mean interitem correlation (unshaded cells): 0.56.

Absence of well-being subscale: mean interitem correlation: 0.51 (lightly shaded cells).

Mean interitem correlation among items from different subscales (darkly shaded cells): 0.30.

(Reprinted with permission from Given, B. A., & Given, C. W. (1993). Family home care for cancer: A community-based model. Grant RO1 N01915. Funded by the National Institute for Nursing Research and the National Cancer Institute.)

rence of these symptoms. However, the correlation pattern in Table 14-11 also shows that item responses within the depressed mood subscale have a much higher correlation with each other (mean inter-item correlation of .56). The same is noted among the absence of well-being items (mean inter-item correlation of .51). Items that belong to different subscales correlate less well (mean inter-item correlation of .30). This pattern is consistent with the conceptual multidimensionality of depression, which posits that depressed mood and the inability to experience pleasure or

enjoy one's life are overlapping, but distinct dimensions of depression.

The CES-D is a well-established measurement scale of depressive symptoms that has a known subscale structure. However, when researchers develop new measurement scales, they go through a complex process of item development.[36] Initially, they cannot be sure whether items that are designed to measure various subdimensions of a complex

---

[36]More details on scale development are given in the next chapter.

concept do, in fact, generate a response pattern among members of the target population that is consistent with the assumed multidimensionality of the instrument. Based on the observed correlation patterns, exploratory factor analysis is used to sort out those items that appear to fall into clearly established subscales.[37] When researchers use established measurement instruments, they can use **confirmatory factor analysis** to test to what extent the subscale structure of the instrument is consistent with the data at hand.[38]

Multi-trait, Multi-method Matrix Methods

Campbell and Fiske (1959) proposed an often praised, but less often employed, approach to establishing construct validity, the **multi-trait, multi-method matrix method.** This method is conceptually related to **factor analysis.** The basic idea is to use at least two different methods of measuring at least two distinct, but related concepts and to use the resulting correlational evidence for construct validation. Suppose we measure burn patients' pain and anxiety using both a self-report standardized questionnaire instrument and nurses' ratings of the patients' pain and anxiety observed at the same time. The four measures yield six correlations: two correlations between the self-reports and the observed scores for the same concept (pain *or* anxiety), two correlations between pain and anxiety using the same measurement method (self-report *or* observation), and two correlations between different constructs *and* different methods (self-report of pain versus observation of anxiety and observation of pain versus self-report of anxiety). Two alternative methods measuring the same concept should yield very similar results, and thus, the highest correlations. This property of "convergence" is contrasted with that of "discriminability," which is the ability of the measurement procedures to discriminate between measures of *different* constructs. Thus, at a minimum, correlations between measures of different constructs (here, pain or anxiety) should be lower than correlations between measures of the same concept, regardless of the method used, and correlations among variables that share neither construct nor method should be the lowest. As with factor analysis, ac-

tual correlation patterns may not produce such clear-cut patterns, but the confirmation of the existence of such patterns increases our confidence that we are indeed measuring the desired concept.

Concluding Remarks on Validity

It is apparent from the previous discussion that the establishment of measurement validity for a particular measurement instrument is a difficult and, to some degree, never-ending process. In practice, one should not make sharp distinctions among content, criterion-related, and construct validity because all of the forms of validation overlap, and any one may be used in any particular instance.[39] All of these validity assessments contribute to a better understanding of the constructs being measured. Further validation occurs when research findings from multiple studies show that the measurement scales behave in ways that conform to the theoretically derived hypotheses and expectations. For instance, if theory suggests that anxious and nervous patients are more likely to experience postoperative pain than patients who are relaxed, and empirical data confirm the existence of a positive correlation between measurement scales intended to measure anxiety and pain, then these empirical results indirectly confirm the validity of the measurement procedures.

When developing new instruments, we think it is quite useful to follow the pithy advice of Stewart and Archbold (1997): "Don't be overconfident about your measures until you have used them in multiple studies. Validity results are full of surprises—and lack of support for your hypotheses may turn out to be an exciting adventure if you can let yourself see where you went wrong."

CONCLUSION

In this chapter, we have focused on ways to judge the quality of measurement procedures. In particular, the twin concepts of reliability and validity were introduced as tools that can be used to set standards and evaluate measurement procedures. Reliability refers to the reproducibility, repeatability, and consistency of measurement procedures. These are essential ingredients for one requirement of scientific evidence: that it can be replicated. Validity is even more fundamental in the sense that testing of theories about relation-

---

[37]If the correlation patterns are not as clear as in Table 14-11, and if many variables ($k > 10$) are involved that are not yet sorted by a possible subscale structure, mere visual inspection of correlation tables may not lead to the discovery of patterns. However, in principle, visual inspection of correlation tables can be considered a simple form of exploratory factor analysis.

[38]Confirmatory factor analysis allows for much more sophisticated testing of particular scale properties than simply testing whether a predetermined item grouping is reproducible in the data. For more details, see Stommel, Wang, Given, and Given (1992).

---

[39]For instance, the use of similar, but distinct constructs to establish discriminability could also be considered a form of criterion-related validity because it involves the use of an "external" criterion.

ships among "real-world" phenomena can occur only if operationalizations, or measurements, of the concepts are adequate empirical representations of the concepts.

Measurement reliability is a necessary, but not sufficient, condition for measurement validity (i.e., for a measurement tool or instrument to be valid, it must possess some minimum of reliability because an instrument that produces only measurement error does not capture any real variation in phenomena). At the same time, the reliability of a measurement procedure (e.g., it produces consistent results on repeated measurement occasions) is not sufficient evidence of its validity. For instance, whether a particular measurement instrument measures anxiety rather than depression cannot be decided simply on the basis of evidence that it produces consistent scores in repeated applications. As discussed, validity considerations are never completely settled. Both researchers and readers must remain alert to the possibility that new evidence may challenge a long-held view about the validity of a particular measurement procedure.

In chapter 15, we will address the major practical steps in evaluating existing measurement tools, focusing on health outcome measures and screening tools. Even if you never engage in empirical research, the ability to judge the adequacy of information about the quality of measurement tools and procedures is an essential skill for anyone who reads research reports.

Suggested Activities

1. Read the article by DeFloor and Grypdonck (2001).
   a. List all procedures mentioned in the article that serve to ensure sufficient measurement reliability.
   b. In your judgment, is the reliability of the outcome measure adequate?
   c. Is the validity of the measurement procedures assessed?
   d. Provide a specific rationale for each of your judgments, with reference to the content of this chapter.
2. Read the article by Friedemann, Montgomery, Rice, and Farrell (1999), and answer the following questions:
   a. List all of the concepts or constructs involved in the theoretic discussion and all of the empirical measurement instruments. Do they correspond?
   b. For each measurement scale that is introduced, determine the type of reliability assessment provided. Are the reliability assessments adequate?
   c. Are measurement validity considerations discussed?
   d. Does the information provided in the article give the reader a sense of how to interpret scores from the various measurement variables?
   e. Provide a specific rationale for each of your judgments.

Suggested Readings

DeFloor, T., & Grypdonck, M. H. F. (2000). Do pressure relief cushions really relieve pressure? *Western Journal of Nursing Research, 22,* 3, 335–350.

Friedemann, M.-L., Montgomery, R. J., Rice, C., & Farrell, L. (1999). Family involvement in the nursing home. *Western Journal of Nursing Research, 21,4,* 549–567.

References

Altman, D. G. (1991). *Practical statistics for medical research.* Boca Raton, FL: Chapman & Hall/CRC.

American Psychological Association. (1994). *Diagnostic and statistical manual of mental disorders* (4th ed.). Washington, DC: American Psychological Association.

Camilli, G., & Shepard, L. A. (1994). *Methods for identifying biased test items.* Thousand Oaks, CA: Sage.

Campbell, D. T. & Fiske, D. W. (1951). Convergent and discriminant validation by the multitrait-multimethod matrix. *Psychological Bulletin, 56,* 81–105.

Cohen, J. (1960). A coefficient of agreement for nominal scales. *Educational and Psychological Measurement, 20,* 37–46.

Collins, C. E., Stommel, M., & King, S. (1991). Assessment of the attitudes of family caregivers toward community services. *The Gerontologist, 31,* 6, 756–761.

Cronbach, L. J. (1951). Coefficient alpha and the internal structure of tests. *Psychometrica, 16,* 297–334.

DeLong, E. R., DeLong, D. M., & Clarke-Pearson, D. L. (1988). Comparing the areas under two or more correlated receiver operating curves: A nonparametric approach. *Biometrics, 44,* 837–845.

Devins, G. M., & Orme, C. M. (1985). Center for Epidemiological Studies depression scale. In Keyser, D. J., & Sweetland, R. C. (Eds.), *Test critiques* (pp. 144–160). Kansas City, MO: Test Corporation of America.

Friedemann, M.-L., Montgomery, R. J., Rice, C., & Farrell, L. (1999). Family involvement in the nursing home. *Western Journal of Nursing Research, 21,4,* 549–567.

Given, B. A., & Given, C. W. (1993). Family home care for cancer: A community-based model. Grant RO1 NR01915. Funded by the National Institute for Nursing Research and the National Cancer Institute.

Hambleton, R. K., & Swaminathan, H. (1994). *Fundamen-*

tals of item-response theory. Thousand Oaks, CA: Sage.

Hamilton, M. (1960). A rating scale for depression. *Journal of Neurology, Neurosurgery, and Psychiatry, 23,* 56–62.

Hammer, A. L. (1988). *Manual for the coping resources inventory (research edition).* Palo Alto, CA: Consulting Psychologists Press.

Knapp, T. R. (1985). Validity, reliability and neither. *Nursing Research, 34,* 3, 189–192.

Knapp, T. R., & Brown, J. K. (1995). Ten measurement commandments that often should be broken. *Research in Nursing & Health, 18,* 465–469.

Kraemer, H. C. (1992). *Evaluating medical tests: Objective and quantitative guidelines.* Newbury Park, CA: Sage.

Landis, J. R., & Koch, G. G. (1977). The measurement of observer agreement for categorical data. *Biometrics, 33,* 159–174.

McCrae, R. R., & Costa, P. T. (1990). *Personality in adulthood.* New York: Guilford Press.

McHorney, C. A., Ware, J. E., & Raczek, A. E. (1993a). The MOS 36-item short form health survey (SF-36): II. Psychometric and clinical tests of validity in measuring physical and mental health constructs. *Medical Care, 31,* 3, 247–263.

McHorney, C. A., Ware, J. E., & Raczek, A. E. (1993b). The MOS 36-item short form health survey (SF-36): II. Psychometric and clinical tests of validity in measuring physical and mental health constructs. *Medical Care, 31,* 3, 247–263.

McNair, D. M., Lorr, M., & Droppleman, L. F. (1992). *Manual for the profile of mood states.* San Diego, CA: Educational and Industrial Testing Service.

Munro, B. H. (2001). *Statistical Methods for Health Care Research* (2nd ed.). Philadelphia, PA: Lippincott.

Norbeck, J. S. (1995). *Scoring instructions for the Norbeck social support questionnaire.* San Francisco: University of California.

Nunnally, J. C., & Bernstein, I. H. (1994). *Psychometric theory* (3rd ed.). New York: McGraw-Hill.

Ornstein, S., Markert, G., Litchfield, L., & Zemp, L. (1988). Evaluation of the DINAMAP blood pressure monitor in an ambulatory primary care setting. *The Journal of Family Practice, 26,* 5, 517–521.

Radloff, L. S. (1977). The CES-D scale: A self-report depression scale for research in the general population. *Applied Psychological Measurement, 1,* 385–401.

Radloff, L. S. and Locke, B. Z. (1986). The community mental health assessment survey and the CES-D scale. Pp. 177–189 in: Weissman, M. M., Myers, J. K. and Ross, C. E. (eds.). *Community Surveys of Psychiatric Disorders.* New Brunswick, NJ: Rutgers University Press.

Shavelson, R. J., & Webb, N. M. (1991). *Generalizability theory.* Thousand Oaks, CA: Sage.

Siegel, S., & Castellan, N. J. (1988). *Nonparametric statistics for behavioral sciences* (2nd ed.). New York: McGraw-Hill.

Spector, P. E. (1990). *Summated rating scale construction: An introduction* [QASS 82]. Newbury Park, CA: Sage.

Stewart, B. J., & Archbold, P. G. (1997). A new look at measurement validity. *Journal of Nursing Education, 36,* 3, 99–101.

Stommel, M., Wang, S., Given, C. W., & Given, B. A. (1992). Confirmatory factor analysis (CFA) as a method to assess measurement equivalence. *Research in Nursing & Health, 15,* 5, 352–360.

Stommel, M., Given, B. A., Given, C. W., Kalaian, H. A., Schulz, R., et al. (1993). Gender bias in the measurement properties of the center for epidemiologic studies depression scale (CES-D). *Psychiatry Research, 49,* 3, 239–250.

Traub, R. E. (1994). *Reliability for the social sciences: Theory and applications.* Thousand Oaks, CA: Sage.

Ware, J. E., & Sherbourne, C. D. (1992). The MOS 36-item short form health survey (SF-36): I. Conceptual framework and item selection. *Medical Care, 30,* 6, 473–483.

Wong, S. L., Edwards, M. J., Tuttle, M. T. (2001). Accuracy of sentinel lymph node biopsy for patients with T(2) and T(3) breast cancers. *The American Surgeon, 67,* 6, 522–528.

Yesavage, J. A., Brink, T. L., Rose, T. L., Lum, O., Huang, V., Adey, M., & Lierer, V. O. (1983). Development and validation of a geriatric depression screening scale: A preliminary report. *Journal of Psychiatric Research, 17,* 1, 37–34.

CHAPTER 15   Outcome Measures for Research and Practice

BROAD PURPOSES OF MEASUREMENT

In this chapter, we focus on the measurement of **outcomes** for research and clinical practice. Consistent with the usage in earlier chapters, we use the term *outcome* when we refer to the intended target or actual result of an intervention. For clinicians and researchers alike, measuring an outcome involves an assessment of the variation and changes in it. For example, a nurse researcher may be interested in finding out whether an educational and social support intervention is effective in reducing the incidence of low infant birth weight (outcome), as measured by the weight of infants at birth (outcome measure).

Although outcomes and outcome measures of various types have received increased emphasis in recent years in nursing and other health-related fields, they are not the only types of measures that are of interest to nurses. In addition to *outcome* measures, *diagnostic* and *process* measures are clinically relevant.[1] As will be described in the following sections, each of these types of measures serves a different purpose.

DIAGNOSTIC AND SCREENING MEASURES

In the last chapter, we discussed the accuracy of biophysiologic tests in terms of their sensitivity and specificity, emphasizing the tradeoff between them. We also introduced the concept of the receiver-operating characteristic curve as a way to describe and compare the quality of two or more diagnostic and screening tests. When a choice must be made among existing tests, there are additional issues to consider. They include the following:

- Technical adjustments
- Understanding of the purpose of the test
- Patient preferences

Technical Adjustments

Regarding technical adjustments, even though sensitivity and specificity (different from the positive and negative

predictive values) do not depend on the prevalence of a disease or condition in the target population, they must be *recalibrated* before they can be used to compare different tests.

🔁 Recall from the discussion of interrater reliability and Cohen's kappa (chapter 14) that some level of agreement between two raters can always be expected to occur as a result of pure random chance. Thus, evidence of interrater reliability requires levels of agreement that go beyond the level expected on the basis of a purely random process.

The principle of comparing test results with "expected" levels also applies to sensitivity and specificity. Even a test that has *no* discriminating power and *randomly* labels test takers as "positive" or "negative" will nonetheless generate some "true-positive" results and some "true-negative" results. The key issue is that for a test to be "legitimate," the test outcomes must agree with the gold standard at a level that goes beyond what can be expected under the assumption of mere random assignment. For technical details, see the relevant literature.[2]

Another technical issue that has not always received sufficient attention in the clinical literature is that any estimates of sensitivity and specificity are just that: *estimates* based on particular study samples (Fleiss, 1981). As such, they are subject to sampling fluctuations as well as selection bias.[3] An important implication for clinical practice is that, if the estimates of sensitivity and specificity of a test come from studies with target populations that differ substantially from the current clinical population, it is useful to be cautious in the interpretation of such tests.

Purpose of Tests

When using a biophysiologic test, an important distinction must be made between a **diagnostic test** and a **screening test.**

Diagnostic Tests

Diagnostic tests are usually ordered by clinicians based on patient complaints or reported symptoms as well as on clinical observations that point in the direction of a suspected diagnosis. Diagnostic tests are most useful when a clinician is uncertain about the diagnosis based on other information, or when a particular test promises to yield significant new information that could change the course of action for the clinician and patient. In addition to assisting in the identification of a disease, diagnostic tests can provide greater

---

[1]These categories are not necessarily mutually exclusive, and a given measure can be conceptualized as belonging to any or all of the categories, depending on the purpose for which it is used. For example, a diagnostic measure, such as HgA_1C monitoring for classifying patients as "diabetic" or "not diabetic" may also be used to document a process (control of diabetes) over time. It can also function as an indicator of intermediate and more distal outcomes (e.g., adequacy of diabetic control) and the likelihood of adverse health events, such as stroke and vascular insufficiency related to the adequacy of diabetic control.

[2]See the lucid discussion in Kraemer (1992).

[3]See chapters 19 and 20 for more detailed information.

specificity about the stage or advancement of a disease, thus providing a better base for appropriate treatment. With diagnostic tests, the likelihood of a positive diagnosis (the disease is present) is usually quite high because the clinical population for whom the test is ordered is usually highly selective, and grounds for "suspicion" of a positive diagnosis already exist. For example, consider the use of needle biopsies of the prostate among men who have already been identified, through digital rectal examination, as having a prostate mass. The likelihood of prostate cancer in men who already have an identified prostate mass is certainly greater than in a population of men who have not been examined for prostate masses.

Screening Tests

In contrast, a screening test is used to discover possible diseases in their early, preclinical (usually asymptomatic) stages. Such screening tests, even if targeted to special population groups, still cover a large number of people, many of whom will *not* have the disease. The fact that screening tests are used in seemingly healthy populations requires careful consideration of the conditions under which they might be usefully applied. For example, consider a recommendation for health care providers to perform blood glucose screenings (via finger stick blood samples that are tested by a glucometer) in shopping malls, with the goal of detecting people who have undiagnosed diabetes mellitus. As we will see, the usefulness of screening a general, untested population in a shopping mall may be quite limited, especially if the screened-for disease or condition has a low prevalence in the targeted population.

Criteria for the Use of Screening Tests. Population-based screening tests, such as mammography and Pap smears, have become common in the American health care system. Yet, as shown by the recent debates about the benefits and liabilities of mammography and prostate-specific antigen testing, the use of screening tests can be quite controversial. A screening test should meet multiple criteria *before* being used with a given target population. Some of these criteria incorporate considerations of patient preferences:

- *The disease that is being screened for must be severe enough, in terms of its mortality and morbidity effects on the population, to warrant a screening program.* Examples of severe diseases for which screening programs are conducted in at least some population groups that are deemed at high risk include several types of cancer, diabetes, HIV, Alzheimer's disease, and clinical depression.

- *The trajectory of the disease includes a preclinical phase during which the screening test can detect the disease, but the patient does not experience any symptoms.* This is essentially a question about the size of the "window of opportunity." For example, mammography may detect breast cancer tumors before they reach a palpable size. However, if a disease develops vary rapidly, such as certain brain tumors, the time between the biologic onset of disease and the appearance of symptoms is very short, and a screening test is of little help.

- *An acceptable treatment is available that can improve disease outcome in patients who have early-stage, presymptomatic disease.* Early detection without an effective treatment is often undesirable. For example, certain types of genetic screening tests are controversial because there is no cure for the disease; one such disease is Huntington's chorea, which eventually causes severe dementia and death. However, some people may consider screening tests useful, even in the absence of a cure, because information about likely future events may help them to make important life decisions about family, work, and retirement.

- *A screening test must be acceptable to the target population (i.e., relatively painless and uncomplicated to administer) so that people who are ostensibly without disease will be willing to undergo testing.* Colonoscopy, breast tissue biopsy, and digital rectal examination are examples of tests that many people find very unpleasant to prepare for or undergo. In addition, certain tests that involve procedures such as general anesthesia, even when done in a way that is purported to be "minimally invasive" (e.g., routine colonoscopy performed with ultra-short-acting anesthesia), may still be perceived by some patients as too risky or not worth the discomfort, despite strong promotion by health care professionals and assertions about reductions in the risk of morbidity and mortality.

- *Screening tests should be cost-effective.* In addition to consideration of the resources needed for a single administration of the screening test, an important cost consideration is the **yield** (frequency of case detection). If few cases are discovered, the test may not be worthwhile. Consider the example of screening for diabetes in shopping malls, which (depending on the population that is accessible at the mall) may yield few true cases of diabetes. That would be the case, for example, if most of the people who frequent the mall and undergo testing are young adults and teenagers.

- *When the positive predictive value (PPV) of a screen-*

ing test is low, relatively few true-positive findings are discovered in the screened population. The many false-positive results would lead to needless additional diagnostic tests, with their accompanying psychological and physical risks. Thus, in addition to low yields, if a test results in many false-positive findings, it can cause real harm. That is why screening programs must incorporate counseling and referral resources, especially for people who undergo screening procedures and "test positive."

• *A good screening test should also result in few false-negative results.* A test is clearly problematic if is not adequately sensitive and therefore misses many members of the population who have the disease. To most people, a negative test result provides a "sense of security." If that sense is violated, it can lead to a serious breach of trust in the health care provider as well as the potential for follow-up lawsuits.

• *High specificity and high sensitivity are not, by themselves, guarantees of a high PPV.* The PPV and the yield of a screening test also depend on the prevalence of the disease in the target population. Consider Research Scenario 15-1, which shows that positive results on a screening test can lead to highly misleading conclusions if one is not careful in the interpretation of the results.

RESEARCH SCENARIO 15.1

Prevalence and Positive Predictive Value in a Screening Test

Consider the following scenario. A relative tells you that she had a positive result on a screening test for a rare disease. She wants to know if the positive test result means that it is likely that she actually has the disease (true-positive result). The disease in question occurs in approximately 100 of 100,000 members of the population. You also learn that the screening test is highly sensitive (96%) and highly specific (97%). Based on this information, which of the following answers is closest to the truth?

(1) Your relative is *quite likely* to have the disease.
(2) Your relative has *a greater than 50/50 chance* of having the disease.
(3) Your relative has *a less than 50/50 chance* of having the disease.
(4) Your relative is *quite unlikely* to have the disease.

Before you read on, provide an answer and a rationale for your answer.

Experience shows that many readers will choose the first answer. The rationale for this answer seems unassailable: the test has both high sensitivity and high specificity, so it must be highly accurate. In fact it *is* highly accurate with an *efficiency* of more than 97%. However, we must also consider the prevalence of the disease to obtain a correct answer. Consider the data in the following table:

Test result	True disease state		
	Disease	No disease	Total
Positive	96	2,997	3,093
Negative	4	96,903	96,907
Total	100	99,900	100,000

The data in the table incorporate the assumptions of the scenario. Of 100,000 members of the target population, 100 have the disease. The test is highly sensitive (96%) because it correctly identifies 96 of the 100 population members who have the disease. It is also highly specific because it correctly identifies 96,903 of the 99,900 population members who do not have the disease (97%). Yet, overall, the test returns 3,093 positive results, of whom only 96 actually have the disease. Thus, the probability that your relative has the disease, *given her positive test result,* is actually 96 of 3,093 or 3.1%. Thus, (4) is the correct answer!

The *efficiency* of a test is defined as the probability that the test will give *correct* results, regardless of whether they are positive or negative. Thus, efficiency amounts to the probability that a test produces true-positive *or* true-negative results. For sample data, efficiency equals the sum of true-positive results and true-negative results divided by the number of individuals tested.

An important implication of this discussion is that few screening programs should be aimed at the *general population* without qualifications or restrictions. For instance, breast cancer among younger women (younger than age 40) is so rare that mammography screening tests for this population produce a high proportion of "false positives" (often because of the higher density of breast tissue in younger women), together with associated harms in that population (e.g., emotional distress, costs and risks of additional testing). Raising the criterion for a positive test outcome could, of course, increase the specificity of the test. However, as we discussed in chapter 14, there is a tradeoff between the specificity and the sensitivity of a test. If we want to avoid labeling people *without* the disease as "diseased," we also run a greater risk of labeling people *with* the disease as "disease-free." Thus, the probability of obtaining false-negative results increases. The only way to lower the probability of false-positive results for *given* levels of sensitivity and specificity of a test is to apply the test to more restrictive target populations, in which the screened disease can be expected to have a higher prevalence. This is, of course, the major reason why so many routine screening tests (including those for common types of cancer) are usually recommended for *older* populations, in which the prevalence rates for many chronic diseases are much higher compared with younger populations.

Evaluating the Effectiveness of Screening Tests. Beyond the efficiency question, the ultimate justification for any screening program is that it actually helps to improve population health outcomes. The usual criterion is that it "saves lives" or leads to a "significant" reduction in population mortality.[4] Yet, even evidence about the effectiveness of screening programs in reducing mortality is not always easy to establish, as illustrated by the current (2002) controversy about mammography (Olsen & Gotzsche, 2001). At first blush, it appears that collecting the necessary evidence would be a straightforward matter of comparing the survival rates of patients whose disease is discovered through the screening program with the survival rates of patients whose disease is diagnosed after the first symptom appears. On further thought, this comparison is actually quite problematic. Even if early detection and early treatment had no survival benefit, one should still expect the screened patients to have *apparently* longer survival times because their disease was detected in the preclinical stage, before symptoms appeared. Yet, a precise estimate of this **lead time,** as it is called, is difficult to come by and to correct for, reducing the usefulness of this comparison (Morrison, 1997).

A similar bias occurs in comparisons between screened and unscreened patients with disease when a screening test identifies high proportions of people who have relatively *benign* disease, making it more likely that the average survival of screened patients appears longer. Finally, even with very large study cohorts, it may not be possible to adjust statistically for all other important factors that affect survival. For example, people who agree to be screened for certain diseases may have different attitudes and life circumstances from those whose disease is detected only when symptoms develop.

That leaves a clinical trial, with large numbers of people randomly assigned to either a "screening" or a "no screening" group, as the only way to produce unbiased evidence about the efficacy of a screening program. A randomized trial in which a *potentially* beneficial intervention is withheld can be ethically justifiable if the efficacy of the screening program is genuinely in doubt, but the researchers would encounter many problems. For example, when doubts arise about established screening programs, such as mammography (Olsen & Gotzsche, 2001), it is difficult to imagine that researchers could enlist sufficient numbers of volunteers because people would be asked to suspend their belief in the effectiveness of a screening program that has been promoted as effective.

In the final analysis, guidelines and recommendations for screening tests are based not only on empirical information about the screening tests, but also on value judgments, including the incorporation of patient preferences. Even if the evidence of a survival benefit is incontrovertible, an individual must still weigh such benefits against the costs of a false-positive result and the quality-of-life issues associated with undergoing treatment. Some patients might, for instance, prefer a shorter survival time with a better quality of life to a longer survival time with a perceived worse quality of life.[5] Ultimately, only the person affected by the decision can, and should, make that decision.

OUTCOME MEASURES

In recent years, the move toward "evidence-based practice" has led to a greater emphasis on **outcome** measures.

---

[4]In principle, a substantial reduction in morbidity or improved quality of life as a result of earlier treatment could also be a justification for a screening program. However, the establishment of reliable evidence to this effect is often quite difficult. As a result, the "benefits" of screening programs are almost always measured in terms of "lives saved." However, there are certain exceptions, such as screening tests for genetic diseases to inform family and other life-planning decisions.

[5]This is the apparent tradeoff for prostatectomy in older men (Duenwald, 2002).

If clinical practice is supposed to make a difference in patients' health status, it must be possible to show the effect empirically (i.e., it must be a measurable phenomenon). Traditionally, it has been more common to evaluate medical and nursing practice in terms of **process** measures[6] (i.e., measures that capture the activities of health providers). For example, one might record how often patients in a burn unit undergo dressing changes or how often mentally unstable patients in the emergency department are referred for psychiatric evaluation. Although process measures play an important role in the legal system (among other things, they indicate whether patient treatment follows accepted practice guidelines), they do not, by themselves, tell us anything about how effective or successful a treatment has been. Evidence-based practice, however, rests on an assumption that the interventions, treatments, and services that clinicians offer do (if they are truly useful) lead to improved patient outcomes. From this point of view, process measures are *input* measures, representing the providers' activities and procedures that should predict at least some variation in patient outcomes, which are the *output* measures.

In the broadest sense, patient outcome measures reflect patient health status, at either the individual or the aggregate (population) level. Traditionally, the most important "health status" outcome has been patient survival or death. It is still considered the single most important criterion for judging the "success" of many clinical interventions or therapeutic efforts, such as chemotherapy or radiation therapy. Yet, the success of many interventions for chronic health conditions, such as diabetes self-care, is not necessarily captured well by survival measures alone. For such diseases, as for most forms of arthritis,[7] survival is almost irrelevant as a benchmark for successful treatment. In these situations, other measures are needed that can detect changes in morbidity, well-being, and quality of life.[8] Furthermore, successful treatment may not always imply the availability of a "cure," but may mean the successful *management* of a chronic disease, with minimal side effects or maintained or improved quality of life. How, then, do we measure variations and improvements in morbidity and health status? Among the many available approaches, one important choice in measurement strategy is that between generic health status measures and **disease-** or **condition-specific** health status measures (Froberg & Kane, 1989a–d; Kane, 1997).

Generic Health Status Measures: SIP and SF-36

Generic health status measures have three central features with the following characteristics:

1. They include generally broad operationalizations of the concept of health.
2. They are multidimensional.
3. They rely on self-report (i.e., they attempt to provide a comprehensive self-assessment of a person's health).

Because health and health-related quality of life are complex concepts, it is not surprising that the measurement instruments that attempt to capture these concepts are also complex. Two of the most prominent global self-assessment measures in the literature are the Sickness Impact Profile (SIP) of Bergner et al. (1981) and the Short Form of the Medical Outcomes Study Instrument (SF-36) of Ware, Snow, Kosinski, and Gandek (1993). Conceptually, both instruments measure multiple dimensions of health (i.e., physical, emotional, and social functioning) as well as pain, and provide an overall assessment of health and well-being. The SIP also includes cognitive functioning as a health domain, and the SF-36 emphasizes vitality as a separate domain. The SIP is the longer of the two instruments, including 136 separate items designed to represent not only the six major health domains listed above, but also 12 more specific subdomains, such as mobility and alertness. Although it is internally consistent, the biggest drawback of the SIP is the length of its interview schedule, which is often an obstacle in clinical research, especially when dealing with sick, elderly, or easily fatigued populations. In response, a shorter version, the SIP68, was developed by deBruin et al. (1994).

Weighting and Scoring of Generic Measures

In recent years, the SF-36 has become the most widely used generic health and quality-of-life measure. It includes eight subscales that can be combined into two more global domains that emphasize physical and emotional health. As with other complex, multidimensional scales, scoring of the SF-36 involves the application of a complex algorithm. Interested readers can consult the manuals and literature for details, although we emphasize one important aspect of such algorithms. With all complex scales that consist of a large number of individual items, the question arises as to how to combine the items into scale scores. With multidi-

---

[6]The widely accepted distinction between process and outcome measures goes back to a classic paper by Donabedian (1966).

[7]In comparison with milder, very common forms of osteoarthritis, certain severe forms of rheumatoid or psoriatic arthritis may be exceptions because of the potential complications, such as major internal organ failure and increased risk of major depression and suicide.

[8]Diabetes and arthritis are examples of such chronic diseases.

mensional scales, there are at least two steps to consider: (1) the combination of individual items into subscales and (2) the combination of subscale scores into overall scale scores.

To illustrate these steps, consider the Center for Epidemiologic Studies Depression Scale (CES-D), which was discussed in some detail in the last chapter (chapter 14). The overall CES-D scale score is simply the sum of the responses to 20 individual items, each of which has the same response scale, scored 0 through 3.

Although it is perfectly reasonable to sum the response scores of internally consistent items, this algorithm implies two important weighting decisions: (1) each *individual* item is an *equally important* indicator of depressive symptoms, but (2) the subscales of depressed mood and somatization (comprising seven items each) should have a *greater* weight in the overall depression scale score than the absence of well-being (four items) and the interpersonal (two items) subscale. Thus, whether intended or not, any combination of multiple items implies the use of a weighting scheme: "default," or equal, weighting requires, in principle, just as much of a theoretic or empirical justification as other weighting schemes. When one combines the subscales of health status measures, one must make a judgment about the *utility,* or *value,* that survey respondents attach to, say, mental health, vitality, or physical functioning. A large body of literature deals with ways to incorporate respondents' judgments into the weighting of items or subscales. Scoring algorithms of complex, multidimensional scales can be quite sophisticated (Ware et al., 1993), and it is incumbent on the user to use the accepted algorithm when aggregating scale scores, unless explicit reasons and evidence are provided to support the use of alternative scoring algorithms.

Issues in the Use of Generic Measures to Assess the Effect of Treatment

Generic or global measures of health provide an assessment of overall health status, but it is less clear to what extent they can be used to assess the effect of treatment or care. A single health status score for a patient tells us very little unless we have a basis for comparison that provides the relevant context. In other words, we need a "baseline" measure against which to judge the posttreatment scores. Yet, what is the appropriate baseline? People usually seek health care because they feel sick or are experiencing some type of symptoms. Ideally, patients seek to return to the state of health that they experienced before the perceived onset of disease. Yet, especially for chronic diseases, the "onset" may not be clearly defined. In addition, even if an event can be singled out that provides a clear marker of the

onset of the current health problem (e.g., an accident that caused acute injuries, a diagnosis of diabetes based on repeatedly elevated blood glucose readings), before this event, the patient's health status already may have been compromised as a result of comorbid conditions or other complications. Most importantly, no reliable retrospective information may be available on the patient's previous health status (Kreulen et al., 2002). Without a baseline measurement, it is hard to determine what health status constitutes a *restoration,* let alone an *improvement,* over the status prior to the treatment.

A second issue is closely related to the baseline problem. To measure the effect of treatment on a patient's health status, one could measure the improvements (i.e., changes in health status) that start when treatment begins and continue for a predetermined interval. Yet, not all changes can be attributed to the intervention itself. For instance, given the occasionally spontaneous ability of the body to heal itself, some improvements in health status could be expected to occur over time, even though they may not be related to any intervention provided by a clinician. This means that simple pretest–posttest designs that provide generic health status measures of outcomes may be ill suited to the evaluation of an intervention effect. As always, control over maturation processes can be achieved only through comparisons of otherwise equivalent (randomly assigned) treatment and control groups (see chapter 3).

Aside from study design issues, the main problem with using generic health status measures to evaluate the effectiveness of treatment is that a global health status measure may not be *sensitive* enough to detect the effects of treatment.[9] Most clinical treatments or interventions are geared toward specific conditions, such as reducing blood pressure, controlling hyperglycemia, or curing a fungal infection. Even if these treatments or interventions are successful, their effect may be too specific to produce more than a small change in overall health perceptions or well-being. The broader the concept of health addressed in an outcome measure, the more difficult it is to tie the outcome to specific treatments or interventions. Global well-being typically has multifaceted sources. In practice, many researchers have

---

[9]Note the two different meanings of "sensitivity" that we have addressed in this chapter. To say that a biophysiologic measurement instrument is "highly sensitive" means that there is a high probability that people who have the disease in question will be identified. In the current context, however, the *sensitivity* of a measurement instrument refers to its ability to register small increments in the underlying condition that is being measured. *Sensitivity,* in this sense, refers to the ability of an instrument to detect small changes. *Both* usages of "sensitivity" are common in the health research literature.

used the more focused subscales of generic health measures, such as the physical functioning subscale of the SF-36 (see Given, Given, Azzouz, & Stommel, 2001a; Kurtz, Kurtz, Stommel, Given, & Given, 2001) to map illness trajectories and treatment effects. However, generic health status measures remain very useful as overall indicators of quality of life as well as in the comparison of large population groups that may include age cohorts, gender groups, or institutionalized populations.

Disease- and Condition-Specific Health Status Measures

Disease- or condition-specific measures address outcomes for specific health problems. In some respects, they appear to be more "natural" gauges of treatment effectiveness than other types of measures. Suppose that a patient comes to a dermatologist with a rash that cannot be cured with over-the-counter drugs. In this case, the criterion for the success of the treatment used by the dermatologist is an obvious one: to make the rash disappear, visibly or by other means of measurement, such as obtaining negative tissue cultures for certain types of cutaneous fungal infections. Other common clinical situations do not necessarily involve cures, but rather effective control of conditions with reference to critical values derived from population norms. For example, the control of diabetes can be gauged with reference to "normal" or "desirable" blood glucose levels, but the underlying disease process that cause diabetes is not cured. In fact, monitoring and managing patients so that they achieve (or remain within the limits of) target norms for many physiologic measures is one of the primary contributions of nurses to successful clinical interventions.[10]

Not all condition-specific measures are tests with readily available, quantitative reference norms. Many condition-specific measures are dependent on either patient self-reports (**symptoms**) or clinicians' observations (**signs**). Nurse researchers have been at the forefront of efforts to measure and quantify patients' experience of symptoms (McCorkle, 1983; Dodd, Miaskowski, & Paul, 2001; Given, Given, Azzouz, Kozachik, & Stommel, 2001b). That such measures are based on subjective appraisals is not a serious objection to their use, especially since subjective well-being is an inherent feature of the concept of health. More problematic is the fact that symptoms often are not condition-specific (e.g., consider the experiences of pain and fatigue), and their etiology may be rooted in co-

morbid conditions rather than the focal disease (Dodd et al., 2001).

With even more justification, the same point can be made about functional status measures. Such measures do not directly address the signs and symptoms of a disease, but instead address their putative functional consequences. Functional status measures are a part of most generic health outcome measures, such as the physical functioning subscale of the SF-36, or measurement may be obtained objectively through a function test.[11] For example, a patient may self-report her or his ability to ambulate, or a family member or clinician may rate the patient's ability. In either case, the ratings are essentially measures of performance or performance capacity, which usually reflects multiple etiologies. For instance, an exercise regimen may improve functional performance in patients with arthritis, but the improved functional performance should not be interpreted as a sign that the arthritis condition itself improved (Atherly, 1997).

The latter example shows that the distinction between generic and condition-specific health outcome measures is rather fluid. The less specific the chosen indicators of health are, the more difficult it is to tie such outcomes directly to a specific disease or treatment (Bessette, Sangha, Kuntz, Keller, Lew, Fossel, & Katz, 1998). However, this does not imply that condition-specific measures are always preferred in the evaluation of health outcomes. The concept of health is inherently multidimensional. As such, it incorporates many domains that might be affected by a disease or treatment. For instance, "full recovery" from surgery after a car accident does not entail only the physical ability to perform daily activities and work-related tasks, but also may include regaining the confidence to resume the full range of activities that the patient performed before the accident. A person who has been traumatized by the experience of a car accident or who has had major surgery that limited the ability to drive may need to rebuild his or her confidence in the ability to drive gradually, over a period of days or weeks. Thus, broader evaluations of health must be part of outcome assessments. The traditional focus on mortality rates or a few specific signs of disease may lead to a mistaken definition of treatment "success" that disregards the effect of illness or treatment on quality of life.

Finally, from a technical point of view, measurement instruments that are geared toward specific outcomes are

---

[10]As always, all monitoring tests and measures are subject to measurement error, and their reliability must be established. See chapter 14.

[11]Some functional measures, such as the Katz Activities of Daily Living (ADL) (Katz, Ford, Moskowitz, Jackson, & Jaffee, 1963), allow flexibility in terms of the source of data (i.e., data collected about function of the patient may be based on either self-report or observations by third parties, including family members or clinicians).

less valuable for comparing different disease populations or treatment modes. If one wants to compare treatment outcomes in men and women, the measurement tools should avoid including indicators of outcomes that are sex-specific, such as vaginal dryness or erectile dysfunction. Likewise, the comparison of chemotherapy, radiation therapy, and surgery, or different combinations of these treatments, in patients with the same cancer diagnosis must be based on outcome measures that are sensitive to the effects of any of these treatments. Thus, a researcher must carefully consider the tradeoffs between generic and condition-specific measures before choosing specific measurement instruments. It is quite common for researchers to use a *combination* of condition-specific and generic health outcomes measures to reap the advantages of both types of measures.

Additional Considerations in Selecting Outcome Measures

Variability and Range of Scores in Different Target Populations

As we have emphasized throughout this text, it is only through comparison that one can make sense out of a finding. This dictum applies *a fortiori* to measurement scales. For example, it means very little to be told that, in a particular sample, the mean CES-D score is 6.5, with a range of 0 to 21. In the context of population norms for the CES-D (i.e., mean, 8–10; range, 0–45), we realize that the sample just described is unusually free of depression. However, if all of the sample members are healthy adults who are 25 to 35 years of age, the finding may be less surprising because this age group tends to show the lowest depression ratings. It is clear, then, that researchers must pay attention to the potential and actual variability of scores in the target population when they select instruments. Suppose an overall quality-of-life measure, such as the SF-36, is used with nursing home residents who are mostly older than 70 years of age. One of the subscales of the SF-36, the physical functioning subscale, asks about the respondents' ability to engage in "vigorous activities such as lifting heavy objects," "climb several flights of stairs," and "walk more than a mile." Among nursing home residents, there may be few persons, even none, who engage in these behaviors, and a few may be essentially confined to bed because of extremely poor physical condition. The result would be a classic "floor effect," such that large numbers of respondents would score very low on the physical functioning subscale, and almost none would reach a "perfect" score of 100, even though such scores are common in the general population. Likewise, a knowledge test may sim-

ply be too easy to discriminate among members of a certain population, and may result in 60%, 70%, or even 80% of test-takers achieving a "perfect" score. Here, we have an example of the "ceiling effect." Another example can be found in Powell, Canterbury, and McCoy (1998). In either case, score variability is restricted because the measurement instrument that is used does not allow for exploring the more extreme manifestations of a phenomenon that may occur in a specific target population, but not in the population referenced in the test.

Norm-referenced Scores. Many health outcome measures are **norm-referenced** (Waltz, Strickland, & Lenz, 1991). That means that their scores are, in a sense, calibrated with reference to the population in which they were developed. The advantage of norm-referenced measures is that they allow us to gauge an individual's "performance," or score, in relation to that of a well-defined group or target population. The crucial issue in choosing such a measure is the relevancy of the target population. Suppose you want to develop a knowledge test for advance practice nurses (APNs). Clearly, given both the training of an APN and the role that APNs are expected to perform, such a test should be more demanding than a test for an entry-level graduate nurse who just completed a basic nursing program. If one were to standardize such a test, one could use the results of tens of thousands of tests *from APN candidates* and assign an arbitrary score, of say, 100, to the mean test score for the total group, with all other scores converted in relation to this test score. Norms are usually expressed in terms of percentile ranks, which indicate an individual's performance relative to that of other members of the target population. For example, a 90th percentile score indicates that a person has performed as well as or better than 90% of the target population. The resulting test would be norm-referenced because it tells us how each new test-taker performs relative to the target population. For a number of clinical tests that are performed to assess the state of patients' health and functioning, such population norms may not be available.

Criterion-referenced Scores. An alternative to norm-referenced scores is **criterion-referenced scores.** These scores essentially rely on external criteria to evaluate a person's performance. In the case of a knowledge test, the criteria may have been established by seasoned practitioners in a particular field. In that case, the test is said to be "content-validated," with the experts establishing the relevant content. In either norm-referenced or criterion-referenced tests or measures, the instruments must generate sufficient variation in scores *within the target population.* Otherwise, measurement scores cannot be used to make the necessary comparisons.

Trait Versus State Measures

An issue that is commonly encountered with health status measures is whether the measure is a **trait** or a **state** measure. The difference is one of flexibility or changeability over time within the individual. A **trait measure** refers to relatively immutable characteristics of individuals that do not change within broadly defined time limits. For instance, when we speak of a "personality trait," we have in mind a collection of psychological and cognitive attributes that are relatively constant, are not situation-specific, and are not easily amenable to change or intervention. For example, we tend to think of generalized (sometimes referred to as "G factor") "intelligence" as such a trait, even though learning and exposure to challenging mental activity can "improve" a person's intelligence scores. To the extent that an individual characteristic is a trait (e.g., a "fearless" or "anxious" personality), it usually cannot be considered an appropriate outcome measure for assessing the effect of an intervention because it is not amenable to change, at least not in response to the usual health care interventions.[12]

Outcome Measures for Institutional Comparisons

Institutional comparisons illustrate the general problem of comparing "naturally occurring" groups. When comparing groups of patients who undergo different treatments or groups of patients who are treated in different institutions or under different practice plans, we encounter the additional problem that the compared groups are not identical in their background characteristics, from physical attributes to social support systems to mental makeup. However, if the inputs differ, so will the outputs.[13] Risk adjustments are often used to address this problem of incomparability. For example, a hospital that admits patients who have particularly serious illnesses may well have higher in-hospital mortality rates than another hospital that admits patients who have "routine" complications. Thus, unadjusted mortality rates (disregarding the severity of specific diagnoses, comorbidities, social backgrounds of patients, age distribution, and so forth) for the hospitals do not provide a valid yardstick for comparing the hospitals' performance. Strictly speaking, the problem of risk adjustment is not a measurement, but a design problem. Risk adjustment is a way to cope with confounding variables.[14]

Measures of Satisfaction

Patient satisfaction measures are often used in studies of interventions that are designed to have an effect on patient health status and quality of life. Such measures are often used for process evaluation when assessing the effect of an intervention. For example, when assessing the effectiveness and economic efficiency of a telephone reminder system for primary care appointments, collecting data on patient satisfaction with the system may enhance the evaluation of the intervention. Information about patient satisfaction can also yield important clues about underlying patient preferences. These preferences can be explored in more depth if patients are found to be dissatisfied with a service or an intervention.

The health-related literature on patient satisfaction is extensive. Various patient satisfaction measures are available, and many of the general considerations for the selection and evaluation of measures apply to patient satisfaction measures. Important additional considerations include: (1) what aspects of satisfaction to measure, (2) the sources and validity of data on satisfaction, and (3) the interpretation of satisfaction measures.

Satisfaction is most often conceptualized as a multidimensional construct that includes distinct aspects of patients' encounters with the health care system. For example, patient satisfaction may be assessed for the interpersonal, technical, and amenity aspects of a health care encounter. Patient ratings or self-report ratings from a variety of other sources (such as family members) may be used to evaluate patient satisfaction with health care delivery and the infrastructure of services. Satisfaction ratings have sometimes been used as markers of the quality of health care, but should not be viewed as either synonymous with quality of care or as valid sources of information about all aspects of

---

[12]One exception is that personality traits could be considered an appropriate outcome measure for a long-term psychotherapeutic intervention that is designed to restructure certain facets of personality. For example, a researcher might conduct a longitudinal study of the effects of a particular intervention on the traits of neuroticism, introversion, and openness to experience, looking for a reduction in neuroticism and increases in extroversion and openness to experience. Likewise, a researcher may be interested in the effects of newer antidepressant medications on "personality," measuring selected "traits" before and after the initiation of drug therapy. However, measuring changes in personality traits that occur as a result of psychotherapy or pharmacotherapy begs the question of what is the appropriate conceptualization of personality "traits."

[13]For example, suppose you compare a graduate of a highly ranked college with a graduate of a college that has open admission. The finding that graduates of the first school tend to do better than those of the second on any number of achievement tests is not necessarily a credit to the school itself. Such a finding may simply reflect the differences in selectivity between the schools. If the highly ranked college admits only students who are academic high achievers, it is not surprising if its graduates do better on academic achievement tests. The relevant question is whether the contributions that the schools make to *improvements* in student achievement are greater in one school than in the other, something that is far more difficult to gauge.

---

[14]For more detail, see the discussion of statistical adjustment and control in chapter 8.

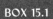

BOX 15.1   Dimensions of Quality Care

For example, in a classic article, Donabedian (1990) described dimensions of quality of care, which include, but go well beyond, patient perceptions of quality. Patients and family members who lack specialized medical training may be able to evaluate most validly the interpersonal and amenity aspects of care, but may not be qualified to evaluate the technical aspects of care. Thus, a patient may feel quite positively toward a provider and be well satisfied with the interpersonal aspects of care, but may not necessarily be receiving high-quality, state-of-the-art health care services. Likewise, a patient may be relatively dissatisfied with a health care provider's interpersonal skills, yet receive medically and technically appropriate care.

quality of care (Box 15-1). As with all multidimensional evaluations and measurements, the relative weighting of each of the dimensions (interpersonal, technical, and amenity) of care in overall patient satisfaction ratings may *vary,* depending on the context of evaluation or the preferences of the patients.

THE SELECTION OF EXISTING MEASUREMENTS

The choice of a measurement instrument usually proceeds in two steps. The first step involves locating measurement instruments, and the second step involves making decisions about their quality and appropriateness for the intended application. In recent years, it has become much easier to search for and locate existing measurement tools. Evaluating the quality and appropriateness of measures for a specific purpose, however, is more challenging. We discuss each step in turn.

Step 1: Searching for and Locating Measurement Tools

As just mentioned, in recent years, it has become easier to locate measurement tools. However, not all of the desired information for a measurement evaluation is always available in an accessible form. If a researcher already knows the name of a specific measurement instrument, such as the Beck Depression Inventory (Beck, Ward, et al., 1961) or the Duke Health Profile (Parkerson et al., 1990), it is easy to use the search features of standard electronic databases (e.g., CINAHL, MEDLINE, PSYCHINFO, HEALTHSTAR) by typing in the name of the instrument. It is more difficult to use these search engines to *find* new instruments for given constructs, such as "anxiety" or "pain," because a search using the general constructs would turn up large numbers of articles that are not con-

cerned with scale development. Still, with a little trial and error, locating measurement articles in professional journals is no longer difficult.[15] In addition, an increasing number of published compendiums of measures for various topics, such as long-term care and nursing, as well as annual reviews in nursing and psychology, present annotated bibliographies and lists of key references and contact information for obtaining additional information about selected measures. It is also useful to use the search features available at key web sites, such as that of the National Institutes of Health, to locate relevant measures and to obtain contact information for the authors of measures (see chapter 23). Personal contact (through e-mail or telephone calls) with individual researchers or specialized research listservs can sometimes yield additional, unpublished information about measures.

Step 2: Assessing the Quality and Appropriateness of Measures

In this and the previous chapter, we have discussed many criteria for judging the quality of measurement scales and procedures. Chief among them are the various forms of reliability, validity, and accuracy. Before selecting a specific tool, one must be able to compare the quality of the tools. This comparison requires the availability of the relevant information in published reports that discuss the measurement properties of the tools. At the very minimum, for psychosocial measurement instruments, a potential user would need to know the following:

- The conceptual and theoretic base for the overall scale construct and its subdimensions, including its similarities to and differences from existing constructs in the literature
- A list of the actual wording of all items in the instrument and their associated response scales

---

[15]See chapter 23 for more detailed information on literature searches.

- Information about the size and composition (subject characteristics) of the study sample that was used to develop and test the measurement instrument
- Psychometric evaluations of the scaling properties, including evidence about the unidimensionality or multidimensionality of the instrument, as determined by factor analyses, and evidence about internal consistency, repeated-measures reliability, and so forth
- Confirmation of the measurement properties in different study samples from different target populations
- If available, empirical relationships of the measurement instrument to existing similar ("convergent") and dissimilar ("discriminant") measures
- If available, evidence about population norms for the measurement scale

For biophysiologic measures, a similar list of considerations applies. A potential user would need information on the following:

- The relationship between the conceptual definitions of a physiologic variable of interest and the biophysical, biochemical, or microbiologic basis for the measurement procedure (DeKeyser & Pugh, 1991)
- The precision, reliability, and variability of the measurement procedure in repeated applications by different personnel, as distinct from biologic or physiologic variability
- Evidence about the *selectivity* of the measurement procedure, for example, its ability to distinguish signals related to the disease under study from unrelated signals
- Evidence about *reference values* and *population norms;* in particular, evidence about the "normal" range of intrapersonal and interpersonal variation

CONCLUSION

It is clear from these lists that the evaluation of measurement tools is a complex task that requires substantial amounts of information. It is not enough to cite a high value for a reliability coefficient or high sensitivity and specificity values as evidence that a measurement tool has all of the desirable qualities. One additional area of evaluation for a measurement instrument, which we have mentioned several times, is that of its prior use with many different and diverse target populations. The measurement properties of measurement scales often *vary* depending on the target population. This is particularly true for psychosocial measures, but also applies to biophysiologic measures (Waltz et al., 1991; Kraemer, 1992). Thus, users

of instruments generally should be skeptical about measurement scales for which evidence is available *only* from a *single, moderately* sized sample. Unfortunately, the measurement properties of such scales often *cannot* be reproduced in new study samples. That is one reason why novice researchers and clinicians alike should, whenever possible, rely on well-established measurement instruments for which a substantial body of evidence is available that describes their reliability, validity, and use in many different population groups.

Ultimately, to make a judgment about the appropriateness and quality of a particular measurement tool, the purposes for using the tool must be kept in mind. As noted earlier, a screening tool and a diagnostic tool must meet different criteria. Likewise, a tool that is sensitive enough to capture *individual* changes in patient outcomes must meet higher psychometric standards than one that is designed to produce accurate estimates of population averages, and so forth. The selection of a particular measurement tool or instrument also involves consideration of the ease with which the data can be collected. We will turn to such considerations in chapter 16.

Suggested Activities

1. Read the articles by Ware and Sherbourne (1992); McHorney, Ware, and Raczek (1993); and McHorney, Ware, Lee, and Sherbourne (1994). Follow the development of the SF-36 from the conceptual discussion to its first psychometric evaluation.
2. Select Friedemann, Montgomery, Rice, and Farrell (1999) or Teel, Press, Lindgren, and Nichols (1999), and focus on the psychosocial outcome measures that the researchers use.
   a. List all of the psychosocial scales used in the article.
   b. Using the summary list for assessing the quality and appropriateness of psychosocial outcome measures in this chapter, list all of the information on the measurement properties of the scales provided in the article. Is the information sufficient and complete enough to allow you to make a reasoned judgment about the quality of the scale?
   c. Select one or two instruments that are referenced in the article, and search for additional published information on the instruments to obtain the following information:
      i. Copies of the questionnaire instruments underlying the scales
      ii. Information on scoring of the interview responses
      iii. Information on the dimensionality of the instru-

ments: Which items form which subscales? Do different studies report the same item groupings into subscales?

iv. The internal consistency and reliability of all subscales as well as the overall scale score, the average inter-item correlations among the sub-scale items, and interscale correlations among the subscales

v. The size and characteristics of the samples used in the development and refinement of the instruments and a description of the population groups to which the instrument has, and has not, been applied

vi. Evidence of the *validity* of the instrument and its subscales, including face validity (do item group-ings and subscale labels make sense to you?) and construct validity (evidence of convergent and discriminant validity in the literature)

d. Based on what you learned from researching the instruments, what are the key strengths and potential limitations of the measure as used in the study listed in the suggested readings?

Suggested Readings

Friedemann, M.-L., Montgomery, R. J., Rice, C., & Farrell, L. (1999). Family involvement in the nursing home. *Western Journal of Nursing Research, 21,* 4, 549–567.

McHorney, C. A., Ware, J. E., & Raczek, A. E. (1993). The MOS 36-item short form health survey (SF-36): II. Psychometric and clinical tests of validity in measuring physical and mental health constructs. *Medical Care, 31,* 3, 247–263.

McHorney, C. A., Ware, J. E., Lee, J. F. R., & Sherbourne, C. D. (1994). The MOS 36-item short form health survey (SF-36): III. Tests of data quality, scaling assumptions, and reliability across diverse patient groups. *Medical Care, 32,* 1, 40–66.

Teel, C. S., Press, A. N., Lindgren, C. L., & Nichols, E. G. (1999). Fatigue among elders in caregiving and non-caregiving roles. *Western Journal of Nursing Research, 21,* 4, 498–520.

Ware, J. E., & Sherbourne, C. D. (1992). The MOS 36-item short form health survey (SF-36): I. Conceptual framework and item selection. *Medical Care, 30,* 6, 473–483.

References

Atherly, A. (1997). Condition-specific measures. In Kane, R. L. *Understanding health care outcomes research* (pp. 53–66). Gaithersburg, MD: Aspen.

Beck, A. T., Ward, C. H., Mendelson, M., Mock, J., and Erbaugh, J. (1961). An inventory for measuring depression. *Archives of General Psychiatry, 4,* 53–63.

Bergner, M., Bobbitt, R. and Carter, W. (1989). The sickness impact profile: development and final revision of a health status measure. *Medical Care, 19,* 787–805.

Bessette, L., Sangha, O., Kuntz, K. M., Keller, R. B., Lew, R. A., Fossel, A. H., & Katz, J. N. (1998). Comparative responsiveness of generic versus disease-specific and weighted versus unweighted health status measures in carpal tunnel syndrome. *Medical Care, 36,* 4, 491–502.

de Bruin, A. F., Diederiks, J. P. M., deWitte, L. P., Stevens, J. A. and Philipsen, H. (1994). The development of a short generic version of the Sickness Impact Profile. *Journal of Clinical Epidemiology, 47,* 407–18.

DeKeyser, F. G., & Pugh, L. C. (1991). Approaches to physiologic measurement. In Waltz, C. H., O. L. Strickland, & E. R. Lenz (Eds.). *Measurement in nursing research* (2nd ed.) (pp. 387–412). Philadelphia: F. A. Davis.

Donabedian, A. (1966). Evaluating the quality of medical care. *Milbank Memorial Fund Quarterly, 44,* 3, 166–206.

Donabedian, A. (1990). The seven pillars of quality. *Archives of Pathology and Laboratory Medicine, 114,* 1115–1118.

Dodd, M., Miaskowski, C., & Paul, S. (2001). Symptom clusters and their effects on the functional status of patients with cancer. *Oncology Nursing Forum, 28,* 3, 465–470.

Duenwald, M. (2002). Putting cancer screening to the test. *New York Times;* October 15, 2002.

Fleiss, J. L. (1981). *Statistical methods for rates and proportions.* New York: John Wiley & Sons.

Friedemann, M.-L., Montgomery, R. J., Rice, C., & Farrell, L. (1999). Family involvement in the nursing home. *Western Journal of Nursing Research, 21,* 4, 549–567.

Froberg, D. G., & Kane, R. L. (1989a). Methodology for measuring health state preferences: I. Measurement strategies. *Journal of Clinical Epidemiology, 42,* 4, 345–354.

Froberg, D. G., & Kane, R. L. (1989b). Methodology for measuring health state preferences: II. Scaling methods. *Journal of Clinical Epidemiology, 42,* 5, 459–471.

Froberg, D. G., & Kane, R. L. (1989c). Methodology for measuring health state preferences: III. Population and context effects. *Journal of Clinical Epidemiology, 42,* 6, 585–592.

Froberg, D. G., & Kane, R. L. (1989d). Methodology for

measuring health state preferences: IV. Progress and a research agenda. *Journal of Clinical Epidemiology, 42,* 7, 675–685.

Given, B. A., Given, C. W., Azzouz, F., & Stommel, M. (2001a). Physical functioning of elderly cancer patients prior to diagnosis and following initial treatment. *Nursing Research, 50,* 4, 222–232.

Given, C. W., Given, B., Azzouz, F., Kozachik, S., & Stommel, M. (2001b). Predictors of pain and fatigue in the year following diagnosis among elderly cancer patients. *Journal of Pain and Symptom Management, 21,* 6, 456–466.

Kane, R. L. (1997). *Understanding health care outcomes research.* Gaithersburg, MD: Aspen.

Katz, S., Ford, A. B., Moskowitz, R. W., Jackson, B. A., & Jaffee, M. W. (1963). Studies of illness in the aged: The index of ADL. A standardized measure of biological and psychosocial functioning. *Journal of the American Medical Association, 185,* 914–919.

Kraemer, H. C. (1992). *Evaluating medical tests: Objective and quantitative guidelines.* Newbury Park, CA: Sage.

Kreulen, G. J., Stommel, M., Gutek, B. A., Burns, L. R., & Braden, C. J. (2002). The utility of retrospective pretest ratings of patient satisfaction with health status. *Research in Nursing & Health, 25,* 3, 233–41.

Kurtz, M. E., Kurtz, J. C., Stommel, M., Given, C. W., & Given, B. A. (2001). Physical functioning and depression among older persons with cancer. *Cancer Practice, 9,* 1, 11–18.

McCorkle, R. (1983). Symptom distress, current concerns and mood disturbances after diagnosis of life-threatening disease. *Social Science Medicine, 17,* 431–438.

McHorney, C. A., Ware, J. E., & Raczek, A. E. (1993). The MOS 36-item short form health survey (SF-36): II. Psychometric and clinical tests of validity in measuring physical and mental health constructs. *Medical Care, 31,* 3, 247–263.

McHorney, C. A., Ware, J. E., Lee, J. F. R., & Sherbourne, C. D. (1994). The MOS 36-item short form health survey (SF-36): III. Tests of data quality, scaling assumptions, and reliability across diverse patient groups. *Medical Care, 32,* 1, 40–66.

Morrison, A. S. (1997). Screening. In Rothman, K. J., & S. Greenland. (Eds.), *Modern Epidemiology* (2nd ed.) (pp. 499–518). Philadelphia: Lippincott Williams & Wilkins.

Olsen, O., & Gotzsche, P. C. (2001). *Systematic review of screening for breast cancer with mammography.* Copenhagen: The Nordic Cochrane Center.

Parkerson, G. R., Broadhead, W. E. and Chiu-Kit, J. T. (1990). The Duke Health Profile. *Medical Care, 28,* 1056–72.

Powell, S. S., Canterbury, M. A., & McCoy, D. (1998). Medication administration: Does the teaching method really matter? *Journal of Nursing Education, 37,* 6, 281–283.

Teel, C. S., Press, A. N., Lindgren, C. L., & Nichols, E. G. (1999). Fatigue among elders in caregiving and non-caregiving roles. *Western Journal of Nursing Research, 21,* 4, 498–520.

Waltz, C. H., Strickland, O. L., & Lenz, E. R. (1991). *Measurement in nursing research* (2nd ed.). Philadelphia: F. A. Davis.

Ware, J.E., & Sherbourne, C.D. (1992). The MOS 36-item short form health survey (SF-36): I. Conceptual framework and item selection. *Medical Care, 30,* 6, 473–483.

Ware, J. E., Snow, K. K., Kosinski, M., & Gandek, B. (1993). *SF-36 health survey manual and interpretation Guide.* Boston: The Health Institute, New England Medical Center.

CHAPTER 16   Data Collection Techniques

INTRODUCTION: MEASUREMENT AND DATA COLLECTION

So far, we have talked about measurement instruments, tests, and scales, but have not yet examined the actual activities and procedures involved in collecting data. Data collection and measurement are related, but not identical, concepts. Although measurement requires data collection, data collection for quantitative research does not, in and of itself, constitute "measurement." This may seem counterintuitive, but measurement goes a step further by requiring the use of a **scaling algorithm** (i.e., a standardized procedure for converting observations into numerical scores).[1]

Modes of Data Collection

In research studies and clinical practice activities that involve human subjects, the researcher much choose from three basic modes of data collection. The researcher or clinician can: (1) ask questions, (2) observe events or behaviors, or (3) use physiologic or biologic tests. Two of these modes of data collection—observation and testing—are common to all sciences, including life and social sciences as well as natural sciences.[2] However, the natural science approach to data collection relies exclusively on the *interpretation of observations*. The observations may be indirect and relatively structured, as when they are obtained with calibrated instruments and tests. In contrast, in the social sciences and the applied clinical and health disciplines, such as psychology, sociology, nursing, medicine, and social work, there is the additional option of *asking questions* about behaviors, symptoms, or individual histories. Thus, self-report data constitute an important data source for nurse researchers and other health scientists and clinicians. By comparison, self-report data from human (or any other) subjects are irrelevant to an agriculturalist or a microbiologist as they measure, for example, the height of corn in a field or the density of microbial cultures in a Petri dish.

Advantages of Self-report Sources of Data

The potential advantages of collecting self-report data are often intuitively obvious in clinical practice, but it is useful here to consider some specific advantages of this approach. Clinicians often note the value of understanding a patient's "lived experience" based on conversations with the patient, but there are many other advantages to being able to ask questions of human subjects that go beyond accounts of lived experiences. Interviews (and self-report diaries) are also the main source of information about many health-related *events* and *behaviors*. To see the importance of this type of data collection, just imagine a situation in which a veterinarian could ask an emaciated turtle if and why it stopped eating. If it were feasible, this would certainly aid in finding the potential causes of the turtle's state of health.

Even though many events and behaviors of interest can be observed *in principle,* in reality, practical barriers, such as limited resources, time, and social barriers, can make it very challenging or impossible to observe actual behavior. Thus, if the only source of information about nutritional intake or substance use is observation, researchers might have difficulty obtaining adequate information for the purpose of their study.[3] However, there is a price to be paid for the advantage of obtaining information indirectly through asking questions. In a sense, one might say that the data are "interpreted twice" in that they incorporate both the respondents' interpretations of reality (behaviors, symptoms, attitudes, or values) and those of the researcher. Nonetheless, interviews and their extensions (e.g., health diaries) play a central role in the data collection efforts of nurse researchers. These sources are often the only source of information about health-relevant behaviors. In addition, a key reason for the reliance on asking questions is the substantial emphasis on psychosocial issues in nursing research. In contrast, biophysiologic and observational data collection have played a more limited role in nursing research, especially before about a decade ago, even though both types of measures are a prominent part of clinical practice. However, research that relies on multiple data sources is becoming more common and, in our view, will be increasingly important in the future.[4]

TYPES OF INTERVIEWS

When researchers consider collecting information through interviews, they must first decide how structured they want

---

[1]Here, we use the term *observation* in its broadest sense, referring to *any* type of data collection. For the remainder of this chapter, we use the term in the narrow sense of perceiving and recording external events.

[2]The classification of applied practice disciplines, such as nursing, varies across academic settings. Sometimes nursing is conceptualized as a "natural science" or a "social science," but more often, it is classified as a "life science" and almost always as a "health science." These terms are relevant in this text insofar as they link to references about the specific types of research methods that are used in a variety of disciplines.

[3]See chapter 11 for a detailed discussion of what kind of information can be gathered in surveys.

[4]To consider this idea further, it may be interesting to review the nursing research priorities of the National Institute for Nursing Research as described on their web site, available at: *http://www.nih.gov/ninr*. Note the prominence of *both* psychosocial and biophysiologic priorities.

their interview to be. Interview styles can vary substantially in degree of structure. A highly **structured interview** is one in which all of the questions are predetermined and interview respondents are asked to make choices among fixed response categories. In addition, the administration of the interview instrument is standardized as far as possible, including a predetermined sequence of asking questions and using interviewers that follow the same rules of administration. This style of highly structured interviewing is most conducive to measurement because it is relatively easy to convert fixed response categories into numerical scores.

In contrast, less structured interview styles allow respondents to answer questions in their own words. Such open-ended responses are more difficult to categorize and may sometimes defy attempts to subsume them meaningfully under a few numerical codes. Yet, differences in the degree of structure of an interview often go beyond the emphasis on fixed response categories. They also include the responsiveness of the interviewer to the flow of the interview. In a completely flexible, **unstructured interview,** the interviewer may not even write out any predetermined questions other than a list of *broad topics* to be covered. In somewhat less flexible, **semistructured interviews,** the interviewer may use a predetermined set of questions, but their sequence would depend on the course of the individual interview. In addition, certain **standardized probes** may be incorporated systematically into the interview to clarify comments made by study participants. For example, the interviewer may ask, "Can you tell me more about what you mean when you say your pain 'travels'?" In general, the less structured an interview is, the more the respondents influence its shape and content. Each style of interviewing has its place in health research (see Box 16-1 for a list of advantages and disadvantages). The focus of this chapter is on structured interviews that use fixed response categories. Unstructured interviews are discussed in detail in chapter 18.

The Development of a Structured Interview Schedule

In this section, we will discuss **interview schedules** or questionnaires across various modes of administration (i.e., face-to-face or personal interview, telephone interview, mailed or online questionnaire). Many, but not all, principles of questionnaire construction apply, regardless of the mode of administration. The development of an interview schedule (questionnaire) is an *art* in the sense that good instruments are largely the result of experience, and (not uncommonly), trial and error. Fortunately, researchers and clinicians need not, and should not, start every time

"from scratch," in considering how to formulate questionnaire items. There are now many excellent guides on how to write questions[5] as well as publicly available examples of questionnaires.[6] Yet, quite often, one still encounters questionnaires in surveys that were put together "from scratch," even though this approach is likely to yield at least some mistaken or uninterpretable data because of design limitations. The reasons for this are complex, but can include several key factors: (1) lack of awareness that "asking questions" is not as straightforward as it may seem and, in fact, requires careful planning and testing; (2) concern about the adequacy or quality of existing measures for use with a particular patient population; and (3) awareness that a newly created instrument or an existing questionnaire may not be optimal, but a lack of skills and resources to develop a better instrument.

Fortunately, substantial experience in questionnaire development has been accumulating in a number of disciplines, ranging from the social sciences to marketing to health research. A number of conventional rules and maxims have been distilled from this collective experience. If these conventions are followed, the chances of obtaining quality information through a structured interview are increased substantially. Although a detailed discussion is beyond the scope of this book, in the next sections of this chapter, we consider some of these general principles and provide examples with respect to the following areas: (1) conceptual preparation and organization, (2) sources for new questionnaire or survey items, (3) principles for formulating individual items, (4) principles for choosing answer categories and response scales to individual questions, and (5) preliminary evaluation of individual items.

Conceptual Preparation and Organization

A good questionnaire should have a conceptual and theoretic focus that is apparent to the respondent or study participant. As a function of informed consent standards (see chapter 24), the study participant should understand what the researcher "is after." At times, this may require a "preamble" or clarifying introductory statement to a set of questions, such as: "We are trying to understand how your illness has affected you and your family financially. For this reason, I am going to ask you several questions about income, health insurance, and health care expenditures. All information you give us is absolutely confidential and is

---

[5]Converse and Presser (1986) provide a short, succinct guide that helps researchers to avoid most of the common mistakes in questionnaire construction. Sheatsley (1983) is also very useful.

[6]One easily accessible source is the questionnaires for the federal surveys conducted by the National Center of Health Statistics (NCHS), which can be downloaded from the NCHS web site, available at: *http://www.cdc.gov/nchs/.*

BOX 16.1   Advantages and Disadvantages of Structured Interviews

Advantages

- Structured interviews yield the *same* answer categories *across* cases or time, facilitating *comparison.*
- Structured instruments do not require efforts to formulate verbal responses, increasing the *ease* of response.
- Summary and analysis of findings is easier when dealing with limited and standardized response categories.
- Structured interviews are the method of choice for mailed and online interviews. Requiring respondents to *write* open-ended responses on a questionnaire or in an online survey increases the demands on their time and literacy skills and is likely to reduce response rates.
- Structured interviews are also the preferred method for computer-aided telephone interviewing because open-ended responses (or the later transcriptions of taped interviews) must be typed in by the interviewer or transcriber.
- Structured interviews are essential for large-sample studies. Interpretive analysis of narrative texts is inherently limited to small samples (N < 100).*

Disadvantages

- Structured interviews require more work in the preparation stage. All questions and response categories must be finalized before the interviews commence.
- In structured interviews, all relevant alternative responses must be anticipated and listed. Otherwise, respondents are pressed into giving wrong answers, or refusals and missing responses are increased.
- Structured interviews require extensive *pretesting,* especially of the question items, which are hypothesized to form unidimensional or multidimensional measurement scales.
- Structured interviews are of *limited usefulness as tools of exploration.* The use of predetermined questions and fixed response categories severely restricts the possibility of unanticipated findings or information.
- Structured interviews cannot easily accommodate the language of the target population. The format conventions of structured interviews might appear "alien" to members of a target group, thereby reducing the likelihood of useful results.

Structured interviews perform *less well* when the emphasis and purpose of the study are on *exploration* of a phenomenon or a subject area about which relatively little is known. Such a situation suggests the necessity of small-scale, open-ended pilot studies (perhaps including both individual and focus group interviews) before an instrument for large samples can be developed.

*For more on this topic, see Chapter 21.

---

being asked to give us a better understanding of the financial situations of patients like you."

In general, careful qualifiers such as this should be considered for survey questions if they address topics that would be viewed as sensitive by many people. Examples include questions about finances, religion, sexuality, emotional health, smoking, and the use of alcohol or illicit substances. Even though every section of the actual questionnaire may not contain such an explicit introduction, a researcher should be prepared and able to justify every item in the instrument. Some overall considerations about questionnaire items include:

- What does a particular item attempt to measure?
- What is its relationship to the study concepts?

- Would its omission seriously impair the fulfillment of the study objectives?

To answer these central questions, it is important to have explicit research goals and survey objectives. These goals and objectives should be written down before questions are being formulated. Usually, one would start with a list of the major concepts and content areas that the questionnaire should cover. For example, in a study of family caregivers, the objectives may be defined in terms of information gathering with respect to broad conceptual areas of interest, such as the mental health of the caregiver; the psychological reactions of the caregiver; the physical and mental functioning of the patient; and the involvement in tangible care by the primary caregiver, other family members, nonfamily informal helpers, formal care services, and so forth. Each of these broad conceptual areas may be covered with one or more established instruments, such as the Center for Epidemiologic Studies Depression Scale (CES-D), as an indicator of "mental health."[7] Whenever possible, all major study concepts should be represented by multiple questions or items so that their reliability and validity can be established or confirmed.

An important feasibility concern with this approach, however, is that it can easily lead to long, and sometimes burdensome, interview schedules. The best way to shorten a questionnaire is to concentrate on a few concepts that can be addressed with a relatively limited number of instruments and questions. As a general principle, questionnaires should not be loaded up with many untested items in the hope that they will somehow be useful. Sometimes this "shotgun" approach is tempting to use, especially when there may not be subsequent opportunities to collect data, but it should be avoided for both theoretic and practical reasons. Questions that have not been pretested often produce unanticipated, and sometimes undesirable, response patterns. For example, the items may not correlate with other items as expected, or they may produce unexpectedly "lopsided" responses that show little variation.[8] These common problems demonstrate why the development of *new* measures or questionnaire items should be approached cautiously.

Sources for New Questionnaire and Survey Items

This section concerns the selection and development of *individual* items. Ideally, for the reasons we have already mentioned, untested items usually should be introduced only in pilot studies or in studies focused on instrument development.[9] Because the usefulness of a question or item depends not only on the way it is formulated, but also on what kinds of response patterns it tends to produce, structured items require pretesting with potential respondents. In some instances, pilot testing *with members of the target population* is essential. For example, if a nurse researcher wants to develop a new standardized measure to compare sex-specific cultural beliefs about using formal health care services, an essential first step would be to determine, with both men and women, if the measure has at least content validity for both groups. Depending on the special characteristics of the target population, certain questionnaire items may have little or no relevance for the respondents, or may even offend some of them. Even in the case of apparently "straightforward" questions about the socioeconomic characteristics of study participants, a researcher is usually better off using already developed and tested questions, such as those developed by the U.S. Census Bureau.[10] If federal questionnaire formats are used for some of the background questions, an important added advantage is that (in the analysis stage) comparisons between one's own data and those from nationally representative samples are facilitated.

With these caveats in mind, to test new concepts or study new population groups about which little is known or published, new questionnaire items often must be developed. Before new items are actually administered to a pilot sample of study subjects, at a minimum, they should be examined for their content validity and the appropriateness of the language used for the target population for which the questions were developed. The primary sources for initial content validation are often clinical and research experts who are familiar with the clinical problems as well as the target populations. It is also desirable to consult with experts in survey research and question formulation.

Additional experts needed for questionnaire development include "cultural insiders." This is especially important when a researcher is studying groups from a substantially different culture.[11] Key informants, or members of the target population who are interested in the research, can provide valuable help with wording as well as insights into the appropriateness of the questions. For example, a researcher may learn that the members of a particular community may refer to the experience of depression as "having no get-up-and-go" or "having nerves," but that describing the same experience as "depression" or "feeling down" in

---

[7]The appropriate measure depends on how concepts such as *mental health* are defined, and this definition is central to conceptualizing what should be included in a survey. For example, if *health* is defined, as per the World Health Organization, as "more than the mere absence of disease," the CES-D scale, which measures depression, would be an incomplete measure of mental health in that the absence of a positive score (a positive score indicates depression) would not be sufficient to assess the person as mentally "healthy." This type of conceptual thinking about what is to be measured may result in a decision to include a positive measure of mental health or well-being in addition to a depression measure that indicates a lack of mental health well-being.

[8]See the section on evaluating individual items.

[9]There are certain exceptions. For example, one "questionnaire" that is quite familiar to nurses is the NCLEX-RN examination that is taken for registered nursing licensure in the United States. The NCLEX-RN routinely includes a certain number of untested or experimental items that are being tested for possible use on future administrations of the NCLEX-RN. Likewise, educators sometimes include a certain number of untested items on course examinations for students. However, the spirit of these exceptions is still to provide pilot testing of the items in the ways we discussed earlier.

[10]Instruments available from the NCHS or the Census Bureau can be used as a starting point.

[11]Cultural groups may be defined in many different ways, such as by ethnicity or race (e.g., Hispanics, African Americans, Chinese Americans) or by social class or occupation (e.g., truck drivers, stockbrokers, farmers).

a questionnaire item may provoke negative reactions in study participants. In fact, if a term such as "depression" is not socially acceptable or is not commonly used in a particular population, respondents might even be irritated or puzzled by the question. For this and other reasons, many survey researchers now use **focus groups** that consist of members of the target population to generate ideas for and formulations of question items (Morgan, 1988).[12] Even though, at this stage, the emphasis is still on item generation, discussions with a few members of the target population can also be used to obtain their reactions to a preliminary formulation of a question item.

Principles for Formulating Individual Items

No amount of wizardry in the analysis and interpretation of data can fully compensate for significant problems with the design of a questionnaire. As has already been mentioned, when a researcher constructs a questionnaire, the first decision is whether to use existing items or instruments or to generate new ones. If a questionnaire contains sections that represent items from standardized scales, these items should be left unchanged as far as possible.[13] Still, it is worth remembering that language is a "living thing" that can be viewed as a constantly changing historical artifact. That means that the same words may have different meanings, both over time and across different population groups. For example, if a particular word used in a standardized scale has different meanings for different generations of respondents, then it is important for the research team to consider the need for changes.[14] However, changing the wording on an established instrument is likely to have at least some effect on its reliability and validity. Generally, making changes in an established instrument should be done only when the reasons are compelling (e.g., the old format gives flawed results with the intended target population), and any such change requires testing and reestablishing reliability and validity with the new format.

Earlier, we emphasized that the generation of new questionnaire items is substantially conceptual work. When a question or statement is formulated, it is intended to solicit information about the concept of which the item is a possible indicator. Beyond these issues of content validity, there are also the *mechanics* of asking questions. In particular, newly generated questionnaire items, regardless of content area, must be examined with respect to their *reading level, clarity,* and *acceptability* to the target audience.

Writing Easily Understood Questions: Simplicity Is King. Many survey researchers recommend that the wording of most questionnaire items should be compatible with a sixth- to eighth-grade reading level (Fowler, 2002). Although the average educational level in the target population obviously makes a difference in what kinds of questions may be asked, even among highly educated respondents, simpler questions and statements are preferable to more complex ones. Readability is essentially a function of the complexity of sentences and the length and frequency of usage of particular words. Several widely used methods are available to measure the reading level of printed materials. Aside from indices for reading levels, more fundamental considerations apply to writing survey items. For example, Fry (1968) proposed basic ways to assess the readability of a text. Translated into item construction, the following guidelines are suggested:

- *Avoid the use of jargon.* **Jargon** refers to the specialized languages common to members of many occupational and professional groups. Health professionals commonly use terms such as "digestion," "hypertension," "contagious," or "tissue," not to speak of "psoriasis," "appendectomy," or "myocardial infarction." However, the meaning of these words may be unclear to many members of the general public. Even such seemingly common words as "digestion" and "hypertension" are not necessarily well understood, and they should be either replaced by everyday terms, such as "high blood pressure," *or explained or defined* in simpler terms. Avoiding jargon is not always easy because a researcher's very familiarity with these terms can blind him or her to the fact that someone else may be unfamiliar with them. Again, testing of question items with members of the target population is an indispensable step in the development of items with appropriate language.

- Avoid negatives and double negatives. **Negatives** are qualifiers that change the meaning of a word or sentence, but may be easily overlooked (Holden, Fekken, & Jackson, 1985). In a survey of nutritional habits and attitudes, parents might be asked to agree or disagree with a statement such as "children should *not* be allowed to get more food unless they have eaten all the food on their

---

[12]This qualitative approach to data collection is discussed in more detail in chapter 18.

[13]Researchers sometimes make small adjustments in standardized instruments. For instance, because of the fit with a study design, a question stem may be changed to refer to the time "since you were discharged from the hospital" instead of "the past 2 weeks." On occasion, such format changes can jeopardize comparisons of standardized scores.

[14]One item in the SF-36 asks respondents how much of the time they felt "full of pep" during a particular period. Although this terminology may be perfectly appropriate for many older Americans, it may produce puzzlement or even a certain amount of derision in a younger population.

plate." Because of the negative qualifier, respondents could potentially be confused by this question and give an incorrect, and possibly misleading, response. To avoid this problem, the researcher could reformulate the statement as "children should eat all the food on their plate before getting more," and reverse the coding for agreement or disagreement. Furthermore, when worded negatively, items with response categories that require agreement or disagreement can sometimes be confusing because *disagreement* with a negatively worded statement in effect amounts to a **double negative** (Sheatsley, 1983). For example, a statement such as "I never or rarely get distressed over changing wound dressings," in combination with a negative response, such as "strongly disagree," produces the awkward combination of, "[I] strongly disagree [that] I never or rarely get distressed. . ." Chances are good that many respondents will be confused. Involuntary double negatives occur most often as a result of combining a question or statement stem with the response categories. If one reads aloud *both* the stem and the response categories, it is usually easy to discover such problems.

- Whenever possible, *questions should be short and succinct*. Nothing contributes more to the confusion of a respondent than long-winded questions. There are no precise cutoff points but, as a rule of thumb, questions or statements that contain fewer than 20 words are preferred. In most cases, this can be achieved by breaking up longer, more complex questions into several shorter ones. When evaluating the complexity of items, the wording of questions should be geared to the literacy level of the least educated respondent who is likely to be included in the study sample.

- *Address only a single, clearly delineated problem in each question.* Consider a **double-barreled** question such as this one: "Are you currently on a diet or exercising?" A person who *is* on a diet, but is *not* exercising might have a hard time answering such a question.

- *Avoid ambiguity in the wording of questions.* Many ordinary words are open to multiple interpretations and meanings. If the intended meaning cannot be gleaned from the context, additional clarifying definitions may be necessary. An example that appears in the sociodemographic section of many health surveys is the question on "income." It may refer to personal income, earned income (from wages and salaries only), household income, gross income, net income, and so on. Asking a respondent about income, but leaving it up to him or her to define its meaning, is likely to result in measurement error.

- Although clarity and succinctness are important, *occasionally, questions are too brief.* Instead of simply asking: "Age?" or "Sex?," it is better to ask "What is your age?" or "What is your sex?" If nothing else, the usual standards of courtesy would seem to necessitate this approach.

Considering the Value Connotations of Language When Formulating Questions. So far, our comments have dealt with issues of clarity and ease of understanding. However, words, phrases, and sentences often carry *value connotations* and may be emotionally charged, or the information sought may be *socially sensitive.* For this reason, writing high-quality questionnaire items that can produce unbiased information also requires a substantial amount of social awareness of subtle nuances of language, including different usages in different target populations. Clinicians and health researchers often deal with behaviors and attitudes that many people are reluctant to discuss. Prominent examples are the use of legal and illegal substances, general risk-taking behavior, and sexual activities. To gather accurate information about sensitive issues, the cardinal rule is to avoid passing judgment and to use words and phrases that describe the behaviors or attitudes in question in neutral, factual terms. Examples of specific strategies include the following:

- *Provide context for the behavior.* For instance, as part of a questionnaire on teenage risk-taking behavior, a question about school truancy could be introduced with a factual statement about what percentage of students in the school district have missed classes or school days, with or without permission. Such context reduces the likelihood that the respondent would fear being singled out if he or she answered truthfully. However, as we emphasized in the chapter on survey research (chapter 11), we should not be so unrealistic as to believe that we can always get unbiased answers to questions about illegal, or even socially undesirable, behavior.

- *Avoid leading questions that suggest a particular answer.* Consider the question: "Should nurses receive higher compensation for the hard work they do?" This type of question is unlikely to elicit the respondent's true opinion about support for higher nursing salaries because the phrase "hard work" already implies what should be done.

- *Avoid questions that ask about preferences without a realistic context of choice.* For example, the unqualified question, "Should older Americans receive drug benefits under Medicare?" elicits substantially greater agreement than the question, "Would you be willing to pay more taxes so that older Americans can receive drug benefits under Medicare?"

- *Counterbalance one-sided value questions with examples of different positions.* It is important to avoid giving the impression that the researcher favors certain values and positions over others. For example, a questionnaire on public support for the deinstitutionalization of the mentally ill would need to ask questions that address both the positive and the negative potential consequences of deinstitutionalization.

- *Avoid inflammatory or emotionally charged language.* In practice, this may not always be easy. The real problem with the exhortation to use socially and emotionally neutral language is that it can be difficult to anticipate what words or statements will be offensive to a particular population. For instance, the mere mention of the word "condom" in a survey of teenagers' sexual behavior may offend some respondents. In the end, there is no substitute for knowing the target audience well enough to avoid at least major missteps in question formulation. Thus, pretesting with members of the target population is the key to well-designed new question items.

Translation of Questionnaire Items. The translation of questionnaire items into another language is a special case of being sensitive to, and aware of, the language requirements of minority groups. In the 21st century, health researchers and clinicians cannot afford to ignore whole population groups whose primary language is not English, a growing segment of the population (Lange, 2002). Clinicians and researchers work in a world that has become increasingly international and multicultural. Although fluency in a common language remains the best guarantee for avoiding misunderstandings in the interaction between patient and provider, the translation of questionnaire items and of complete standardized instruments requires more than just a fluent translator. Anyone who is familiar with more than one language knows that words in one language almost never correspond directly to words in another language. Meanings and connotations, even of words for even seemingly concrete concepts, such as "wood," are never quite the same because their usage may differ in any two languages. Thus, translating an instrument that is designed to measure "anxiety," "depression," or "quality of life" from one language into another, even if done by a skillful translator who is familiar with both languages, is at best a difficult task.

One standard technique is to have items translated by one person and back-translated by another skillful interpreter (Brislin, 1970). If the results are not recognizable, then there is obviously a problem. Yet, even if they are, problems remain. An "anxiety" scale that is recreated in another language is essentially a *new* measure, and its validity and reliability in the context of the new language must be proven. Sometimes, the very concept at issue has a different meaning. For instance, the English word "anxiety" usually translates into the German word "angst," but the two have different connotations. *Angst* connotes a much stronger emphasis on fear of some particular thing, whereas *anxiety* is a more generalized feeling that is less directed toward any specific object. The counter-translation issue is also illustrated by this example, because the common understanding of the word "angst," as used in the United States, for example, is more closely akin to a depressive state that also has a significant component of anxiety. Any reader who is fluent in another language will be able to come up with similar examples.

These brief comments on translation are meant as a note of caution, but are not meant to suggest that it is impossible to recreate standardized scales in other languages. The translation of standardized instruments requires high levels of language skills and must always proceed from the basic assumption that the validity and reliability of the translated instrument must be reestablished in the new context (Lange, 2002).

Principles for Choosing Answer Categories and Response Scales to Individual Questions

In structured questionnaires, item generation includes not only the question stem, but also the predetermined, or **closed-ended,** answer categories. Closed-ended answer categories essentially present the respondent with a limited, given set of alternatives. Although most people find it easier to respond to predetermined choices rather than formulating their own responses, fixed response categories work only if they are constructed in a way that does not feel "forced." Answer categories may not be workable for respondents if they do not fully represent the spectrum of views among the study participants.

When choosing or constructing answer categories for closed-ended responses, two questions require immediate attention: "How many response categories are needed?" and "What level of measurement do the response categories represent?" The first question usually involves making a choice between binary, or dichotomous, responses on the one hand or three or more response categories on the other. Especially if the interview is conducted verbally, a respondent would rarely be asked to choose from more than 12 categories, unless a written, prepared checklist can be used, and this type of checklist may also allow for multiple responses (see Box 16-2 for examples). Most response categories[15] in structured questionnaires are either *categorical,* dividing respondents into mutually exclusive groups, or *ordinal,* asking respondents to indicate degrees of agreement (as in Likert-type response scales) or to rate their preferences with respect to multiple objects or actions. *Interval-level* response categories are less common in questionnaires, except as grouped response categories. For example, respondents could be asked to indicate their age in years, without response categories, or they could be provided with **grouped interval categories,** such as "less than 10," "11 to 20," "21 to 30," and so forth. Box 16-2 offers several examples for each type of response category.

Beyond levels of measurement and numbers of categories, a few principles are helpful for the construction of workable response categories:

- *Answer categories must be conceptually unidimensional and mutually exclusive.* Here is a counterexample that violates the principles of unidimensionality and exclusivity: In a clinical study, patients were asked to choose among the following living arrangements: "with family," "in own home," "in apartment complex," and "with in-laws." The obvious problem is that the response categories mix the conceptual dimension of "relationship to co-residents" with "type of housing," resulting in nonexclusive categories. For example, a person may live *both* "with family" *and* "in an apartment complex."
- *Answer categories should exhaust all possible choices or provide an "other" category.* For example, asking caregivers to list "children within the household" excludes children living elsewhere who could be a potential source of support. If an instrument includes a question about comorbid conditions, next to the most common conditions, such as heart disease, cancer, and hypertension, respondents should be expressly asked about "other" comorbid conditions and allowed to list them.
- *Response categories should produce "well-distributed" response patterns.* In general, categories that produce an absolute number of responses of less than N = 5, or less than half of the sample, N, divided by the number of categories, are not very useful in the analysis stage. For example, with a study sample of N = 160, any variable that potentially divides the sample into five groups should result in a minimum of 16 cases in the least frequent response category (160/5 $\times$ 1/2 = 16).

- *Grouped interval-level response categories must be realistic in terms of the distribution of values in the target population.* For instance, the use of household income categories such as "$0 to $19,999," "$21,000 to $39,999," "$40,000 to $59,999," and "$60,000 to $79,999" may not be appropriate if the target population is rural elderly persons, many of whom live in households with incomes of less than $40,000. As mentioned before, useful response categories often require prior knowledge of the target population.
- *Knowledge of the likely distribution of cases in the target population is often a prerequisite for a realistic choice of an "other" category.* For instance, unless study samples are very large, asking about specific cancer diagnoses other than breast, lung, prostate, or colorectal may not yield any positive responses. On the other hand, asking only about breast cancer and lumping all other types of cancer into an "other" category may yield a lopsided distribution in favor of "other."
- *Grouped interval-level response categories should either avoid open-ended upper or lower categories or provide follow-up questions.* For example, household income categories on a survey may include "$0 to $9,999," "$10,000 to $19,999," "$20,000 to $29,999," and so forth, with "$60,000 and over" as the final option. In this situation, it would not be possible to calculate a mean based on category means (e.g., $5,000, $15,000), because the open-ended upper category covers a potentially very large range. Under these conditions, it is not even possible to guess the approximate median value within the upper category.
- *In items that require respondents to indicate agreement or disagreement, Likert-type response scales that include neutral categories may lead to a ritualized response set if many members of the target population prefer not to reveal their true preferences ("fence sitters").* In such situations, it may be preferable not to provide a middle, or neutral, category. However, if many respondents genuinely prefer a neutral category, they may consider the remaining categories forced. In that case, the effect on nonresponse must be monitored.
- *Another type of response set problem is the "acquiescence response."* This problem occurs when respondents display a tendency to agree with all statements, regardless of their content. This is more common among respondents who have little education, among some ethnic minority groups, and among study participants who feel intimidated or are unwilling for other reasons to share their true opinions (Lange, 2002). One way to reduce response set patterns is to break up the

---

[15]See chapter 13 for a more detailed discussion of levels of measurement.

BOX 16.2   Examples of Formats for Items in Structured Questionnaires

Binary or Dichotomous items
What is your sex? (Circle one)
    Female (1)
    Male (2)
Were you hospitalized (stayed overnight in a hospital) during the last year? (Circle one)
    Yes (1)
    No (2)

Multiple mutually exclusive categories
What is your religious affiliation? (Circle one)
    Catholic (1)
    Protestant (2)
    Jewish (3)
    Other (4)

Multiple response item or checklist
The following shows a list of chronic health problems. Do you currently suffer from any of these health problems?
(On the lines provided, please check off ALL that apply to you)
    Heart problems (such as angina or heart murmur) _____
    Cancer _____
    Arthritis _____
    Diabetes (high blood sugar) _____
    Hypertension (high blood pressure) _____

Ordinal scales
Likert (ordinal) rating scale
(On the lines provided, check the answer that applies to you)
During the past 4 weeks, I felt sad.
(1) Strongly disagree _____
(2) Disagree _____
(3) Neutral _____
(4) Agree _____
(5) Strongly agree _____

Preference rating
Information about feeding your child can come from different sources. Listed below are people and media from whom or which you may get your information about how to feed your child. Please number from 1 to 10 the source you listen to the most (1) and the source you listen to the least (10) when deciding how to feed your child. Use each number only once.
Example:
    _4_ Grandparent
    _2_ Sister
    _____Friends _____Parents _____Doctor _____Clinic nurse _____Nutrition educator _____Newspaper/magazine
    _____TV _____Books _____Web _____Other (Specify)

Grouped interval–level scale
Considering all your earnings from your work activity, place a checkmark on the line that indicates how much income (before taxes) you earned during the last calendar year.

≤ $4,999_____	$5,000–$9,999_____	$10,000–$14,999_____	$15,000–$19,999_____
$20,000–$24,999_____	$25,000–$29,999_____	$30,000–$34,999_____	$35,000–$39,999_____
$40,000–$44,999_____	$45,000–$49,999_____	$50,000–$54,999_____	$55,000–$59,999_____
≥ $60,000_____	(If over $60,000, please indicate approximate amount: _____)		

monotony of response scales through reverse coding. The four positive well-being items in the CES-D scale (see chapter 14) offer an example of this strategy.

- *Sometimes the number of response categories can be enlarged to overcome respondents' reluctance to choose extreme categories.* For example, income categories that include "artificially" low ranges for the target sample may make it easier for low-income respondents to indicate their true household income because they need not identify with the lowest category.

There are many other technical details that belong in a specialized text on questionnaire construction. Examples include the use of labels, intermittent labeling, or numbers on a rating scale; and the proper construction of skip patterns (i.e., when subsequent items are asked of subsets of respondents who meet a condition defined by the response to an earlier question [Fowler, 1995]). Writing questionnaire items is not inherently difficult and involves a fair amount of common sense. However, it also requires experience and knowledge of the evidence available on what has been shown to work.[16]

Preliminary Evaluation of Individual Items

As has been emphasized, questionnaire construction requires careful forethought, development, and pretesting. Even if all of the conventional rules are followed, there is no guarantee that the questionnaire items will provide unbiased, information-rich responses. Ultimately, only testing with samples from the target population will provide evidence about the measurement properties of new items. Fortunately, several readily implemented tests can provide useful information about the quality of questionnaire items.

Probably the first test of the quality of a questionnaire item is comparison of its individual response rate with those of other items on the questionnaire. If a particular item results in an unusually high proportion of missing responses, say, more than twice the average missing response rate for all other questionnaire items,[17] one should take note: Is there something peculiar about the wording, the choice of response categories, and so forth, that might have led to misunderstandings? Is there a bias in response rate by subgroup? For example, are the missing responses uniform across the sample, or do the nonrespondents show particular characteristics? Suppose female respondents,

but not male respondents, skipped a particular question. In this case, one would certainly need to investigate the reasons for this bias. A large proportion of missing responses may also be a sign of having tapped into a socially sensitive area. For instance, questions about income and financial status uniformly produce lower response rates than most other kinds of questions.

Another simple preliminary test for a questionnaire item involves looking at its frequency distribution. An item that results in extremely low variation in responses is generally problematic: it does not discriminate (differentiate, or show differences) among subjects of the target population, and thus may not be useful. There are several common reasons for lopsided response patterns (and their corollary: low endorsement levels for other categories). These include: (1) the social desirability of a preferred answer, (2) ceiling or floor effects (see chapter 15), and (3) disregard for the underlying population distribution when grouped categories were used. As these examples show, much of questionnaire construction involves trial and error, going back and forth between item writing and preliminary empirical testing.

Scale Development

So far, we have considered the development of individual questionnaire items more or less in isolation.

> In previous chapters (chapters 14 and 15 in particular), we described strategies for selecting and evaluating whole instruments or scales.

Here, we briefly discuss the development of items that are intended to form new composite scales that measure complex concepts.

In general, we do not recommend that clinicians or novice researchers attempt to develop new psychosocial instruments, especially if resources (e.g., knowledge, skills, time, access to study populations) are less than optimal. Scale development is a complex process, calling not only for specialized research knowledge and skills, but also sometimes for substantial resources.

> As a general rule, scale or instrument development should *not* be part of the same study in which the newly developed instrument is used to test a substantive hypothesis concerning the effectiveness of some intervention. As mentioned in chapters 2 and 4, the process of validation of a new measurement scale should be separate from the use of the measure.[18]

---

[16]For further information about constructing questionnaires, see Sudman and Bradburn (1982), Sheatsley (1983), Converse and Presser (1986), and Fowler (2002).

[17]The denominator of a response rate for an individual item is calculated on the basis of *eligible* respondents for that item (i.e., it considers skipping patterns).

---

[18]Many researchers incorporate the testing of some new items for measures into larger studies. This is usually done because of feasibility factors, such as limited time, money, and ability to collect data from study participants. However, for the reasons indicated, it is problematic.

BOX 16.3   Steps in the Development of a New Measurement Scale

- A conceptual and theoretical exploration of the dimensions of the construct
- A review of existing literature on related constructs
- Selection and definition of all possible target populations
- Initial exploratory discussions involving members of the target population, possibly including focus group discussions
- Writing of the first batch of items designed to be indicators of each conceptual dimension of the construct
- Proofreading of items by experts in the fields and members of the target population
- Administration of the questionnaire to a large *sample* of the target population to be followed by exploratory factor analysis (*minimum* of 5 subjects per item, preferably 10 subjects per item)
- Selection of items into unidimensional subscales based on exploratory factor analysis
- Selection of final subscale items after reliability analysis of each subscale
- Efforts to validate construct through exploring its relationship to other constructs (convergent and discriminant validity)
- Resubmission of "final" items to a *second, independent* sample for confirmatory factor analysis
- Establishment of "factorial invariance" among target population groups of interest
- Establishment of factorial invariance over time (if scale is used for analysis of change; requires repeated measures on same subjects)
- Establishment of population norms using *representative* samples of target populations

A study in which both measurement procedures and substantive hypotheses are at stake cannot provide convincing evidence against a hypothesis. That is, if the results do not confirm the hypothesis, there remains the possibility that the measurement procedures were faulty. Thus, whenever possible, it is important to validate the measures first, before using them in a study in which they will be counted on to provide credible evidence for or against a hypothesis.

In Box 16-3, we provide a list of the major steps that are necessary for the development of a new standardized measurement scale. Many of the initial steps were already discussed in this chapter in terms of the development of individual items. The additional evaluation of an item that is hypothesized to form a measurement scale with other items entails an examination of the empirical relationship of its response pattern to those of the other items. All of the issues (discussed in chapter 14) concerning the internal consistency and dimensionality of an instrument and its subscales are also pertinent to this examination. In general, until the factor structure of a new scale has been con-

firmed on at least a second, independent sample,[19] the instrument must be considered "under development."[20] For an introduction to scale development and the psychometric criteria that individual items must meet, see DeVellis (1991). A comprehensive discussion of the psychometric techniques involved can be found in Nunnally and Bernstein (1994).

Modes of Collecting Interview Data

Once the questionnaire is written, a decision must be made about the preferred mode of administration. The most fundamental choice is between the following options: (1) relying on verbal interactions between interviewers and respondents and (2) asking respondents to complete written questionnaires. If personal interviews are used, interviewers may establish contact with respondents either face-to-face or via telephone, whereas written questionnaires can be filled out in group settings, may be mailed in, or may be administered on computer screens, including distribution over the Internet.

---

[19]At a *minimum,* "confirming a factor structure" means providing evidence that the same items form the same subscales. As discussed in chapter 14, there are also more sophisticated indicators of factorial invariance.

[20]As we have emphasized, in a certain sense, all measures should be viewed as "works in progress" because their psychometric properties can change, depending on the target population, and sometimes as a function of time and society itself.

Strengths and Weaknesses of Face-to-Face and Telephone Interviews

All interviews, whether conducted face-to-face or via telephone, involve the verbal exchange of information between interviewer and respondent, which must be recorded to become usable data. Especially for studies with large sample sizes, interview information is now increasingly collected with computer-aided telephone interviewing (CATI) or computer-aided personal interview (CAPI) systems. These systems allow interviewers to enter respondents' answers directly into a computer that is programmed to guide the interviewers through the questionnaire. For small-scale clinical studies, CATI and CAPI systems may not be cost-effective, and so it is more common to record the interview responses on hard copies of the questionnaire. The responses are then entered into a computer using the data entry interface of various standard software programs.[21]

Face-to-Face Interviews. Among the different modes of collecting interview data, the face-to-face, or in-person, interview is in many ways the "gold standard." In all of the following circumstances, face-to-face interviews tend to perform best: if the questionnaire material is complex and requires frequent feedback from the interviewer, if the questions include open-ended responses interspersed with standardized interview formats, and if the presentation of the material must be varied with the use of visual aids as well as verbal reassurance (Rossi, Wright, & Anderson, 1983; Streiner & Norman, 1995).

In contrast, telephone interviews may not always be suitable for the frail, the very sick, or the very young, all of whom are frequent target groups in health care research. Elderly patients are sometimes more reluctant to participate when contacted exclusively via telephone.[22] The presence of a "live," skilled interviewer provides respondents with reassurance, and face-to-face interviews usually achieve the highest response and completion rates (Fowler, 2002).

A further advantage of face-to-face interviewing is that because the respondent becomes known to the interviewer, substitution of other respondents for the desired or designated respondent is difficult. Respondents are also observed during the interview, and these observations can provide additional clues about the respondent (Fowler &

Mangione, 1990). The physical presence of an interviewer makes it comparatively easy to ask clarifying questions and also allows for mixing verbal and visual stimuli, as when using cards with printed response categories.

However, face-to-face interviews are not always the best way to ask questions. In particular, respondents may feel embarrassed if they are asked to answer questions about socially sensitive topics, such as risk-taking behavior, sexual dysfunction, urinary problems, and so forth. In such situations, a mode of questioning that avoids direct personal confrontation is preferred. Face-to-face interviewing also tends to be the most expensive mode of administration, especially when combined with a complex sampling scheme. It is simply not realistic or defensible to draw a random sample from a geographically widely distributed target population, say, all registered nurses in a particular state, and to send interviewers to meet with all selected respondents. The travel costs alone for such a project would be very large.[23] However, in many clinical research situations, personal interviews may be a less costly option and may also improve response rates. For example, interviewing postsurgical patients while they are still in the hospital may sometimes be easier than waiting until after discharge, when telephone interviews are the only cost-effective interview method available (Minnick & Young, 1998). On the other hand, in recent years, it has become the case that many postsurgical patients are too ill to participate in interviews while they are still hospitalized. Thus, a researcher must think very carefully about what barriers to data collection may exist in a clinical research setting. Likewise, time constraints during patient visits to primary care providers may preclude data collection as part of a primary care visit. In other instances, data collection may be better carried out in settings in which people spend enough time to complete the necessary instruments, even if these settings are outside the formal health care system.

Telephone Interviews. Supported by the development of CATI, telephone interviewing is now the preferred mode of data collection in large-scale studies. It is also frequently used for follow-up interviews with patients who are undergoing treatment for serious medical problems, such as cancer or heart disease. When skillfully used, telephone interviewing is a flexible tool that can achieve response rates similar to those of face-to-face interviewing. Its obvious advantage is that the interviewer does not need to travel to the respondents' locations, drastically reducing

---

[21]In chapter 23, we discuss some of the issues involved in coding and data entry.

[22]There are also sampling frame problems with telephone interviews: not all population groups are equally accessible through the telephone. For further discussion, see chapters 19 and 20.

[23]For this reason, the NCHS often uses modified sampling designs, such as cluster sampling. See chapter 20 for more detail.

the costs of interviews. However, new problems for telephone interviewing lurk on the horizon. One evolving trend that may adversely affect response rates for telephone surveys is the increasing use of unlisted cellular telephone numbers and screening technology for incoming telephone calls. Especially in younger populations, a number of potential study participants may not have traditional telephone service and may not necessarily provide their mobile telephone numbers for inclusion in medical records. In addition, the increased volume of direct marketing via telephone may lead at least some potential survey respondents to avoid answering the telephone if they believe that a marketer may be calling them.

Concerning the implementation of a complex interview schedule, telephone interviews have a few limitations that must be considered. The most obvious limitation is the lack of visual contact, reducing the interviewer's ability to gauge the condition of the respondent and eliminating the use of visual clues to facilitate questioning. One consequence is that telephone interviews are less well adapted to managing lengthy, complex response scales. Take, for example, a standard Likert response scale with five or more choices, such as "strongly disagree," "disagree," "neutral," "agree," and "strongly agree." The need to repeat these choices *every time a new question is asked* can be tedious for the interviewer and potentially annoying for the respondent. In a face-to-face interview, holding up a simple cue card can easily solve this problem. In fact, it is much easier to visually process a list of multiple alternatives than to listen to the same information being read; furthermore, it is likely that the respondent will forget the first few items by the time the interviewer reaches the end of an extensive list. In general, more than in face-to-face interviews, telephone interviews work best when the questions are short and the response categories are simple to follow. Unless there has been previous personal contact, it may be difficult for an interviewer to establish rapport and trust with a respondent over the telephone. As a result, respondents may be reluctant to answer sensitive questions. However, a skilled telephone interviewer can overcome many of these problems.

Interviewer Training. In large-scale surveys and panel studies that use several, if not dozens, of different interviewers, researchers must attempt to standardize the administration of interviews, whether conducted face-to-face or by telephone. This can be achieved only through well-organized training sessions and monitoring of the multiple interviewers to address such issues as how to ensure that: (1) questions are asked in a standardized format, (2) questions for clarification by the respondent are handled in a standardized fashion, (3) response and retention rates are

uniformly high across interviewers, and (4) researchers receive feedback information from the interviewers about problems encountered with the interview schedule or with particular respondents. See the specialized literature for more detailed information (Collins et al., 1998; Fowler & Mangione, 1990; Ribisl, Walton, Mowbray, Luke, Davidson, & Bootsmiller, 1996).

Self-administered Questionnaires

Self-administered questionnaires do not involve an interviewer, but rely on the respondent to provide written responses. For that reason alone, they are not always the best method for collecting information: some people may be less accustomed to writing or uncomfortable with writing. This problem can be especially pronounced in target populations that are seriously ill or have low literacy skills. Self-administered questionnaires are least appropriate if they contain many open-ended questions; such questions impose the greatest writing burden on respondents. In addition, handwritten responses may be quite difficult to decipher or interpret, adding another potential source of error.

This is not to say that self-administered questionnaires cannot provide advantages over interviews. When response categories are highly standardized, it is often easier and faster to mark the most appropriate response category than to respond verbally to the same item. In general, questions that are followed by checklists, including those that allow for multiple responses, are particularly easy to deal with in written format. However, if response categories change from question to question, the advantage of this format disappears because the respondent is forced to pay greater attention when filling out the questionnaire. Self-administered questionnaires also appear to afford the respondent some kind of "anonymity" when answering sensitive questions. Many respondents find it easier to respond to such questions on paper than when facing an interviewer.

Compared with interviews, a disadvantage of written questionnaires is that misunderstandings are difficult to correct. In an interview situation, a respondent who is unsure about the meaning of a particular question may ask for an explanation. On a written questionnaire, such questions go unanswered, or the respondent simply marks an answer without much conviction that it reflects his or her actual thinking. In general, because of the lack of interaction between an interviewer and a respondent, there is less feedback from respondents about problems that they encounter. For instance, an interviewer can determine whether a respondent has problems with language or has a mental disability such as dementia, and can probe for reasons for nonresponse to particular items.

Without an interviewer, there is also less control over how the responses are completed (Fowler, 2002). One issue concerns the sequencing of questions. Even though a questionnaire may have been constructed with the questions placed in a particular sequence, there is little to prevent a respondent from answering items out of sequence.[24] Likewise, there is no way to control how much time a respondent takes to contemplate answers; there is also no way to prevent lengthy interruptions. That could mean, for example, that questions on a standardized scale designed to probe the "current" level of anxiety may be completed hours apart.

Finally, the need for a clear, easily understood format for a self-administered questionnaire limits the complexity of conditional responses (skipping patterns) that can be introduced on a written questionnaire.[25] Problems of control also concern the identity of the respondent. When questionnaires are mailed to home addresses or are posted on the Internet, it is impossible to ensure that the targeted persons will be the actual respondents.

One advantage of self-administered questionnaires is that they offer a relatively inexpensive way to collect data. This is certainly the case when questionnaires are administered to captive audiences in institutional settings, such as hospital wards, nursing homes, or schools. In addition, if administered in a group setting (in a school class or during lunch hour in a nursing home), anonymity can be preserved, some control over the timing can be maintained, and feedback questions can be addressed.

Mailing questionnaires is also a relatively inexpensive way to collect information, certainly when compared with telephone or face-to-face interviews. On the other hand, mailing questionnaires to home addresses generally results in lower response rates compared with telephone or face-to-face interviews. However, this disadvantage can often be partially offset with certain strategies, including: sending a cover letter with an endorsement from an authority that is well-established among members of the target population (e.g., including a letter from a state nursing association addressed to all registered nurses in that state); focusing on a topic of general interest to the target population; providing an advance mailing or notice of arrival of the questionnaire; providing financial compensation for the time spent completing a survey, such as including a token dollar in the mailing; enclosing a stamped return envelope; and using a short questionnaire (Fowler, 2002).

From a cost perspective, distributing questionnaires via the Internet is a promising new avenue for surveying large numbers of selected target populations. However, only approximately half of the U.S. population currently has Internet access. This means that, depending on the target population, one could encounter a potentially severe sampling bias built into the sampling frame.[26] The other unresolved issue concerning the distribution of survey material via the Internet involves the privacy rights of holders of e-mail accounts. The current debate about the regulation of "spam" (unsolicited commercial e-mail messages) is likely to have a bearing on electronic mailing of surveys as well.

DIARIES AND LOGS

In the chapter on survey research (chapter 11), we emphasized that interviews may at times overtax the ability of a respondent to accurately recall past events or behavior. In addition, in panel studies that involve repeated interviews, it is often difficult to time the interviews to coincide closely with the pivotal health or illness events of interest for data collection purposes. Whenever the behaviors in question occur on an irregular basis or take a large variety of forms, it is difficult for interview respondents to recall and adequately reconstruct such behavior, especially if the information sought covers an extended period. Consider, for example, an interview question such as: "During the last 2 weeks, how often did you eat chicken or other poultry?" Many people, with the exception of vegetarians, would find it difficult to answer such a question with accuracy. In general, interview questions about nutrition, physical activities, or medication use may require prodigious memories, unless they refer to short periods, such as the 24-hour recall of food intake. On the other hand, a "mere" 24-hour recall can be quite unrepresentative of a person's "typical" eating habits (Willett, 1997).

In situations such as these, researchers have sometimes used diaries and activity logs as an alternative way to collect self-report data. The potential advantage of diaries or activity logs is that they provide the flexibility to deal with the variable timing of events and experiences. For instance, study participants could be instructed to record a certain event of interest every time it occurs, or shortly thereafter, or they could be instructed to make a daily entry into the

---

[24]This disadvantage applies to hard copies, but with computerized or Internet versions of written questionnaires, control of the question sequence is maintained.

[25]This limitation does not extend to computerized or Internet versions of written questionnaires, because they can easily be programmed to direct the respondent through all skipping patterns.

[26]For a discussion of the importance of an unbiased sampling frame, see chapter 19.

diary, indicating whether the event occurred. For example, Stinson (1997) used a fatigue diary to document fatigue in pregnant women who were members of the military. They recorded this data during a 2-week preterm period. Kesmodel and Olsen (2001) asked pregnant women to record their alcohol intake during a 2-week period using daily reporting. Daily activity logs have also been used to record self-reported physical activity (Wu & Pender, 2002) as well as outcomes in clinical trials and intervention studies of incontinence (Malone-Lee, Walsh, Maugourd, et al., 2001; Dougherty, Dwyer, Pendergast, Boyington, Tomlinson, Coward, Duncan, Vogel, & Rooks, 2002) and cry-fuss behaviors of babies (Kramer, Barr, Dagenais, Yang, Jones, Ciafani, & Jane, 2001). In these studies, the behavior recorded occurs intermittently and may vary substantially from one day to the next. In addition, the timing of its occurrence is hard to predict.

The distinction between "diaries" and "activity logs" is *fluent* (some researchers use the terms interchangeably), and it essentially hinges on the rules and specificity for data entry. Like interviews, diaries can run the gamut from completely unstructured reports of self-expression (e.g., personal histories) to highly structured activity logs that are accompanied by detailed instructions on when and how often to make an entry as well as what to record, focusing on a set of predetermined activities. Essentially the same issues arise as in the choice between structured and unstructured interviews. Less structured diaries may be a better exploratory tool, but require study participants to have a higher level of literacy and more advanced language skills. Highly structured activity logs, which may include readily available checklists for events and their timing, may be much easier to complete. However, the demands of participation can be substantial in a study that uses self-monitoring (Dougherty et al., 2002) or daily reporting (Kesmodel & Olsen, 2001). As a consequence, studies that use diaries often have high attrition rates. When studies use both diaries and interviews, the subset of respondents that returns the diaries is often substantially smaller than the interview sample (Kramer et al., 2001). Thus, the use of diaries and activity logs tends to be limited to more literate and highly motivated populations (Willett, 1997). However, this technique can still be highly useful as a device to validate interview information (Kesmodel & Olsen, 2001). If the goal is to reconstruct detailed accounts of specific health-related activities, including nutrition patterns, over an extended period, diaries may be the only feasible method to obtain such information, despite the lower response and participation rates associated with their use.

ELECTRONIC DATA COLLECTION METHODS

Recently, new technologies have been used to augment participant-recorded data in diaries and activity logs. For example, to remind study participants to record information in diaries or activity logs, some researchers have used electronic devices to signal to study participants when they should record their activities. The timers are most often set to a preestablished time sequence, for example, every 4 hours between 8:00 AM and 8:00 PM, but can also be programmed to prompt participants at random intervals. Likewise, electronic timers on medication containers can be programmed both to signal the medication user to take medication and to record when a medication container has been accessed. Finally, electronic devices can be used to record people's activity. Just as pedometers, which have been available for a number of years, are used to record walking distance, the newer electronic devices can record more detailed information about the timing and relative amounts of activity. Still, the extent to which people are willing to accept such devices as part of a research project may vary substantially. In addition, many behaviors that are of interest to health and nurse researchers, such as nutrition, are not easily monitored with such electronic devices.

OBSERVATIONS

Patient observation is a primary source of information for clinicians, but observational methods are less commonly used in research, even though there is a distinct tradition of using such methods in nursing and health care research.[27] There are many reasons for this, most of which can be reduced to three main issues: (1) the accessibility of behaviors and other phenomena to observation, (2) the relationship of observers to the observed, and (3) the methods of recording observations and converting them to "data."

Accessibility of Behaviors and Other Phenomena to Observations

Any cursory browsing of clinical journals, with their ubiquitous photos of patients' physical conditions, attests

---

[27]In earlier chapters (chapters 8–12), we used the term "observational studies" in the sense of *nonexperimental studies*. In such studies, researchers "observe" variables, which means that they do not manipulate them. However, such variables may be based on self-reported interview data. In this section, we refer to "observations" in the narrower sense of a *data collection mode*, which is contrasted with self-reports as another data collection mode.

to the importance of observations in clinical practice. Nurses and physicians alike make inferences about a patient's condition based on skin coloration, perspiration, breathing sounds, and so forth. In addition to observations of physiologic characteristics, clinicians rely on observations of patients' behavior to obtain information about patients' "true" state of health. These observations occur within the privileged relationship between providers and patients. Because the confidentiality of this relationship is legally and socially protected, patients are often willing to reveal information about themselves that they would not necessarily reveal in other situations. Researchers who observe subjects are in a less protected relationship and may need to work harder to earn the trust of study participants (see chapter 24 for additional discussion about covert observation).

If the primary outcome variables of concern are physical or behavioral, observations seem to be a logical choice for data collection. Although we can, and often do, *ask* people about their symptoms and behavior, in some situations, this may not be an optimal or even a feasible strategy. In particular, when there is good reason to believe that human subjects will not or cannot give truthful verbal responses, observations may be the only way to obtain accurate records of behavior. This situation occurs most often when the subjects cannot provide answers to questions of interest. Examples include very young, preverbal children; people experiencing moderate or severe dementia; delirious patients; and barely conscious accident victims. Whenever the focus is on the behavioral interaction patterns themselves, rather than on the interpretation of such interactions by one or all of the participants, observations also appear to be preferable to self-reports. By the same token, observational methods are problematic in studies that focus on mental processes, although they can certainly play a useful supporting role. Nevertheless, inferring the existence of particular emotions, attitudes, values, or preferences, based on observations of behavior alone, is quite risky (Kerlinger, 1986). To be credible, such observations must be supplemented with self-report data.

Probably the single biggest limitation to observational methods as a means of collecting data is the fact that only *current* behaviors and symptoms can be observed. More specifically, *the observer must be present when a symptom is visible or a behavior occurs*. That simple fact ensures that many health-relevant behaviors can never be observed directly by researchers because potential subjects would often be unwilling to allow researchers to intrude into their private lives to observe the relevant behaviors. In addition, the need for observers to be present also

means that studies that use observational methods cannot be retrospective.

The Relationship of Observer and Observed

Participant Observation

With respect to the role of the observer, the major choice is that between participant and nonparticipant observation. **Participant observation** implies that researchers or observers become part of, and active participants in, the social networks and interaction patterns that are being studied. Through immersion in the social world and participation in the social roles of the target group, the goal of participant observation is to achieve a greater level of understanding than would be available to a passive bystander. At its most extreme, participant observation entails concealment of the role of the researcher. In that case, researchers participate in social groups *as if* they were group members or occupied well-defined social roles within the group.[28] The main claim in support of this clandestine approach to observation is that it is intended to minimize intrusion into the "normal" social intercourse, thereby reducing the potential for bias, as when people, conscious of being observed, start play-acting for the observer or audience. It is common for people who are aware of being observed to change their behavior. Consider the differences in responses that might be obtained when adolescents are interviewed about their sexual behavior with or without their parents present. However, although almost everyone plays to an audience (Goffman, 1961), this is not by itself a strong methodologic argument for concealing an observer within the study population. An observer must take on *some* role identity if he or she wants to observe behaviors, and depending on which role is adopted, people will reveal different aspects of their realities.[29] In this sense, no observation is unbiased: *reactivity to the presence of an observer is always part of any relationship between observer and observed*.

Participant observation requires observers to "go with the flow" to avoid betraying their identity. Thus, this method of observation is compatible with qualitative approaches to research: it is necessarily less structured and occurs in naturalistic environments. The conduct of observers who use participant observation poses several

---

[28]There is obviously an ethical issue of deception involved here. See chapter 24 for an additional discussion of the use of deception in research.

[29]Imagine a researcher who is studying interaction patterns in an emergency department. He or she could be introduced as a visiting physician, a nurse, or a hospital administrator, and would likely see different "slices of life," depending on the assumed role.

ethical and methodologic challenges. Chief among the latter are the problems of recording observed behaviors. Recording behavior more or less simultaneously as it unfolds would be impossible because it would uncover the observer's true identity. Thus, a substantial part of the behavior must be recorded in "field notes," from memory.[30]

Nonparticipant Observation

As the name indicates, a **nonparticipant** observer does not participate in the social interactions of the subjects being observed, at least not in the sense of being a regular member of the group. However, the distinction between participant and nonparticipant observation is quite fluid, and it depends on the degree of social interaction between observer and observed as well as on the explicitness of the observer or researcher role. Ideally, a nonparticipant observer attempts to fade into the background and hopes to be able to devote all of his or her energies to the process of observation. In some situations, minimizing obtrusiveness may be considered an act of concealment; however, in most cases, nonparticipant observers introduce themselves as such, but attempt to be as unobtrusive as possible. To a large degree, the distinction between participant and nonparticipant observation is less important in public settings, such as a primary care clinic waiting room. Observing behavior in a public space, even if the observer pretends to be just another patient in the clinic, does not necessarily violate norms and expectations for privacy protection, as would be the case for family or friendship relationships.

From a methodologic point of view, the main advantage of nonparticipant observation is that the observer or multiple observers can concentrate on observation without being drawn into the ongoing action, allowing for stricter standards of observation and recording. However, to the extent that the observed individual considers nonparticipant observers obtrusive, the price is a distorted picture of the usual interaction patterns.

Units of Observation

The English word *observation* encompasses two meanings: (1) "the act and practice of noting and recording facts and events" and (2) "the data so noted and recorded" (*Webster's Unabridged Dictionary,* 1983). In other words, it refers to both the process and its outcome. Using "observation" in the latter sense, the most important question that a researcher who is using observational methods must ask is, "What is the observational unit that is to be observed?"

The broadness or narrowness of an observational unit can be defined in terms of both time and content (Waltz et al., 1991).

At one extreme, researchers can choose *naturalistic inquiry* and *ethnographic research*. These approaches often involve participant observation by a single observer in real-life situations. The observer relies on field notes as the primary mode of recording and interpreting observed events. This approach tends to be diffuse in the sense that it is rarely focused on one or two specific behaviors that are singled out for observation. Observations of this kind are said to be **molar,** meaning that they invariably span a substantial time interval, during which whole sequences of action may take place. At the other extreme are highly structured, or **molecular,** observations of short duration that may capture only parts of naturally occurring sequences of action. Such observations usually focus on a few predetermined actions and involve a single or multiple independent observers, each using a predetermined checklist or scaling device to rate the observed phenomena and behaviors.

Similar to the choices in interview formats, the preference for less structured (molar) observations or more structured (molecular) observations is largely one of purpose. When exploration is the primary goal, the researcher needs to make sure that nothing important is missed during the observation period. This calls for extended and unstructured observations. When the goal is measurement of outcomes in intervention studies, the observations must be amenable to conversion into a standardized scoring system so that intervention and control groups can be compared. Only highly structured observations are amenable to a scoring algorithm.

Timing of Observations

All observations occur during a specific time (i.e., they have a beginning and an end). In clinical practice, the length of an encounter between provider and patient is usually determined by the complexity of the clinical problem, but is also influenced by social norms, economic incentives, and work rules. In research projects, which are also subject to resource constraints, contact time with study subjects must be deliberately planned. If observational methods are used, decisions about contact time involve the following questions:

- How *long* should a given observation period last?
- Should the length of the observation period be standardized across study participants?
- How *often* should patients be observed (i.e., how many distinct observation periods, per subject, are involved)?

---

[30]See Atkinson and Hammersley (1994) for further information.

- What mechanism should be used to select or trigger observation periods?

Beginning with the last question, observations in research studies are often triggered by specific events. These events may be critical thresholds that initiate an observational cycle, for example, observing patients' behavior for 2 hours after they take an antipyretic or once their fever exceeds 99°F. Events are often defined in terms of meaningful complexes of action with natural boundaries, such as interactions during mealtime (Tulviste, 2000), bathing episodes (Clark, Lipe, & Bilbrey, 1998), or treatment sessions (Bowers, 1999). Sometimes it is difficult to define the *boundaries* of the "event." Although mealtimes and bathing episodes are relatively easy to circumscribe, the process of "bonding" between a mother and a newborn baby, for example, has no clearly defined boundaries.

The decision about when and how often to observe study participants is a sampling decision. Especially when a study uses highly structured, molecular observations of short duration, it is important to select observation times that provide a representative sample of the behavior or behaviors in question. This can be accomplished through either systematic sampling (e.g., 3-minute observations performed every 10 minutes) or random sampling of time slots from a longer period during which the researcher has access to the study participants.[31] The advantage of this approach is that it is likely to yield an unbiased count of the occurrence of behaviors; its limitation is that the sampled time segments may not coincide with the real-life events to be observed. This is also an issue when considering the length of a single observation period, which may vary substantially from study to study. Even when the focus is on structured observations of particular actions, the useful length of a single observation period is largely determined by the typical time boundaries of the actions involved (e.g., observing nursing students giving an injection or doing a physical examination).

Recording Observations and Converting Them to Data

To be useful in research, observations must be recorded and converted into a format that allows researchers to analyze and interpret the data. When the ethnographic approach is used, observations are recorded in field notes that describe and interpret the observed behaviors and events.[32]

Highly structured observations for intervention studies are usually converted into *numerical codes* that are generated by the observer to record the following: (1) the absence or presence of specific events, behaviors, or health-related hazards on a checklist (Tortolero, Bartholomew, Tyrrell, Abramson, Sockrider, Markham, Whitehead, & Parcel, 2002) or (2) ordinal ratings that characterize the strength or severity of a particular behavior (Bowers, 1999). In either case, the feasibility of the coding scheme depends to a large degree on its reliability (i.e., independent observers must come to the same conclusion about what they observe).[33]

To a substantial degree, agreement among different observers is easier to reach if the description of the observed events or behaviors requires observational, rather then interpretive, language. Consider the difference between recording "a muscle movement around the mouth" versus "a smile" or "a smirk." The classification of the movement as "a smirk" requires the observer to make a certain interpretive leap, and agreement on this interpretation is harder to achieve than agreement on observed physical movements.

As mentioned earlier, if observations are to be recorded at the time they are made, the observers usually must be nonparticipants (i.e., somewhat detached from the ongoing interaction), and their observer role must be accepted by the persons who are being observed. This is less of a problem in clinical interactions, where a patient often expects the clinician to make notes and record observations during an examination. However, the demands of a research protocol that contains highly specific instructions for structured observations may be difficult to combine with the role of an advanced practice clinician whose primary purpose is to gather information relevant to diagnosis, treatment, and patient care.

In recent years, video cameras have become a frequently used assistive device to document events and behaviors. The great advantage of such documentation is that it provides a record that can be viewed by multiple observers after the documented events have transpired. Thus, unlike participant observation, in which the field notes composed by the observer are the only record, video records offer the opportunity to "verify" interpretations by having them reviewed independently. In addition, video records can be used to probe alternate observational coding systems and evaluate their interrater reliability (Bowers, 1999). Yet, as with the use of any technology, the use of video cameras to record the behaviors of study participants poses methodologic and ethical questions.

---

[31]See chapters 19 and 20 for details on sampling.

[32]Field notes are discussed in chapter 18.

---

[33]For the evaluation of interrater reliability, see chapter 14.

As a general principle, unless the site of recording is clearly marked as a *public* space, video recordings require the consent of the recorded subjects.[34] In addition, if the recording will be shown in public, individual consent of the subjects should be obtained, both for taping and for use of the recording. From a methodologic point of view, video technology can also be problematic. The presence of live observers may change the behavior of the observed participants, and the presence of video cameras and their perceived intrusiveness may have a similar reactivity or observer effect (Bowers, 1999). Furthermore, a video recording should not be considered an unquestionably objective document of what transpires in a particular setting. As any camera operator knows, for any given scene, there are many choices to be made and angles from which to shoot the action. Which participants of an interaction appear in the foreground or background, which speakers are seen in close-up view, and so forth, reflect *decisions* that affect the final video document as well as the interpretation of an event by secondary observers or viewers. To date, we know of no study that has systematically explored how multiple, different video records of the same situation may affect viewers' conclusions and interpretations of the observed behaviors and actions.

The collection of observational data, particularly data based on structured observations that can be converted to measurement scales, is one of the less developed areas of nursing research. Although it is not easy to devise reliable observational methods that can be replicated across settings, the promise of such methods is that they represent a step away from self-reports, which either involve respondent bias or cannot be obtained if the potential respondent is incapacitated. For research involving mentally ill, very frail, or very young participants, observations, in conjunction with biophysiologic tests, are often the only source of information available.

ISSUES IN THE DATA COLLECTION OF BIOPHYSIOLOGIC MEASURES

Although nursing is a clinical discipline, biophysiologic variables have played a less prominent role in nursing research, with nursing theory and research primarily focused on psychosocial variables. Yet, there is a distinct research tradition interested in biophysiologic outcomes that involve such topics as biophysical measures, such as blood pressure, body temperature, or forced expiratory

---

[34]See chapter 24 for a detailed discussion of consent issues.

volume; skin breakdown; biochemical measures of serum hormones or electrolyte levels; microbiologic measurements from culture tests for the presence of bacteria; and microscopic tests for the presence of viral infections (Carroll, 2000; Gift & Narsarage, 1998, 2000; Liehr, Meininger, Mueller, Chandler, & Chan, 1997; Maguire, 1999). In addition, the application of biophysical tests or the collection of relevant specimens is a major part of the clinical activities of nurses.

Biophysiologic measurement can be considered a special form of highly structured observation. Most biophysiologic measurement involves the use of calibrated measurement instruments, such as scales, microscopes, electrocardiogram monitors, and sphygmomanometers. Although health professionals use such devices and usually leave the calibration to technicians, the accuracy and reliability of measurement depends on the activities of clinicians. Clinicians monitor the use of technical measurement devices for malfunctioning and ensure that the application of the devices and the interpretation of results follow standardized procedures. Thus, it is essential to remember that having a well-calibrated instrument does not guarantee that measurement will be reliable. In fact, haphazard application of a calibrated instrument can be just as much a source of measurement error. Thus, rules for standardizing the application of a technical measurement procedure are just as important for reliability as the technical quality of the instrument. Consider, for example, the measurement of blood gases in an umbilical cord.

►CLINICAL RESEARCH IN ACTION
Collecting Arterial and Venous Cord Blood

Cottrell and Shannahan (1987) collected arterial and venous cord blood from the clamped segment of the cord, using syringes that had been flushed with 1000 units/mL of heparin solution. The syringes were capped, and the collected specimen was immediately chilled in ice slush and sent to a laboratory, which used a specific commercial blood gas analyzer to obtain results. This is a simple example of an effort to standardize the procedures for collecting a particular specimen so that all patients who are being compared undergo more or less the same measurement procedures.

CONCLUSION

Data collection encompasses all of the procedures and activities that lead to the generation of data. With the current emphasis on psychosocial and behavioral processes in nursing research, self-report data, in the form of interviews, written responses to questionnaires, or diaries, are by far the most important sources of information. Nevertheless, distinct traditions of relying on observational and biophysiologic data have also been present in nursing research. Although biophysiologic tests are generally calibrated and their application is standardized, both interviews and observations can run the gamut from unstructured data collection to highly structured measurement protocols. As emphasized before, the amount of structure associated with study design, measurement, and data collection procedures is primarily a function of the emphasis on exploration versus hypothesis testing. The former requires openness and flexibility in study procedures; the latter is best served with standardized procedures that can be replicated in different settings and with different samples.

Although testing and confirming the propositions and theories of any empirical science ultimately depend on the compatibility of the propositions with the data, not all empirical studies must rely on newly collected data. In fact, in nursing and the broader health sciences, empirical tests are sometimes based on data that were collected for other purposes, ranging from vital statistics to insurance files and from large-scale federal surveys to routine clinical data. In the next chapter, we turn to some of the issues involved in the secondary analysis of existing data.

Suggested Activities

1. Access the web site of the National Center of Health Statistics (NCHS), available at: *http://www.cdc.gov/ nchs/about.htm*. Download the questionnaire of the latest version of the Health Interview Survey.
2. Examine the sociodemographic portion of the interview, and propose a simplified version that could be used for a small-scale clinical study that you might consider for the clinical setting that you are familiar with. The key to simplification is to:
   a. Eliminate categories that do not apply to your target population.
   b. Alternatively, collapse existing categories or propose additional ones that are compatible with the federal categories so that you can compare distributions in the small-scale clinical study with those in the federal data.
3. Read the article by Kesmodel and Olsen (2001) that compares four methods of self-reporting alcohol intake among pregnant women. In the absence of a gold standard, how might the accuracy of any of these methods be established?
4. Visit the National Institute for Nursing Research web site, available at: *http://www.nih.gov/ninr*. Review the

nursing research priorities that are described, and note which priorities involve psychosocial versus biophysiologic phenomena.

Suggested Readings

Converse, J. M. & Presser, S. (1986). *Asking questions: The handcrafted questionnaire*. Thousand Oaks, CA: Sage.

Fowler, F. J. (1995). *Improving survey questions*. Thousand Oaks, CA: Sage.

Kesmodel, U., & Olsen, S. F. (2001). Self reported alcohol intake in pregnancy: Comparison between four methods. *Journal of Epidemiologic Community Health, 55*, 738–745.

Lange, J. W. (2002). Methodological concerns for non-Hispanic investigators conducting research with Hispanic Americans. *Research in Nursing & Health, 25*, 3, 411–419.

Ornstein, S., Markert, G., Litchfield, L., & Zemp, L. (1988). Evaluation of the DINAMAP blood pressure monitor in an ambulatory primary care setting. *The Journal of Family Practice, 26*, 5, 517–521.

References

Atkinson, P., & Hammersley, M. (1994). Ethnography and participant observation. In Denzin, N. K., & Y. S. Lincoln (Eds.), *Handbook of qualitative research* (pp. 248–261). Thousand Oaks, CA: Sage.

Bowers, L. (1999). A critical appraisal of violent incident measures. *Journal of Mental Health, 8*, 4, 339–349.

Brislin, R. W. (1970). Back-translation for cross-cultural research. *Journal of Cross-Cultural Psychology, 1*, 185–216.

Carroll, M. (2000). An evaluation of temperature measurement. *Nursing Standard, 14*, 44, 39–43.

Clark, M. E., Lipe, A. W., & Bilbrey, M. (1998). Use of music to decrease aggressive behaviors in people with dementia. *Gerontological Nursing, 24*, 7, 10–17.

Cottrell, B. H., & Shannahan, M. K. (1987). A comparison of fetal outcome in birth chair and delivery table births. *Research in Nursing & Health, 10*, 237–243.

DeVellis, R. (1991). *Scale development: Theory and applications*. Newbury Park, CA: Sage.

Dougherty, M. C., Dwyer, J. W., Pendergast, J. F., Boyington, A. R., Tomlinson, B. U., Coward, R. T., Duncan, R. P., Vogel, B., & Rooks, L. G. (2002). A randomized trial of behavioral management for continence with older rural women. *Research in Nursing & Health, 25*, 1, 3–13.

Fowler, F. J. (1995). *Improving survey questions*. Thousand Oaks, CA: Sage.

Fowler, F. J. (2002). *Survey research methods* (3rd ed.). Thousand Oaks, CA: Sage.

Fowler, F. J., & Mangione, T.W. (1990). *Standardized survey interviewing*. Newbury Park, CA: Sage.

Goffman, E. (1961). *Encounters: Two studies in the sociology of interaction*. Indianapolis: Bobbs-Merrill.

Holden, R. R., Fekken, G. C., & Jackson, D. N. (1985). Structured personality test item characteristics and validity. *Journal of Research in Personality, 19*, 386–494.

Kerlinger, F. N. (1986). *Foundations of behavioral research* (3rd ed.). New York: Holt, Rhinehart & Winston.

Kesmodel, U., & Olsen, S.F. (2001). Self reported alcohol intake in pregnancy: Comparison between four methods. *Journal of Epidemiologic Community Health, 55*, 738–745.

Kramer, M. S., Barr, R. G., Dagenais, S., Yang, H., Jones, P., Ciofani, L. & Jane, F. (2001). Pacifier use, early weaning, and cry/fuss behavior: A randomized trial. *Journal of the American Medical Association, 286*, 3, 322–326.

Lange, J. W. (2002). Methodological concerns for non-Hispanic investigators conducting research with Hispanic Americans. *Research in Nursing & Health, 25*, 3, 411–419.

Liehr, P., Meininger, J. C., Mueller, W., Chandler, S. P., & Chan, W. (1997). Blood pressure reactivity in urban youth during angry and normal talking. *Journal of Cardiovascular Nursing, 11*, 85–94.

Maguire, P. D. (1999). Skin protection and breakdown in ELBW infants: A national survey. *Clinical Nursing Research, 8*, 3, 222–234.

Malone-Lee, J. G., Walsh, J. B., Maugourd, M.-F. (2001). Tolterodine: A safe and effective treatment for older patients with overactive bladder. *Journal of the American Geriatrics Society, 49*, 6, 700–705.

Minnick, A., & Young, W. B. (1998). Comparison between reports of care obtained by postdischarge telephone interview and predischarge personal interview. *Outcomes Management for Nursing Practice, 3*, 1, 32–37.

Nunnally, J. C., & Bernstein, I. H. (1994). *Psychometric theory* (3rd ed.). New York: McGraw-Hill.

Ribisl, K. M., Walton, M. A., Mowbray, C. T., Luke, D. A., Davidson, W. S., & Bootsmiller, B. J. (1996). Minimizing participant attrition in panel studies through the use of effective retention and tracking strategies: Review and recommendations. *Evaluation and Program Planning, 19*, 1–25.

Rossi, P. H., Wright, J. D., & Anderson, A. B. (1983). *Handbook of survey research*. Orlando, FL: Academic Press.

Sheatsley, P. B. (1983). Questionnaire construction and item writing. In Rossi, P. H., J. D. Wright, & A. B. Anderson (Eds.), *Handbook of survey research* (pp. 195–230). Orlando, FL: Academic Press.

Stinson, J. (1997). *Association of fatigue and preterm birth in active duty military*. Bethesda, MD: Triservice Nursing Research Program.

Streiner, D. L., & Norman, G. R. (1995). *Health measurement scales: A practical guide to their development and use* (2nd ed.). Oxford, UK: Oxford University Press.

Sudman, S., & Bradburn, N. (1982). *Asking questions*. San Francisco: Jossey-Bass.

Tortolero, S. R., Bartholomew, L. K., Tyrrell, S., Abramson, S. L., Sockrider, M. M., Markham, C. M., Whitehead, L. W., & Parcel, G. S. (2002). Environmental allergens and irritants in schools: A focus on asthma. *Journal of School Health, 71*, 1, 33–38.

Tulviste, T. (2000). Socialization at meals: A comparison of American and Estonian mother-adolescent interaction. *Journal of Cross-Cultural Psychology, 31*, 5, 537–556.

Weeks, M. F., Kulka, R. A., Lessler, J. T., & Whitmore, R. W. (1983). Personal versus telephone surveys for collecting household health data at the local level. *American Journal of Public Health, 73*,12, 1389–1394.

Willett, W. C. (1997). Nutritional epidemiology. In Rothman, K. J., & S. Greenland. *Modern Epidemiology* (pp. 623–642). Philadelphia: Lippincott Williams & Wilkins.

Wu, T.-Y., & Pender, N. (2002). Determinants of physical activity among Taiwanese adolescents: An application of the health promotion model. *Research in Nursing & Health, 25*, 1, 25–36.

CHAPTER 17   Analysis of Existing Data

INTRODUCTION

In the last chapter, we focused on methods to collect original (new) data that are designed to shed light on research problems or hypotheses. There are many reasons for collecting original data. The main advantages are the ability to: (1) select or develop the desired measures that best address the concepts of interest; (2) exercise control over the data collection process, including training of data collectors and quality control; and (3) implement prospective study designs, including experimental and quasi-experimental designs, which usually provide stronger evidence about causal inference.

There are also several important reasons for not collecting original data. If appropriate data are already available that can shed light on the research problem, new data collection efforts could be considered unnecessary, and a waste of resources. Furthermore, beyond the often substantial expenses involved,[1] new data collection also requires specific expertise and skills in research design, measurement, interviewing, sampling, and other areas. Finally, data collection for clinical research projects is usually at least somewhat intrusive. Data collection tends to disrupt institutional routines and day-to-day clinical practice; it also requires the consent of study participants as well as thorough review of the study design and procedures by institutional review boards.[2]

Although the collection of new data may be difficult to implement in clinical care settings, there are few settings in society that are as "data rich" as clinical sites, where routine data collection is very much a part of everyday practice. Furthermore, all advanced industrial countries have a dense network of public and private agencies that are engaged in an ongoing effort to collect information on health and illness in the population. For example, consider the following partial listing of data collection efforts, all of which can be useful in clinical research:

- Birth and death certificates
- Disease registries
- Medical records
- Pathology reports
- Autopsy results
- Insurance records and claim files
- Records of professional licensing boards
- Institutional data on hospitals, nursing homes, and clinics
- Census data
- National health surveys
- Existing data from past research studies

Given the immense improvements in information technology that have occurred during the last two decades as well as the substantially reduced costs of collecting information, efforts to collect and integrate clinical data have intensified. Increasingly, clinics and primary care practices use computerized information systems and collect a host of routine data, including diagnostic and treatment information, social and financial characteristics of patients and their families, records of provider–patient interactions and visits, records of referrals and prescriptions, and information on compliance with treatment. Such data are also potentially useful for many types of clinical research, and constitute the focus of discussion for the remainder of this chapter.

PRINCIPAL ISSUES IN CONDUCTING RESEARCH WITH EXISTING DATA

It is useful to distinguish among several types of research conducted with existing data. The first is **secondary data analysis,** which was defined by Polit and Hungler (2001) as involving, "the use of data gathered in a previous study to test new hypotheses or explore new relationships." Note that this definition refers to data from a previous *research study*. Thus, the secondary data analyst builds on the design, sampling, and data collection decisions of the original research team, but focuses on variables and relationships that were not considered before. A secondary analyst may also devise new measurement scales from the existing indicator items in the data set, and may select and analyze only a specific subset of the original data sample.

A slight variation on the theme of secondary analysis of already collected research data is the **secondary analysis of large data sets** made available (often publicly) to the research community for analysis purposes. The federal surveys conducted by the National Center of Health Statistics are good examples. These data collection efforts differ from the usual research study in that they are intended,

---

[1]In many cases, these expenses are substantial enough that they cannot be met without special grant or contract monies that are provided by public or private sources.

[2]Depending on the nature of the research, because of potential conflicts of interest, many clinical agencies require that institutional staff (who are not associated with the research as investigators) approach potential study participants for consent. For vulnerable populations, the institutional review board may require the patient's individual health care provider to obtain the patient's consent for study participation. Over the last several years, regulations for informed consent procedures have become increasingly stringent. The net effect is that the needed resources (e.g., staff time) have increased substantially with regard to obtaining consent for original data collection. Because of concerns about privacy and confidentiality, the use of existing data is also subject to review by institutional review boards, but these reviews are usually expedited because direct patient contact and interventions are not involved. See chapter 24 for more on these issues.

from the outset, to appeal to a broad array of secondary analysts with diverse research interests. Thus, they are not designed to answer specific research hypotheses, but to address broadly defined areas of interest that often address national health concerns and policy questions. Another extension of the secondary analysis approach is the analysis of data that represent a *compilation* of data from several research studies.

The secondary analysis of research studies should be distinguished from the **analysis of data from clinical or administrative records** that are often collected routinely. These kinds of data are collected for purposes other than research, usually for clinical care, quality improvement, and accounting purposes. This means that the data collection efforts are rarely organized with the goal of implementing a particular research design, and this has implications for the types of research questions that can and cannot be addressed with these data sources. A final type of study that uses existing data is an **ancillary study,** which mixes some new data collection with existing data records from previous research or nonresearch sources.

Key Principles Concerning the Use of Existing Data

A few general principles guide the use of existing data for research purposes. These principles are "general" in that they apply to a wide range of studies that rely on existing sources of data.

Formulate Research Questions or Hypotheses

The first steps in secondary data analysis are identical to those in any research project. Researchers start with formulating specific research questions or hypotheses after a review of the relevant literature or existing clinical evidence.[3] Because secondary analysts often use existing data for purposes that were not originally intended or even anticipated by the data collectors, they cannot rely exclusively on the problem formulation and rationale for the original study: they essentially "invent" new purposes for the use of the existing data, which is an act of imagination and creativity.

Select Data Sets to Address the Questions and Hypotheses

The process of formulating research questions and hypotheses may have started before any specific data sets

were considered. In that case, the researcher must search for appropriate data sets that "speak to" the problems formulated. At a minimum, this involves finding data sets that contain adequate measures of the dependent and independent variables considered in the research problem as well as measures of potential confounding variables that are important to control for, given the current state of knowledge in the chosen area. If more than one data set is accessible that meets these characteristics, study design and sampling become additional considerations in choosing the "best" data set available.

Understand the Constraints When Formulating Questions or Hypotheses

Often, secondary analysts start with an existing data set to which they have convenient access.[4] In that situation, the formulation of the research problem or hypotheses is constrained by the information available in the data set.[5] Usually, a potential analyst would study the code book (see chapter 23) or other documentation that describes the information available in the data set, before formulating research questions or hypotheses.

Avoid "Data Dredging"

The analysis of existing data without prior specification and formulation of a research problem or hypotheses is controversial. In "data dredging" approaches, the data are examined to search for relationships among variables, and the patterns that are discovered are described. Although describing the patterns in an existing data set is not necessarily controversial,[6] controversy may occur if plausible-sounding explanations for the patterns are constructed *post hoc,* without regard to the approach used. The usual intent of hypothesis formulation (especially when the goal of the study is to test causal or theoretically specified relationships between variables) is to provide an *a priori* guide to the analysis by specifying which relationships to test for. In contrast, the data dredging approach (Hulley, Cummings, Browner, Grady, Hearst, & Newman, 2001) is objectionable, mainly because it does not really "test"

---

[3]See chapter 23 for more details on the use of literature in the formulation of a research problem.

[4]A common example is that of a graduate student who uses data collected by his or her faculty mentor or thesis advisor.

[5]This is often considered a "disadvantage" of secondary analysis, but the difference between this method and primary data collection is not always large. When researchers collect primary data, they also make compromises concerning what data to collect, usually because of resource or accessibility considerations.

[6]In exploratory descriptive studies, including qualitative studies, the data exploration approach may be very useful. However, in reports of the research findings, this information should be qualified with regard to the goals of the analysis.

anything; it is merely an account of patterns found in a particular study sample. This approach is particularly problematic when results are reported selectively. To see the differences in approaches, consider the examples of an exploratory or descriptive approach and a data dredging approach to the same data set (presented in Box 17-1).

Look for Linkages to Other Data Sets that May Contain Relevant Variables

It has become increasingly common to link data sets if, as separate data files, they do not provide answers to the research questions. For example, Stommel, Given, and

---

BOX 17.1   Example of Data Exploration and Description versus Data Dredging

Example of data exploration and description

Suppose that a researcher uses existing data about the health status, educational level, and age of a population of diabetic patients to provide a profile of the characteristics of this population. The researcher prepares descriptive data for the clinic providers, considering information about:

1. Average age (including range and standard deviation)
2. Health status (number and type of health problems and their severity)
3. Educational level (number of years of education)

The researcher also computes the bivariate correlations among the key variables, and finds that age is positively related to the number and types of health problems (older patients have a greater number and more types of health problems) and marginally and inversely related to education (older patients have lower levels of education). It is also found that health status and educational level are significantly related (patients with lower levels of education tend to have larger numbers of health problems).

The researcher presents all of the findings to the clinic providers as a profile of the patient population. The researcher is careful to note the following during the presentation of the findings: the limitations of the existing data set, the lack of *a priori* hypotheses. The researcher also cautions against causal interpretations of the statistically significant correlations.

The researcher is asked by a person who is attending the presentation to speculate about what theories or causal relationships might underlie the study findings and what implications there might be for clinic policies. The researcher provides a brief discussion of the rationale for "not going beyond the data," before providing possible explanations for the observed correlations. The rationale includes identifying what conditions would need to be present to permit a rigorous scientific examination of causal relationships or hypothesis testing (refer to chapters 3–5 on experimental design) as well as indicating that it would be premature to base policy decisions on the limited analysis that was done. However, the description of the characteristics of the population may be useful to clinicians in thinking about the possible needs of the population for clinical care. The researcher concludes the presentation by discussing recommendations for possible future research that could address questions raised by audience members.

Example of data dredging

Suppose the same data are analyzed, but the analyst has the computer search for every statistically significant bivariate correlation among the variables in the data set. Several of these involve race and ethnicity and various health status measures. The researcher now searches the literature and finds a couple of articles in which other researchers report that members of minority groups are less likely to comply with treatment recommendations. Now, the analyst presents the results as confirmed theory about causal relationships between the variables, without mentioning that the theory was not tested or confirmed, but represents an ad hoc explanation of an originally unsuspected relationship. When asked about the policy implications, the researcher states that clinicians "should focus on improving compliance rates among minority patients because the lack of compliance causes greater health problems in these groups." When asked by a skeptical audience member about the possible role of patient finances, insurance, education, and transportation in obtaining access to health care (refer back to Chapter 9 for the role of confounding and control variables on observational studies), the researcher admits that these variables were not examined in the analysis, but "could be important to think about." Audience members might leave the presentation wondering whether any useful knowledge was gained from the resources invested in the data analysis project.

Given (2002) linked information from a state Bureau of Vital Statistics to data from an existing panel study to predict subsequent mortality and survival rates among patients with cancer, based on variables measured in the panel study. Of course, any such linkage requires a set of common identifiers in all data sets that are being linked.[7]

Examine the Limitations of Existing and Available Data Sets

After the formulation of the research question and the choice of the data set, analysts must spend considerable time familiarizing themselves with the particular characteristics (including limitations) of the data set. This process requires a thorough study of the data collection and measurement procedures that were originally used as well as the scope of the data collection effort that went into the data file. For instance, if a researcher uses Medicare claims files to document elderly patients' use of formal health care services over a period of a year or so, he or she must recognize that some services, such as an extended nursing home stay or outpatient medications, are not covered by Medicare. In principle, most services that are paid for out-of-pocket or through additional private insurance may not be part of the Medicare record. Almost any given data set is limited in one way or another through the use of definitions of cases, services, or diagnoses that may not be identical to those of the original researcher. (Orsi, Gray, Mahon, Moriarity, Shepard et al., 1999) If such limitations cannot be remedied (e.g., through linkages with other data sets), they must be clearly stated, and their implications for the findings must be discussed in the final research report.

Investigate the Purposes and Procedures for Data Collection

For all data sets, but especially in the case of routine, non-research data collection efforts, it is essential to understand why the data are collected, who collects the data at the source, and if common standards are used to decide when to report a particular piece of information. One example of the importance of the purpose for data collection is the use of insurance claim files to obtain information on patient treatment. Such files generally are not assembled for the purpose of providing a complete treatment picture, but instead are meant to list all *billable* services. It is important to remember that reliability in data collection is not always a high priority, especially if the files are assembled for purposes other than research.

SECONDARY ANALYSIS OF RESEARCH STUDIES

Reanalysis of data from a past research study is an approach that is commonly used in published research reports. Secondary analyses are frequently, but not exclusively, based on data from survey studies. This is, in part, the result of the fact that surveys, in contrast to experimental studies, often contain multiple measures that are not all tightly integrated into the study objectives. This feature often leaves room for additional exploration and analysis. For example, as was mentioned earlier, in the case of the national surveys conducted by the National Center of Health Statistics (NCHS), such as the National Health Interview Survey (NHIS), the National Health and Nutrition Examination Survey (NHANES), and the National Medical Care Expenditure Survey,[8] versatility of use is a feature that is built in by design. These surveys are conducted and the data are collected from the start with the anticipation that secondary analyses will be undertaken (Korn & Graubard, 1999).

Typically, secondary analyses of existing research data have a new focus, choose new outcome variables, and are largely driven by a new conceptual framework or set of hypotheses. Such secondary analyses are often conducted by new analysts who were not part of the original research team. However, they may also be undertaken by the original researcher who collected the data (Herron, 1989). Thus, the main principle is that secondary analysis starts with a new idea or concern that is translated into a new research problem, but evidence relevant to this new problem is sought in existing research data.

For example, Khanh, Roosa, Tein, and Lopez (2002) used data from an existing panel study to examine the relationship between acculturation and proneness to problem behaviors in Hispanic youth. As is typical for a secondary analysis, the available measures for the main concepts in the analysis are not always ideal from a conceptual point of view. In this case, the analysts used three proxy measures of acculturation: (1) immigrant status (whether the secondary school student was born in the United States), (2) the primary language spoken at home (Spanish or English), and (3) the language used to complete the survey (Spanish or English). The researchers showed that the three items were internally consistent (highly correlated) and cited other research that used similar proxy measures. As in many other secondary analyses, these researchers concentrated on a subset of the originally collected data: their

---

[7]Linking separate data sources also requires the consent of the study participants if they are individually identifiable.

[8]See chapter 11 for more information on these surveys.

focus on Hispanic secondary school students led to the exclusion of more than 50% of the participants in the original study.

Wolinsky, Krygiel, and Wyrwich (2002) conducted an analysis of data from the Longitudinal Study of Aging, which is a supplement to the NHIS, and used survey data on 2,254 elderly men (70 years of age and older) to predict hospitalization for prostate cancer. This study is a good example of how linking multiple data sets can help to widen the analytic possibilities, because the information on hospitalization came from Medicare claim files (*International Classification of Diseases, 9th revision, Clinical Modification* [ICD-9-CM] discharge diagnosis codes) and the mortality data came from the National Death Index. In many ways, such linkages among existing data sets are the "wave of the future" for health services research.

Linkages of a different sort are provided by comparisons of nationally representative cross-sectional surveys, such as the NHIS.[9] For instance, Makuc, Breen, and Freid (1999) used data from five annual administrations of the NHIS, spanning the years 1987 to 1994, to track improvements in mammography screening among low-income African American and European American women, aged 50 to 64 years, as well as possible reasons for the observed changes. The collection of nationally representative data of this kind from interviews conducted in approximately 45,000 households for each year of data collection clearly goes beyond the monetary and organizational resources available to individual researchers. A similar example is provided by the analysis of Hewitt, Devesa, and Breen (2002), which estimated the prevalence of using Pap tests among women who are at high risk for cervical cancer. The data for this analysis came from the 1995 National Survey of Family Growth, which included nearly 11,000 women aged 15 to 44 years.

Secondary analysis of large-scale federal surveys and panel studies has become a growing field of specialization among nurse researchers (Moriarty, Deatrick, Mahon, Feetham, Carroll, Shepard, & Orsi, 1999). The use of such data offers several important advantages.

- As mentioned earlier, these studies provide information on nationally representative samples. This type of information is almost impossible for individual researchers to collect, especially when the sampling design requires accurate information on population subgroups, such as minorities or regional or state populations.

- The studies conducted by the NCHS are often performed with the latest, most sophisticated survey techniques, including computer-aided telephone interviewing and computer-aided personal interview systems (see chapter 16). In addition, some of them combine survey data with biophysiologic data on the respondents, as in the NHANES.

- For secondary analysis, NCHS studies have the additional advantage of providing analysts with extensive information about study and sampling design as well as code books and written computer codes for major statistical analysis packages (e.g., SAS, SPSS). In this context, it is interesting to think about how quickly computer and information technologies have changed in recent years. For example, all a researcher needs to analyze the public use files of the major surveys conducted by NCHS is access to a personal computer with the appropriate software. Even 15 years ago, this type of analysis capability was not readily available for mainstream health services research.

- A final advantage of the use of data files that are available to the public is that published analyses can be challenged or supported by the results reported by multiple analysts who are using the same data. This adds to the desired transparency of data analysis, ensures quality, and increases confidence in the validity of the results.

The disadvantages of using national data sets are the inevitable limitations in the kinds of data and variables collected; changes in the foci of data collection depending on prevailing policy, which may make longitudinal comparisons more difficult; and the time lapse between data collection and the release of public use data, which often takes more than a year. In addition, the analysis of most nationally representative sample surveys requires a certain level of technical and analytic sophistication. To obtain representative study samples that are still "affordable,"[10] such surveys invariably use complex cluster sampling techniques in which thousands of study participants are enrolled and are sometimes recontacted after several years for panel interviews. The analysis of data from such studies requires the use of statistical techniques that take into account the complex weighting and variance estimation problems associated with cluster sampling designs (Korn & Graubard, 1999; Kneipp & Yarandi, 2002).

---

[9]Recall that the NHIS is not a panel study, which would follow the same individuals over time, allowing for analysis of individual changes. It is a repeated cross-sectional survey that uses different (nationally representative) samples at each data collection time. Such data can be used to track population trends.

---

[10]*Affordable* is a relative term. Data from nationally and regionally representative samples, with thousands of study participants, invariably cost millions of dollars.

Secondary analysis of existing research data necessarily implies a retrospective research approach.[11] Thus, multivariate analyses that attempt to control for a variety of confounding variables are the prevailing approach to analyzing such data. Although it is possible to analyze data obtained from an experiment retrospectively, secondary analysis usually focuses on new questions that were not formulated at the time the data were collected. Thus, experimental studies are usually reanalyzed only if possible errors in the initial analysis are detected. However, secondary analysts sometimes use data from experimental, or intervention, studies and focus on subsidiary issues that involve observational, or nonintervention, variables.

THE USE OF EXISTING MEDICAL AND INSURANCE RECORDS AND OTHER CLINICAL DATA SETS

Different from the secondary analysis of research data, the analysis of clinical data sets is more complicated from a research design point of view. In general, rather than having to accept the research design as a *fait accompli* (as with secondary analysis of past research studies), with clinical data, the researcher still must decide how to use the data within a researcher-chosen study design. In principle, the choice of study designs is still open, and research based on clinical records can be both retrospective and prospective, including even experimental designs. For instance, Lantz et al. (1995) tested the efficacy of physician letters and telephone calls as reminders to improve participation in screening programs for breast and cervical cancer among low-income women. The outcome data for this study were obtained 6 months after the intervention, using medical claim files. However, it is far more common that studies that involve clinical records use a retrospective design. As discussed in chapter 9, clinical records are almost tailor-made for case–control studies, in which researchers attempt to use past patient records to uncover antecedents of current illnesses or conditions.

As with the collection of original data, the use of clinical records involves decisions about the sampling of study participants and the periods for which collected data are assembled. This requires, for example, the development of specific inclusion and exclusion criteria, so that the researcher can decide which observations in the data set belong to the targeted population (Brown, Pedula, & Bakst, 1999). Clinical data are an immensely valuable source of information for researchers because they contain individual-level information on patients' diagnoses, comorbidities, prescribed treatments, visits, compliance, and family and social characteristics. For the recruitment and determination of eligibility of patients, clinical records, such as admission and discharge records, are indispensable in most clinical research, even if it is focused on self-report data (see chapter 19 for more information on practical sampling issues). In addition to recruitment, it is quite common to use clinical records as the source for diagnostic and treatment information and to combine this information with self-report data obtained directly from patients. For example, Given, Given, Azzouz, and Stommel (2001) and Kurtz, Kurtz, Stommel, Given, and Given (2002a, 2002b) used treatment information about surgery, chemotherapy, and radiation therapy obtained from medical record audits as predictors of psychosocial outcome variables (depression, physical functioning), based on self-report interview data. Finally, many studies are based exclusively on the records of clinics, insurance companies, or disease registries. This is a common strategy that is used by health services researchers who use insurance or health maintenance organization (HMO) data to gain access to large numbers of patient records with which to study questions of quality of care (Schneider, Zaslavsky, & Epstein, 2002) or who link disease registries with vital records to study disease outcomes (O'Malley et al., 2002).

VALIDITY CONSIDERATIONS FOR EXISTING DATA

As mentioned earlier, when researchers use existing data, particularly routinely collected clinical data, they must consider a variety of data quality (validity) issues that arise from the fact that the original data collection is not researcher-controlled. These considerations include the following:

- *Completeness.* Records of existing data may be incomplete or missing entirely, particularly in studies in which no in-person contact occurred for data collection. One important problem in the use of medical or patient records is how to interpret the absence of information. Suppose that one record of a patient with diabetes contains information on smoking status or an entry on complaints about sleep disturbances, whereas the record of another patient with diabetes does not. Should the absence of entries about smoking or sleep disturbances be interpreted to mean that the second patient is neither a smoker nor experiences sleep disturbances, or does it mean that the provider did not ask these questions

---

[11]See chapter 11 for more detailed discussion of "retrospective" designs.

during the visit or did not record the answers? In a study with researcher-controlled data collection, such issues can be clarified in advance, and data collectors can be instructed to pose certain questions explicitly. When using existing records, the researcher must at least attempt to learn the organizational rules for data entry and quality control. Although it would seem that standardized recording procedures are likely to enhance the quality of data, this is often true only to a limited extent in clinical settings. For example, in a hospital where nursing staff use a standard protocol to assess pain and administer various types and doses of pain medications based on pain ratings, such data are often missing for patients within a short period after surgery; at other times, entries in patient records are based on inferences in situations in which the patient cannot provide a self-report of the level of pain. When data are missing, the only recourse, other than dropping a case, is the adoption of a procedure for the imputation of missing values (see chapter 16 for an overview and suggested readings).

• *Coding.* The data may or may not be coded in a way that is fully usable for the purposes of a given secondary data analysis, and it may not be possible to retrieve the information that is needed through recoding of the data. This is often the case for the many varieties of medical records that do not make extensive use of standardized measures. For example, a medical record may contain the entry "Hispanic" for the race of an individual, even though the federal category of "Hispanic" refers to an ethnicity that may include any race. Furthermore, diagnostic codes, such as ICD-9 codes, are sometimes used mistakenly because the person entering the code is not sufficiently familiar with the relevant classification system. If trained chart abstractors are used to transcribe the information, such errors can often be corrected based on other information in the record.

• *Accuracy and use of multiple data coders.* If computerized records are not available, the use of "chart abstracters" or staff to collect and code certain existing data from medical records is a common, but expensive, strategy. In addition to the cost involved, this approach poses substantial quality control issues, necessitating great care in the training and monitoring of the chart abstracters. To obtain high-quality data for a complex analysis, the training and monitoring process is usually substantial. It requires extended practice and a formal plan that includes procedures for dealing with ambiguities in coding as well as routine assessments of interrater reliability among the coders.

• *Choice and application of coding categories.* The cod-

ing scheme must be specific enough to yield interpretable categories and to be free of unreasonable ambiguity about what is to be coded; yet, it must also be able to accommodate the need to collapse the likely variety of record entries into fewer categories without "violating" the meaning of the record entries. For example, consider medical record entries that are based only on patient self-report and that *might* indicate the presence of depressive symptoms. Because only a subset of patients would directly report that they feel "depressed," a coding scheme is needed that includes provisions for other types of patient comments that *may* refer to depression. For example, a coding manual for older adults may include as possible indicators of depression phrases such as "nerves" or "no get-up-and-go." A particularly clear example of the occasional ambiguity that occurs in coding unstandardized entries in clinical records is the coding of "fall" events in inpatient settings. Although it seems intuitively obvious that staff members who are recording observations in a medical record would know whether a patient has fallen, in many instances, it remains unclear whether the patient actually fell, sat down on the floor, or had an event that occurred while walking that should "count" as a fall. Another common source of ambiguity in abstracting handwritten clinical records is the handwriting itself. There can be substantial obstacles to the correct interpretation of entries if the handwriting is illegible or if the recording clinician uses abbreviations that are not known to third parties.

• *Reliability.* Problems can occur with the reliability of data recorded in medical records. For example, there may be omissions or errors in the recording of weight, medications and dosages, or chief complaints and patient symptoms. In addition, medical records often include narrative entries from multiple clinicians, including those of different disciplines. Charts, which may contain notes written by nurses, physicians, and social workers, also reflect the differing viewpoints and concerns associated with these professions and the patients' reactions to them. For example, a patient who is admitted to a psychiatric unit after a suicide attempt may report being currently suicidal to one type of health care provider, but not to another. A nurse and a physician who see the same patient within 10 minutes of each other may record different ratings for a patient's current level of pain. Even entries of "simple" measures, such as the weight of a patient recorded in a primary care clinic, may show suspicious volatility over time. In addition, the date of a procedure may be recorded incorrectly. In short, medical and other clinical records, like any other data, are subject to error.

As always, using multiple data sources can help to detect and reduce such errors.

- *Accuracy of computer-based data files*. For some studies that rely on existing data sets, the data already exist as computer files. For data that are collected as part of a research study conducted by an experienced, National Institutes of Health (NIH)-funded researcher, it is often a straightforward process to obtain information from the study investigator about the data management procedures as well as sufficient documentation so that the data can be used for statistical analyses. However, many clinical data sets are not designed for research purposes, and may lack essential features of quality control. For example, data entry into computerized medical or pharmacy records of a health care organization may occur directly in the presence of patients, or staff members may enter the data from paper medical records. In this instance, the computerized records may represent both primary and secondary data, without the analyst necessarily knowing which type of data the records contain. In either instance, such data are collected as part of routine clinical practice, which usually does not entail the use of double-entry procedures to ensure high levels of accuracy.[12] Except for some basic "data cleaning" procedures,[13] the researcher usually must accept the data as they are, because no outside sources are available to check the reliability of most entries. If serious errors are suspected and sufficient funds are available, it may be possible to audit all or a random selection of the paper records that served as the basis for the computer files. However, in most cases, the original records are not available or, at least, not accessible. Finally, the proprietary software that is used for many institutional records may not be designed to produce output files in formats that can be easily analyzed with statistical software. In particular, raw data files in so-called ASCII formats can be read only with the help of code books that sometimes need to be created.

Compared with collecting one's own data, the use of existing data is often advantageous and less resource-intensive. However, analysts of existing data must guard against naïve acceptance of data as more or less error-free, especially if they are already in electronic form. All of the issues of reliability and validity in measurement that researchers must confront when collecting their own data also apply to existing data, except that the data collection procedures can no longer be improved after the fact. However, the basic principle of reliability checking, using multiple information sources, can also apply to the use of existing data.

META-ANALYSIS

Meta-analysis is a method used to summarize and statistically evaluate the *results* of several, and often many, research studies. It should be distinguished from secondary data analysis because it does not usually involve reanalysis of the original data. Meta-analysis goes beyond the traditional narrative literature review, which uses no formal method of weighting different study results based on the quality of the study, sample size, and possible adjustments for confounding variables (Greenland, 1998). For instance, a simple count, such as "seven studies found that reminders sent to patients significantly reduced no-show rates, but three studies did not show such an effect," should not necessarily be taken at face value as a statement of the preponderance of the evidence. In the extreme, suppose the three studies with negative findings are all randomized intervention studies with large study samples and the seven studies with positive findings all rely on small convenience samples without random assignment to control groups. In that case, a simple count of "positive" and "negative" study findings would be highly misleading. Thus, one might question whether there are ways to combine the information from several studies without resorting to an arbitrary weighting system (e.g., 10 points for an experimental design, 4 points for observational design).

There is general agreement that meta-analysis can be an important tool to formalize the evaluation of results from multiple clinical trials (Sacks et al., 1987); however, the use of this technique in combining results from observational studies has been questioned (Shapiro, 1994). A further controversy concerns the use of "standardized effect sizes" as the common metric across the studies, a practice that is common in the social sciences, but not in epidemiology (Greenland, Schlesselman, & Criqui, 1986). Next, we provide a brief description of the uses and assumptions of meta-analysis. The interested should consult the literature for further details.

Basic Principles of Meta-Analysis

Suppose you are interested in obtaining an approximate estimate of the effects of reminders on no-show rates for

---

[12]In NIH-funded studies, the standard for assuring the accuracy of data entry is the double-entry system (or equivalent). This system has become standard for all other types of research, regardless of the funding source or funding status. See chapter 23 for more details.

[13]See chapter 23 for more details.

primary care office visits. In the simplest case, both the outcome and the primary independent variable are dichotomous: an individual patient does or does not show up for the office appointment and he or she did or did not receive a reminder. In that case, the effect size could be modeled as an odds ratio, comparing the odds of being a no-show in the reminder group with the odds of being a no-show in the no-reminder group. Now, suppose you discovered 50 studies that report results that are cast either in terms of odds ratios or in terms of frequency tables that can be converted to such odds ratios.[14] These studies are likely to vary with respect to: (1) sample size, (2) study design, and (3) number and type of control or confounding variables used in the analysis. To begin with the third point mentioned, before the various odds ratio estimates from the different studies can somehow be "thrown together" and "averaged," the meta-analyst would need to determine if the odds ratio in a particular study has been adjusted for known confounding variables. To the extent that this has not been done, results from studies that have controlled for a particular confounding variable may be used to estimate this adjustment effect, which can be applied to the unadjusted effect size estimates.[15]

Assuming that "comparable" effect sizes are available for each of the studies included, the meta-analyst must decide how much evidential weight to give to each of the individual studies. A logical choice to use is the inverse of the standard error of each individual study estimate of the adjusted odds ratio: $1/se_i$.

Recall from chapter 3 that the standard error of a statistic is an estimate of its sampling fluctuation. In other words, if sample estimates of a population parameter vary a great deal from sample to sample, the statistic has a large standard error, indicating the relative lack of precision. Statistics that have relatively small associated standard errors vary less from sample to sample; thus, the estimates are more precise. Using the inverse of the standard error as a weighting factor means that, in the overall estimate of the average effect size, across all studies, more precise estimates have greater weight and less precise estimates have less weight. In chapter 3, it was also noted that the size of a

standard error is, to a considerable degree, influenced by the sample size, with larger study samples producing smaller fluctuations in estimates than smaller samples. Thus, using the inverse of the standard error implicitly gives greater weight to studies with larger samples.

One principal strategy to deal with study design effects (e.g., differences in effect size estimates depending on whether the estimates come from experimental or nonexperimental studies) is to use regression models to predict effect size. Design indicator variables are part of the prediction equation. This way, one can estimate the systematic differences in effect sizes based on the design of the study from which the estimates are derived. Many other technical issues are involved in meta-analysis, for example, what criteria to use for inclusion or exclusion of a study and how to deal with alternative measures of the same concept (e.g., different measures of depression or anxiety). Details are available in the specialized literature. For a lucid application of meta-analysis to the examination of race as a possible predictor, or even cause, of breast cancer mortality, see the study by Newman, Mason, Cote, Vin, Carolin, Bouwman, and Colditz (2002).

►CLINICAL RESEARCH IN ACTION
Examples of Studies Using Secondary Data Analysis
Example 1

Clarke, Frasure-Smith, Lesperance, and Bourassa (2000) published the results of a secondary analysis of data from multisite clinical trials, the Studies of Left Ventricular Dysfunction (SOLVD) Prevention and Treatment Trials. Although the trials were designed to test the efficacy of a particular enzyme inhibitor in patients with low left ventricular ejection fractions, the data also included 1-year follow-up and baseline measures of functional impairment (i.e., ability to perform instrumental activities, such as running errands, driving a car, or participating in social activities such as visiting friends) as well as baseline measures of social and psychological characteristics. In addition, the data included information on clinical diagnoses and comorbid conditions. The secondary analysts relied on the public use data from the clinical trials, but focused on the psychosocial predictors of functional impairment, regardless of the assignment of a patient to the treatment or the placebo group in the original clinical trials. More precisely, treatment versus placebo assignment is treated as one of the control or possible confounding variables. Other confounding variables include clinical attributes, such as left ventricular ejection fraction, the presence of heart failure at baseline evaluation, classification ratings based on the New York Heart Association functional class, and the presence of three comorbid condi-

---

[14]The usual approach to finding such studies would be through electronic literature searches, using CINAHL or MEDLINE, for example. However, in preparation for a meta-analysis, it would also be worthwhile to search for unpublished studies, because of a likely "publication bias" in favor of studies reporting positive results (Greenland, 1998). Some meta-analysis experts take the strong position that unpublished studies should be included, if possible. See chapter 22 for more on literature searches.

[15]Technical details can be found in Greenland (1998).

tions at baseline (i.e., diabetes, chronic obstructive pulmonary disease, stroke). Controlling for these factors as well as for age, the researchers focused on measures of social integration (i.e., marital status and visits from friends or relatives), mood disturbance (using the Profile of Mood States),[16] and socioeconomic status (i.e., education, occupation, minority status) as predictors of functional impairment in instrumental and social activities 1 year after the baseline measures. The analysis is conducted only with the subset of patients who were enrolled at U.S. trial sites (to obtain sufficient numbers of minority participants). Of these patients, a sample of N = 2,993 participated in the 1-year follow-up. It is clear that it would be very difficult to obtain funding for a purely observational study[17] with such a large sample of patients who share a single diagnosis (left ventricular ejection fraction of 35% or less). A secondary analysis of clinical trial data is a cost-effective way to examine the effect and role of psychosocial factors in predicting functional impairment.

Example 2

The research by Simmons, Peterson, and Hale (1999), focusing on the background characteristics of persons who attempted suicide, is an example of a small-scale study based solely on clinical records. These researchers conducted a chart review of 145 persons who presented to the emergency department at the county's only hospital as "suicide attempts" within a 7-month period. Using a template based on previous research, the researchers collected demographic information (i.e., sex, age, occupation), social support information (i.e., availability of social support, living arrangements), and clinical information (i.e., previous suicide attempts and previous counseling) to construct a descriptive profile of the persons who attempted suicide. Despite missing information, especially concerning social support and previous clinical contact, the study clearly shows the promise of using information from charts, accessible in particular clinical settings, to profile population groups at risk for suicide. The study also exemplifies some missed opportunities. Although it is interesting to learn that more than two-thirds of suicide attempts were made by women, more than 40% were made by persons between 10 and 24 years of age, and one-third of the persons were unemployed, this information would be much more informative if placed into the proper comparative perspective. With a little more effort, a descriptive study such as this could be turned into a case–control study. For instance, using county-level population data available from the Census Bureau's web site, one might discover that in the general (nonsuici-

dal) population, say, only 22% are between 10 and 24 years of age. In that case, the odds of being suicidal are roughly 2.4 times higher among young persons between the ages of 10 and 24 years.[18] Similar comparative statements could be made about many other potential risk factors. For instance, to evaluate whether the level of social support (or lack thereof) is a risk factor for persons who attempted suicide, one could compare the charts of patients who made suicide attempts with those of other age- and sex-matched patients who came to the same emergency department. Another way to extend the research of Simmons et al. would be to compare the characteristics of persons who attempted suicide with those of people who "successfully" committed suicide, given that the researchers had data from the coroner's office for the same period. In short, although the use of clinical records for research purposes requires care and effort to check the reliability of records with respect to the information sought, studies based on such records are promising avenues for clinical research and are within the reach of many clinicians.

CONCLUSION

In this chapter, we have introduced and discussed the uses of existing data. Important advantages and challenges are associated with the use of secondary data. Key advantages include:

- Relative cost-effectiveness, either because the data are already collected or because they are being collected as part of an ongoing project
- Access to large population-based records, such as insurance files
- Access to diagnostic and treatment information that is not available through self-reports
- Relative timeliness in obtaining results

Key disadvantages include:

- Limited control or no control over the research design
- Lack of quality control and standardized approaches to data collection
- Occasionally intractable problems with reliability

Nonetheless, analysis of existing data is an attractive option for researchers in nursing and other health-related fields for several reasons: (1) the development of computer

---

[16]The Profile of Mood States (McNair et al., 1971) is a widely used psychosocial instrument in nursing research.

[17]For many years, NIH has emphasized moving behavioral research from observational study designs to intervention studies.

[18]Recall that the odds ratio is a symmetric measure: $(40/60)/(22/78) = (40/22)(60/78) = 2.36$. Given that Simmons et al. (1999) report a county population of about 225,000 residents, the age structure of the total population and that of the nonsuicidal population are virtually identical. For more on odds ratios, see chapter 9.

and information technologies has improved the access to databases; (2) the challenges associated with collecting original data in clinical settings have increased because of concerns about protecting human subjects; and (3) fewer resources are needed to analyze existing data.

In this chapter, we have focused exclusively on the secondary analysis of quantitative data, in part because it constitutes the bulk of secondary analysis. In principle, there is no reason why secondary analysis could not also be conducted with qualitative data (e.g., reanalysis of transcripts from unstructured interviews). However, qualitative researchers usually do not approach data "to test new hypotheses or explore new relationships." In comparison, the purpose of reanalysis or reinterpretation of a narrative text, for example, is more likely to be to confirm the "correctness" of an interpretation. In other words, this type of analysis is more akin to a confirmation of interrater reliability than to secondary analysis. These issues will be discussed in the next chapter.

Suggested Activities

1. Read both of the articles discussed in the Clinical Research in Action section of this chapter. Critique the articles with respect to the discussion of secondary data analysis.
   a. How did the authors address the issue of data quality?
   b. How were the research questions or hypotheses determined in each study?
   c. Which study (if either) could provide better evidence of causal relationships? Justify your rationale with reference to specific aspects of the methods used.
2. Read the article by Newman et al. (2002), which describes a meta-analysis. Identify the key elements of the analysis as discussed in the meta-analysis section of this chapter.

Suggested Readings

Clarke, S. P., Frasure-Smith, N., Lesperance, F., & Bourassa, M. (2000). Psychosocial factors as predictors of functional status at 1 year in patients with left ventricular dysfunction. *Research in Nursing & Health, 23,* 3, 290–300.

Newman, L. A., Mason, J., Cote, D., Vin, Y., Carolin, K., Bouwman, D., & Colditz, G. A. (2002). African-American ethnicity, socioeconomic status, and breast cancer survival: A meta-analysis of 14 studies involving over 10,000 African American and 40,000 White American patients with carcinoma of the breast. *Cancer, 94,* 11, 2844–2854.

Simmons, N., Peterson, J. W., & Hale, C. (1999). Surveillance of suicidal behavior in Kitsap County, Washington: A retrospective study. *Public Health Nursing, 16,* 5, 337–340.

References

Brown, J. B., Pedula, K. L., & Bakst, A. W. (1999). The progressive cost of complications in type 2 diabetes mellitus. *Archives of Internal Medicine, 159,* 1873–1880.

Clarke, S. P., Frasure-Smith, N., Lesperance, F., & Bourassa, M. (2000). Psychosocial factors as predictors of functional status at 1 year in patients with left ventricular dysfunction. *Research in Nursing & Health, 23,* 3, 290–300.

Given, B. A., Given, C. W., Azzouz, F., Stommel, M. (2001). Physical functioning of elderly cancer patients prior to diagnosis and following initial treatment. *Nursing Research, 50,* 4, 222–232.

Greenland, S., Schlesselman, J. J., & Criqui, M. H. (1986). The fallacy of employing standardized regression coefficients and correlations as measures of effect. *American Journal of Epidemiology, 123,* 203–208.

Greenland, S. (1998). Meta-analysis. In Rothman, K. J., & S. Greenland (Eds.), *Modern epidemiology* (pp. 643–673). Philadelphia: Lippincott Williams & Wilkins.

Herron, D. G. (1989). Secondary analysis: Research method for the clinical specialist. *Clinical Nurse Specialist, 3,* 2, 66–69.

Hewitt, M., Devesa, S., & Breen, N. (2002). Papanicolaou test use among reproductive-age women at high risk for cervical cancer: Analyses of the 1995 National Survey of Family Growth. *American Journal of Public Health, 92,* 4, 666–669.

Hulley, S. B., Cummings, S. R., Browner, W. S., Grady, D., Hearst, N., & Newman, T. B. (2001). *Designing clinical research* (2nd ed.). Philadelphia: Lippincott Williams & Wilkins.

Khanh, T. D., Roosa, M. W., Tein, J.-Y., & Lopez, V. A. (2002). The relationship between acculturation and problem behavior proneness in a Hispanic youth sample: A longitudinal mediation model. *Journal of Abnormal Child Psychology, 30,* 3, 295–309.

Kneipp, S. M., & Yarandi, H. N. (2002). Complex sampling designs and statistical issues in secondary analysis. *Western Journal of Nursing Research, 24,* 5, 552–566.

Korn, E. L., & Graubard, B. I. (1999). *Analysis of health surveys.* New York: John Wiley & Sons.

Kurtz, M. E., Kurtz, J. C., Stommel, M., Given, C. W., & Given, B. A. (2002a). Predictors of depressive symptomatology of geriatric patients with colorectal cancer: A longitudinal analysis. *Supportive Cancer Care, 10,* 494–501.

Kurtz, M. E., Kurtz, J. C., Stommel, M., Given, C. W., & Given, B. A. (2002b). Predictors of depressive symptomatology of geriatric patients with lung cancer: A longitudinal analysis. *Psycho-Oncology, 11,* 12–22.

Lantz, P. M., Stencil, D., Lippert, M. T., Beversdorf, S., Jaros, L. and Remington, P. L. (1995). Breast and cervical cancer screening in a low-income managed care sample: The efficacy of physician letters and phone calls. *American Journal of Public Health, 85, 6,* 834–836.

Makuc, D. M., Breen, N., & Freid, V. (1999). Low income, race, and the use of mammography. *Health Services Research, 34,* 1, 229–239.

McNair, D. M., Lorr, M., & Droppleman, L. F. (1971). *Manual for the Profile of Mood States.* San Diego: Education and Industrial Testing Service.

McNair, D. M., Lorr, M., & Droppleman, L. F. (1992). *Ed-ITS manual for the Profile of Mood States.* San Diego: Educational and Industrial Testing Service.

Moriarty, H. J., Deatrick, J. A., Mahon, M. M., Feetham, S. L., Carroll, R. M., Shepard, M. P., & Orsi, A. J. (1999). Issues to consider when choosing and using large national databases for research on families. *Western Journal of Nursing Research, 21,* 2, 143–153.

Newman, L. A., Mason, J., Cote, D., Vin, Y., Carolin, K., Bouwman, D., & Colditz, G. A. (2002). African-American ethnicity, socioeconomic status, and breast cancer survival: A meta-analysis of 14 studies involving over 10,000 African American and 40,000 White American patients with carcinoma of the breast. *Cancer, 94,* 11, 2844–2854.

O'Malley, C. D., Prehn, A. W., Shema, S. J. & Glaser, S. L. (2002). Racial/ethnic differences in survival rates in a population based series of men with breast carcinoma. *Cancer, 94, 11,* 2836–2843.

Orsi, A. J., Grey, M., Mahon, M. M., Moriarty, H. J., Shepard, M. P., & Carroll, R. M. (1999). Conceptual and technical considerations when combing large data sets. *Western Journal of Nursing Research, 21,* 2, 130–142.

Polit, D. F., & Hungler, B. P. (2001). *Nursing research: Principles and methods* (6th ed.). Philadelphia: Lippincott Williams & Wilkins.

Sacks, H. S., Berrier, J., Reitman, D. (1987). Meta-analysis and randomized controlled trials. *The New England Journal of Medicine, 316,* 450–455.

Shapiro, S. (1994). Meta-analysis/shmeta-analysis. *American Journal of Epidemiology, 140,* 771–778.

Schneider, E. C., Zaslavsky, A. M., & Epstein, A. M. (2002). Racial disparities in the quality of care for enrollees in Medicare managed care. *Journal of the American Medical Association, 287,* 10, 1288–1294.

Simmons, N., Peterson, J. W., & Hale, C. (1999). Surveillance of suicidal behavior in Kitsap County, Washington: A retrospective study. *Public Health Nursing, 16,* 5, 337–340.

Stommel, M., Given, B. A., & Given, C. W. (2002). Depression and functional status as predictors of death among cancer patients. *Cancer, 94,* 10, 2719–2727.

Wolinsky, F. D., Krygiel, J., & Wyrwich, K. W. (2002). Hospitalization for prostate cancer among the older men in the longitudinal study on aging, 1984–1991. *Journals of Gerontology, 57A,* 2, M115–M121.

CHAPTER 18 Qualitative Approaches to Data Collection and Interpretation

INTRODUCTION

In this chapter, we focus on approaches to data collection and analysis in qualitative research studies.

As emphasized in chapter 12, qualitative approaches to research constitute a distinct and valuable complementary approach to the quantitative research methods that are more commonly used in nursing and other health-related research. Qualitative and quantitative approaches differ in nontrivial ways with regard to certain philosophic assumptions that have implications for the research methods (design, sampling, measurement, data collection, data analysis) used.[1]

Here, we turn to a review of some of the methods used in qualitative data collection and interpretation, together with some important general considerations for the use of these methods.[2]

Notice that we refer to "data collection and interpretation," not "measurement." Recall that the goal of measurement is to assign numbers to the characteristics and attributes of objects according to a rule system that is, as far as possible, context-free. That is, the measurement procedure is to yield the same results across time, location, and users, as long as the underlying reality remains unchanged. In contrast to the standardized measurement tools that are used in quantitative research studies, qualitative research studies most commonly use less structured, nonstandardized, and reactive methods of data collection that necessitate different approaches to data analysis and the interpretation of study findings.

On the surface, the use of qualitative research methods may appear "easier" than quantitative research methods. First, seemingly little preparation is required to start a qualitative study. There appears to be: (1) no need to worry about the reliability and validity of measurement tools, (2) no need to pilot test the instruments, (3) no need to determine in advance the size of the study sample required, and (4) no need to specify a complex study design in advance. Furthermore, qualitative studies seem to require fewer resources (in time, money, and personnel) because they usually involve smaller numbers of study participants. Also, during the analysis stage, the researcher does not need to rely on the mastery of increasingly sophisticated quantita-

tive statistical procedures and does not necessarily need to acquire the computer skills needed to operate specialized software programs used for quantitative data analysis.[3] In comparison, on the surface, qualitative research may seem much more straightforward.

Real-Life Example: Assumption about Qualitative Research

A number of years ago, one of the authors had a conversation with a fellow graduate student, who was eying (with apparent distaste!) the ever-increasing, many-inches-thick, "quantitative" computer printouts. The author had generated these printouts, which contained the statistical analyses of her dissertation data set (based on more than N = 250 study participants). During the conversation, the fellow student (who had recently started doctoral study) mentioned that she was thinking of using a qualitative (phenomenologic) approach for her dissertation research. As a rationale for her choice of methods, she mentioned the following: (1) it takes more time to recruit and obtain data from the larger samples that are often used in quantitative research, and (2) quantitative research methods are mathematically and statistically more sophisticated; therefore, data analysis would be more difficult than in qualitative research.

There are two misunderstandings encompassed in this rationale. The first is an assumption that research proceeds from the means (i.e., research methods) to the ends (i.e., research problems), rather than the other way around. Instead of focusing on a substantive research problem that is a high priority for research or clinical practice, the problem is defined in terms of the methods that are preferred. The second misconception is the assumption that qualitative research is relatively easy and less time-consuming, an assumption that many well-experienced and respected qualitative researchers know to be far from reality.

As the fellow student soon discovered, there are a variety of methodologic challenges associated with doing high-quality qualitative research. In addition, when study participants report on their "lived experiences," this tends to generate large volumes of narrative text, even in small study samples. Thus, the amount of work needed to properly analyze and interpret the data can far exceed the much more straightforward analysis of numerical data, which is done with standard statistical analysis software. Quantitative research approaches tend to require more work in the earlier stages of research, but are comparatively

---

[1]See chapter 12, Box 12-1, for an overview of the philosophic and methodologic distinctions between qualitative and quantitative research paradigms. A discussion of qualitative sampling designs and associated sampling issues is presented in chapter 21.

[2]A detailed, in-depth discussion of particular qualitative research methods is beyond the scope of this book. Consult the resources included in the list of suggested readings for additional information about particular qualitative research methods. For an excellent basic discussion of the process aspects of doing qualitative research, see Polit and Hungler (1999).

[3]In recent years, qualitative data analysis has been increasingly performed with specialized, computer-based software programs. This trend has followed the realization that computers can be of great help in the development of more rigorous, sophisticated approaches to qualitative data analysis.

less time-consuming in the analysis stage.[4] In contrast to a quantitative research process, in a qualitative study, it often takes substantially longer to analyze the data in a way that produces high-quality results and substantive interpretations of the study findings. For this, and other methodologic reasons that are described later in this chapter, it may actually be more difficult to use qualitative research methods in a rigorous way that will assure valid results. However, if the problem fits the method, the potential benefits of doing qualitative research are also considerable and are often well worth the extra time and effort.

As we discussed in chapter 12, when the research goal is to produce a rich, in-depth understanding of phenomena or concepts, qualitative approaches are indispensable. In such situations, one would not want to rely solely on quantitative approaches.

DATA SOURCES IN QUALITATIVE RESEARCH

In chapter 12, we introduced several qualitative research approaches and briefly discussed the multiplicity of data sources used in this research tradition. In chapter 16, we emphasized that, compared with quantitative research, data collection in qualitative research is relatively flexible, unstructured, and responsive to context.

Data produced through qualitative methods tend to better fit the descriptive research goals of nonexperimental studies, as opposed to the hypothesis testing objectives that are primarily associated with experimental and quasi-experimental study designs. However, within experimental studies, researchers sometimes supplement information on quantitative outcome variables with qualitative observational data.[5] The reason for this is that the information obtained from the use of standardized outcome measures does not always provide a complete picture when evaluating the effects of an intervention. Very often, process evaluations that include detailed descriptive information, for example, about the circumstances under which an intervention is acceptable to people or information about quality-of-life issues, are also an important part of the evaluation

of an intervention. In addition, researchers must remain open to the possibility of unanticipated consequences from interventions. It is in these areas where qualitative data can make valuable contributions to knowledge obtained from clinical interventions. For example, in testing a nursing intervention to foster disease management skills among people who have a chronic health condition, it may be discovered that the intervention works substantially better for some patients, but not for other subgroups of patients. Thus, patients may be interviewed and qualitative data collected to gain a better understanding of the differences in the effects of the intervention.

The sources of qualitative data vary widely, depending on the specific type of research that is done, but most often include the following:

- Narrative text recorded verbatim from unstructured or semistructured one-to-one or group-level (e.g., focus group) interviews
- Field notes and other records based on observations of behavior
- Archival records of various sorts, including written texts (e.g., newspaper articles as well as medical, clinical, and insurance records) and nonnarrative records (e.g., photographs, video and audio records)

Although qualitative data sources include a very broad array of data types and records, many of them could also serve as the basis for quantitative measurement. The basic distinction is that, in quantitative measurement, the goal is to convert existing data, via a coding algorithm, into a numerical data file, which is then analyzed statistically to find or test for relationship patterns among variables. In qualitative research, the primary goal is interpretation of meaning. Thus, it is more common in qualitative research that data are not reduced to numerical formats because numerical data are not directly amenable to the interpretative methods of qualitative analyses.[6] More specifically, "reduction" of the data to numbers is considered unhelpful because the essential meanings of the information may be lost. In line with its emphasis on human motivation and meanings, language, in the form of narrative texts by study participants (transcripts of interviews or verbal interactions) or observational and interpretive notes by observers (field notes), plays a prominent role in qualitative analysis.

---

[4]Statistical analysis performed with modern computers is not more complex and time-consuming when the study sample is large. For example, statistical analyses can be done just as quickly if the sample size is N = 900 instead of N = 250.

[5]In nursing research, it has become more common to include multiple approaches to data collection (quantitative and qualitative).

[6]Many programs for qualitative data analysis rely on textual analysis algorithms that incorporate quantitative analysis strategies for categorized data. These programs can often detect rich patterns that a human could not detect by engaging in interpretive content analysis without the help of computers.

Matching Data Collection with the Research Goals

As in quantitative research, the specific types of data collected in a particular qualitative research study depend on the questions that the research is designed to address as well as on the characteristics of the target population. Consider the following example. When the verbal abilities of members of a special target population are limited, as in the case of persons with severe levels of dementia, observational methods might be preferred over interviews or verbal interactions. However, certain qualitative research traditions tend to rely heavily on particular data collection techniques. For example, for the most part, phenomenologic and hermeneutic inquiry, as well as other closely related types of qualitative research, use unstructured interviews to understand lived experiences. The same can be said about grounded theory and various approaches to content analysis. Ethnographic research of various sorts relies heavily on observation of behavior, although other methods of data collection, such as interviews and the study of cultural symbols or artifacts, may also be used. Historical research emphasizes the analysis of archival records, but may also use interviews as a source of data, such as "first-person" or "survivor" accounts of era-specific living circumstances or historical events. In addition, nonnarrative materials, such as historic artifacts, may also be studied, and the analysis and interpretation of the significance of the materials may be published as part of the research. Like historical research, case studies use a wide variety of data sources, including interviews with key informants, organizational documents, and archival material (Yin, 1994). Although the data used in qualitative research may be gathered separately from individuals or simultaneously from groups of individuals, qualitative researchers, especially those of the ethnographic tradition, display a preference for collecting information in group settings, instead of in sequential one-on-one interviews. This preference reflects the generally greater emphasis on context and naturalistic observations in qualitative research.

USES AND TYPES OF INTERVIEWS

In chapters 11 and 16, we addressed many of the issues involved in conducting interviews, but in those chapters, the general emphasis was on highly structured interviews that use predetermined questions and fixed response categories. Information derived from interviews also plays a central, and sometimes dominant, role in qualitative research, but qualitative researchers generally use less structured interview techniques.

As discussed in chapter 16, interview techniques can be conceptualized along a continuum from very flexible, responsive, and unstructured approaches to predetermined and highly structured techniques. The amount of structure involved in an interview depends not only on the degree to which the questions and answers are fixed and documented in the questionnaire instrument, but also on the rules of execution, which determine how much control the researcher exerts while collecting data in an interview. Factors include the level of standardization of the measures, the sequencing of questions, and the data collection procedures.

Structured Interviews

In chapter 16, we discussed the features of fully (or highly) structured interviews. In this type of interview, the responses to both questions and probes can be converted to numerical categories, and there are a finite number of categories (usually determined *a priori*) into which responses are coded. In structured interviews, the specific categories for coding responses are already known, or predetermined. There are standardized scoring rules, and published psychometric data are often available regarding the reliability and validity of the interview technique for its established purpose.

To better understand the "flavor" of a highly structured interview, it may be useful to review a prominent example of a structured interview for psychiatric diagnostic purposes. See Research Scenario 18-1.

Qualitative Approaches to Interviews

Qualitative researchers tend to have research goals that show the limits of structured interviews. For instance, a structured probe leaves the interviewer in control of the content and form of the interview. Yet, if the goal of the interview is not just to gather a few specific pieces of information, but to understand the point of view of the research participant, the initiative and control over the interview situation must, at least partially, shift to the participant. This can be accomplished only by loosening the interview protocol or, in short, by turning an "interview" into something that more closely resembles a "conversation" or a "dialogue."

In practice, researchers use a large variety of interview techniques to "steer" the interviewee in certain directions, while leaving room for spontaneous redirection by the

DSM-IV

In the Structured Clinical Interview for DSM-IV (SCID-IV), interview responses are mutually and exclusively coded into predetermined categories and a scoring algorithm is used to determine whether the responses are consistent with given psychiatric diagnoses. The SCID-IV (see the general description in First, Spitzer, Gibbon, et al., 1995) is based on criteria for the diagnosis of mental disorders as defined in the *Diagnostic and Statistical Manual of Mental Disorders,* 4th edition (DSM-IV).

This interview also makes use of **structured probes,** which are limited exploratory devices that are used to clarify or obtain additional information about a given interview response by presenting the respondent with fixed choices that can easily be converted to numeric codes. An example of a probe used in the SCID involves the determination of whether a potential somatic symptom of depression, such as weight loss, may be the result of another condition. For example, a probe would be incorporated to find out whether the patient had an acute or chronic illness that could account for weight loss, or if the patient was trying to lose weight. Depending on the patient's response, weight loss would be coded in a way that it either counts or does not count as a symptom in the diagnosis of depression.

interviewee. For our discussion, it is useful to distinguish between **semistructured interviews,** which are more commonly used as exploratory devices in preparation for quantitative research approaches, and **unstructured interview** techniques, which are the preferred method in qualitative research approaches. The **focus group** session is one particular interview format that involves group responses rather than separate individual responses. Its implementation incorporates interview techniques that tend to vary from semistructured to fairly unstructured.

Semistructured Interviews

A semistructured interview includes standard questions that are asked of all study participants throughout a predetermined time for data collection. However, the coding cat-

egories for the responses to the questions are not fixed in advance. Instead, they are derived from the study participants' answers, which are grouped into meaningful categories. With semistructured interviews, data analysis typically occurs after the data are collected, still with the goal of providing a level of standardization to the analysis of responses to the questions that are asked of all participants. In contrast, in some qualitative research approaches, preliminary judgments and analysis take place concurrently with data collection. These judgments inform decisions about subsequent data collection.

Semistructured interview approaches to data collection are used in many nursing research studies in which the goal is to explore or describe a phenomenon or concept that is not yet well defined theoretically. Probes in semistructured interviews may take the form of very general questions, such as, "Could you tell me more about that?" However, in some cases, the probes may be more specific, such as, "Were you trying to lose weight, or did any physical illness cause you to lose weight?" However, unlike with a structured probe, study participants usually are not asked to choose from among a set of fixed responses. Consequently, psychometric evaluation of the reliability and validity of a semistructured interview is more difficult because the responses of different study participants must be cast into a standard format. However, interrater reliability estimates can be computed for the coders, or raters, who group the responses into categories for analysis. Research Scenario 18-2 gives an example of a semistructured interview.

Focus Group Interviews

Focus group interviews have become an increasingly popular form of qualitative group interview in health care research.[7] For this technique of data collection, study participants meet in small groups, typically 6 to 12 people, to discuss a series of predetermined "focus" questions that are provided by the researcher. Unlike questions in semistructured interviews, which can be quite specific, questions used in focus groups usually orient the discussion toward a particular topic of interest to the researcher. Focus group members are chosen primarily because they are believed by the researcher to have some specialized knowledge or expertise that is relevant to the topic. In other words, group members are usually viewed as **key informants.**

Focus Group Procedures. Procedurally, focus groups depart from the usual interview format, which divides the interacting parties into two groups: those who ask ques-

---

[7]Focus group interviews were originally pioneered by sociologists, but are now widely used in marketing research. See Morgan (1988) for more detail.

Mental Health and Allergies

An example of a semistructured interview can be found in Wills (1997). In this study, people who experienced mental health problems, especially depression and anxiety, were compared with people who had allergies or asthma to determine to what extent the two groups differed in terms of the factors they considered when making decisions about accepting medications for treatment. All study participants were asked a standard set of questions, and standardized probes were used to further explore their responses. However, coding categories for the responses were not known *a priori* and were derived from the interview data. Responses to questions were coded with a global (binary) coding scheme, for example, whether particular considerations were mentioned versus not mentioned. As part of the data analysis plan, the interrater reliability of the coding scheme was established as well as the predictive validity of the questions for assessing personal values and the likelihood of medication use.

tions (interviewers) and those who answer them (respondents). Instead, the pivotal characteristic of focus group "interviews" is that the researcher relies on the interaction among group members as a mechanism to illuminate the topic. Thus, the role of the interviewer is transformed into that of a **moderator.** One of the functions of the moderator is to keep the group discussion on the focus questions and to avoid unrelated conversational tangents. An additional observer from the research team may also be present, and is usually seated outside, but near, the group, to record notes on the behaviors and interactions in the focus group. Focus group sessions vary in length, depending on the characteristics of the group members and the focus questions. The sessions are usually audiotaped and may sometimes be videotaped, depending on the purposes of the research. Transcripts of the discussions that occur during the sessions are the main data that are generated by the focus groups.

The focus questions are used to define and delineate a predetermined topic. The purpose of these questions is to initiate group discussions and elicit in-depth information from the focus group participants. As long as group membership is balanced, in the sense that no single group member dominates the discussion, group interaction can foster a sense of openness that is sometimes harder to achieve in a one-on-one interview situation, in which individuals tend to feel "put on the spot" (Morgan, 1988). In addition, the ideas and contributions of various group members usually stimulate other members to explore a topic further than they would outside the group context. Compared with the traditional interviewer role, the moderator exercises much less control over the situation. This is desirable when the main research purpose is to elicit new and unanticipated information. However, occasionally, a moderator may need to display considerable skill and ingenuity in dealing with "unruly" or "domineering" group members, who can easily turn the advantages of group interaction into a liability.

Focus groups are used as an exploratory technique for topics about which relatively little is known. For example, they have been used as an initial step in the design of a survey instrument to generate ideas about the relevant conceptual dimensions of a broad theoretic concept (Collins, Stommel, & King, 1991). Focus groups may also be used as part of a process evaluation for a clinical nursing intervention or as an instrument of validation of study results that have been obtained previously through a quantitative survey. For example, a subset of study participants, who participated in two variations of an experimental intervention and rated the intervention as "highly effective" on a numerical rating scale, may be interviewed in focus groups to assess their views of the effectiveness of the interventions, including the specific reasons for rating the interventions as "highly effective."

Focus groups are most often constituted by the researcher, and often occur in a setting of the researcher's choice. However, in many types of community-based research, the researcher gathers information in advance about the best meeting locations for the study participants. Researchers must consider the implications of choosing a particular setting or settings for their focus group sessions. Depending on the target populations, the selected study participants may feel uncomfortable in certain settings. For example, people who are experiencing serious mental illnesses may wish to avoid meeting in public locations because they are concerned about the stigma they may incur if seen by others. Likewise, in a study of barriers to the use of clean needles among people who use illicit drugs, certain locations (e.g., a school, a church) may not necessarily be a good choice for a focus group meeting. Other barriers to the use of certain meeting locations, such as transportation issues, should also be carefully assessed in advance.

Focus Group Composition. The selection of focus group members requires careful decisions to optimize the usefulness of the focus group. In general, if a researcher wants to foster free-flowing discussions, it is best to assemble a fairly homogeneous group (Morgan, 1988). For instance, a group that includes people with widely varying levels of education (e.g., less than high school to graduate degrees) may be dominated by the more verbal group members (who are likely to be those with higher levels of education). Thus, if the target population for the focus group interviews is caregivers of patients with dementia, it may be useful to set up several focus groups, each relatively homogeneous with respect to educational level. Similar issues may arise concerning the sex or age composition of focus groups.

Given the usual size of focus groups, they can never be considered fully representative of a larger target population. Thus, from a sampling point of view, selection bias probably cannot be avoided.[8] In addition, the need for more or less homogeneous discussion groups is incompatible with the requirements of generalizability because the latter would usually require a rather diverse group membership.[9] Although obtaining a "representative" sample of a target population is not a useful goal in focus group research, the recruitment of study participants is usually based on theoretic and practical considerations. For example, a researcher may decide to constitute caregiver focus groups, deliberately selecting group members only from among spouse caregivers or child caregivers. Such a selection would be justified, given the substantial evidence in the literature that these two groups of caregivers face different sets of problems (Kahana, Biegel, & Wykle, 1994).

There is a consensus in the literature that, for most purposes, groups of 6 to 10 members are optimal (Morgan, 1988; Stewart & Shamdasani, 1990). Smaller groups usually run the risk of not being able to sustain an extended discussion on a given topic, in part, because these discussions demand too large a contribution from each member, especially if they continue for 1 or even 2 hours. On the other hand, when groups have more than 10 members, there is a tendency for some members to "hide," or for subgroups" or "parties" to emerge that may complicate discussions.

Strengths and Weaknesses of Focus Group Research. To summarize, focus group research has distinct advantages and limitations.

The advantages include:

- Focus groups are an efficient tool for exploring a topic.
- Although the moderator determines the "focus," focus groups allow for a considerable degree of group direction and member-volunteered information. Compared with the role and influence of the interviewer, the moderator is less involved in guiding the responses of study participants.
- Data emerge from a synergistic group process that gives group members a chance to prompt or enhance their own thinking on the subject in response to other group members' contributions.
- Researchers can support their interpretation of the focus group data with ancillary observations obtained, and possibly videotaped, during the group sessions.
- Data obtained with the use of focus groups are often rich and may provide excellent "food for thought" for future research, as in the case of instrument development.
- Focus groups are a flexible mechanism for data collection, and they are appropriate for addressing a wide variety of topics.

Potential and actual limitations of focus groups include:

- Because of the small size of focus groups and the nature of group member selection, the findings typically cannot be generalized to larger target populations.
- Group processes and interactions may have undesirable effects, such as domination by one member or "shutting down" of group members in response to the behavior of other participants.
- As with all narrative transcripts of unstructured interviews, the data generated in focus group sessions may be extensive and challenging to interpret, classify, or code into distinct **themes,** or key issues.
- Some group members may be reluctant to reveal their "true" opinions in a group context, especially if they are concerned that others in the group do not share their opinions.

Additional information, especially about the practical steps involved in conducting focus groups, can be found in Morgan (1988) and Stewart and Shamdasani (1990).

Unstructured Interviews

As the name suggests, the *unstructured interview* is the least planned, most flexible interview procedure. Such interviews do not use closed-ended response formats, nor do they even use a standard set of questions. To place qualitative methods along the dimension of how much of the data generated are volunteered by the study subjects as opposed to being re-

---

[8]Issues of selection bias and sampling principles are discussed in chapters 19 through 21.

[9]Recall the discussion in chapters 4 and 5 of the tradeoff between design (internal) validity and generalizability.

quested by the researcher, unstructured interviews clearly tend toward the *volunteer* end of this dimension.[10] In the extreme, not even the topic of the conversation is fully determined by the researcher. In such cases, a researcher might enter the interview situation with a broad "agenda" or with a set of "objectives," but he or she would be willing to change the topic in response to the comments and preferences of the study participant. This situation creates an interesting tension. Researchers usually initiate the talk with the study participants because they want to know something specific about or from the persons involved. At the very least, researchers enter the interview situation with a "mental map" that defines their objectives based on the original focus of the research problem. Thus, they cannot truly give up all control over the content of a conversation; otherwise, a discussion about the role of a caregiver might, for instance, turn into a talk about gambling or music, if those are the topics that interest the study participants. Thus, although researchers strive to maintain a conversational style in unstructured interviews, these interviews are still forms of communication that are directed by a researcher who is interested in obtaining certain information. In keeping with the general intent to reduce the researcher's control over the interview situation, unstructured interviews preferably take place in settings that are familiar to the interview subjects. Likewise, within very broad limits, the length of unstructured interviews can vary substantially among study participants because the participant's personality, volubility, or laconism shapes the content of the interview.

Studies in the phenomenologic tradition of qualitative research rely most heavily on unstructured interview approaches for data collection. In all phenomenologic studies, the main concern is understanding the lived experiences of the study participants. In keeping with the philosophic assumptions underpinning this type of qualitative research, when gathering data, the phenomenologic researcher wishes to avoid imposing a certain reality (of many possible co-constructed realities) on the study participant. In this view, the unstructured process of interviewing is thought to be necessary to allow for maximal flexibility in exploring a person's subjective experience. The use of any prestructured categories (preconceptions) is viewed as potentially hindering the process of evolving, co-created meaning that occurs within the context of the interview. See Research Scenario 18-3.

This type of interview process has two potential strengths. One is the hope that study participants are more

RESEARCH SCENARIO 18.3

Living with a Urinary Catheter

An example of an unstructured interview process can be found in Wilde's (2002) study of the experience of living with a urinary catheter. Interviews began with questions about the experience of using a urinary catheter, its effect on daily activities, and participants' views of the catheter in relation to themselves. These questions provided the "map" for the interview process, incorporating the broad objectives for the study. Additional interview questions were then derived from the ongoing analysis and reflection of the data, with a goal of clarifying and elaborating on the basis of interpretations of the initial interview.*

*Additional details about the methods of this study are discussed in the last section of this chapter, "Clinical Nursing Research in Action: Examples of Qualitative Research Studies."

likely to "reveal" themselves in unstructured interviews, providing "unfiltered" personal views of their experiences. In unstructured interviews, study participants are not asked to rely on, or even accept, the language conventions and categorizations provided by the researcher. This point goes beyond the strategies discussed in chapter 16 for arriving at closed-ended response categories that do not feel "forced" to the respondents and that reflect the prevailing range of views and opinions in the target population. Some qualitative researchers would argue that the use of any set of predetermined questions, even if derived after extensive pretesting with members of the target population, imposes explicit preconceptions. Thus, only an approach that allows interview participants to use their own language should be viewed as a "bias-free" account of their experiences.

The second strength of an unstructured interview is its potential to provide a rich, highly specific perspective of experience. Much more than any structured interview, unstructured interviews, at least in the hands of a skilled interviewer, can often provide information on the "contextual flavor" of experiences. In contrast, the "artificial" constraints imposed by the responses to a researcher-determined interview protocol are viewed as reductionistic.

There are counterarguments to a strong position that alleges "bias" in more structured approaches to interviews. When researchers summarize and interpret the narrative

---

[10]This classification was originally proposed by Becker (1958).

transcripts from unstructured interviews, when they abstract "themes" and code the material into "categories," they inevitably impose a conceptual framework, or at least emphasize some, but not other, conceptual themes that "strike them" as more important. As mentioned earlier, it is inevitable that researchers have preconceptions and personal biases. In our view, scientific objectivity cannot be based solely on the efforts of individual scientists to purge their minds of preconceptions, but it is supported through the openness of the process of discussion and the replicability of study results. This idea underscores the importance of using well-established outside or external peer review mechanisms for the review of research, including data collection, analysis, and interpretation of research findings. In qualitative studies, for example, a key standard for data quality rests on the ability of another person or researcher to arrive at the same substantive interpretation of a data set as the first researcher.

Although unstructured interviews can yield substantial benefits for research, as we will discuss below, a central challenge to obtaining the potential benefits of less structured approaches is the establishment and assessment of criteria for data quality. As with any other type of research, researchers are (and must be) centrally concerned with whether they are reporting the "truth" in their results and in the interpretation of the results.

FIELD NOTES

Researchers in the ethnographic tradition are less wedded to the exclusive analysis and interpretation of narrative texts that represent literal transcripts of unstructured interviews or dialogues. Instead, their primary source of data is the field notes that contain accounts of their research conducted in naturalistic settings. Ethnographic research is observational in the sense that anything that can be observed, watched, or listened to may be recorded by the researcher in the field notes. Although field notes often contain short characteristic remarks or statements by the study participants, the notes typically are not extended transcripts of long conversations. Instead, they contain the following:

- Descriptions of persons in the observed setting. These descriptions may include their physical appearance, manner of speaking, social background (if revealed), style of interacting, or anything that can be used to provide insights into the study participants.
- Short quotations or verbal exchanges that are meant to indicate the "language," "flavor," or "tone" of verbal communications in a particular setting. Because these

quotations are usually filtered through the observer's memory, they are not always literal quotations, unlike, for example, transcripts of audiotapes.
- Descriptions of the physical setting itself. Such descriptions are meant to illuminate the context of the social interactions that are described. For instance, the layout of a physical setting may favor some types of communication and hinder others (e.g., when different groups of workers are divided by a glass wall).
- Descriptions of events, activities, and interaction patterns that occur in the setting. For instance, in a work setting, an observer might notice who talks with whom or who avoids whom, and how these interaction patterns promote or impede the workflow.

Composing field notes that are truthful reflections of the events and actions observed is difficult and requires practice. In many situations, it is not possible to take notes while the action takes place. In that case, notes must be written from memory. Depending on the setting observed, say, a busy emergency department, even within a half hour of observation, there is likely to be enough material to fill 20 to 30 pages. Even if it is possible to take notes while observing, the occasional "onrush" of events and happenings will force the note taker to be selective. Field researchers must experiment to find out how long they can observe a setting and still be able to recall detailed events. The field notes should be composed as soon as possible after the observations take place. The observer should write the field notes before he or she has any discussions with other persons that might influence his or her perceptions (Hammersley & Atkinson, 1995).

Field notes are composed on several levels, traditionally denoted as **observational notes, theoretic notes, methodologic notes,** and **personal notes.** The following remarks and examples are intended only to convey the "flavor" of these different levels of note-taking. For extended discussions, see the literature (Fetterman, 1998; Atkinson, Coffey, Delamont, Lofland, & Lofland, 2001).

Observational Notes

Observational notes are attempts to describe people, events, or interactions in neutral language that adheres to observable details. For example, observational notes describing an afternoon in an emergency department may contain descriptive sentences and sentence fragments like these: "slow day at the emergency department, with four nurses working the shift," "several instances of patients not recognizing their names when announced over the loudspeaker," "when asked about the bruises on her arms and shoulders, the patient appeared to make up a far-fetched story of how a saucepan fell out of her kitchen cabinet and hit her," and so forth. Although all of the examples describe events and occurrences that can be observed, it is clear that observational notes cannot be completely divorced from interpretive inferences. For example, a statement such as "an excited patient approached the counter" both describes the event and contains an inference about an emotional state that is not directly observable.

Theoretic Notes

Theoretic notes represent the first deliberate attempts at conjecture about the larger meaning of particular events. For instance, the notes might elaborate on an observation like this one: "The work relations among the personnel are friendly, but not smooth. There are frequent requests for clarification, questions about where equipment is stored or what papers to fill out, etc. Is this a sign of frequent turnover among personnel?"

Methodologic Notes

Methodologic notes are often written in the form of reminders to the observer to follow up on an observed pattern. They may also contain comments about successful and unsuccessful approaches to the fieldwork. For instance, after the conjecture cited in the previous example of a theoretic note, the field notes may contain the following reminder: "Examine staffing patterns over the last month." A methodologic note may also contain a warning such as: "Whenever Dr. X enters the floor, fade into the background. He obviously resents my being there and induces others to put up their guard. Better that he doesn't see me."

Personal Notes

Personal notes contain reflections and comments about personal and emotional reactions to the fieldwork. Personal notes can be considered a special type of methodologic note because their purpose is to clarify to the observer how his or her reactions influence and possibly bias the observations and their interpretation. For example, a personal note may read like this: "I never could stand watching people in pain, especially children. When the orthopedist pulled the broken leg of a 6-year-old boy to reset it, all I saw was the boy writhing in pain, and I forgot about everybody else in the room."

As these examples show, field notes cannot claim to be "raw data" in the same sense as audio or video records.

They are descriptions of events from the point of view of the observer. Although several observers may watch or listen to audio and video records or compare their transcripts independently, field notes are the only record that is left after the observed events have passed. No other method of data collection requires the researcher to place this much trust in a single observer. This raises the question of how to ensure and evaluate the quality of the data.

CRITERIA FOR DATA QUALITY: CONFIRMABILITY, DEPENDABILITY, CREDIBILITY, AND TRANSFERABILITY

As mentioned earlier, one of the most important methodologic challenges for qualitative research concerns the criteria used to evaluate the quality of the data obtained. Particularly for the less structured types of qualitative research, reliability and validity standards have often been challenged by the research community as less than rigorous. This issue is further complicated by the difficulty involved in describing complex research procedures in a way that makes the data collection methods as well as data analysis and interpretation fully "transparent" to others. In part, the lack of procedural description in published reports results from the frequent need to streamline the report of an entire study (including background, methods, results, and interpretation of results) to approximately 15 pages of typewritten text,[11] for the purposes of publishing the research in a journal. Thus, devoting substantial space to the description of procedures may reduce the presentation of results so much that the central goal (i.e., presenting rich, detailed, holistic data that come close to capturing the essence of the lived experience of study participants) is jeopardized.

In contrast with quantitative data analysis, qualitative data analysis has fewer conventions and less standardized steps for interpretation. Although qualitative researchers use many different types of research approaches, including many specific procedures for analyzing data (Crabtree & Miller, 1992), a defining feature of most qualitative research is that data collection, analysis, and interpretation usually occur simultaneously, or at least within very close time frames. Thus, collection of data and interpretation of the findings are often closely intertwined.

In contrast, with the quantitative approach, the measurement and interpretation of data are viewed as quite separable processes. Testing of measurement instruments

---

[11]Depending on the specific requirements of a particular journal, the acceptable page length of a manuscript submitted for review for publication may be either less than or more than 15 pages, but would rarely exceed 30 pages.

occurs independently, followed by data collection, which is followed by data analysis. By quantitative standards, the intertwining of measurement and interpretation is problematic because it does not provide adequate control of the measurement process. Yet, many qualitative researchers see a great deal of "control" or "structure" as counterproductive, given their research goals of producing context-rich descriptions.

In other chapters, we mentioned that a key standard or convention for judging the quality of research methods and the validity of research results is *replicability*. Replicability, as a criterion for data quality, means that the readers of a research report should expect to see enough information about the data collection methods and study design so that these methods could be used again (replicated) in a similar study.[12] Such information is an essential element that allows researchers to broaden the generalizability of study results to other target populations that were not part of the original study, to refine the findings by exploring the conditions under which they hold, and to challenge findings as "flukes" if they cannot be replicated by any other researcher.

In contrast, many types of qualitative research have been viewed as inherently nonreplicable.[13] Thus, some qualitative researchers have proposed other criteria for gauging the quality of their data, although this position is somewhat controversial among researchers. For example, some researchers believe that replicability is an absolute standard that should apply to all types of research studies, in all branches of science, because it is the only means for other researchers to know if the methods used worked in a given study and if the results can be confirmed in other studies. Nonetheless, four other criteria or standards proposed by Lincoln and Guba (1985) are now widely referred to and used to assess qualitative data quality: (1) confirmability, (2) dependability, (3) transferability, and (4) credibility.

Confirmability

One standard for data quality in qualitative studies is **confirmability.** Confirmability is conceptually similar to interrater reliability assessment that is used in quantitative research studies. The goal of confirmability assessment is to determine whether two or more researchers can agree on the decisions made during the study on what data to collect and how to interpret the data, including the implications or relevance of the study findings for a practice field, such as nursing. Qualitative researchers seek to establish confirmability through the use of **audit trails,** in which approaches to data collection, decisions about what data to collect, and decisions about the interpretation of data are carefully documented, so that another knowledgeable researcher can arrive at the same conclusions about the data as the primary researcher. The construction of an audit trail for a qualitative research study is not much different from the standard procedures followed in a quantitative study, in which all information, key decisions, and associated rationales are tracked and carefully recorded throughout all stages of the research process. Carefully documented audit trails provide important context for data analysis and interpretation, and are essential for the protection of human subjects, as required by institutional review boards (see chapter 24).

Dependability

A second standard for assessing the quality of qualitative data is **dependability.** Dependability is most conceptually similar to the concept of test–retest and internal consistency reliability in quantitative research approaches, and refers to how stable or unstable the data patterns tend to be over time or occasions. In some qualitative studies, a technique called **stepwise replication** is used to assess the internal consistency of the data. For example, a researcher may have another researcher or a consultant do some independent data collection and analysis for a portion of the data. The data and analyses are then checked for comparability and similarity, and discrepancies are resolved. Two different researchers might gather data at two different times, comparing the results in a way that is similar to the procedure for stepwise replication. Just as with quantitative research approaches, however, it is very important for the researcher to consider in advance what types of data are likely to remain stable versus less stable over the course of the study, as a function of the nature of the phenomena themselves. For example, the lived experience of pain, as reported by people who are recovering from a selected surgical procedure, may vary considerably, depending on the time that elapses between the surgery and the interview.

Transferability

A third standard for assessing the quality of qualitative data is **transferability.** Transferability is conceptually similar to generalizability (external validity) in quantitative stud-

---

[12]Because of the usual space limitations in professional journals, not all of the information necessary for study replication may be reported, but one would expect the authors to provide whatever additional information is needed for credible replication.

[13]Often, the price of flexibility is that the study methods cannot be repeated, even if they are explicitly recorded.

ies, which refers to the extent to which findings can be generalized to other situations and target populations. **Thick description,** a very detailed description of the nature of the study participants, their reported experiences, and the researcher's observations during the study, is used to provide sufficiently detailed information on the study, such that interested others could gauge the extent to which the findings might apply in another population or setting.

Credibility

A final standard for judging the quality of qualitative data is **credibility.** Credibility standards involve performing specific activities that increase the trustworthiness of the reported findings. Lincoln and Guba (1985) described specific procedures for aiding the believability of qualitative research findings. These include: (1) prolonged engagement and persistent observation, (2) peer debriefing, (3) member checks, and (4) triangulation techniques. **Prolonged engagement** is the researcher's substantial level of immersion in the research process, such that the researcher becomes truly engaged with the research, establishes valid and meaningful relationships with study participants, and is open to the deeper meanings that unfold during the process of research. Although this is an important issue for the researcher, there is no way for a *reader* of a study to know if the researcher's engagement was sufficiently prolonged and if his or her observations were persistent enough. **Peer debriefing** is the interaction of the researcher with others who are experienced in the research methods used (e.g., research colleagues, consultants for the study) and provide guidance for research design, data collection, and data analysis. Peer debriefing could be regarded as concurrent confirmability because it involves the review and creation of a consensus about how to proceed. **Member checking** is a process in which the researcher invites study participants to review, add to, or otherwise revise transcripts of their study responses, or to correct the researcher's interpretation of the meaning of the data. This process of external validation greatly enhances the credibility of a researcher's interpretations. It can be considered akin to pilot testing of quantitative instruments with members of the target population (see chapter 16). **Triangulation** is the use of multiple data sources to examine and validate conclusions about meanings. It contains elements of journalistic standards for verifying stories using additional sources of information. It can also refer to a strategy in which multiple researchers examine the data set separately from each other to validate or provide alternative interpretations of the study results.

▶CLINICAL RESEARCH IN ACTION
Examples of Qualitative Research Studies
Example 1

In 2002, Wilde published a report of a phenomenologic study of the lived experience of living with a urinary catheter. The study was funded by a National Research Service Award granted by the National Institute of Nursing Research. The main goal of the study was to address the question: "What is it like to live with a long-term indwelling urinary catheter?" (p. 14). The problem was justified as clinically significant and in need of study, because of the anticipated increase in urinary catheter use as well as the dearth of information about patients' instrumental and coping skills for managing long-term use of a catheter. Increased catheter use was assumed to occur as a result of aging of the population; this population is expected to grow over the next few decades. Relevant literature was reviewed and showed that catheter use may cause coping problems for patients (e.g., skills deficits in knowing how to manage catheter care, social stigma, sexual issues). Nurses' need to recognize the substantial effect of catheter use on patients was also discussed as well as how the knowledge obtained through the study could improve nursing care.

A phenomenologic approach to studying the research question was chosen to ". . . uncover the hidden dimensions in the lived experience of urinary catheterization, experiences not easily accessible to conscious awareness" (p. 16). The rationale for not using structured interviews or surveys to obtain information for the study was based on the assumption that people would not be able to self-report experiences that they did not consciously recognize. The researcher stated that, "A phenomenologic approach, on the other hand, brings everyday knowledge to conscious awareness for examination and interpretation." This rationale for the use of a phenomenologic approach could be criticized on the basis that any type of interview approach, structured or unstructured, relies on self-reporting by the study participant. Thus, the deeper claim here—that a phenomenologic interview approach would be able to coax information from study participants that they are not fully aware of—would need to be substantiated. That is, because both unstructured phenomenologic and structured quantitative approaches to interviews depend on self-report data gathered from study participants, claims that either approach can bring barely conscious experiences to the level of conscious awareness would require supporting evidence.

For this study, a sample of N = 14 participants was selected through a purposive sampling technique.[14] The philosophic and methodologic features of a particular type of phenomenologic research (Merlau-Ponty, 1967 & van Manen, 1997) were discussed as the foundation for the methods used in the study. The author described general steps in the

---

[14]Sampling design and sampling issues will be discussed in further detail in chapter 21.

data collection process, including starting with thinking carefully about her own experiences with urinary catheters in preparation for interviewing the study participants. The one-to-one interviews with study participants were audiotaped in the participants' homes. Some general aspects of the interview process were described, such as the use of a "short interview schedule" and some preset questions (e.g., what the patient experienced in relation to catheter use). The interview procedure included encouragement of the participants ". . . to do most of the talking and to tell what the experience was like in their own words" (p. 17). Seven study participants were interviewed a second time, to ". . . clarify and expand on ideas that were emerging through analysis of the data" (p. 17). This could be viewed as evidence of credibility in terms of prolonged engagement and persistent observation of the data. The author analyzed the data, and two other "experienced qualitative nurse researchers" reviewed portions of the transcripts and provided methodologic support. This could be interpreted as evidence of support for dependability of the data analysis, and also as evidence of credibility, in terms of peer debriefing. A qualitative data software program (MARTIN) was used to "manage" data, but specifically how the data were analyzed, with the program or otherwise, is not fully explained. The author indicated that, "an interactive process was used to create an internal dialogue between me and the text from interviews." Furthermore, the author used examples of quotes from patients to illustrate the "embodied knowledge about urine flow" that was uncovered, in addition to the specific vulnerabilities of the patient related to "urine flow." The information presented in the article about data collection and analysis was somewhat general, possibly due, at least in part, to length restrictions for the article. In this context, evidence for overall confirmability of the study was somewhat limited.

The author did, however, attempt to enhance the credibility of the interpretations through member checking (i.e., the author restated what she had heard to the study participants during the interviews, and a few participants also read the summaries of the written transcripts). However, it is notable that most of the study participants declined to read the text of their interviews because of "poor eyesight or lack of interest." Still, the participants did, ". . . answer questions about subject matter and clarified what was not clear from the transcripts" (p. 19).

The main finding of the study was that, "Living with a urinary catheter was found to be like living with the forces of flowing water" (p. 19). The discussion section provided detailed information about key themes for the negative impact of mishaps with urinary catheters, drawing specific examples from participants' stories. Implications for nursing were presented, including the need to provide patients with guidance for living with catheters (e.g., the sensations and experiences that may occur in association with catheter use). In terms of the transferability criterion for quality assessment of the data, the level of description in the article was quite "thick," such that others could understand a fair amount about the participants who made up the study sample. This aspect of the study report addressed the transferability aspect of qualitative data quality.

Example 2

Dallas and Chen (1998) used a descriptive focus group approach to describe the lived experience of fatherhood among five African American adolescent fathers. The goal of the study was to ". . . describe unmarried, low-income, African American adolescent fathers' lived experience of fatherhood" (p. 211). The need for the study was justified on the basis of the claim that little is known about the experience of fatherhood among African American adolescents. The clinical significance of adolescent fatherhood experiences was not well elaborated or justified in the background section of the article, but the authors did cite a study in which, ". . . pregnant African American adolescents who cited their babies' fathers as important sources of support demonstrated strong fetal attachment" (p. 211). The use of a qualitative naturalistic inquiry approach to the research was justified on the basis of the flexibility of the design in promoting, "...indepth descriptions of the phenomena of interest" (p. 212). The use of a focus group was justified on the basis of the efficiency of data collection and the use of an adolescent sample, in which a sensitive topic was discussed.

Procedurally, two separate focus groups were conducted, with N = 2 and N = 3 adolescent fathers, respectively, because the researchers were unable to schedule all five fathers for a focus group at the same time. The sample size for focus groups in this study is quite small,[15] and the authors indicated that they had difficulty recruiting study participants. The authors stated that, "A prepared question route drawn from research literature on African American adolescent fathers elicited the participants' perceptions concerning their paternal behaviors" (p. 213). It was also noted in the article that the first author conducted the focus groups and was trained in focus group techniques. The focus group sessions were audiotaped, and the researcher transcribed and analyzed the data from the transcripts. In addition, the researcher who moderated the focus groups, ". . . wrote brief descriptive summaries that included thoughts and feelings about the focus group interviews, descriptions of the participants, and sketches of the seating arrangements" (p. 213). This information was used as part of an audit trail in support of the confirmability of the study findings, but the use of the information in data analysis was not explicitly addressed. The use of member checking was not reported for this study. Overall, the confirmability of the study data was low, based on the limited description of the methods in the article.[16]

With regard to data analysis, the article reported that data reduction, display, and conclusion drawing occurred,

---

[15]As noted earlier, focus groups usually include 6 to 10 individuals, and sometimes more.

[16]See also the note about limitations to the length of manuscripts in the description of the Wilde (2002) study as a possible factor in the brevity of descriptions of study methods.

and nine predetermined behavioral domains that were identified by the authors in an earlier research project served as the basis for initial coding of transcripts. A computer software program (Ethnograph) was used to, ". . . add codes and retrieve text-based data" (p. 213). Although the description of the study methods was quite brief, it appears that the authors used a semistructured process for data collection and analysis. Some structure was provided by the use of standard questions for the focus groups as well as the use of predetermined coding categories for data analysis. Control was also provided through the use of a computer program for assistance with coding and data reduction as well as the recoding of transcripts until *intrarater* reliability reached 94% to 100% for coding. A potential limitation of the methods of this study was the lack of peer debriefing or *interrater* assessments for data coding (i.e., the article provided limited evidence of confirmability and dependability in the coding and analysis of study findings).

The main results of the study were organized according to seven key themes that emerged from the data analysis:

1. Barriers to fatherhood
2. Value of fatherhood
3. Transition to fatherhood
4. Competencies of fatherhood
5. Role-set relationships
6. Social norms of fatherhood
7. Father–child contact

Each theme was described in detail in the results section of the article. The authors provided "thick" descriptions of defining attributes, descriptions of what the fathers did and did not discuss in the focus groups, and quotes from the fathers that were illustrative of the themes. The in-depth descriptions of the themes are a strength of this article, providing evidence of consideration of transferability issues.

The discussion section of the article provided commentary about the specific new knowledge generated by the study, including the influences of the children's grandmothers on the fathers, barriers to involvement of the fathers with their children, the fathers' connectedness with their children despite barriers, and a finding that the fathers did not identify health care providers as sources of information about pregnancy and parenting. The study also discussed specific implications of the findings for nursing, such as the usefulness of involving grandmothers and the fathers' parents to communicate needed health information and the use of the school setting and school staff to gain access to the adolescent fathers. Finally, the discussion of the implications of the findings was tied to existing literature, enhancing the credibility of the interpretations of the findings.

CONCLUSION

In this chapter, we introduced and discussed some of the qualitative approaches to data collection. As we have re-

peatedly emphasized, researchers make tradeoffs when they choose one method of data collection over another. How the tradeoffs are made is largely a question of the goals of a particular study. When compared with the formal measurement models used for quantitative scaling (see chapters 13 and 14) and the efforts to standardize data collection procedures for quantitative measures (chapter 16), qualitative data collection appears to lack rigor and objectivity. However, it would be erroneous to conclude that clinical research can "do without" the flexible methods provided by qualitative research approaches. The main reasons for this are:

- Every quantitative psychosocial measurement tool that is population-normed and has been shown to have a high degree of validity and reliability originally took shape through a process of exploration and trial and error. Qualitative exploratory methods are indispensable for this process of scale development.
- Because language is constantly changing, which means that it is bound by its historical context, by necessity, language-based measurement tools undergo changes that may affect their reliability and validity. Thus, language-based measurement tools ultimately must evolve with the language or risk losing their usefulness.
- Not all phenomena of interest to clinicians can be studied with standardized, context-free measurement tools. Sometimes the study of context is the primary objective of the research. For instance, interactions between clinicians and patients are a cornerstone of clinical practice; understanding the dynamics of such interactions requires the very emphasis on context that quantitative methods eschew.

However, although qualitative research is indispensable, it can be criticized for placing too much trust in the credibility and integrity of the individual researcher. In the ordinary scientific canon, methods that produce results that cannot be replicated may be heuristically useful, but they do not meet the standards of objectivity, which demand that results can be corroborated by other independent researchers. Using both qualitative and quantitative methods in a truly complementary and developmental fashion is still rare, in part, because researchers not only are specialists in certain subject areas, but also may be specialists in particular methods. Thus, they may lack the specific training to "cross over" to using different methods. Nonetheless, a number of examples show how qualitative and quantitative approaches can be used to mutual advantage (Beck, 1993; Beck and Gable, 1997; Beck and Gable, 2000; Beck and Gable, 2001). High-quality research studies rely more and more on the work of teams whose members bring diverse and complementary sets of knowledge and skills.

Now that we have dealt with many of the complexities involved in research design (Parts II through IV) and measurement and data collection (Part V), we turn to the final key issue that every empirical clinical research study must address: Among all of the possible human subjects who can be approached for study participation, who should be chosen and how should that be done? The question of sample selection will be discussed in the next three chapters (Part VI).

_____

Suggested Activities

1. From the reference list or the list of suggested readings in this chapter or in chapter 12, select a few articles to read that report the results of different types of qualitative research studies. For each study, evaluate the extent to which the four criteria for data quality in qualitative research studies (credibility, confirmability, dependability, transferability) were met or at least addressed.

2. For the same two articles, summarize the potential ethical issues involved in the study and critique the way in which they were addressed. Refer to chapter 24 as needed.

3. Consider a research idea that is of interest to you and could involve the use of an interview technique. What type of interview technique (structured, semistructured, unstructured) would you use to address this research question? Provide a rationale for your choice, discussing both your reasons for choosing a particular interview technique and your reasons for rejecting other interview options.

4. Read the four articles by Beck listed in the suggested readings.
   a. Show how the conceptual underpinnings developed in the qualitative portion of the research illuminated the final quantitative instrument.
   b. Document all forms of validation and reliability tests that were undertaken until the final form of the instrument was achieved.

_____

Suggested Readings

Atkinson, P., Coffey, A., Delamont, S., Lofland, J., & Lofland, L. (Eds.). (2001). *Handbook of ethnography.* Thousand Oaks, CA: Sage.

Barnard, A., McCosker, H., & Gerber, R. (1999). Phenomenography: A qualitative research approach for exploring understanding in health care. *Qualitative Health Research, 9,* 212–226.

Beck, C. T. (1997). Developing a research program using qualitative and quantitative research approaches. *Nursing Outlook, 45,* 6, 265–269.

Beck, C. T. (1993). Teetering on the edge: A substantive theory of postpartum depression. *Nursing Research, 42,* 1, 42–48.

Beck, C. T. (1993). Postpartum depression screening scale: Development and psychometric testing. *Nursing Research, 49,* 5, 272–283.

Beck, C. T. (1993). Comparative analysis of performance of the postpartum depression screening scale with two other depression instruments. *Nursing Research, 50,* 4, 242–249.

Cote-Arsenault, D., & Morrison-Beedy, D. (1999). Practical advice for planning and conducting focus groups. *Nursing Research, 48,* 280–283.

Crabtree, B. F., & Miller, W. L. (1999). *Doing qualitative research.* Thousand Oaks, CA: Sage.

Denzin, N. K., & Lincoln, Y. S. (2000). *Handbook of qualitative research* (2nd ed.). Thousand Oaks, CA: Sage.

Fetterman, D. M. (1998). *Ethnography: Step-by-step* (2nd ed.). Thousand Oaks, CA: Sage.

Gomm, R., Hammersley, M., & Foster, P. (Eds.). (2001). *Case study method: Key issues, key texts.* Thousand Oaks, CA: Sage.

Hammersley, M., & Atkinson, P. (1995). *Ethnography: Principles in practice* (2nd ed.). New York: Routledge.

Kahana, E., Biegel, D. E., & Wykle, M. L. (Eds.). (1996). *Family caregiving across the lifespan.* Thousand Oaks, CA: Sage.

Krueger, R. A., & Casey, M. A. (2000). *Focus groups: A practical guide for applied research* (3rd ed.). Thousand Oaks, CA: Sage.

Morrison, R. S., & Peoples, L. (1999). Using focus group methodology in nursing. *Journal of Continuing Education in Nursing, 30,* 62–65, 94–95.

Morse, J. M., Swanson, J., & Kuzel, A. J. (2001). *The nature of qualitative evidence.* Thousand Oaks, CA: Sage.

Roper, J. M., & Shapira, J. (1999). *Ethnography in nursing research.* Thousand Oaks, CA: Sage.

Sharts-Hopko, N. C. (2001). Focus group methodology: When and why? *Journal of the Association of Nurses in AIDS Care, 12,* 89–91.

Stewart, D. W., & Shamdasani, P. N. (1990). *Focus groups: Theory and practice.* Thousand Oaks, CA: Sage.

_____

References

Atkinson, P., Coffey, A., Delamont, S., Lofland, J., & Lofland, L. (Eds.). (2001). *Handbook of ethnography.* Thousand Oaks, CA: Sage.

Beck, C. T. (1993). Teetering on the edge: A substantive theory of postpartum depression. *Nursing Research, 42,* 1, 42–48.

Beck, C. T. (1997). Developing a research program using qualitative and quantitative research approaches. *Nursing Outlook, 45,* 6, 265–269.

Beck, C. T. (2000). Postpartum depression screening scale: Development and psychometric testing. *Nursing Research, 49,* 5, 272–283.

Beck, C. T. (2001). Comparative analysis of performance of the postpartum depression screening scale with two other depression instruments. *Nursing Research, 50,* 4, 242–249.

Becker, H. S. (1958). Problems of inference and proof in participant observation. *American Sociological Review, 23,* 6, 652–660.

Collins, C. E., Stommel, M., & King, S. (1991). Assessment of the attitudes of family caregivers toward community services. *The Gerontologist, 31,* 6, 756–761.

Crabtree, B. F., & Miller, W. L. (Eds.). (1992). *Doing qualitative research.* Newbury Park, CA: Sage.

Dallas, C. M., & Chen, S. C. (1998). Experiences of African American adolescent fathers. *Western Journal of Nursing Research, 20,* 210–222.

Fetterman, D. M. (1998). *Ethnography: Step-by-step* (2nd ed.). Thousand Oaks, CA: Sage.

First, M. B., Spitzer, R. L., Gibbon, M., & Williams, P. (1995). *Structured clinical interview for DSM-IV Axis I disorders (patient edition [SCID-I/P, Version 2.0]).* New York: New York State Psychiatric Institute.

Hammersley, M., & Atkinson, P. (1995). *Ethnography: Principles in practice* (2nd ed.). New York: Routledge.

Kahana, E., Biegel, D. E., & Wykle, M. L. (Eds.). (1996). *Family caregiving across the lifespan.* Thousand Oaks, CA: Sage.

Lincoln, Y. S., & Guba, E. G. (1985). *Naturalistic inquiry.* Newbury Park, CA: Sage.

Merleau-Ponty, M. (1962). *Phenomenology of Perception.* New York, NY: Routledge & Kegan.

Morgan, D. L. (1988). *Focus groups as qualitative research.* Newbury Park, CA: Sage.

Polit, D. F., & Hungler, B. P. (1999). *Nursing research: Principles and methods (6th ed.)* Philadelphia, PA: Lippincott Williams & Wilkins.

Stewart, D. W., & Shamdasani, P. N. (1990). *Focus groups: Theory and practice.* Newbury Park, CA: Sage.

van Manen, M. (1997). From meaning to method. *Qualitative Health Research, 7,* 345–369.

Wilde, M. H. (2002). Urine flowing: A phenomenological study of living with a urinary catheter. *Research in Nursing & Health, 25,* 14–24.

Wills, C. E. (1997). Young adult medication decision making: Similarities and differences among mental versus physical health treatment contexts. *The Journal of Nursing Science, 2,* 59–72.

Yin, R. K. (1994). *Case Study Research: Design and Methods. (2nd ed.).* Thousand Oaks, CA: Sage Publications.

THE VOCABULARY OF SAMPLING

In this chapter, we focus on **sampling,** the process by which particular subsets of members of larger groups are selected. Although we address sampling in this chapter as a specific research activity, we believe that it is important to see sampling in a broader context. Sampling is actually an everyday human activity that occurs when we make observations or gather information. For example, what we "know" about the world is based on sensory input (sight, sense, smell, touch), direct interpersonal contact, reading materials, media exposure, and so forth. Daily experiences such as these make up only a tiny proportion of the universe of all *possible* sensory effects, personal contacts, reading materials, or media messages. Yet, most people take for granted that their information about the world is mostly accurate. In everyday life, people routinely make assumptions (in the form of broad generalizations) about the nature of reality based on typically small and highly selective sets of experiences. For example, consider how many people would agree with the statement, "I pretty much understand what human beings are like," even though they may, over their whole lifetime, become well acquainted with only a small number of people out of a world population that numbers in the billions.

Although casual generalizations are often useful and adaptive for efficient functioning in daily life,[1] in research, we must ask the question: To what extent is it possible to systematize the process of generalizing from limited sets of experiences (or limited amounts of information) to larger universes? Both researchers and readers of research reports usually want to know about the broader applicability of the sampled observations. We are rarely interested in just the cases or observations at hand, but want to know if what we learn about them can be confidently projected ("generalized") to larger populations of interest.

Consider the example found in Research Scenario 19-1, which compares the experience of an advance practice nurse (APN) who sees clients in a particular clinic with the experience of a police chief who is familiar with the number and types of accidents reported to the police department. Whose experience should be considered an "accurate" reflection of the scope of teenage drinking?

RESEARCH SCENARIO 19.1

How Much of a Problem is Teenage Drinking in the Community?

Suppose that an advance practice nurse (APN) and a police chief who serve together on a community planning board are debating the extent to which teenage alcohol use is a problem in their community.

The APN, who works in a small family practice clinic, observes that a substantial number of the teenagers she sees in the clinic are in need of follow-up care for injuries incurred during motor vehicle accidents. She believes that many of these injuries are alcohol-related because more than half of the teenagers she sees indicate that they were "maybe drinking too much" when they had their accidents. Based on this clinical experience, the APN believes quite strongly that drinking and driving among teenagers is a problem of substantial magnitude in the community served by her clinic. At tonight's planning board meeting, she brings up the idea of a community public awareness campaign regarding teenage drinking.

At this point, the police chief raises the concern that drinking and driving might actually be a "minor" problem in the local community. He cites alcohol use statistics from other similarly sized townships in the state, and indicates that the local community's statistics are actually much lower compared with the other townships. He cites figures from police department accident reports to justify his viewpoint. On that basis, he questions the need for a community awareness campaign.

Who is most likely to have the "more accurate" data, the APN or the police chief?

Neither of these two sets of databases should be exclusively relied on as 100% valid reflections of teenage drinking behavior in the community. In both cases, judgments about what is a "minor problem" versus a "problem of substantial magnitude" are based on biased samples and different comparison groups.[2] For instance,

---

[1]*Heuristics* ("shortcut" information processing strategies that assist in discovery) and *biases* (errors in judgments that occur as a result of the use of heuristics) are concepts that are important to clinical decision-making among advance practice nurses. Both concepts address the fact that clinical judgments are based on incomplete information, with its attendant problems of bias and generalization in assessing the state of the patient. A full discussion of heuristics and biases is beyond the scope of this chapter, but see Sox, Blatt, Higgins, and Marton (1988) for a "classic" discussion of this topic and Gigerenzer, Todd, and the ABC Research Group (1999) for an alternative view.

[2]The term *bias* means different things to different people. As we will see in this chapter, a sample is considered "biased" if it tends to systematically overrepresent or underrepresent a characteristic of the population from which the sample was drawn. In statistical inference, we talk of "unbiased estimators" if their "expected values," or means of all estimates produced by the estimators, equal the true population values.

because of the neighborhood in which the clinic is located and the types of payment that the clinic accepts, the youth seen in the clinic might come from a middle-class social stratum of the town, representing neither very poor nor very well-off families. On the other hand, at least some of the youth seen in the clinic may have been involved in car accidents that families tried to settle privately to avoid increasing their insurance premiums. Such cases would not be represented at all in the police department data. In addition, police departments often base judgments about the magnitude of accident rates on comparisons with the number of accidents reported in other communities of similar size. This example introduces the following central idea: *Conclusions drawn about the nature of reality depend greatly on how the data were selected (sampled) from the relevant universe (population).* One person's conclusions about a given subject matter may vary greatly from another person's conclusions simply because they base their judgments on different samples of observations.

Samples and Populations

Now we are ready to turn to a more formal discussion of samples and populations and introduce some related vocabulary. A **sample** is defined as any **subset** of cases or observations drawn from a larger **population** of cases or observations. The population constitutes the **universe** of interest. Thus, **sampling** is the process of selecting a particular subset from a larger population or universe. **Generalization** involves taking the sample information and drawing inferences about the characteristics of the population from which the sample is drawn.

Defining the Population

These seemingly simple, straightforward definitions entail a number of challenging and philosophically intriguing questions. The first challenge is to consider a suitable definition of the "population" involved in a problem. The term *population,* used without any qualifier, may lead the reader to think in terms of *human populations.* Although the major focus of health care research is people, "populations" may consist of other elements as well.

For example, in chapter 11, we mentioned the concept of a *unit of analysis.* It was noted that many data sets that are routinely assembled in hospitals and clinics use units such as "visits" or "admissions" as their basic data unit.

In addition, hospital administrators or insurance companies may be interested in information about the out-comes of certain medical "procedures," whereas researchers might be interested in "Lamaze classes," the safety regulations at "nursing homes," or the success of "diabetes education programs." Samples drawn from populations made up of each of these units of analysis must contain the same units or elements as the particular populations to which the researcher wants to generalize. For example, a health educator who selects a sample of different Lamaze classes might be interested in generalizing to all Lamaze classes offered in a local community, township or county, state, or the United States. Similarly, insurance companies might be interested in comparing the outcomes for selected procedures, with the goal of generalizing to all such procedures performed on patients enrolled in a certain health plan. Thus, a **population** is the universe of all of the units or elements to which we want to generalize.

Population Characteristics

As implied in the above discussion, before researchers choose specific sampling procedures, they must define the elements or units that they want to study as well as the universe of such elements or units. Usually, this process is referred to as the definition of the **target population.** In the examples just provided, it would be quite important to specify clearly that the target populations are aggregates (e.g., Lamaze classes) or procedures (e.g., appendectomies), but not individual persons, before determining how to sample from these populations. As it turns out, definitions of target populations are often quite imprecise, especially with respect to the dimensions of *time* and *location.* For example, when researchers speak of "depression in patients recovering from myocardial infarction" (Ziegelstein, 2001) or "effects of pacifier use on weaning" (Kramer, Barr, Dagenais, Yang, Jones, Ciofani, & Jane, 2001), they are implicitly referring to **infinite** (or open-ended) populations of patients or mothers and their babies. In neither case would a researcher want to claim that the findings pertained only to, say, Americans, or only to persons born within the last 60 years.

Yet, in practice, researchers draw their samples from **accessible populations** that are often **finite.** Accessible populations may be defined in terms of their geographic location (e.g., all patients diagnosed with cancer in a particular city) or institutional affiliation (e.g., all students enrolled in public high schools, all patients in a particular hospital) or personal characteristics (e.g., all patients with diabetics who are older than 65 years of age and do not have dementia). In addition, accessible populations are always, at least implicitly, defined in terms of the *observation period* chosen by the researcher. This is because tar-

Sampling from Finite, Accessible Populations

Suppose you are interested in drawing a sample of all patients treated for a hip fracture at a particular hospital between January 1, 2001, and December 31, 2002. Your study goal is to describe the specific outcomes of clinical care provided for hip fracture. This is clearly a well-defined, finite population, for which every member can potentially be enumerated using the medical and financial records of the hospital. As we discuss in later sections of this chapter, there are probability-based sampling techniques that allow a researcher to draw unbiased samples from this type of population. As a result, the researcher can have a high level of confidence that the selected sample accurately "represents," or "looks like," the accessible population.

geted populations (e.g., depressed patients who are recovering from myocardial infarction, mothers and babies) vary in number and composition as new members are added and others are removed. Research Scenario 19-2 illustrates these concepts.

As this example shows, the accessible population and the broader target population can differ from each other in important ways. The patients at the hospital may be the population of patients to which you have access, given your resources and familiarity with the "gatekeepers" at the institution. However, this accessible population of patients with hip fracture may not be representative of the target population of all patients with hip fracture, which is likely to be the population of interest to you and the readers of your report. This is an important issue concerning the generalizability[3] of clinical studies, namely, the drawing of inferences to patients in other hospitals or institutions, states, or countries, or even to future populations of patients.

In most instances, because of resource limitations, researchers must recruit study participants from a less-than-optimal, accessible population that may differ in important respects from the ideal target population. Yet, even the best sampling technique cannot bridge the gap between an ac-

cessible population and an ideal target population. The same point can be made about generalizations to future cases. Given that any sample drawn from an accessible population is bound by time, when generalizations are made about future cases, there is an implicit assumption that the process that generated the observed patterns in the currently accessible population will remain unchanged. Of course, such assumptions are not always warranted. Particularly for phenomena that are affected by social or technologic change over relatively short periods, research results from one decade ago may not hold up in future investigations. For example, in the early decades of the 20th century, smoking was an activity engaged in by relatively affluent, privileged members of society. Now, however, smoking is more widespread among less educated, poorer members of society (Link, 1995). For a biologic example, consider the fact that resistance of certain bacteria to antibiotics has been increasing in recent years. Because resistance to antibiotics is a moving target, so to speak, studies of antibiotic-resistant organisms in people must be updated continually, requiring resampling of the relevant populations so that clinical practice guidelines for antibiotic therapy for infectious diseases can keep pace with a changing world.

Now that we have shown the importance of time and geographic distribution in defining accessible populations, a key conclusion can be drawn from this discussion: *Populations exist in specific locations of the space–time continuum; thus, they necessarily undergo changes as a function of time and space.* As a result, from a sampling point of view, it matters very much how *stationary* (stable) or *unstable* a population is. For an example, see Research Scenario 19-3.

In summary, the populations from which we obtain samples are usually limited in terms of time and geographic distribution. Although sampling procedures are available to assure that representative samples are obtained from these accessible populations, any inferences *beyond* the location and time parameters involved in defining the population are hazardous because they are *not* based on a mathematical or statistical algorithm associated with a formal sampling procedure.[4]

From Target Populations to Obtained Samples

To the extent that researchers are interested in the broader applicability of their findings, they would like to be able to draw study samples that allow them to make inferences

---

[3]In experimental studies in particular, *generalizability* is often referred to as "external validity" of the study results.

[4]Recall from the earlier discussion in this chapter that the key advantage of formal sampling techniques (as described in this chapter) is that they systematize and remove bias in generalizations from samples to populations.

RESEARCH SCENARIO 19.3

Sampling from Changing Populations

The U.S. Census Bureau estimated that on July 1, 2001, the state of Michigan had a population of 9,990,817 residents (U.S. Census Bureau, 2002). However, in Michigan, in 2001, each hour 15 to 16 babies were born and almost 10 deaths were recorded. There was also a modest net outmigration (people moving, mostly to other states) of more than nine persons per day. This example illustrates that a human population as large as that of a U.S. state is not exactly stable. Any attempt to enumerate *precisely* the population at a given time will inevitably be less than 100% accurate because it is impossible to perform the complete enumeration and report the results within just a few minutes! However, for most practical and research purposes, the state population is "stable enough," with an annual net change of less than 1%. In fact, the Census Bureau customarily uses the midyear (July 1) as the reference day for its population estimates.

get population. When researchers identify diabetes as a risk factor for heart disease, for example, they mean to refer to *all people with diabetes,* diagnosed or not, American or Mexican, rich or poor, and so forth. Similarly, to state that depression is a "common" mental health problem among patients recovering from myocardial infarction is to make an *unconditional* statement that potentially applies to all myocardial patients, past, present, and future. In general, when researchers investigate such problems as the acceptability of using arm span measures as substitutes for body height measures in clinical situations (Brown, Whittemore, & Knapp, 2000), they intend to come up with rules that are broadly applicable (i.e., rules that hold "across the board," not just among the studied subjects). Thus, researchers usually have ideal target populations in mind when they posit causal linkages, make predictions, or describe patterns.

However, as we have already seen, in real-life research, it is not feasible to study such open-ended, potentially infinite populations. Thus, we move from ideal target populations to **study populations** that are accessible to the researcher, at least in principle, if there are sufficient resources. These accessible study populations are more limited in time and space (e.g., all people involved in motor vehicle accidents during June 2002) and are also defined (and thus further delimited) in terms of specific **inclusion** and **exclusion criteria.**[5] It is from these accessible study populations that researchers attempt to draw their study samples. Unless the study populations are quite small

[5]See the discussion of practical sampling issues.

about the target populations of interest. The process of drawing study samples involves at least four major stages that are successively less general and inclusive. As seen in Figure 19-1, the most general level is that of the ideal **tar-**

Target Population:	Accessible Study Population:	Approached Sample:	Obtained Sample:
Ideal population to which the researcher would like to generalize	Population often fixed in time and space from which the actual sample is drawn	Subset of the accessible study population that is selected to be in the study sample	Members of the approached sample who consent and actually participate in the data collection

FIGURE 19.1 From target population to obtained study sample

enough resources are available to enroll all members of the study population, researchers adopt one or another sampling scheme that specifies which members of the accessible population will be targeted for recruitment. This is defined as the **approached sample.**

Finally, *drawing* samples is one thing, but having all members of the targeted sample *participate* in the study is quite another issue. Especially in health care research, where the sample units are human beings, aggregates of human beings, human organizations (e.g., hospital wards), or observations on human beings (e.g., admissions, visits), the final study sample can be assembled only from among those who provide active consent to participate.[6] Not all approached members of an accessible study population will actually give consent and participate in the data collection process (Neumark et al., 2001). In fact, sometimes response rates (i.e., number of participants/number of approached study subjects) are quite low, occasionally less than 50%. Thus, it is ultimately the **obtained sample** on which the study results and conclusions rest.

As illustrated in this discussion and in Figure 19-1, with each step in the sampling process, from target population to accessible population, from accessible population to approached sample, and from approached sample to obtained study sample, there is the potential for a loss of generalizability. However, researchers can do many things to minimize this loss. As we will see, the choice of inclusion and exclusion criteria influences how "close" the accessible population comes to the ideal target population. Likewise, the choice of sampling techniques influences the extent to which the approached sample truly reflects the characteristics of the accessible population. The researcher's level of success in reducing nonresponse also affects the extent to which the obtained sample can be considered a fair representation of the intended study sample. We will elaborate on each of these issues in later sections of this chapter.

TYPES OF SAMPLING PROCEDURES

After a researcher clearly defines a study population, he or she must determine how to select potential subjects or units from this population (i.e., which specific sampling procedure to use). In the next section, we will introduce several common techniques for drawing samples from larger populations. Beyond the fact that populations themselves—and thus the samples drawn from them—may change over

time, the very process of drawing samples introduces another source of variation and uncertainty, which is referred to as **sampling fluctuation.** Depending on the aims of the study, some sampling techniques are better than others in the sense that they may minimize systematic selection biases. However, a common feature of all sampling techniques is that individual samples will more or less differ from each other, even when obtained from the *same* population. These sampling fluctuations occur even when the populations from which the samples are drawn do not change at all (i.e., they consist of identical elements or units during the time the samples are drawn). In this section, we will address the extent to which this may be problematic for making inferences about the nature of the population.

Probability Versus Nonprobability Sampling

A major choice with respect to sampling procedures is that between **probability** and **nonprobability sampling procedures.** Probability sampling is a sampling procedure that relies on some type of random selection process. The essential feature of probability sampling is that *the researcher gives up control over which particular population members will be selected for inclusion in the study sample.* In this sense, a random, or probability, selection process is *impartial:* it does not favor the selection of any *individual* population member over others. It is important to differentiate the impartial selection of individual sample members from other aspects of the sampling procedure, over which the researcher may exert control. For example, when using probability sampling, researchers still determine the *sample size* or the *sampling ratio* (sample size/population size), or they may even use more complex sampling schemes in which different population subgroups are sampled at different ratios.

In contrast, nonprobability sampling procedures are distinguished by the lack of random selection procedures. As a result, inferences drawn about populations on the basis of sample results cannot be based on mathematical theories of probability. Therefore, such inferences remain, at some level, more "subjective" than those based on probability samples. However, it should not be concluded from this statement that health researchers always prefer probability sampling to nonprobability sampling. Which type of sampling is most desirable or most useful is driven largely by the nature of the research question. If the aim of a study is to obtain accurate information about large segments of the population, then probability sampling is preferred, if not essential, for drawing valid conclusions. For example, surveys conducted by the National Center for Health Sta-

---

[6]Distinctions between active and passive consent for study participation will be discussed in chapter 24.

tistics (NCHS) rely on complex probability sampling techniques to be able to draw valid conclusions about health and illness in the U.S. population and subgroups of the U.S. population (NCHS, 2002).

In typically smaller-scale clinical studies, limited access to relevant study populations is a likely obstacle to obtaining unbiased information about relevant target populations. The lack of probability sampling may be less of a problem. Even if a researcher obtained a good probability sample *that reflects the characteristics of the accessible study population,* this may not be of great interest to a reader who is concerned with the applicability of the findings to larger target populations. A further problem in health care studies is that obtained samples often underrepresent patients who have the most severe illness, either by design (exclusion criteria) or because these patients are unable or unwilling to participate in research.

As an example, the sample described in Research Scenario 19-4 may provide a fairly good reflection of the underlying *study* population. Yet, the research question really aims at a much larger *target* population of patients who have had a myocardial infarction. The problem stems from the fact that the three-hospital study population may not be a particularly representative subset of the larger target population of patients who have had a myocardial in-

farction. Thus, although probability sampling may produce unbiased samples of particular study populations, it cannot help researchers to generalize from accessible study populations to the often much broader target populations of interest. Given this reality, confidence in the generalizability of study findings also relies on extrastatistical considerations, such as the confirmation of particular study results in other studies that draw samples from different study populations.

Major Types of Nonprobability Sampling

Most published nursing and health-related research, particularly clinical research, is based on nonprobability samples. The key reason for this is the practical difficulty of obtaining probability samples from many target populations. As a result, it is sometimes difficult to gauge the extent to which findings from a particular study are applicable to broader populations. As noted earlier, it is often the replication and confirmation of findings in other studies that leads to greater confidence in the generalizability of a pattern of relationships. Researchers have come to distinguish among four major types of nonprobability sampling: convenience sampling, snowball sampling, quota sampling, and purposive sampling. These sampling types are described in the sections that follow.

Convenience Sampling

Convenience sampling is, by far, the most common approach in clinical studies. At first glance, the term *convenience sampling* would seem to imply a lack of effort on the part of the researcher to assemble the study sample. Although convenience sampling does involve using the most accessible subjects for a research study, often, there are no feasible alternatives, given the resource constraints that apply to almost any research project. The main problem with convenience sampling is that members of such a sample may have some characteristics, often unrecognized, if not explicitly studied or thought about, that distinguish them from the overall target population. Box 19-1 shows some of the key ways in which convenience samples are obtained. These examples all involve a substantial element of *self-selection.* Even if a researcher succeeded in getting *all* of the patients in a clinic's waiting room to participate in a small survey study conducted on a particular day, the patients present may have chosen to come that day for reasons that make them different from the next day's patients. For example, staff at a clinic located near an automotive plant may see different patients depending on the shift patterns in the nearby plant, and so forth. Beyond such subtle

RESEARCH SCENARIO 19.4

Sampling from Accessible Populations

Suppose a researcher wants to study the relationship between the following two variables:

1. Severity of a myocardial infarction (independent variable)
2. Likelihood of referral to cardiac rehabilitation on discharge from the hospital (dependent variable)

Having access to three large hospitals in the county in which the researcher lives, he can approach a true probability sample of all patients discharged from these hospitals after a myocardial infarction within a given year (let's say a sample of 250 patients is obtained from among 1,354 patients discharged from these hospitals after a myocardial infarction).

BOX 19.1   Examples of Convenience Sampling

- Advertising for study participants in a newspaper
- Asking for volunteers at a public meeting
- Enrolling study subjects on a first-come, first-served basis
- Interviewing patients in a clinic's waiting room
- Sampling caregivers from caregiver support groups
- Interviewing any group with a specific health condition or illness, such as tonsillitis or chronic back pain, seen in a particular practice setting

---

differences, patients in private practice clinical settings are almost always more likely to have health insurance coverage than those who do not have a regular health care provider, whereas patients in certain hospital emergency departments may include a disproportionate number of people who lack health insurance. Thus, in the broader sense, the use of accessible clinical populations almost always involves some form of convenience sampling. If no prior information about the characteristics of the ideal target population is available, a circumstance that is not unusual in nursing and health care research, it may be difficult to gauge the extent to which the studied sample is unique rather than representative of broader populations.

Snowball Sampling

Snowball sampling, sometimes called "network sampling," is a special type of convenience sampling that is occasionally used in health care research, especially in qualitative research studies. The hallmark of snowball sampling is that early study participants are asked to help identify or recruit further study participants who meet the study criteria. Researchers adopt this approach in cases of special populations that are very difficult or impossible to locate otherwise, in part, because of a lack of available or appropriate population registries or lists. A common situation is the study of people whose experiences or characteristics are subject to stigma or disapproval in society at large, such as homeless people or those whose behaviors set them apart from most of society (e.g., prostitutes, persons with substance abuse or dependence). In such cases, the only way to accumulate a larger sample of subjects may be to ask each identified subject to act as a "referral agent" for additional subjects.

Quota Sampling

Quota sampling is another nonprobability approach. Although it is still mentioned in almost any research methods text, this type of nonprobability sampling has fallen out of favor and is rarely used in health care studies. However, occasionally, it might provide an improvement over straight convenience sampling, and it can also be considered a form of purposive sampling (discussed later). The main idea behind quota sampling is this: A researcher may know (based on Census Bureau or NCHS data) the distribution of certain key attributes in the target population of interest, such as the proportion of female patients who have diabetes or the proportion of patients with diabetes who receive Medicaid. Knowing these population proportions, the researcher may decide to select study participants such that the proportions of female and Medicaid patients in the sample mirror the population proportions exactly.

Similar to purposive sampling, the merit of this approach is that it deliberately generates variation in subject characteristics that may otherwise be missing in unqualified convenience sampling. However, quota sampling shares two fundamental weaknesses with matching in cohort studies (chapter 9).

1. To be feasible, quotas may not involve more than a few subject characteristics. If the quota scheme is complex, few subjects will be found who can fit into cells that are predetermined by the particular subject characteristics (e.g., think of having to find a 40-year-old woman who has diabetes and receives Medicaid).
2. As with matching, quota sampling does not guarantee, or even address, the representativeness of samples with respect to population characteristics that are not built into the quota categories.

Yet, despite these limitations, quotas may represent an easily implemented improvement over pure convenience sampling, as when a researcher tries to ensure that an underrepresented group in a local clinical sample is oversampled. In some cases, this approach is used in federally funded studies that involve convenience samples. These studies may have quotas of sex or race categories to meet the inclusion requirements for federal funding.

Purposive Sampling

Purposive sampling, sometimes called "judgmental sampling," is a type of sampling in which a researcher more or less handpicks cases. However, the primary goal in purposive sampling is not so much to generate a sample that is "representative" of a larger target population as it is to represent certain subject characteristics that are considered relevant to the investigation. For instance, a researcher may use clinicians' judgments about key stages of illness experience in the trajectory of a particular disease to select sample subjects that have the appropriate characteristics. In particular, this could involve the purposive selection of both "typical" and "extreme" cases to cover the range of manifestations of the disease. Likewise, when testing new measurement instruments for the first time (say, a self-report depression scale designed for use with adolescents), it makes sense to select both highly depressed and happy persons to evaluate the sensitivity of the instrument in identifying differences among subjects. Used in this way, purposive sampling is a way to implement the "known groups" approach to construct validation of a newly developed measure.[7] Clearly, in this situation, generating sufficient variation, rather than representativeness, is of foremost concern.

As we will see in chapter 21, purposive sampling has much in common with the sampling approaches used in qualitative studies. Although this sampling approach has the potential for serious sampling bias in the sense that the sample may not be considered a mirror image of the target population, that may not be the most important issue. When the researcher's primary concern is generating variation with respect to a key characteristic, rather than obtaining samples that are representative of larger target populations, purposive sampling fulfills an important and useful research function.

When we judge the adequacy of a sampling procedure, our judgments should consider not only the feasibility and resource-intensiveness of alternative sampling techniques, but also the overall goal of the study. The particular sampling strategy used is strongly driven by the aims of the research. For example, in a pilot study, it rarely makes sense for a researcher to waste time and resources obtaining a sample that is "representative" of the ultimate target population. In addition, representativeness is of concern only if there is reason to believe that the findings from a particular study sample will not necessarily apply to other study populations. For example, consider the fit of school furniture to schoolchildren's body dimensions (Parcells et al., 1999). If a child in a particular school experiences discomfort and posture problems when popliteal height exceeds the stool's seat height by more than 2 inches, there is no strong reason to believe that this finding would not be replicated in another school. In the final analysis, only when the express purpose of a study is to obtain accurate information on a well-defined target population does it make sense to use sampling techniques that can deliver the required evidence.

Major Types of Probability Sampling

If the representativeness of a study sample is a major focus in a research problem, nonprobability sampling should be avoided whenever possible. Nonprobability sampling provides *no formal way to estimate the probability of error* in making inferences about the target population. Thus, we cannot gauge how confident we should be in our inferences about the study population. In contrast, with probability sampling, researchers use sample selection techniques that make use of the results of formal statistical sampling theory.[8] Although many probability sampling procedures are used, all are based on the principle that sample units are selected from target populations according to a random selection process. With these processes, the selection of any *individual* sample unit cannot be predicted, but the *probability* of its selection, or sampling chance, is predetermined.[9] Probability sampling procedures are usually divided into four major categories: simple random sampling, stratified random sampling, cluster sampling, and systematic sampling. Each procedure is discussed in the next section.

Simple Random Sampling

Simple random sampling is the least complex approach to probability sampling. With this type of sampling, *each* population member has an equal chance of being selected. The sample elements or units are chosen randomly from a list that represents all elements or units of the accessible population. This list is often referred to as the **sampling frame.** For instance, if the sample is drawn from a finite population, as in the previous example of all patients with a hip fracture treated in a particular hospital during a 2-year period, it would be possible to obtain a list of all members of that population. Suppose that this list contains all 1,354 patients who were treated for hip fracture at this hospital, as previously indicated. If the researcher has resources for studying only 200 of them,[10] he or she might adopt the following sample selection procedure:

- All patients on the list or sampling frame are numbered from 1 to 1354.
- Using a random number table, patients are selected from the list.

---

[7]Issues of measurement validity are addressed in chapter 14.

[8]Key principles of sampling theory and the underlying probability theory will be described in chapter 20. Two classic texts on the subject are Deming (1950) and Kish (1965).

[9]For more detail, see chapter 20.

[10]The choice of appropriate sample size is influenced not only by the resources available to a researcher, but also by considerations of accuracy of the resulting sample estimates. The principles of determining sample sizes will be discussed in chapter 20.

- Whenever one of the assigned four-digit numbers (0001–1,354) comes up in a four-digit column, that case is selected proceeding from top to bottom until 200 patients are selected (see Appendix C).

- Because each number less than 1,355 in the random number table has the *same* probability of occurring, the resulting random sample can be considered an "equal probability" or "simple random" sample.

Stratified Random Sampling

Stratified random sampling is a straightforward extension of simple random sampling. Members of the target population are divided into **strata,** which are mutually exclusive subgroups identified on the basis of a stratification variable. Usually, the stratification variable divides the target population into subgroups that are thought to differ on, or be otherwise relevant to, the research outcomes investigated. Once the strata are identified, simple random sampling procedures are applied *separately* within each stratum. Why complicate matters in this way? One advantage is that this procedure *guarantees* that a predetermined number of cases from each identified population subgroup or stratum will appear in the sample, something that simple random sampling cannot ensure. However, in most cases, stratified random sampling is used when a researcher wants to apply *different* selection probabilities within each stratum. This makes sense when the underlying population groups are highly unequal in size. For instance, 14% of Michigan's residents are African American, whereas only approximately 1% of the population is Native American. Thus, a simple random sample of 1,000 Michigan residents would likely contain about 140 African Americans and only 10 Native Americans. As a result, not enough cases would be included in the sample to allow the researcher to say anything with confidence about these minorities. However, one could vary the sampling ratio (or probability of selection) among the various strata, such that each group contributes an equal number of sample subjects. In this way, one would still obtain a probability sample, but the unequal sampling ratios in the different strata would guarantee the inclusion of sufficient numbers of sample members from the smaller population groups.

Cluster Sampling

Cluster sampling is a type of sampling that is useful for large-scale surveys, for which a complete listing of the population elements is not feasible or possible, and for which the population may be widely dispersed. Cluster sampling involves multiple or successive stages, and is also referred to as **multistage sampling.** For example, suppose you want to survey high school students in the United

States who have a current diagnosis of asthma. Because asthma is a very common health condition in the United States, the overall population size is very large. A cluster sample design could start with a list of all school districts in the United States (more than 20,000). From this list, researchers could randomly select a sample of 100 school districts, from each of which they would obtain a list of all high schools. In a second stage, the researchers would draw a random sample of high schools from the school district lists. In a third stage, the researchers might draw random samples of various sizes from lists of students at each selected school. At each stage, different sampling ratios are applied, a fact that must be taken into account when the data are analyzed. Such studies are complex and resource-intensive, but they would be the only way to obtain representative samples of U.S. high school students with asthma because there is no "master list" from which a sample could easily be drawn. Many NCHS surveys use this approach to sampling (Cox & Cohen, 1985).

Systematic Sampling

Systematic sampling refers to selecting, from a population list or "sampling frame," every nth case, where n is the inverse of the sampling ratio. Thus, to select a sample of 500 cases from a target population of 10,000, the sampling ratio would be 1/20, and every 20th case would be selected. This process is equivalent to probability or random sampling, *if* the first case is chosen randomly and the **sampling interval** of n (the distance between the cases selected) does not correspond to a systematic, recurring characteristic of the population elements.[11] Although systematic sampling is simple to perform, it is almost always better to use a random selection procedure based on random number sequencing. Given the current availability of computers, this is easily accomplished in many clinical settings. This way, the systematic ordering in a sampling frame will not lead to problems with systematic bias.

PRACTICAL SAMPLING ISSUES

When implementing a sampling plan, researchers must settle a host of practical issues, many of which are specific to the research project. However, certain sampling issues must be addressed in all research studies. First and fore-

---

[11]Occasionally, computerized lists of persons may be subject to ordering schemes unknown to the researcher. Suppose a list of high school students is alphabetically ordered *within* the classes that they attend. In this case, selecting every 20th or 30th student from such a list may disproportionately select students whose name starts with a certain letter, say, "A." In turn, such a selection procedure could exclude entire ethnic groups with names that never start with "A."

most among them is identifying the accessible **study population,** which may differ from the **target population** in systemic, yet unavoidable ways.

Inclusion and Exclusion Criteria

When researchers prepare to recruit study subjects, they usually start by formulating a set of **inclusion and exclusion criteria.** Such criteria are used to define who is *eligible* to become a study participant and who is not. In clinical studies, inclusion and exclusion criteria, combined with the selection of clinical sites for recruitment, provide the precise, operational definition of the *study* population. Study populations often differ from the *target* population to which the researchers would like to generalize. The systematic definitional difference between the two may be viewed as a nonsampling (or presampling) bias.

Consider the following list of inclusion and exclusion criteria that researchers might use in a study of patients with acute coronary symptoms. After the researchers obtain permission from the institutional review boards of three or four hospitals to review admission records (to determine likely diagnoses) and to contact patients briefly for consent while they are still in the hospital, before any further information can be collected, the researchers establish the following list of *inclusion* criteria:

- Symptoms such as severe discomfort in the anterior chest (substernal region), back, epigastrium, jaw, neck, shoulders, elbow, forearm or wrist, or upper arm (between the elbow and the shoulder) *as well as* a slightly elevated troponin level, with a troponin T level or troponin I level greater than 1.5 times the limit of normal (i.e., ≥ 2 ng/mL), indicating unstable angina, and normal levels of ST-MI or AMI
- *Or* elevated enzyme levels: creatine kinase MB1 or MB2 level greater than 2 times the upper limit of normal (i.e., ≥ 12 ng/mL) or creatine kinase MB index greater than 2%

In addition, some patients who meet these criteria will be *excluded* if they also have any of the following characteristics:

- Renal failure
- Inability to speak English
- Inability to complete a brief in-hospital interview because of the severity of illness
- Dementia or another physical or mental condition that prevents him or her from participating in interviews

Decisions about the broadness or narrowness of such eligibility criteria are not always easy to make. To optimize the ability to generalize study findings to prospective target populations, it is clearly preferable to have *broad inclusion criteria* and *minimal exclusion criteria*. However, this may not always be feasible. For instance, in the previous example, the researchers who were interested in patients with acute coronary symptoms decided to exclude patients with dementia, simply because these patients may not be able to participate in the interview self-reports used in the study. Yet, some patients with coronary symptoms also simultaneously have dementia. Clearly, a rule that excludes patients with dementia, or any other comorbid condition, restricts the generalizability of the findings, even before the actual sampling strategy is chosen.

If a comorbid condition occurs frequently (e.g., heart disease among patients with diabetes), its use as an exclusion criterion may result in a study population that differs substantially from the target population that was originally envisioned. Likewise, the requirement to accept only patients who have a sufficient command of English limits generalizability, sometimes in ways that appear arbitrary with respect to the research problem, as in the case of finding an effective drug or clinical intervention. Yet, researchers routinely use such exclusion criteria, primarily because it would be too difficult or resource-intensive to include certain subgroups in the study. For instance, the inclusion of non-English speakers requires the use of translators and interpreters, and the use of telephone interviews requires study participants to be able to hear and speak. Readers of research reports should be "on the lookout" for exclusion criteria, especially if they are "external to" the problem at hand (i.e., they have nothing to do with the disease or illness progression).

Sampling Frames

When researchers draw samples from populations, they implicitly or explicitly use **sampling frames** to select members of the population for inclusion. In the broadest sense, a sampling frame is a symbolic representation of the target or study population. It is either an existing list of all, or at least many, members of the target population, or a set of procedures that allow the researcher to access the members of the target population. An example is random-digit dialing, which implicitly defines the target population as members of the resident population that can be reached by telephone.

Technically, the easiest way to draw probability samples is to start with a detailed list of members of the target population that can serve as the sampling frame. Obviously, researchers should consider the quality of a population list before they start using it. As the questions in Box 19-2 indicate, lists of population members might

BOX 19.2 Questions about Population Lists That Serve as Sampling Frames

- What are the inclusion criteria that get a person on the list, and what are the exclusion criteria that prevent a person from being on the list?
- How often is the list updated to reflect changes in the population?
- What data collection techniques were used to obtain information about population members?

differ in systematic ways from the target populations. For instance, mailing lists of professional organizations may be updated once a quarter or even less frequently, resulting in zero probability for the most recent members to be included in a study that targets these members. Because health insurance information includes only billable services, it may be a less than perfect source of data for a study of other patient contacts. Medical records may not contain complete accounts of all services performed, all diagnostic information, and so forth. Thus, the use of sampling frames implicitly may lead to a redefinition of the study population as one that differs from the target population in characteristic ways. In a way, sampling frames have their own inclusion and exclusion criteria, and the investigator should clarify them before using a sampling frame.

Timing of Data Collection

Most of the time, when people think of study samples, they mean subsets selected from a population of sampling units. In health care research, this is usually a subset of individual persons (sampling units or units of analysis) drawn from a larger population of similar persons. Earlier, we noted that populations are usually defined in terms of a space–time continuum (i.e., they *change* both in geographic distribution and over time). Among other factors, the sampling process must take into account the time involved.

There are actually two timing issues to consider. One is that populations change over time. As a result, a sample of patients who have a myocardial infarction and are representative of the population of patients with myocardial infarction in 1990 may differ in many ways from another sample that is representative of the population of patients with myocardial infarction in 2000. More important in health care studies is the sampling of clinical populations in particular settings. Such populations may vary markedly, depending on the timing. For instance, patients who come to a hospital emergency department during the day are likely to include a much larger percentage of uninsured persons who are seeking nonemergent care compared with patients who come to the same emergency department at night. College students who are enrolled during summer terms differ systematically from those who are enrolled during fall and spring terms. Study samples that are obtained on weekdays are likely to differ from those obtained on weekends, even if both are ostensibly drawn from the same target population. In short, sampling bias can arise when investigators do not consider the effect of the timing of data collection on the accessibility of various population segments.

Another reason why the timing of observations is also a sampling issue is that observations of the same sampling units may vary, simply because they were made at different times of the day, month, or season. The same set of subjects can be interviewed or observed at many different times. As emphasized in the chapters on measurement (chapters 13 and 14), *any* data set, whether a sample or a well-defined population of subjects, is always a *sample of observations* selected from a population of infinitely many observations that could have been obtained on the same subjects.

In that sense, researchers are always concerned with inferences beyond the data at hand (e.g., they hope that the obtained blood pressure or anxiety scores represent the true scores for the individuals observed).

Proper sampling of observations is particularly important in studies that aim to reconstruct study participants' activity schedule or time commitment to care tasks. Limitations in respondents' recall ability may suggest the need for short recall periods (e.g., think of recalling all of the foods you ate yesterday as opposed to last month), short recall periods are less likely to represent general food consumption and nutrition patterns.

Nonresponse

From a practical point of view, few issues have a greater potential for sampling bias than nonresponse. Even a sample of members of the study population that has been selected and approached, based on a well-defined probability algorithm, can turn into an unrepresentative obtained sample if many of the approached and targeted members of the study population refuse to participate in the study. Thus, an obtained study sample is always, to some degree, a self-selected sample because study participants must consent to participate before they can be studied. Few tasks are more important for viable, representative samples than obtaining high participation rates and maintaining high retention rates among study subjects (Collins et al. 1990; Ribisl et al. 1995).

►CLINICAL NURSING RESEARCH IN ACTION
Examples of Sampling Procedures

Although experimental studies always involve random *assignment* of subjects to experimental (intervention) and control groups, they often do not use random sampling or random selection from a well-defined target population.

Example 1

One example is the study by Clark and Lester (2000), which tested three experimental and control group interventions on caregiver self-care behaviors, appraisal, and perceived burdens and satisfaction. The comparison groups involved the following:

- A group that watched a video on caregiver self-care behaviors
- A group that watched the video and then participated in a structured discussion
- A control group that participated in an interaction unrelated to self-care

Recruited caregivers were randomly *assigned* to one of these three conditions or groups, but were enrolled as a convenience sample of "97 female caregivers actively caring for an elderly dependent in the community for a minimum of 6 hours a week." These caregivers were recruited by telephone from home health agencies, churches, and community elder care agencies, presumably within the communities adjacent to the researchers' university. They also met additional eligibility criteria, such as being at least 40 years old. Although the authors provided some descriptive information on the ethnic composition of this sample as well as age, educational background, and marital status, there is no sense that these caregivers represented any larger population of caregivers.

Example 2

As part of a randomized trial of the effectiveness of primary care provided by either nurse practitioners or primary care physicians, Mundinger et al. (2000) recruited 1,316 study participants "consecutively" at one urgent care center and two hospital emergency departments. The participants met the following criteria: They had no regular source of care, kept their initial appointment, and planned to stay in

area for at least 6 months. Furthermore, patients with chronic conditions, such as asthma, diabetes, or hypertension, were "oversampled," because such patients are likely to benefit from regular primary care. Consent was provided by 1,316 subjects, who were randomly assigned to either a nurse practitioner provider (n = 806) or a physician provider (n = 510). Over a 2-year period, 3,397 adult patients were screened to obtain the sample of 1,316 subjects. However, it is not clear how many of these screened patients were eligible to be included in the study and how many eligible subjects refused to participate. Thus, the reader cannot calculate the response rate: (number of participants)/(number of eligible subjects approached by the researchers).

The comment that study participants were recruited "consecutively" suggests that the researchers intended to enroll all eligible subjects in the recruitment settings, an approach to sampling that is not uncommon in clinical studies. In principle, if the response rate is not too low and the recruitment period is long enough to gain a representative cross-section of the clinical population, this approach to sampling makes sense.

In contrast, the process of "oversampling" of patients with chronic diseases was not adequately explained. For example, did it involve a formal stratification of the study population, with differential and fixed sampling ratios, favoring the selection of patients with chronic diseases? Or was the oversampling done in a less systematic way, depending on point-of-contact decisions by the recruiter? As in many reports on clinical trials (DeFloor & Grypdonck, 2000; Moore & Dolansky, 2001; Naylor, Brooten, Campbell, Jacobson, Mezey, Pauly, & Schwartz, 1999), the emphasis was on design validity (i.e., showing the reader that the study tested the efficacy of an intervention by comparing it with an alternative intervention in another [control] group that can be considered "equivalent" in its initial characteristics).

The concern for generalizability is clearly secondary in many reports of clinical trials. Even if Mundinger et al. (2000) had been able to assemble a study sample that was truly representative of the clinical population *in these settings,* proper statistical inference would not have allowed them to generalize beyond the particular settings. In other words, the gain in generalizability from the point of view of the reader would not have been great. For this reason, generalizability of causal hypotheses is rarely accomplished through statistical inference from large population-based samples, but through replication with study populations in different settings.

Example 3

In survey and cohort studies, the concern with sampling generalizability is often greater than in clinical trials. Especially when the research is aimed at providing descriptive information about the prevalence of a disease or the distribution of health-related behaviors in a target population, it is important to use some form of probability sampling to obtain unbiased estimates of population characteristics. For example, in their study of risk factors for sudden infant death syndrome, Willinger, Hoffman, Wu, Hou, Kessler, Ward, Keens, and Corwin (1998) were concerned with determining "the typical sleep position of infants younger than 8 months in the United States," an objective that requires a careful approach to sampling. These researchers used data from the National Infant Sleep Position Study, which relied on telephone screening of randomly selected households that had a high probability of having an infant. The list from which the households were selected was purchased from a commercial research institute and assembled based on "birth records, infant photography, and infant formula companies."

For practical reasons, random screening of selected households from among all households would be far too time-consuming, because only a small fraction of all households contain infants younger than 7 months of age at any given time. Because the eligibility of a household for the study (having a resident infant born within the last 7 months) can be determined only through a household member's interview response to the question about whether an infant lives there, precise response rates could not be determined. The calculation of response rates requires a comparison of participating households and all eligible households. Nonetheless, approximate response rates, based on the assumption that refusals have the same overall eligibility rate as respondents, could be calculated, and exceeded 80% in all 4 years of data collection (1993–1996). However, given the sampling frame (i.e., purchased telephone lists of households gleaned from birth records, infant photographers, and infant formula companies), it is not surprising that minorities, poorer households, and those headed by younger mothers were underrepresented in the sample. Overall, the study report by Willinger et al. (1998) represents a model of how to report on a study's approach to sampling and how to evaluate suspected sampling biases.

Example 4

Mintzes, Barer, Kravitz, Kazanjian, Bassett, Laxchin, Evans, Pan, and Marion (2002), in their study of the effects of direct consumer advertising by pharmaceutical companies, provided an example of cluster sampling, an approach to sampling that makes sense when direct sampling frames or lists of the target populations of interest are not available. In their two-stage approach to sampling, the researchers identified primary care physicians in Vancouver, Canada, and Sacramento, California, and then interviewed a total of 1,431 (683 in Sacramento and 748 in Vancouver) adult patients in these practices. From the information provided, it is difficult to say to what extent the primary care practices were representative of all such practices in these two cities. Thus, although 61% of the patients, who were approached at predetermined days within these practices, responded to the survey, it is unclear how many practices were approached and refused participation. Although the sampling procedures in this study did not provide a basis for statistical generalizability to all primary care patients in the two cities compared, the data shed light on the effects of patient requests for advertised drugs on the prescription habits of the physicians involved.

CONCLUSION

Most survey studies reported in the health care literature are not based on large probability samples. Such studies are still valuable, however, because they can suggest interesting relationships (Mintzes et al., 2002; Stommel et al., 1998; Fischbacher, Bhopal, Unwin, Walker, White, & Alberti, 2001; Bradley, Smith, Long, & O'Dowd, 2002). Yet, any claim of generalizability to a defined target population must be tempered by the recognition that nonprobability samples do not allow one to make the necessary statistical inferences. Readers should be alert to the occasionally large mismatch between the implied claim to generalizability in the title (e.g., "Needs of Chinese Families of Critically Ill Patients") and the data on which the research report is based. For example, in this case, the study was based on a convenience sample of 37 Chinese family members and 45 registered nurses (Leung, Chien, & Mackenzie, 2000). Although the study provides a valuable contribution to knowledge, the sampling is limited and the findings would need to be confirmed with additional research.

Suggested Activities

1. Select one or two articles from the reference list that are not discussed in detail with regard to sampling in this chapter. For each study:
   a. Identify the specific type of sampling used.
   b. Identify the inclusion and exclusion criteria used.
   c. Describe the strengths and weakness of the sampling strategy used.
   d. Suggest feasible improvements to the sampling strategy used.
   e. Characterize the completeness of the description of the sampling process.
2. Describe several specific examples of research topics that would be best studied by the following methods. Justify your selections of *specific* sampling strategies by referring to the study aims and feasibility considerations.
   a. Probability sampling
   b. Nonprobability sampling
3. After referring to chapter 24, discuss feasible and ethical ways to reduce common forms of sampling bias in relation to the examples of research topics that you identify for question 2.

References

Bradley, F., Smith, M., Long, J., & O'Dowd, T. (2002). Reported frequency of domestic violence: Cross-sectional survey of women attending general practice. *British Medical Journal, 324,* 271–274.

Brown, J. K., Whittemore, K. T., & Knapp, T. R. (2000). Is

arm span an accurate measure of height in young and middle-aged adults? *Clinical Nursing Research, 9,* 1, 84–94.

Clark, M. C., & Lester, J. (2000). The effect of video-based interventions on self-care. *Western Journal of Nursing Research, 22,* 8, 895–911.

Cox, B. G., & Cohen, S. B. (1985). *Methodological issues for health care Surveys.* New York: Marcel Dekker.

DeFloor, T., & Grypdonck, M. H. F. (2000). Do pressure relief cushions really relieve pressure? *Western Journal of Nursing Research, 22,* 3, 335–350.

Deming, W. E. (1966). *Some theory of sampling.* (Reprint of 1950 edition published by John Wiley & Sons.). New York: Dover.

Fischbacher, C. M., Bhopal, R., Unwin, N., Walker, M., White, M., Alberti, K. G. M. M. (2001). Maternal transmission of type 2 diabetes varies by ethnic group. *Diabetes Care, 24,* 9, 1685–1686.

Given, B. A., Keilman, L. J., Collins C., & Given C. W. (1990). Strategies to minimize attrition in longitudinal studies. *Nursing Research, 39, 3,* 184–186.

Gigerenzer, G., Todd, P. M., & the ABC Research Group. (1999). *Simple heuristics that make us smart.* New York: Oxford University Press.

Kish, L. (1965). *Survey sampling.* New York: John Wiley & Sons.

Kramer, M. S., Barr, R. G., Dagenais, S., Yang, H., Jones, P., Ciofani, L., & Jane, F. (2001). Pacifier use, early weaning, and cry/fuss behavior: A randomized trial. *JAMA, 286, 3,* 322–326.

Leung, K., Chien, W., Mackenzie A. E. (2000). Needs of Chinese families of critically ill patients. *Western Journal of Nursing Research, 22,* 7, 826–840.

Link, B. G. (1995). Social conditions as fundamental causes of disease. *Journal of Health and Social Behavior, 36,* 80–94.

Mintzes B., Barer M. L., Kravitz R. L., Kazanjian A., Bassett K., Laxchin J., Evans R. G., Pan R., & Marion S. A. (2002). Influence of direct to consumer pharmaceutical advertising and patients' request on prescribing physicians: Two site cross-sectional survey. *British Medical Journal, 324,* 278–279.

Moore, S. M., & Dolansky, M. A. (2001). Randomized trial of a home recovery intervention following coronary artery bypass surgery. *Research in Nursing & Health, 24,* 93–104.

Mundinger, M. O., Kane, R. L., Lenz, E. R., Totten, A. M., Tsai, W-Y, et al. (2000). Primary care outcomes in patients treated by nurse practitioners or physicians: A randomized trial. *Journal of the American Medical Association, 283, 1,* 59–68.

Naylor, M. D., Brooten, D., Campbell, R., Jacobson, B. S., Mezey, M. D., Pauly, M. V., & Schwartz, J. S. (1999). Comprehensive discharge planning and home follow-up of hospitalized elders: A randomized clinical trial. *Journal of the American Medical Association, 281,* 7, 613–620.

NCHS: National Center for Health Statistics. (2002). Available at: http://www.cdc.gov/nchs/NCHS-Surveys and Data Collection Systems-National Health Interview Survey.htm.

NCHS: National Center for Health Statistics. (2003). http://www.cdc.gov/nchs/express.htm Surveys and Data Collection Systems page with link to National Health Interview Survey.

Neumark, D. E., Stommel, M., Given, C. W., & Given, B. A. (2001). Research design and subject characteristics predicting nonparticipation in a panel survey of older families with cancer. *Nursing Research, 50, 6,* 363–8.

Parcells, C., Stommel, M., & Hubbard, R. P. (1999). Mismatch of classroom furniture and student body dimensions: empirical findings and health implications. *Journal of Adolescent Health, 24, 4,* 265–273.

Ribisl, K. M., Walton, M. A., Mowbray, C. T., Luke, D. A., Davidson, W. S., & Bootsmiller, B. J. (1996). Minimizing participant attrition in panel studies through the use of effective retention and tracking strategies: Review and recommendations. *Evaluation and Program Planning, 19,* 1–25.

Sox, H. C., Blatt, M. A., Higgins, M. C., & Marton, K. I. (1988). *Medical decision making.* Boston: Butterworth-Heinemann.

Stommel, M., Given, C. W., & Given B. A. (1998). Racial differences in the division of labor among primary and secondary caregivers. *Research on Aging, 20, 1,* 242–257.

U.S. Census Bureau. (2002). Available at: *http://eire. census.gov/popest/data/states.php*

Willinger, M., Hoffman, H. J., Wu, K. T., Hou, J. R., Kessler, R. C., Ward, S. L., Keens, T. G., & Corwin, M. J. (1998). Factors associated with the transition to non-prone sleep positions of infants in the United States. *Journal of the American Medical Association, 280,* 329–335.

Ziegelstein, R. C. (2001). Depression in patients recovering from a myocardial infarction. *Journal of the American Medical Association, 286, 13,* 1621–1627.

CHAPTER 20

The Logic of Statistical Inference After Probability Sampling

STATISTICAL INFERENCE AFTER PROBABILITY SAMPLING

As mentioned in chapter 19, sample information can be used to draw statistical inferences about population characteristics only if the sample selection is based on some type of probability or random selection procedure.

Depending on the complexity of the sampling plan and the particular statistical estimator[1] in question, the mathematics of statistical inference can be quite involved. However, the basic principles of statistical inference are not, and understanding the underlying logic is quite useful for understanding the conclusions that can be drawn validly about a population on the basis of observed sample values. The statistical concepts are the same as those introduced earlier in the text, when we discussed causal inferences after random assignment (see chapter 3).

Sampling Illustration of the Properties of Statistical Estimators

To see how statistical inference based on probability sampling works, consider some hypothetical data (Table 20-1). Suppose that the 11 people (ID column) whose age is given (X_i column) represent the entire "population" to which we want to generalize on the basis of sample information. If the sampling process is truly random, we can draw conclusions about the age of the target population (the population from which the sample was drawn) with specifiable levels of confidence. In Table 20-1, the mean age for this population is $\mu = 23$.[2] Now we draw *all possible* simple random samples of size n = 2, n = 3, n = 4, and n = 5 from this population. For instance, for the two-person samples, we draw 1 and 2, followed by 1 and 3, 1 and 4, and so on, until we reach 10 and 11. Each time we draw a sample, we compute the sample mean age, resulting in the following sample means:

$$\bar{X}_{1-2} = (18 + 19)/2 = 18.5 \; \bar{X}_{1-3} = (18 + 20)/2 = 19 \ldots$$
$$\bar{X}_{10-11} = (27 + 28)/2 = 27.5$$

In this example, there are 55 distinct combinations of such two-person samples and, with simple random sampling, each of these samples is equally likely to be selected.

Now, we repeat this procedure and compute sample means for all samples of size n = 3 that can be drawn from this population. Analogous to the procedure for samples of size n = 2, we obtain the following mean sample ages for samples of size n = 3:

$$\bar{X}_{1-2-3} = (18 + 19) + 20)/3 = 19, \bar{X}_{1-2-4} = (18 + 19 + 21)/3 = 19.33 \ldots \bar{X}_{9-10-11} = (26 + 27 + 28)/3 = 27$$

Using the formula for **combinations** presented in chapter 3: N!/n!(N-n)!, where *N* represents the target population size and *n* represents the sample size, we see that it is possible to draw 165 distinct random samples of size n = 3, to draw 330 distinct samples of size n = 4, and to draw 462 distinct samples of size n = 5. For all samples, we would use a computer to calculate the sample mean ages. Now, look at the distributions of the mean ages ($\bar{X}$ values) for each of the distinct sample sizes. When we compute and plot these frequency distributions of sample means, we obtain their **sampling distributions** (Figure 20-1).

Figure 20-1 shows that these four sampling distributions of mean ages in samples drawn from the same study population share two important characteristics: (1) they are symmetric around the centers (or means) of the distributions, and (2) the means of the sampling distributions are all equal to the population mean of 23. This pattern of results shows what should happen if the statistical estimator is **unbiased.** When the mean of the sampling distribution of a statistical estimator equals the population mean, then the estimator is considered *unbiased*.[3]

With very small samples (N < 30), the sampling distributions are symmetric only if the underlying population distribution is also symmetric. However, as the samples grow in size, the sampling distributions for the sample means become more and more symmetric, regardless of the population distribution. They approach the shape of the normal distribution when N > 120. Figure 20-2 shows the shape of the normal, bell-shaped curve, which is symmetric around its mean.

As mentioned in chapter 3, this process is referred to as the **central limit theorem.** Its significance is that sampling distributions of means take on the symmetric shape of a normal distribution, *even if the underlying population distribution has a different shape.*

---

[1]A *statistical estimator* is a formula that is used to estimate a population parameter based on observed sample values. For example, we use the sample mean (the sample statistic) to estimate the population mean (the population parameter). A particular sample value for the estimator is called an *estimate*.

[2]We are using the Greek symbol μ, not $\bar{X}$, to indicate that we are referring to a population mean, not a sample mean.

[3]A statistical estimator also may have other desirable properties. For example, such an estimator is considered *efficient* if it has the least variance among all unbiased estimators. It is considered *consistent* if the sample statistic converges toward the population parameter as the sample size grows. The sample mean has all of these properties.

Subject ID	X$_i$ (age)	X$_i$ − $\bar{X}$	(X$_i$ − $\bar{X}$)^2
		TABLE 20.1 Hypothetical Age Distribution in a Population of 11 Persons	
1	18	18 − 23 = −5	25
2	19	19 − 23 = −4	16
3	20	20 − 23 = −3	9
4	21	21 − 23 = −2	4
5	22	22 − 23 = −1	1
6	23	23 − 23 = 0	0
7	24	24 − 23 = 1	1
8	25	25 − 23 = 2	4
9	26	26 − 23 = 3	9
10	27	27 − 23 = 4	16
11	28	28 − 23 = 5	25

$\Sigma X_i = 253$; $\bar{X} = \Sigma X_i / N = 253/11 = 23$

$\Sigma (X_i − \bar{X})^2 = 110$; $s^2 = 110/11 = 10$
$s = \sqrt{10} = 3.16$

Although the examples in Figure 20-1 show sampling distributions that are derived from very small samples, this tendency toward "normality" is already visible. For example, the sampling distribution for samples of size n = 5 is already very close in shape to a normal distribution. Yet, the underlying population distribution is actually uni-formly flat because each age occurs only once in the population data, which are seen in Table 20-1.

We can use this information about the shapes of the sampling distributions to draw inferences about population means. As seen in this example, the means of the four sampling distributions are the same: they equal the popu-

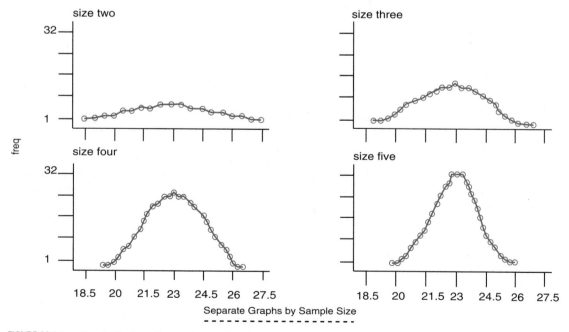

FIGURE 20.1 Sampling distributions of means for samples of size two, three, four, and five

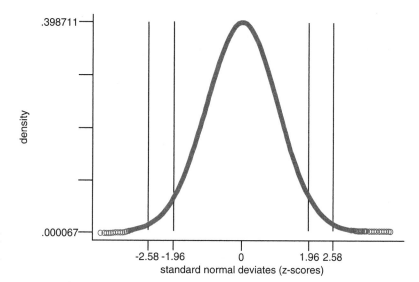

FIGURE 20.2 Standard normal distribution N(0,1) with two-tailed cut-off points for alpha = .05(+/−1.96), .01(+/−2.58)

lation mean of 23. However, as the samples increase in size,[4] the standard errors associated with the sampling distributions become smaller and smaller, decreasing from 2.14 (for samples of n = 2) to 1.10 (for samples of n = 5). This result is consistent with intuitive expectations: when samples increase in size, sample estimates of means are likely to be closer to the true population mean. In other words, given the greater accuracy of population estimates that are obtained from larger samples, the means fluctuate less around the true population mean (i.e., their

standard errors become smaller). We can use this fact when we estimate population means from sample means. For instance, the data shown in Table 20-2 for the graphs in Figure 20-1 indicate that, for samples of n = 2 drawn from this population, 95% of all sample means lie between 21.5 and 24.5. However, for samples of n = 5, 95% of all sample means lie between 22.2 and 23.8, clearly a narrower band. According to the same principle, if we increase the sample size, most of the sample estimates for larger samples will fall closer and closer to the true population value. This principle forms the basis for statistical inference.

---

[4]The **standard error** is the standard deviation of a sampling distribution.

TABLE 20.2   Summary Statistics for Sampling Distributions in Figure 20-1

		Sample Size			
		n = 2	n = 3	n = 4	n = 5
N of samples drawn		N = 55	N = 165	N = 330	N = 462
Mean		23.0	23.0	23.0	23.0
Median		23.0	23.0	23.0	23.0
Mode		22.5	23.0	23.0	22.8
Standard error		2.14	1.64	1.32	1.10
Skew		.000	.000	.000	.000
Range	Minimum	18.5	19.0	19.5	20.0
	Maximum	27.5	27.0	26.5	26.0
Percentile	.05	21.5	21.8	22.0	22.2
	.95	24.5	24.2	24.0	23.8

DRAWING INFERENCES ABOUT POPULATION PARAMETERS: CONFIDENCE INTERVALS

Most of the target populations that health and nurse researchers are interested in are much larger than the hypothetical population of 11 subjects in the previous example. For instance, a cancer registry may contain the names of thousands of patients who were diagnosed with cancer within the last year, or an up-to-date list of registered nurses in a large state may hold more than 10,000 names. In principle, we could use the same procedure demonstrated in the previous section, drawing all possible random samples of a given size, or at least a very large number (say, thousands), from such populations. This would allow us to empirically construct the sampling distribution of the statistic, following the principles we illustrated for the example of age. Thus, to find the proportion of patients with diabetes among patients newly diagnosed with cancer, we could draw 3,000 random samples of size n = 200, compute the proportion of diabetics in each sample, and construct a sampling distribution of these sample proportions.

This would be a tedious and resource-intensive undertaking that is, as it turns out, wholly unnecessary. We do not have to go through with this exercise because we know from the central limit theorem that the sampling distributions for means and proportions take on the shape of the normal distribution, as long as the samples are reasonably large (n > 120).[5] This is an important result because the normal distribution has a number of characteristics that make it easy to use in statistical inference.

Properties of the Normal Distribution

As shown in Figure 20-1, the normal distribution is a symmetric distribution with values spread (distributed) around its mean, which also coincides with the **median** of the distribution. The median of the distribution divides the distribution exactly in half, such that 50% of its values lie below the median and 50% lie above it. With the normal distribution, the mean also coincides with the **mode,** which is the most frequently occurring value in the distribution.

In all normal distributions, 95% of the values lie within ± 1.96 standard errors of the mean, and 99% of all values fall within 2.58 standard errors of the mean (see Figure 20-2). In other words, because we can rely on the fact that the sampling distribution of sample means is normal when

samples are reasonably large, we also know that 95% (99%) of all sample means lie within ± 1.96 (2.58) standard errors of the true population mean. This fact is usually expressed more formally as follows: Probability ($\mu - 1.96$ s.e. $< \bar{X}_i < \mu + 1.96$ s.e.) = .95, where $\bar{X}_i$ is a sample mean, μ is the true population mean, and *s.e.* is the standard error associated with the sampling distribution of the mean. This equation simply says that 95% of all sample means of randomly drawn samples will fall within ± 1.96 standard errors of the true population mean, which is the same as saying that the probability that a sample mean will fall within these limits is .95.

Normal Distributions and Confidence Intervals

Consider the inequality inside the brackets ($\mu - 1.96$ s.e. $< \bar{X}_i < \mu + 1.96$ s.e.). A few simple algebraic manipulations will provide an even more interesting result:

$$\mu - 1.96 \text{ s.e.} < \bar{X}_i < \mu + 1.96 \text{ s.e.} \mid \text{subtract } \mu$$

$$-1.96 \text{ s.e.} < \bar{X}_i - \mu < +1.96 \text{ s.e.} \mid \text{subtract } \bar{X}_i$$

$$-\bar{X}_i - 1.96 \text{ s.e.} < -\mu < -\bar{X}_i + 1.96 \text{ s.e.} \mid \text{multiply by } (-1)$$

$$\bar{X}_i + 1.96 \text{ s.e.} > \mu > \bar{X} - 1.96 \text{ s.e.}^{[6]}$$

At first blush, this transformation may not look like much, but the result is both remarkable and useful. If we plug this result back into the original probability equation, we get the following: Probability ($\bar{X}_i + 1.96$ s.e. $> \mu > \bar{X}_i - 1.96$ s.e.) = .95. In words, if we take *any* random sample (N > 120) and compute a sample mean on a variable of interest (e.g., mean age, mean systolic blood pressure, proportion of patients with diabetes), then there is a 95% probability that the limits defined by the observed sample mean ± 1.96 standard errors of the sampling distribution will contain the true population mean. In other words, *with a single random sample, we can have 95% confidence that the true population mean lies within ± 1.96 standard errors of its observed sample mean.* This previous derivation shows how we can calculate a specific **confidence interval** or **confidence limits** that are uniquely associated with the normal distribution. If we believe that a 95% confidence interval does not provide enough certainty, we can trade the degree

---

[5]See Bulmer (1979) for the mathematical derivation of the central limit theorem.

[6]You may be familiar with the result from algebra that multiplying an inequality by a negative number reverses the inequality sign. For example: $-4 < -2$ I if multiplied by (-1) yields: $4 > 2$.

TABLE 20.3		Change in Confidence Limits for Population Estimates of Mean CES-D Scores Depending on Confidence Level and Sample Size				
Sample Size (n_i)	Sample Mean $(\bar{X}_i)$	Sample Standard Deviation (SD_i)	Estimated Standard Error (s.e.)	90% Confidence Interval ($\pm$ 1.64 s.e.)	95% Confidence Interval ($\pm$ 1.96 s.e.)	99% Confidence Interval ($\pm$ 2.58 s.e.)
$n_1 = 150$	14.5	8.4	.69	$13.37<\mu<15.63$	$13.15<\mu<15.85$	$12.72<\mu<16.28$
$n_2 = 300$	13.8	9.1	.53	$12.93<\mu<14.67$	$12.76<\mu<14.84$	$12.43<\mu<15.17$
$n_3 = 600$	14.1	8.7	.36	$13.51<\mu<14.69$	$13.39<\mu<14.81$	$13.17<\mu<15.03$
$n_4 = 1200$	14.2	8.8	.25	$13.79<\mu<14.61$	$13.71<\mu<14.69$	$13.56<\mu<14.85$

of certainty against the accuracy or tightness of the limits. As already mentioned, with limits based on the normal curve, there is a 99% probability that the true population mean will lie within $\pm$ 2.58 standard errors of the observed sample mean. To make practical use of these facts, we need just one more piece of information: an estimate of the magnitude of the standard error.

Standard Error of the Mean

The **standard error of the mean** is calculated by dividing the observed sample standard deviation, s, by the square root of n, which represents the sample size: $s\sqrt{n}$.[7] Standard errors of other statistics (e.g., medians, correlations, odds ratios, regression coefficients) are more complex to derive, but share a fundamental feature: *they vary inversely with sample size.* Thus, as the sample size becomes larger, the standard errors of sample statistics become smaller. An important practical implication of this relationship is that it is always possible to increase the sample size until the required level of accuracy is attained. As a result, although the need for greater confidence in our population estimates requires us to widen the confidence interval, we can compensate by increasing the sample size, thereby reducing the size of the standard error.

---

[7]Most basic statistics textbooks provide a discussion and examples of calculating the standard error. See Munro (2001) for additional discussion. The rationale for the formula that we presented for the standard error can be demonstrated as follows: a sample mean is really a sum of n independent random variables (i.e., each of the cases whose values are used to compute the sample mean is independently and randomly selected). Formally, we can rewrite: $\bar{X} = (1/n)(X_1 + X_2 + \ldots + X_n) = (1/n)X_1 + (1/n)X_2 + \ldots + (1/n)X_n$. However, the variance of a sum of independent random variables is the sum of their variances (Σs_i^2), and the variance of a variable multiplied by a constant (here, 1/n) equals the variance of the variable times the square of its constant: $(1/n^2) s_i^2$. Because we have n variances involved in the mean, we get $n \times (1/n^2) s_i^2$ or $(1/n) s_i^2$. The square root of this expression is the sought-after expression for the estimated standard error: $s \div \sqrt{n}$.

Relationships among Confidence Intervals, Sample Sizes, and Standard Errors

The relationships among confidence intervals, sample sizes, and standard errors are shown in Table 20-3. Assume that four random samples of sizes n = 150, n = 300, n = 600, and n = 1200 are drawn from the same population of patients who are newly diagnosed with cancer. All sample respondents complete the self-report Center for Epidemiologic Studies Depression Scale (CES-D; Radloff, 1977; Devins & Orme, 1983). Mean CES-D scores are reported for each of the four samples in the second column of Table 20-3. Although the respondent samples come from the same population, the observed sample means differ because of the usual sampling fluctuation; this fluctuation also affects the observed sample standard deviations for the CES-D scores, which are listed in the third column of Table 20-3.

Because we estimate the standard error of the sampling distribution of means by the equation s.e. = $s\sqrt{n}$, it is easy to see that the estimates vary directly with the size of the observed sample standard deviations. However, the variation in the sizes of the standard error estimates is mostly linked to the term in the denominator ($\sqrt{n}$); therefore, as the sample size increases, sampling fluctuation decreases, which is expressed in the declining size of the standard errors. Given the large sample sizes, we can safely assume that the sampling distributions have the shape of normal distributions. Based on what we have said about the properties of normal distributions, we know that 90% of all sample means will fall within $\pm$ 1.64 standard errors, 95% of all sample means will fall within $\pm$ 1.96 standard errors, and 99% of all sample means will fall within $\pm$ 2.58 standard errors. In other words, the more certain or confident we want to be about our population estimates, the wider the confidence limits we must use. This is shown in Table 20-

3, by following the confidence limits within any given row, going from left to right. However, when we observe the confidence limits within a given column from top to bottom, we see a narrowing of these limits, because of the declining standard errors associated with increased sample size. As we will see, this tradeoff between sample size and accuracy of prediction is also the basis for deciding how large a study sample should be used.

USE OF SIGNIFICANCE TESTS VERSUS CONFIDENCE LIMITS (INTERVALS)

In this book, we have considered two ways of making statistical inferences. In the discussion of the logic of inference for experimental studies or clinical trials, we were primarily concerned with significance testing; however, in this chapter, we have emphasized the establishment of confidence intervals. Significance testing and confidence intervals are closely related: *A finding is considered "statistically significant" if the observed sample value falls outside the established confidence limits.* Although a bit cumbersome, and also less informative, we could apply the language of significance testing to the situation of drawing inferences about population values based on information from random samples, by referring back to Table 20-3.

Illustration of Significance Testing Versus Confidence Intervals

Suppose we start with the following "straw man" or "null hypothesis" about the population value: the four samples are drawn from a population of patients who are newly diagnosed with cancer, in which the true mean CES-D score is no higher than 12. The evidence soundly refutes our null hypothesis, in that the lower confidence limits estimated from all four samples at all three confidence levels are clearly higher than this assumed population value. Thus, the probability is extremely low that these samples come from a population in which the true population mean CES-D score is 12.

For example, consider the confidence limits with the lowest boundary, which is based on the 99% confidence interval for the sample $n_2 = 300$. Based on the evidence from this sample, we are 99% confident that the true population mean lies somewhere between 12.43 and 15.17 (i.e., there is only a 1% probability that the sample comes from a population with a mean less than 12.43 or larger than 15.17). Because the normal distribution is symmetric, we can go even further: the probability that this sample comes from a population in which the true population mean is *smaller* than 12.43 is .5% or $p \le .005$. Thus, we would *reject* the null hypothesis and would call the result *statistically significant.* In other words, the chance that the observed sample evidence is consistent with the population mean assumed in the null hypothesis is very small. Therefore, the patients whose data are shown in Table 20-3 are likely to represent another population of patients who have average CES-D scores considerably higher than 12.

The reader might object that the previous effort to recast statistical inferences about population values in terms of the language of significance testing is rather artificial. How much easier and clearer it is to make a statement such as: "We are 95% confident that a population value of interest falls within specified limits." Indeed, the language of confidence intervals is often preferable in reporting research results because it provides the reader with a range for the most likely population values. Statisticians usually recommend that researchers report the confidence limits for their estimates rather than simply state that the observed result is "statistically significant." The recommendation to report confidence intervals is useful for interpreting the *clinical* significance of study findings as well. The reason is simple. Statistical significance only tells you that, with a specified probability of being correct, you can reject the null hypothesis. However, what is not clear from a report of statistical significance is the magnitude of the population parameter. Thus, if someone tells you that the Pearson's r correlation between a depression measure and a physical functioning measure is statistically significant, all you know is that it is highly likely that it differs from zero in the population. In other words, the level of depression and the level of physical functioning vary together to *some* degree, but it is not clear how strong this relationship is. In contrast, if someone tells you that the 95% confidence limits for this correlation are $-.5$ and $-.4$, then you know that there is a 95% probability that the population correlation lies somewhere between $-.5$ and $-.4$. This is a much more informative statement than saying that you are quite confident that it differs from zero.

Unfortunately, it is still common in many health-related journals, including nursing journals, to read that a particular coefficient or statistic is statistically significant, without being given the confidence limits.[8] The language of significance testing has its historical origin in the development of analysis techniques for experimental data.

---

[8]In at least some instances, authors' presentations of study results are constrained by journal formatting instructions or editorial policies.

As we have seen in chapters 3 and 4, in such experiments, we are interested in establishing the effectiveness of an intervention. Thus, we start with the null hypothesis of "no effect" and determine whether the sample results show large enough differences between experimental and control groups to allow us to reject the null hypothesis of no effect. If so, we call the result statistically significant.

Even in a report on an experimental study, it would be useful to go beyond a statistically significant finding and indicate the range of magnitude for the effect (Greenland, 1990). For example, suppose that there is a clinically significant difference between two groups (control versus experimental) on an intervention outcome measure of interest, such as depression. Without knowing the magnitude of the group difference, it would be impossible to say whether the statistically significant finding has any clinical significance. In many instances, research results that are statistically significant are not necessarily clinically significant. Yet, in the end, one would alter existing clinical practice only if the change is thought to make a "material difference" in clinical practice (i.e., if it is clinically significant).

APPLICABILITY OF STATISTICAL INFERENCE IN EMPIRICAL RESEARCH AND ITS INTERPRETATION

Statistical Versus Clinical Significance

As the discussion in the previous section emphasizes, placing undue emphasis on statistical significance or "p values" can result in neglecting clinically useful information about the magnitude of effects or relationships. To recap, from both a theoretic and practical or clinical point of view, we are interested in the *magnitude* of effects. For instance, we want to know how much we lower the risk of heart disease if we switch to a low-calorie, low-fat diet. Likewise, before we change the clinical guidelines for the treatment of diabetes, we want to know *how effective* these new guidelines are in helping patients with diabetes to control their glucose levels. These questions lead us to a further discussion of the distinction between clinical and statistical significance.

To say that a finding is statistically significant is to use specialized, technical language to express the idea that the finding is unlikely to be the result of mere chance events. More specifically, a statistically significant finding merely indicates that the observed sample result differs sufficiently from the population values stipulated in the null hypothesis such that mere sampling chance is unlikely to have produced this difference. Yet, we know from the discussion of confidence limits that confidence intervals become smaller when study samples become larger. In other words, with large samples, even small differences between hypothesized population values and observed sample values would result in statistically significant differences. Given a sufficiently large sample, differences that are quite small and would not be considered clinically significant nonetheless may be statistically significant.

Thus, statistical significance is not a sure guide to finding "theoretically important" or "clinically relevant" relationships. If the study sample is large enough, even trivial effects may be statistically significant. In the evaluation of study findings, statistical significance provides only a preliminary test. If a finding is statistically significant, we may examine it further to determine whether it is of sufficient magnitude to warrant further attention, or we may examine the causal status of the relationship. In itself, statistical significance does not establish either the theoretic or the clinical importance of a finding. On the other hand, the repeated absence of a statistically significant relationship between two variables of interest (via multiple replication studies) should persuade us "that there is nothing there," and we may disregard this difference in the future. Thus, statistical significance may be considered a necessary, but certainly not sufficient, condition for clinical significance. The fact that the term *significance* is used in both its statistical, technical meaning and its everyday meaning of "importance" has led to untold confusion.

Applicability of Statistical Inference

Another question about the interpretation of statistical significance tests and confidence intervals concerns the applicability of statistical inference in many research situations. Recall that statistical inference is based on the underlying assumption that data are, at least in part, generated by some kind of random process. In two important situations, researchers deliberately introduce a random process into their studies: (1) when they randomly assign subjects to different treatment combinations in experiments or clinical trials and (2) when they randomly select subjects from larger populations. What about nonexperimental studies that are based on convenience samples? Is the logic of statistical inference applicable in this situation? Does it make sense to talk about a statistically significant relationship between two or more variables when the data were not randomly selected from a clearly defined target population? The answer is yes, but it is important to understand the source of the random process to interpret these findings correctly.

Consider again the classic case of statistical inference that is made after random assignment (chapter 3). Here, the main source of randomness in the data is the random assignment process. In this case, a statistically significant effect is one that is unlikely to have been produced by mere random assignment. Hence, we can be relatively confident that the observed treatment effect is "real." Now, consider a survey or cohort study that is based on probability sampling. Suppose that a difference is found between smoking rates in men and women. In this case, a statistically significant difference between men and women indicates that mere random sampling is unlikely to have produced this difference. Thus, it can be considered "real" in the population from which the sample is drawn. Finally, consider a convenience sample of patients with cancer who are enrolled in various clinical settings. Suppose that we find a statistically significant relationship between the intensity of pain experienced by these patients and their self-rated depression scores. How are we to interpret statistical significance in this situation?

The answer is that all data, even those based on convenience samples, should be viewed as partially generated by random forces. Recall the discussion of measurement issues (chapters 13–15) as well as the discussion of generalizability in chapter 19. Any observed value of a variable represents only a single instance of all possible observations that could have been made on the same subjects. In addition, most variables that describe physiologic or psychological characteristics of patients (e.g., blood pressure, anxiety), vary "naturally" over time. Furthermore, even if the underlying reality is stable, mere measurement error, errors in data collection, and errors in data entry would produce different sample data on different occasions. Given these possible sources of error and uncertainty, it would not be unreasonable to consider any data as partially generated by random fluctuations. If we accept this interpretation, it makes sense to apply the logic of statistical inference to data obtained from a convenience sample. A statistically significant relationship (e.g., between pain intensity and depression) in a convenience sample could be interpreted to mean that this result is unlikely to be the result of vagaries in measurement or natural fluctuations in these phenomena. Although this is a legitimate interpretation, in this situation, statistical inference cannot be used to make inferences beyond this particular sample of subjects.

STATISTICAL POWER AND DETERMINATION OF SAMPLE SIZE

Probably the single most frequently asked question of a statistician is: "How many subjects do I need in my study

sample?" Unfortunately, there is no simple rule that can be applied across the board. The answer depends in part on the goals of a particular study, the researcher's willingness to accept the risk of a wrong answer, and prior information about the variability of the major measures used. Although there are good texts (Kramer, 1990; Cohen, 1993) and software applications (Ex-Sample, PASS) that are devoted to this topic, many readers of clinical research reports find the intricacies of sample size calculations difficult to grasp. In this section, we discuss some general principles of sample size calculations that are useful for thinking about the sample sizes needed for research projects and evaluating the adequacy of the sample size in research reports.

The question of appropriate sample size most commonly comes up in the following situations:

- *Before data collection,* when the researcher must determine how large a sample is required to test a hypothesis adequately
- *When reading a research report in which a hypothesis of interest could not be confirmed.* In this situation, the reader must ask this question: Can the absence of an expected finding be trusted, or is it likely to be the result of a study sample that is too small to show the desired effect?
- When researchers want to *conduct a secondary data analysis.*

In secondary data analysis, the data have already been collected, so the sample size is fixed. Yet, before the data are used for further analysis, researchers should determine whether the sample size is large enough to show the existence of an effect or relationship of a given size. Answers to all of these questions are based on the same statistical reasoning. Specifically, they depend on the interplay of four variables:

1. The magnitude of the **effect size** or relationship (δ) in question
2. The **significance level** (Type I error or α) that the researcher is seeking or is willing to accept
3. The **power** of the statistical test ($1 -$ Type II error or [$1 - \beta$]) that the researcher desires or is willing to accept
4. The **sample size** (**n**)

If the magnitude of three of these variables is fixed (or known), then the magnitude of the fourth can be determined. Thus, if we know the desired effect size and have settled on an acceptable significance level and power of the test, we can calculate the sample size required. Similarly, if we know the sample size and have settled on the significance level and power, we can calculate the magnitude of the effect size that can be detected in the study, and so forth. To understand the reasoning, we will briefly review each of the four concepts.

Effect Size

The concept of an effect size is relatively straightforward, although the determination of its magnitude is sometimes complicated and may even appear arbitrary. When a researcher starts an intervention study or a clinical trial, he or she must think about the minimum intervention effect that should be considered adequate for the trial to be called a "success." Similarly, in an observational (cohort) study in which the intent is to discover risk factors for a particular disease, the researchers and clinicians must determine the minimum level of relative risk that they consider practically relevant. It is critical for the study to detect an effect of the identified magnitude.

These kinds of questions about meaningful effect sizes are not really of a statistical nature. Rather, they are substantive clinical questions that draw on past evidence and clinical experience. For instance, is a behavioral intervention that is aimed at reducing depression in postoperative patients worthwhile if it reduces a standardized depression score by one, two, or three points? Should we consider a correlation between diastolic blood pressure and an anxiety score of 0.3 too weak to bother about, or is it large enough to be considered clinically relevant? Answers to such questions may sometimes appear arbitrary; in such cases, researchers tend to rely on well-cited conventions about what to consider a small, medium, or large effect (e.g., see Cohen, 1993). Yet, very often, clinicians and researchers can draw on a stock of experience and research to help them determine what magnitude of an observed effect should be considered clinically relevant. Even if no such stock of knowledge exists, the questions remain important to ask before a study begins. If we cannot state the minimum criterion for a successful intervention, then almost any result, short of a complete absence of effect, could be declared a "success."

When we try to put an actual number on an effect size, we quickly realize that effect sizes can be expressed in many ways, depending on the metric in question and the specific test statistic used to express the effect size. For instance, in the chapters on experimental designs (chapters 3–5), we have seen that treatment effects, or differences between experimental and control groups, are often expressed as differences between the mean scores for these groups.[9] Of course, not all effect sizes are expressed in terms of mean differences.

As we have seen in our discussion of the Analysis of Variance (ANOVA) in chapter 5, if the comparison involves three or more groups simultaneously, it is easier to use the ratio of explained to unexplained variance as a measure of effect size (also known as eta^2)

Likewise, for regression models, we might use the R^2 value as an indicator of explained variance. For dichotomous outcome variables, we might use odds ratios or relative risk ratios, or we might be interested in a simple correlation between two variables as our measure of effect size.[10] Because "effect sizes" can be expressed in terms of many different measures, it is useful to be able to express them in standardized form so that they can be translated from one form into another. The details are provided in the specialized literature and software programs mentioned earlier (see especially Cohen, 1993). Here, we are more concerned with the fundamental ideas underlying power analysis and calculations of sample size.

Type I Error and Significance Level

We already discussed Type I and Type II errors in the context of statistical decision-making in experimental studies after random assignment (chapter 3). Recall that, after random assignment, differences between treatment and control groups are, in part, subject to unavoidable sampling fluctuations.

Thus, even if the null hypothesis in an experiment is true (i.e., the treatment has no effect whatsoever) we should not expect the observed treatment and control group means to be *exactly* equal. In fact, if we conducted the same experiment many times with different random splits of subjects into treatment and control groups, the observed mean differences between the treatment and control groups would be *normally distributed around the true mean difference* or effect size.[11] If we can assume that the sampling distribution of mean differences is approximated by the area under a normal curve, we also know that 90% of all sample mean differences will fall within $\pm$ 1.645 standard errors, 95% of all sample mean differences will fall within $\pm$ 1.96 standard errors, and 99% of all sample mean differences will fall within $\pm$ 2.576 standard errors of that distribution.[12] Thus, if the null hypothesis is correct and an intervention has no

---

[9]Recall that the computation of mean scores requires outcome variables measured at the interval or ratio level.

[10]Several good introductory texts on statistics provide detailed explanations of these statistical measures (e.g., Altman, 1993; Munro, 2001).

[11]If the magnitudes of the standard errors involved are unknown and must be estimated from the sample, we substitute the *t* distribution for the normal distribution. Otherwise, the same argument still holds.

[12]These facts follow from the shape of the area enclosed by the normal curve. The exact numbers are calculated with integral calculus. For convenience of use, probabilities associated with various cutoff points on the normal curve are often tabulated or incorporated into statistical software programs.

effect, the true mean difference between the treatment and control groups equals zero. Furthermore, although observed differences vary as a result of sampling fluctuations, we know that 95% (99%) of the observed differences will fall within ± 1.96 (2.576) standard errors of zero. Thus, if an observed study outcome lies *outside* these confidence limits, we would normally reject the null hypothesis, because mere random assignment produces differences this large in fewer than 5% (1%) of all study samples. Yet, if we adhere to these confidence limits, we will occasionally reject the null hypothesis even when it is true. This means that we would commit a Type I error. The probability or risk of a Type I error is established by the decision about the appropriate "significance level." If we set α at .05, we are on record for rejecting the null hypothesis any time that an observed study outcome is outside the 95% confidence limits for the null hypothesis. If we want greater confidence in our inference that an intervention is effective, we can adopt a more stringent decision rule: reject the null hypothesis only if the observed sample results lie outside the 99% confidence interval. In that case, we set α at .01, meaning that we allow for a 1% probability of committing a Type I error. If that is so, why would we not want to minimize Type I errors and set α at .001, or even smaller? The answer is that we must also pay attention to another error in inference, known as **Type II error.** When a Type II error occurs, the researcher concludes that a difference between the intervention groups does *not* exist, when in fact it does.

Type II Error and the Power of a Statistical Test

Under the conventional decision rule of setting the significance level at α = .05, we would reject the null hypothesis every time a sample outcome differs from zero by more than 1.96 standard errors. Otherwise, if the observed sample difference is *less* than 1.96 standard errors, we accept the null hypothesis and conclude that the intervention is not effective.

Suppose we know that the size of the standard error of the mean difference is 2.219. We can express the true effect size (−8 mm Hg) in terms of standard error units: on average, the intervention reduces blood pressure by −3.605 (−8/2.219) standard errors. This situation is shown in Figure 20-3. The normal distribution on the left is centered on the true mean difference of −3.605 standard errors. Yet, our decision rule is to reject the null hypothesis whenever an observed sample difference is outside the 95% (1 − α) confidence limits around zero. In particular, if the observed difference is more than Z_α = 1.96 standard error units less than zero,[13] we reject the null hypothesis of no effect and accept the intervention as effective. Now, this

RESEARCH SCENARIO 20.1

Reducing Diastolic Blood Pressure through Exercise

Suppose an experiment with a 3-month physical exercise intervention is effective in reducing diastolic blood pressure among patients with hypertension. This implies that the true difference in mean outcomes between the intervention and control groups can no longer be equal to zero. Let's say that the intervention reduces diastolic blood pressure an average of 8 mm Hg. However, because of the use of random assignment, any observed sample difference will vary randomly around this true mean difference. Thus, if the study were repeated a very large number of times, 95% (99%) of all observed mean differences would fall within 1.96 (2.576) standard errors of the true absolute difference of −8 mm Hg.

chosen cutoff point for determining the effectiveness of the intervention is *also* Z_β = 1.645 (−(1.96−(−3.605))) standard error units above the true mean difference of −3.605. However, we know from the normal distribution that 10% of all sample mean differences will be larger than Z_β = 1.645 standard errors above the true mean. In other words, if the true mean difference is 3.605 standard errors below zero, our decision rule to accept the null hypothesis whenever the observed sample mean difference is within the 95% confidence limits of the assumed null hypothesis value of zero leads to a Type II error rate (β = .10) of 10%.

At the same time, this decision rule will correctly lead to the rejection of the null hypothesis whenever an observed sample mean difference *is less than* the stipulated −1.96 standard errors from zero. Because the sample means are actually drawn from a distribution that centers around a true mean of −3.605 standard errors below zero, our decision will be correct 90% of the time. In other words, the power of the test (1 − β) is .90, or 90%. This example shows that *the power of a statistical test is the probability of inferring a treatment effect when there is one.* Naturally, we would like the power to be as large as possible. However, the distance between the hypothesized noneffect (μ_0 = 0) and the true mean difference effect (μ_t = −3.605) is divided into two regions that are demarcated by a single boundary: Z_α = Z_β. The symbol Z_α is used to indicate the number of stan-

---

[13]Although the 95% confidence interval is two-sided, we do not have to worry about the upper limit of +1.96. It is 5.565 standard errors above the true mean difference; the probability of such a sample outcome is practically nil.

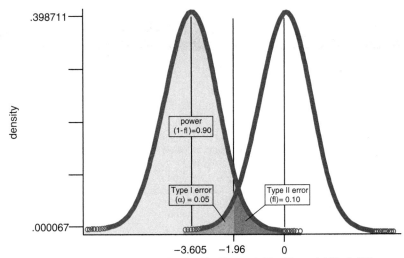

FIGURE 20.3 Trade-off between significance level and power null-hypothesis: mean = 0; alternative hypothesis: mean = −3.605.

Rejection region for Ho: Z=a < -1.96 = Zb < +1.645−3.605

dard errors, counting from μ_0, whereas Z_β indicates the number of standard errors, counting from μ_t. Together, they cover the distance between μ_t and μ_0 ($\mu_0 - \mu_t = Z_\alpha + Z_\beta$ or $3.605 = 1.96 + 1.645$). Shifting Z_β implies simultaneously shifting Z_α because the total distance remains the same. Thus, if we increase the rejection region for the null hypothesis, located to the left of $Z_\alpha = Z_\beta$, or if we increase the power of the test ($1 - \beta$), we also increase α, the probability of committing a Type I error. Other things being equal, there is a direct tradeoff between Type II and Type I errors, or a direct tradeoff between the significance level and the power of a test (Table 20-4). As we will see, however, other things are not necessarily equal.

The Role of Sample Size in Mediating among the Effect Size, Significance Level, and Power of a Test

We expressed the effect size in terms of standard error units, but we have already seen that standard errors vary inversely with sample size because large sample estimates are more accurate. That means that a given effect size, such as a mean difference between the treatment and control groups, equals fewer standard error units for sampling distributions from small samples and more standard error units for those from large samples. This fact shows the connection among sample size, effect size, power, and significance levels. We now express the relationships among these four variables in alternative versions of the same equation (shown in the following list), progressing from a particular set of values to a more general formulation:

1. $\delta = 3.605$ (s.e.)

This equation simply expresses formally that, in the example of the hypertension intervention study, we defined the effect size, or the true mean difference between treatment and control groups, in terms of 3.605 standard errors below zero. Zero represents the null hypothesis (no effect).

2. $\delta = 1.645$ (s.e.) $+ 1.96$ (s.e.)

This equation divides the effect size into two regions. According to our decision rule based on a significance level of $\alpha = .05$, we will reject the null hypothesis whenever an observed sample difference is more than $Z_{\alpha} = 1.96$ standard errors *below* zero. Alternatively, if an observed sample difference differs from zero by *less* than 1.96 standard errors, it must also be *more* than 1.645 standard errors (Z_β) *above* the true mean of −3.605 standard errors. In this case, we accept the null hypothesis.

3. $\delta = Z_{\alpha}$ (s.e.) $+ Z_{\beta}$ (s.e.)

We now restate the same principle in more general terms. Instead of using specific numbers for Z_α (e.g., 1.96 for $Z_{.05}$) and Z_β (e.g., 1.645 for $Z_{.10}$), corresponding to the specific levels of $\alpha = .05$ and $\beta = .10$, we use the general Z scores, which represent the unit normal variates that correspond to any level of Type I or Type II error (or power) that we choose.

4. $\delta = Z_{\alpha} (\sigma \sqrt{2/n}) + Z_{\beta} (\sigma \sqrt{2/n})$[14]

---

[14]Recall that the standard error of a *single* mean is defined as the population standard deviation divided by the square root of the sample size: σ/n. However, in this example, we need the standard error of a *difference between two means*. The variance of such a difference is simply the sum of the two variances: $\sigma^2 + \sigma^2 = 2\sigma^2$. The standard deviation is as follows: $\sigma \sqrt{2}$. The corresponding standard error is then: $\sigma \sqrt{2}/\sqrt{n}$ or $\sigma \sqrt{2/n}$.

TABLE 20.4 Statistical Decision-Making

		True State of Affairs	
		Null hypothesis is false: the intervention *is* effective	Null hypothesis is true: the intervention *is not* effective
Conclusions based on evidence from a statistical test	Null hypothesis is rejected: the observed mean difference lies outside the critical value (is statistically significant)	Correct inference (true-positive result) → Power of test $(1 - \beta)$	Type I error → Significance level or α level
	Null hypothesis is accepted: the observed mean difference lies inside the critical value (is *not* statistically significant)	Type II error or β level	Correct inference (true-negative result)

Here, we replace the standard error by its estimate, the ratio of the population standard deviation divided by the square root of the sample size n. In this formula, *sample size* refers only to one of *either comparison groups,* with total sample size N = 2n. Now, this expression contains all four variables needed to calculate the sample size or power for a given mean difference or effect size.

Calculation of the Required Sample Size

To calculate the required sample size, we rearrange the equation $\delta = Z_\alpha (\sigma \sqrt{2/n}) + Z_\beta (\sigma \sqrt{2/n})$ so that the sample size n is shown as a function of the effect size δ, the standard deviation of the effect size σ, and the normal cutoff points that correspond to the significance level α and the power $1 - \beta$. This equation looks like this: $n = (Z_\alpha + Z_\beta) \times 2\sigma^2/\delta^2$.[15] Because in this case, the effect size, δ, represents the mean differences between intervention and control groups, it can be restated as $\delta = \mu_i - \mu_c$, or the difference between the mean of the intervention group (μ_i) and that of the control group (μ_c).

Suppose we want to test whether a behavioral intervention can reduce CES-D scores by at least four points. From previous studies, we estimate that the standard deviation of CES-D scores in the target population is $\sigma = 8$. Furthermore, we set the significance level at a conventional value of .05; thus, $Z_\alpha = Z_{.05} = 1.96$. We also require the test to be powerful enough so that we have at least an 80% chance of de-

tecting a reduction in CES-D scores by four points. Because $1 - \beta$ is set at .80, $\beta = .2$ and $Z_\beta = Z_{.20} = .84$. Substituting the specific values in the equation, $n = (Z_\alpha + Z_\beta) \times 2\sigma^2/\delta^2$, we get: $n = 2 \times (1.96 + .84)^2 \times 8^2/ 4^2 = 63$. Thus, the total required sample size, including both treatment and control groups equals N = 2n = 126. In other words, if we want to have an 80% chance of detecting a four-point reduction in CES-D scores as a result of our intervention, and if we tolerate no more than a 5% probability of a Type I error, then we must obtain a sample of at least 126 subjects, evenly divided between treatment and control groups.[16]

To recap, to calculate the required sample sizes for experiments in which subjects are randomly assigned to two groups, we can use the following equation: $n = (Z_\alpha + Z_\beta) \times 2\sigma^2/\delta^2$. Then, we substitute the appropriate values for Z_α, Z_β, σ, and δ to obtain the desired sample size, n. In practice, it is easier to use tables that list the required sample sizes as a function of Z_α, Z_β, and the *standardized* effect size (δs). Because variables may have different population standard deviations, tabulations of required sample sizes would seem to require many different tables. However, if we standardize the effect size, a single table can be used to accommodate different variables. Because the standardized effect size is $\delta s = \delta/\sigma$, we can always convert back to δ by multiplying δs by σ.

In the depression intervention example, $\delta = 4$ and $\sigma = 8$; thus, $\delta s = 0.5$, or the standardized effect size is equal to one-half. Table 20-5 shows the total sample size requirement for several standardized effect sizes,[17] including .2,

---

[15] $\delta = Z_\alpha (\sigma \sqrt{2/n}) + Z_\beta (\sigma \sqrt{2/n})$
I factor $\sqrt{2n} \to \delta = (Z_\alpha + Z_\beta) \times (\sigma \sqrt{2/n})$
I multiply by $\sqrt{n} \to \delta \times \sqrt{n} = (Z_\alpha + Z_\beta) \times (\sigma \sqrt{2})$
I divide by $\delta \to \sqrt{n} = [(Z_\alpha + Z_\beta) \times (\sigma \sqrt{2})]/\delta$
I take the square $\to n = (Z_\alpha + Z_\beta)^2 \times 2\sigma^2/\delta^2$

---

[16] In an actual study, we would also need to take into account likely subject attrition before settling on a final recruitment number.

[17] Calculations were performed with the procedure "sampsi" in the STATA release 7.0 software package.

TABLE 20.5		Total Sample Size* as a Function of Effect Size, Significance Level, and Power						

		Standardized effect size						
		.2	.3	.4	.5	.6	.7	.8
Significance level α = .10 (two-tailed)								
Power (1 − β)	.50	272	122	68	44	32	24	18
	.60	362	162	92	58	42	30	24
	.70	472	210	108	76	54	40	30
	.80	620	276	156	100	70	52	40
	.90	858	382	216	138	96	70	54
	.95	1084	482	272	174	122	90	68
	.99	1578	702	396	252	176	130	100
Significance level α = .05 (two-tailed)								
Power (1 − β)	.50	386	172	98	62	44	32	26
	.60	490	218	124	80	56	40	32
	.70	618	276	156	100	70	52	40
	.80	786	350	198	126	88	66	50
	.90	1052	468	264	170	118	86	66
	.95	1300	578	326	208	146	108	82
	.99	1838	818	460	294	206	150	116
Significance level α = .01 (two-tailed)								
Power (1 − β)	.50	664	296	166	108	74	56	42
	.60	802	356	202	130	90	66	52
	.70	962	428	242	154	108	80	62
	.80	1168	520	292	188	130	96	74
	.90	1488	662	372	240	166	122	94
	.95	1782	792	446	286	198	146	112
	.99	2404	1070	602	386	268	198	152

*Total sample size (N = 2 × n), where n = size of either treatment or control group.

commonly considered a "small" effect; .5, a "medium" effect; and .8, a "large" effect (Cohen, 1993). The table also shows the effects of varying significance levels and desired power on required sample size. As is easily seen, when moving from the left to the right column entries in each row, to detect larger effect sizes, one generally needs smaller samples, holding significance levels and power requirements constant. On the other hand, if effect size and significance levels are held constant, sample size requirements *increase* when researchers desire *greater* power. Finally, holding effect size and power constant, sample size requirements also increase when a researcher requires more stringent (i.e., lower) significance levels. All of this makes sense. If we want to increase the confidence in our inference, or reduce the probability of making Type I and

Type II errors, we need larger samples. Clearly, tradeoffs and compromises are an inherent aspect of all calculations of sample size.

Calculation of the Power of a Test

When sample size is fixed, the calculation of power can be based on the same equation that is used for sample size calculations, $n = (Z_\alpha + Z_\beta) \times 2\sigma^2/\delta^2$, except that the equation must be recast to solve for Z_β. Recall that, for the normal distribution centered on the true effect size, Z_β is the cutoff point for rejection of the null hypothesis $(1 - \beta)$, indicating the power of the test, and acceptance of the null hypothesis, (β) indicating the size of the Type II error that the researcher is willing to accept. Solving this equation for

Z_β yields: $Z_\beta = (\delta \sqrt{n})/(\sigma \sqrt{2})^- Z_\alpha$. Because the standardized effect size is δ/σ, we can rewrite this equation as: $Z_\beta = (\delta s \sqrt{n/2}) Z_\alpha$. On a normal curve, the area below Z_β represents the probability of accepting the research hypothesis which, when it is true, is also known as power or $(1 - \beta)$.

Table 20-6 provides power calculations for several combinations of effect sizes, significance levels, and given sample sizes. For instance, if researchers want to test an intervention effect, the magnitude of which, they believe, translates into a moderate standardized effect size of .5, and if they cannot hope to enroll more than 70 subjects in their study, their study will at best achieve a power of 55.2% if they adhere to the conventional significance level of .05. In other words, the probability that they will find a statistically significant effect, if there is one, is only .552.

Note again that power increases with increased effect size, which means that it is easier to discover larger rather than smaller effect sizes. Power also increases with sample size. Finally, the table shows the tradeoff between Type I and Type II errors or its obverse, the power of the test: when effect size and sample size are held constant, a decrease in α (the probability of a Type I error) also leads to a decrease in power $(1 - \beta)$.

▶CLINICAL RESEARCH IN ACTION
Example of Insufficient Sample Size

Ward et al. (2000) conducted a randomized experiment to test whether a nursing intervention that provided individually tailored sensory and coping information about pain and

---

TABLE 20.6 Power as a Function of Effect Size δ, Significance Level, and Total Sample Size*

		δ (standardized effect size)						
		.2	.3	.4	.5	.6	.7	.8
Significance level a = .10 (two-tailed)								
Sample size	20	.134	.175	.232	.302	.382	.469	.558
	50	.184	.283	.410	.549	.683	.797	.882
	70	.216	.350	.512	.673	.797	.900	.956
	100	.264	.443	.639	.812	.912	.968	.991
	200	.410	.683	.882	.971	.995	.999	1.000
	500	.723	.956	.998	1.000	1.000	1.000	1.000
	1000	.935	.999	1.000	1.000	1.000	1.000	1.000
Significance level a = .05 (two-tailed)								
Sample size	20	.073	.103	.146	.201	.269	.347	.432
	50	.109	.186	.293	.424	.564	.697	.807
	70	.133	.241	.387	.552	.709	.834	.917
	100	.170	.323	.516	.705	.851	.938	.979
	200	.293	.564	.807	.942	.989	.999	1.000
	500	.609	.918	.994	.999	1.000	1.000	1.000
	1000	.885	.997	1.000	1.000	1.000	1.000	1.000
Significance level a = .01 (two-tailed)								
Sample size	20	.018	.029	.047	.073	.109	.156	.216
	50	.031	.065	.123	.210	.315	.460	.600
	70	.041	.093	.183	.314	.474	.638	.780
	100	.058	.141	.282	.470	.664	.822	.923
	200	.123	.325	.600	.831	.952	.991	.999
	500	.367	.782	.971	.999	1.000	1.000	1.000
	1000	.721	.985	.999	1.000	1.000	1.000	1.000

*Total sample size (N = 2n), where n = size of either treatment or control group.

analgesic side effects would improve pain management in women with gynecologic cancers. Specifically, they tested if, and to what extent, the intervention made a difference in six outcome measures:

1. A measure of the presence of patient-related barriers to pain management
2. A pain intensity scale
3. A measure of the adequacy of pain management
4. A measure of the severity of medication side effects
5. A measure of the interference of pain with life
6. An overall quality-of-life measure

A repeated-measures, two-group randomized design was used, with one pretest, or baseline, and two follow-up posttests. As discussed in chapters 3–5, the chapters on research design, this is a strong design for testing the causal effects of an intervention. A total of 43 subjects initially consented to participate and were randomized to the intervention group (n = 21) and the control group (n = 22). Of this group, 33 participated in the first posttest and 27 participated in the second posttest.

The study results showed a lack of statistically significant differences on five of the six outcome measures. The authors discussed possible reasons for the lack of an expected intervention effect, including floor effects, in which most responses on variables tended to be clustered at the low extremes of the scales. The authors concluded that lack of statistical power as a result of the small sample size was not a strong explanation for the lack of statistical significance on the basis that a clinically meaningful effect should have been found, even with a small sample. However, the argument for the expectation that clinically meaningful effects can be detected in small samples may not be very strong, and this study provides an excellent opportunity to show the usefulness of power calculations after a study has already been done. To illustrate these calculations, we concentrate on one of the five nonsignificant outcome measures in this study, the quality-of-life measure. The researchers used the Functional Assessment of Cancer Therapy-General Form (FACT-G), which is a quality-of-life measure that sums responses to 29 Likert-type rating questions, scaled on a 5-point (0–4) response scale (Cronbach's α = .88), with higher scores indicating greater quality of life and a possible range of scores of 29 to 116.

On the first posttest measure, involving 15 intervention group responses and 18 control group responses, a FACT-G mean score of 78.46 (standard deviation, 19.97) was found for the intervention group and 76.98 (standard deviation, 18.83) for the control group. This difference was reported as not statistically significant; the specific significance level was not reported in the article. At the pretest, the intervention and control groups had the following means and standard deviations for this quality-of-life measure: 76.79 (20.73) in the intervention group and 76.64 (13.54) in the control group. Thus, there appears to have been a small improvement in the mean scores within the intervention group (78.46 − 76.79 = 1.67) and a less than one-point increase in the control group (76.98 − 76.64 = .34).

Why are these differences not statistically significant? Researchers might test for the intervention effect in two ways. After random assignment, the pretest could be disregarded, with the researchers concentrating only on the posttest and comparing the posttest mean of the intervention group (78.46) with that of the control group (76.98). Alternatively, the researchers could take advantage of the greater efficiency of the repeated-measures design by comparing the change scores in the intervention group (1.67) with those in the control group (.34).

With either option, it is important to consider what mean difference resulting from the intervention would be considered clinically meaningful. Cohen's convention is that a standardized effect size of δs = .8 should be considered "large." Because the authors reported an estimated population standard deviation for the FACT-G from previous literature of 15.86, this would translate into an unstandardized effect size of δ = 12.69, because $\delta s = \delta/\sigma$. Using this large effect size, we could address the question of statistical power with the following: (1) a sample of size N = 33, with n = 15 in the intervention group and n = 18 in the control group; and (2) a conventional significance level set at α = .05. What would be the power of the test to detect a standardized effect size (mean difference) of .8? From Table 20-6, we know that the answer must lie somewhere between .432 and .807 because the total sample size of N = 33 lies between 20 and 50. Precise calculations would yield a power of .629.[18] In other words, even for a large mean difference (δ = 12.69) between the posttest scores of the intervention group and the control group, there would be only a 62.9% chance of detecting this difference in a study of the sample size reported in the article. For a medium effect size of δs = .5 (or δ = 7.93), the power would decline to .299, and for a small effect of δs = .2 (or δ = 3.17), the power would decline to .088. Thus, there is a credible possibility that the lack of statistically significant effects is the result of sample size limitations. Although the power improves with the repeated-measures design and is .893, .517, and .126, respectively, only the detection of large effect sizes could have been expected in this study.[19] Because attrition leads to even smaller numbers (n = 27) in the second posttest sample, there is further loss of power.

We can also reverse the power question and ask what sample size would have been required to show, say, a medium effect size of δs = .5 (or unstandardized δ = 7.93)? If we again assume the conventional significance level of α = .05 and power of 1 − β = .80, to detect this effect we can use Table 20-5 to find the required total sample size of N = 126, with n = 63 in each arm. Although a repeated-measures

---

[18] Cohen (1993) considers .80 a conventional low-end power level.

[19] Calculations were performed with the STATA procedure "sampsi." For a full explanation, see Frison and Pocock (1992).

design would improve efficiency and require only a total sample size of N = 66, with n = 33 in each arm, we can conclude that the actual sample size used in this study would not have been large enough to discover moderate effect sizes. Only fairly substantial effects would have had a chance to be detected.

CONCLUSION

In this chapter, we have taken a somewhat formal approach to statistical inference in the form of significance testing, confidence interval construction, and power analysis. Underlying all three of these concepts are two simple principles: (1) it is assumed that the generation of the data involved some probability procedure or random process, as exemplified by random selection or sampling, random assignment, or possibly measurement error; and (2) sample estimates of population parameters fluctuate or vary less when samples become larger.

Significance testing, although ubiquitous in the applied health care and nursing literature, tends to be a less informative tool of statistical inference than confidence interval construction. When a sample result is classified as "statistically significant," all we know is that the sample result is an unlikely event if we assume that the null hypothesis is true. This approach to significance testing is most useful when we are testing specific, meaningful (null) hypotheses, such as whether an intervention group mean differs from a control group mean or whether a correlation differs from zero. Yet, even in such a situation, it is more informative to obtain the actual range of estimates for population parameters.

Power analysis is most helpful in the planning stage of a study, particularly an experimental study. It helps us to decide how large a sample we need to test a desired effect size, and it clarifies the tradeoffs among Type I and Type II errors of inference, effect size, and sample size. However, we are often in a situation in which neither clinical experience nor past research can provide a good guide for determining what is a meaningful effect size. In that situation, a researcher may be tempted to use power analysis to "justify" a predetermined sample size by changing effect sizes until they predict the "need for" the predetermined sample size. One way to guard against this kind of sleight of hand is to establish general guidelines for the magnitudes of meaningful effect sizes, as has been done by Cohen (1993). Power analysis is generally less useful in descriptive or observational research because the focus is less often on specific effect sizes. In addition, descriptive or observational research tends to be more exploratory, with researchers simultaneously interested in multiple relationships. In that situation, the required sample size should be large enough to show the smallest relationship on which a researcher wants to focus.

In the last two chapters, we focused on quantitative approaches to sampling. In this tradition, the main concern is to devise sampling procedures that yield samples that are objective, unbiased reflections of the populations from which they are drawn. The purpose of using random or probability procedures in quantitative sampling is to exclude the possibility that investigator judgments and biases will affect the sample selection. In contrast, in qualitative sampling, investigator judgments are at the heart of the sampling process. These issues will be discussed in the next chapter.

Suggested Activities

1. Read Ward et al. (2000). Use Table 2 to calculate medium effect sizes for the other outcome variables listed.
   a. Concentrate only on the mean comparison between the two posttest scores.
   b. Convert the medium standardized effect size of $\delta s = .5$ into an unstandardized effect size for each variable. You can obtain an unstandardized effect size δ by multiplying the δs by the *smaller* of the standard deviations in either the treatment or the control group.
2. If we adopt a significance level of $\alpha = .01$, we want to be very sure that the intervention is effective and also requires substantial power (.90). Use Table 20-5 to determine how large a total study sample would be required to detect these medium effect sizes.
3. Researchers conduct an intervention study among postsurgical patients to test the effectiveness of postdischarge telephone calls to reduce the use of the emergency department after hospitalization. They find a "statistically significant" difference, with the intervention group using the emergency department less often. Do they need to perform a power analysis?
4. Using data from a convenience sample, researchers find a "statistically significant" correlation between a measure of depression and a measure of compliance with treatment regimens: more depressed patients are less likely is to comply with treatment. What does it mean to say that the correlation is "statistically significant"?

Suggested Readings
Ward, S., Donovan, H. S., Owen, B., Grosen, E., & Serlin, R. (2000). An individualized intervention to overcome

patient-related barriers to pain management in women with gynecologic cancers. *Research in Nursing & Health, 23,* 393–405.

References

Bulmer, M. G. (1979). *Principles of statistics.* New York: Dover.

Cohen, J. (1993). *Statistical power analysis for the behavioral sciences* (2nd ed.). Hillsdale, NJ: Lawrence Erlbaum.

Devins, G. M., & Orme, C. M. (1986). Center for Epidemiologic Studies depression scale. In Kayser, J. D., Sweetland, R. C. (Eds.), *Test critiques,* Vol. 2. (pp. 144–160). Kansas City, MO: Test Corporation of America.

Frison, L., & Pocock, S. (1992). Repeated measurements in clinical trials: Analysis using mean summary statistics and its implications for design. *Statistics in Medicine, 11,* 1685–1704.

Greenland, S. (1990). Randomization, statistics, and causal inference. *Epidemiology, 1,* 421–429.

Kraemer, H. C., & Thiemann, S. (1987). *How many subjects? Statistical power analysis in research.* Newbury Park, CA: Sage.

Lipsey, M. W. (1990). *Design sensitivity. Statistical power for experimental research.* Thousand Oaks, CA: Sage.

Radloff, L. S. (1977). The CES-D Scale: A self-report depression scale for research in the general population. *Applied Psychological Measurement, 1,* 385–401.

StataCorp. (2001). *STATA statistical software, Release 7.0.* College Station, TX: Stata Corporation.

CHAPTER 21   Qualitative Approaches to Sampling

APPROPRIATENESS OF PROBABILITY SAMPLING FOR QUALITATIVE RESEARCH

In the last two chapters, we discussed the rationale, basic principles, and limitations of probability sampling. We closed the discussion with the remark that, in qualitative studies, investigator judgments play a pivotal role in the sampling process.

Another way to say this is that sampling of study participants in qualitative studies tends to be purposeful (Patton, 1990). This poses the question: Why is probability sampling usually not considered an appropriate strategy for case sampling in qualitative research?

On the face of it, probability sampling seems to be an *ideal* choice for induction-oriented research approaches. Although the conversion of verbal responses into quantitative *measures* may be faulted for being reductionistic and limiting the richness of expression,[1] the application of the mathematical probability calculus to the problem of *sampling* has the undeniable virtue that it is a "presupposition-less" approach. It is the only approach to sampling in which the researcher *gives up control* over the selection of individual study participants or other sampling units. In this sense, probability sampling is the only technique that does not rely on *preconceived* notions or criteria that drive the selection of individual sampling units.

The alternatives to probability sampling are convenience sampling and some form of purposeful sampling (the latter being much preferred in qualitative research). However, purposeful sampling inevitably involves the use of researcher-imposed selection criterion.[2] So, why is it the preferred approach to sampling in qualitative research? To answer this question, we must revisit some of the limitations of probability sampling.

The strongest argument against probability sampling in qualitative research is a technical one: precision in statistical inference depends largely on sample size.[3]

Yet, as we have seen in earlier chapters (chapters 12 and 18), study samples in qualitative research are usually quite small, ranging from studies of 2 to 3 persons to maybe 30 to 40.

The reason is simple: the strategies for interpretive analysis that are used in qualitative research, such as analyses of narrative texts or interpretations of social interactions on videotape, require a level of immersion and time commitment that make it impossible for a single researcher to deal with more than a handful of cases. However, the benefits of probability sampling can be realized only if the sample estimates are reasonably accurate. For instance, even if a researcher had somehow drawn a simple random sample of 10 patients undergoing dialysis from all such patients in the United States during a given year, population estimates based on samples of 10 patients would vary so substantially from one sample to the next that, for all practical purposes, such "estimates" would not provide useful information. In short, although estimates based on small random samples may be unbiased, the lack of precision in the estimates outweighs any potential advantages associated with the lack of bias.

Next to the technical limitations associated with drawing inferences from very small samples, probability sampling, *if applied to inappropriate sampling units,* appears to be in conflict with the goals of most qualitative research. Whatever their specific approach, qualitative researchers strive to obtain context-sensitive information. Yet, the random selection of *individual study participants* normally results in a study sample of persons drawn from multiple, unrelated social contexts. In other words, random selection breaks up the context of the sample, unless the units of analysis are redefined in terms of whole settings or clusters. With a suitable sampling frame, it is technically possible to randomly select such institutional and social settings as hospital wards, nursing homes, and school classes for inclusion in a study. However, the study of social and institutional aggregates through ethnographic fieldwork is even more time-consuming than the study of individuals with a qualitative research approach. Thus, the number of settings that can be studied ethnographically in a given study is necessarily very small, and meaningful probability samples, representative of larger populations of similar institutional settings, cannot be obtained.

Given these obstacles to using probability sampling, an important question inevitably arises. Are there other ways to generalize beyond a study setting or a particular sample of study participants? Some qualitative researchers have gone so far as to assert that generalization is impossible. We will turn to this question next.

GENERALIZATIONS IN QUALITATIVE RESEARCH

Lincoln and Guba (1985) reject generalization as a research goal, because "local conditions . . . make it impossible to generalize. If there is a *true* generalization, it is that there can be no generalization" (p. 124). If that were literally true, descriptive epidemiology would have to be accused of

---

[1]See chapters 16 and 18 for a more complete discussion.

[2]This topic is discussed in more detail later in this chapter.

[3]Refer back to the discussion of standard errors in chapter 20.

attempting the impossible. Descriptive generalizations, such as "cancer incidence rates rise with age" or "HIV infections are much more prevalent among heroin addicts than in the general population," would be considered statements that cannot be justified on the basis of sample observations. Implicit in Lincoln and Guba's (1985) rejection of generalization is an overly restrictive view of generalization that does not take into account the *statistical* nature of most descriptive generalizations in research. Consider a statement such as: "Mexico (or Italy) is a Catholic country." This statement does not imply that the speaker assumes that *all* residents in these countries are Catholic, only that Catholicism is the dominant religion that has shaped the culture of the country. In the same way, whether quantitative or qualitative in their orientation, researchers often make assertions such as the following:

- *Caregivers of mentally ill care recipients are intent on pursuing (the appearance of) normalcy (Rose, Mallinson, & Walton-Moss, 2002).*
- *Spouses of persons with dementia are a particularly vulnerable segment of the caregiving population (Perry, 2002).*
- *Persons who engage more frequently in spiritual practices enjoy better mental health (Meisenhelder & Chandler, 2000).*

Such statements are not only generalizations in the sense that they characterize a dominant pattern observed in a particular study group, but also are often meant to refer to patterns that hold beyond the particular group of research participants or settings.

This, then, is the crux of the problem of generalization: Every research project collects evidence consisting of a *particular and finite* set of observations. However, these observations are often used to make statements about broad patterns. Such generalizations do not always, and certainly do not only, involve statistical generalization.

Consider the following example. Suppose a study finds that, in a particular state, children in households without private insurance coverage have much lower immunization rates than children in households with private insurance coverage. Unless the study sample is highly unusual and atypical of the general population in that state, there is every reason to believe that this is not just a local pattern.

In this example, two kinds of generalizations are at work. One is strictly statistical: within a state, the usual way to investigate differences in child immunization rates between two subpopulations is to use probability samples so that one can generalize to the state population. The assumption that similar differences in immunization rates be-

tween insured and uninsured children also hold in other states is *not* based on statistical evidence. However, this does not make it an unreasonable assumption. Given established economic theories about the relationship between price and demand for services, ample evidence that lack of health insurance is a major barrier to accessing primary care services, and evidence of lower participation rates of uninsured persons in other preventive health services (e.g., cancer screenings), the finding that, in a particular state, uninsured children have lower immunization rates should be considered strong evidence in favor of a general pattern. The strength of such nonstatistical generalizations depends entirely on the consistency of a particular study finding with well-established principles and theories as well as supporting evidence from related empirical work. If this type of supporting evidence is available, the burden of proof shifts to those who believe that the generalization is unwarranted. Box 21-1 shows different types of generalizations used by researchers.

Certain kinds of nonstatistical generalizations are common in qualitative research as well, although they are not always acknowledged. In most cases, readers of qualitative research accounts make implicit generalizations. Why would a clinician want to read an account of, say, the experience of spouses of patients who undergo heart transplantation (McCurry & Thomas, 2002), unless that account shows patterns that are potentially applicable to his or her own patients? Most nursing and health care research is engaged in generalizations.[4] The goal of this research is to go beyond the description of particular situations and to present results and patterns that are broadly applicable and are seen as relevant by other researchers or clinicians, who typically are not interested in the particular cases described.[5]

APPROACHES TO SAMPLING IN QUALITATIVE STUDIES

Although qualitative researchers usually avoid using the term "generalization," many use sampling criteria that suggest an interest in the broader applicability of their study findings. The very term *sampling* implies that the sample is a subset of a larger population. As always, any effort to draw

---

[4]An obvious exception is strictly historical research. Its main goal is to reconstruct and understand particular historic events and situations. Yet, even here, our interest in historical research often goes beyond the particular events described, which may be seen as "analogies" to current situations, from which we can learn.

[5]Even the traditional case study report in medical journals is not presented for its own sake, but as an example to illuminate a broader pattern.

BOX 21.1   Types of Generalizations

Statistical generalizations

Statistical generalizations are based on finite samples of observations. Such generalizations from observed samples to population units are possible only if the sample selection is consistent with the assumptions of probability theory. Strictly speaking, statistical generalizations can be made only about the populations from which the samples are *actually* drawn. Thus, all statements that extrapolate a pattern or relationship into the future or to some other population whose members are not sampled go beyond the inferences made possible by the mathematics of the probability calculus.

Measurement generalizations

In the domain sampling theory, each indicator item or instance of measurement is viewed as a single selection from all possible indicator items or measurement occasions. Multiple indicators or multiple measurements are thus a sample of all possible measurements. However because we cannot specify the population of all possible indicator items of a concept (such as depression) or all possible measurement occasions, strictly speaking, the generalization is not based on statistical probability theory because no random selection occurred in the first place. In reality, we use nonstatistical criteria to create measurement indicators or select measurement occasions.

Causal generalizations

Causal generalizations are often used in research. However, it is very rare that experiments and clinical trials are based on random *samples* of study participants from larger populations (see chapters 4 and 5). Still, researchers generalize, for example, from the results of a particular drug trial to the efficacy of the tested drug in general. Such causal generalizations are often eminently plausible because they are not only supported by the evidence from a particular trial, but also rest on the identification of a causal mechanism, such as the specific chemical and biophysiologic pathways that make the drug effective. In other words, such evidence gains credence because it is consistent with many other pieces of evidence and established theories in multiple areas.

a sample from a population requires a definition of the relevant population and sampling units. Although most qualitative nursing research appears to focus on individuals as the primary sampling units (e.g., Davis, 2002; Messecar, Archbold, Stewart, & Kirschling, 2002; Moore, 2000; Perry, 2002), ethnographically oriented researchers often choose a setting (Emami, Torres, Lipson, & Ekman, 2002). Others focus on social relationships (Tulviste, 2000), which is in keeping with the goals of understanding context-bound actions.

As in other areas of study design, in qualitative studies, sampling tends to be flexible, and study reports usually provide very short descriptions of the sampling process. Sampling units are often selected serially, either on the basis of *theoretic sampling* (Rose et al., 2002) or through *snowball* or *network sampling* (Ayres, 2000).

As discussed in chapter 19, the latter form of sampling is also used in quantitative studies. It relies on early study participants to suggest the names of other people to be contacted for study participation and is a useful strategy for accessing socially marginal populations for which no sampling frames are available.

Here, we will discuss only theoretic sampling because of its central role in qualitative research.

Theoretic Sampling

Theoretic sampling is a concept used by researchers in the grounded theory tradition (Glaser & Strauss, 1967; Chenitz & Swanson, 1986). As the term suggests, the primary concern is not with obtaining a sample of study participants that is representative of a sample of a particular population, but rather with sampling study participants in a way that covers all aspects of a concept or an emerging theory (see Research Scenario 21-1).[6]

Whether based on initial or emerging theoretic considerations, the goal of theoretic sampling is to seek study participants that help to probe similarities and differences as well as the whole range of phenomena involved. For

---

[6]In the discussion of the domain sampling theory in measurement (chapter 13), we encountered an analogous concern: that the indicators for a theoretic concept, such as depression, fully cover all aspects or dimensions of the concept.

RESEARCH SCENARIO 21.1

Sampling on the Basis of Emerging Theory

Perry (2002), in a study of caregivers of spouses with Alzheimer's disease, discovered the importance of satisfaction with the marriage for the caring process and proceeded to seek new study participants who varied in terms of marital satisfaction. Likewise, this researcher sought to enroll study participants whose husbands "were in the middle and advanced stages" of dementia, because of the implications for care. This decision appears to have been made on prior grounds rather than on the basis of "emerging" theoretical considerations that arose as a result of talking to the first caregivers who participated in the study.

instance, the "process of interpretive caring" (Perry, 2002), with its suggested stages ("seeing the signs, picking up the slack, taking over, rewriting identities, making daily life work"), might be experienced differently by wives who are satisfied with their marriage than by those who are not satisfied.

Theoretic sampling is a form of *purposive sampling* that is very much akin to Cook and Campbell's (1979) deliberate sampling for heterogeneous qualities, a strategy that is also used in the initial stages of scale development for quantitative measures (DeVellis, 1991). For exploratory purposes, it is a very useful approach to sampling. However, like all nonprobability approaches to sampling, it suffers from potential bias in two areas. The first issue is the selection of initial sampling units. Glaser and Strauss (1967) acknowledge that the initial selection of study participants usually rests on prior, if "loose," theoretic considerations of the researcher. The only other alternative is "blind," or haphazard, selection of initial study participants. This type of selection is problematic for theoretic sampling because a serial approach to sampling may be heavily influenced by the initial conditions. If the researcher decides to approach future study participants based on what he or she learned from the initial study participants, then the initial study participants exert a substantial influence on the direction of the investigation.

A different, but also potentially contentious, issue is the timing of the decision to terminate data collection.

Grounded theorists use as their criterion for termination the **theoretic saturation** of a concept or category. This saturation occurs when "the researcher becomes empirically confident that a category is saturated" (Glaser & Strauss, 1967, p. 61). Yet, this "confidence" does not rest on logical exhaustiveness, but on the theoretic acumen, imagination, and sensitivity of the individual researcher. A similar approach to terminating data collection can be found in phenomenologic investigation. As one researcher, examining mental health issues among Southeast Asian refugee women, formulated: "I stopped collecting data when I was able to envision an accurate portrayal of the women's experiences through their descriptions" (Davis, 2000). As often occurs in qualitative research, the individual researcher becomes the ultimate arbiter of validity.

There are many other forms of purposeful sampling, and Patton (1990) provides a comprehensive account of them. Most of these approaches can be divided into two major categories: (1) sampling of heterogeneous sampling units and (2) sampling of homogeneous sampling units.

Sampling of Heterogeneous Sampling Units

The example by Perry (2002) of including wives who are satisfied and those who are dissatisfied with their marriage in their study of dementia caregivers is an instance of **sampling of heterogeneous sampling units.** Rose et al. (2002) provide another example of deliberately seeking heterogeneity in a sample, using both hospital-based and community-based patients in their study of family responses to mental illness. Sometimes researchers sample **extreme or deviant cases** (e.g., sexually abstinent and promiscuous youth) or **disconfirming cases** (cases that do not fit the pattern, such as high academic achievers from poverty-stricken areas), because they are most likely to reveal the factors that explain the differences in outcomes. **Maximum variation** sometimes can be achieved if the study sample for a qualitative study is selected from a large roster of participants in a quantitative study (Butcher, Holkup, Park, & Maas, 2002). In such cases, the information available from the quantitative study can be used to divide cases into extreme strata and to select a stratified random sample that incorporates maximal variation on a number of theoretically relevant criteria.

Sampling of Homogeneous Sampling Units

The opposite strategy is to recruit *homogeneous samples* of study participants.

In chapter 18, we encountered one example of homogeneous sampling of study participants in the recruitment of focus group participants. As we saw, one main attraction of recruiting homogeneous samples for focus group sessions is that it greatly facilitates the group interviewing process.

By definition, homogeneity reduces variance and thus allows the researcher a limited view of the phenomenon of interest. Unless deliberately counteracted by a researcher who searches for heterogeneous cases, overly homogeneous samples are a great danger in qualitative research studies with small samples of study participants. Most clinical research is conducted in particular localities (Chiu, 2000; Im & Meleis, 2000) that fall far short of representing all patients of a particular kind. Many such samples are obtained through a single institutional setting or agency (Foley, Minick, & Kee, 2000; Moore, 2000), which usually acts as a social filtering device.[7] The only way to overcome such limitations is to move beyond a particular setting. Thus, although qualitative research reports often mention efforts to generate heterogeneity with respect to age, ethnicity, or other socioeconomic characteristics, such as occupational background (Benzein, Saveman, & Norberg, 2000; Butcher et al., 2001; Rose et al., 2002), such efforts usually refer to heterogeneity *within* particular settings, not among members of different social settings. Although snowball and network sampling methods are usually not viewed as subcategories of homogeneous sampling, they have a bias toward homogeneity. If researchers rely on informants and contacts to enroll a sample of study participants (Davis, 2000; Davis, 2002; Kennedy, 2000), they run the risk of assembling a sample that is socially more homogeneous than the larger target population. This may be one reason why qualitative research reports often tend to emphasize *major themes,* or *commonalities,* rather than differences and heterogeneity (e.g., Im & Meleis, 2000; Perry, 2002).

CONCLUSION: CRITERIA FOR THE ADEQUACY OF GENERALIZING FROM SAMPLE DATA

Sampling decisions are inescapable in all research. As Miles and Huberman (1984) aptly remarked, "one cannot study everyone everywhere doing everything." Thus, researchers must limit their investigation to a subset of settings, locations, actors, events, and processes. Hence, the problem of sampling: what should we observe?

As soon as we recognize that our observations are only small subsets of all possible observations, we face the possibility of *sampling bias* (i.e., selecting observations that somehow do not present an accurate reflection of reality). In this sense, in both quantitative and qualitative research, sampling and generalizations based on sample observations are always an issue.

Many generalizations in research are *not* based on the formal criteria of statistical inference, which apply only if the observations were selected in ways that conform to the axioms of mathematical probability theory. This is plainly not the case for most qualitative and quantitative research studies. Instead, many scientific generalizations are essentially based on judgments about the transferability of results to new situations or populations. This does not necessarily make them arbitrary. As noted earlier, a causal generalization that is supported by specific evidence from a clinical trial and is consistent with well-established theories and accumulated evidence in related fields may well be justified.

In somewhat the same spirit, the **transferability** criterion proposed by Lincoln and Guba (1985) is related to the goal of generalizability. Lincoln and Guba do not suggest a clear set of criteria according to which one can decide whether "local findings" can be generalized to different contexts and settings. However, they do recommend that qualitative research reports offer "thick description" (i.e., a rich, thorough description of the research setting). The intended purpose of thick description is to help the reader to decide whether there are sufficient similarities and analogies between the setting described in the research report and the setting familiar to the reader to allow the reader to "transfer," or generalize, the findings from one setting to another. Even though it is left to the reader to determine transferability, the acknowledgement of its possibility implies that there are common or "general" patterns of human interaction. Such generalizations presuppose similarity, but not identity. Each human being is unique: no other has the same combination of genetic endowment, physical traits, and social experience. Yet, for example, grieving after the loss of a friend or relative is a common human experience, and we can learn something about this process by studying a subset (or sample) of grieving persons.

---

[7]For example, hospitals or nursing homes tend to draw from ethnically and socially homogeneous area populations.

Suggested Activities

1. Review the papers by Ayres (2000), Benzein et al. (2000), Butcher et al. (2001), Chiu (2000), Davis (2000), Davis (2002), Draucker and Stern (2000), Emami et al. (2000), McCurry and Thomas (2002), Perry (2002), and

Rose et al. (2002). Then create a summary grid that focuses on the following two issues:

  a. Describe all information provided in these articles on sample selection and recruitment procedures.

  b. Summarize all descriptive information on the study sample that details the socioeconomic and clinical background characteristics of the study participants.

2. Do the descriptions of the sampling processes provide a clear understanding of how study participants were recruited from an identifiable target population?

3. Which studies use single settings, and which use diverse settings for recruitment?

4. Using the participant characteristics, such as age, sex, ethnicity, education, and socioeconomic status, do the samples of study participants tend toward homogeneity or heterogeneity?

5. How many studies emphasize the discovery of different social processes for different subgroups of study participants?

6. Do the titles and text claim the existence of generalized patterns supported by the evidence?

Suggested Readings

Ayres, L. (2000). Narratives of family caregiving: Four story types. *Research in Nursing & Health, 23,* 3, 359–371.

Benzein, E. G., Saveman, B.-I., & Norberg, A. (2000). The meaning of hope in healthy, non-religious Swedes. *Western Journal of Nursing Research, 22,* 3, 303–319.

Butcher, H. K., Holkup, P. A., Park, M., & Maas, M. (2001). Thematic analysis of the experience of making a decision to place a family member with Alzheimer's disease in a special care unit. *Research in Nursing & Health, 24,* 4, 470–480.

Chenitz, W. C. & Swanson, J. M. (1986). From Practice to Grounded Theory: Qualitative Research in Nursing. Boston, MA: Addison-Wesley Publishing Co., Inc.

Chiu, L. (2000). Lived experience of spirituality in Taiwanese women with breast cancer. *Western Journal of Nursing Research, 22,* 1, 29–53.

Cook T. D. & Campbell, D. T. (1979). *Quasi-Experimentation: Design & Analysis Issues for Field Settings.* Boston, MA: Houghton Mifflin Company

Davis, R. E. (2000). Refugee experiences and Southeast Asian women's mental health. *Western Journal of Nursing Research, 22,* 2, 144–168.

Davis, R. E. (2002). Leave-taking experiences in the lives of abused women. *Clinical Nursing Research, 11,* 3, 285–305.

Draucker, C. B., & Stern, P. N. (2000). Women's responses to sexual violence by male intimates. *Western Journal of Nursing Research, 22,* 4, 385–406.

Emami, A., Torres, S., Lipson, J. G., & Ekman, S.-L. (2000). An ethnographic study of a daycare center for Iranian immigrant seniors. *Western Journal of Nursing Research, 22,* 2, 169–188.

McCurry, A. H., & Thomas, S. P. (2002). Spouses' experiences in heart transplantation. *Western Journal of Nursing Research, 24,* 2, 180–194.

Perry, J. (2002). Wives giving care to husbands with Alzheimer's disease: A process of interpretive caring. *Research in Nursing & Health, 25,* 3, 307–316.

Rose, L., Mallinson, R. K., & Walton-Moss, B. (2002). A grounded theory of families responding to mental illness. *Western Journal of Nursing Research, 24,* 5, 516–536.

References

Ayres, L. (2000). Narratives of family caregiving: Four story types. *Research in Nursing & Health, 23,* 3, 359–371.

Benzein, E. G., Saveman, B.-I., & Norberg, A. (2000). The meaning of hope in healthy, non-religious Swedes. *Western Journal of Nursing Research, 22,* 3, 303–319.

Butcher, H. K., Holkup, P. A., Park, M., & Maas, M. (2001). Thematic analysis of the experience of making a decision to place a family member with Alzheimer's disease in a special care unit. *Research in Nursing & Health, 24,* 4, 470–480.

Chiu, L. (2000). Lived experience of spirituality in Taiwanese women with breast cancer. *Western Journal of Nursing Research, 22,* 1, 29–53.

Davis, R. E. (2000). Refugee experiences and Southeast Asian women's mental health. *Western Journal of Nursing Research, 22,* 2, 144–168.

Davis, R. E. (2002). Leave-taking experiences in the lives of abused women. *Clinical Nursing Research, 11,* 3, 285–305.

DeVellis, R. (1991). *Scale development: Theory and applications.* Newbury Park, CA: Sage.

Draucker, C. B., & Stern, P. N. (2000). Women's responses to sexual violence by male intimates. *Western Journal of Nursing Research, 22,* 4, 385–406.

Emami, A., Torres, S., Lipson, J. G., & Ekman, S.-L. (2000). An ethnographic study of a daycare center for Iranian immigrant seniors. *Western Journal of Nursing Research, 22,* 2, 169–188.

Foley, B. J., Minick, P., & Kee, C. (2000). Nursing advocacy during a military operation. *Western Journal of Nursing Research, 22,* 4, 492–507.

Glaser, B. G., & Strauss, A. L. (1967). *The discovery of grounded theory: Strategies for qualitative research.* New York: Aldine DeGruyter.

Im, E.-O., & Meleis, A. I. (2000). Meanings of menopause to Korean immigrant women. *Western Journal of Nursing Research, 22,* 1, 84–102.

Kennedy, M. G. (2000). Commentary on Davis, R. E. (2000). *Western Journal of Nursing Research, 22,* 2, 162–164.

Lincoln, Y. S., & Guba, E. G. (1985). *Naturalistic inquiry.* Beverly Hills, CA: Sage.

McCurry, A. H., & Thomas, S. P. (2002). Spouses' experiences in heart transplantation. *Western Journal of Nursing Research, 24,* 2, 180–194.

Meisenhelder, J. B., & Chandler, E. N. (2002). Prayer and health outcomes in church lay leaders. *Western Journal of Nursing Research, 22,* 6, 706–716.

Messecar, D. C., Archbold, P. G., Stewart, B. J., & Kirschling, J. (2002). Home environmental modification strategies used by caregivers of the elders. *Research in Nursing & Health, 25,* 3, 357–370.

Miles, M. B. & Huberman, A. M. (1984). *Analyzing Qualitative Data: A Sourcebook for New Methods.* Beverly Hills, CA: Sage Publications.

Moore, L. W. (2000). Severe visual impairment in older women. *Western Journal of Nursing Research, 22,* 5, 571–595.

Patton, M. Q. (1990). *Qualitative evaluation and research methods.* Newbury Park, CA: Sage.

Perry, J. (2002). Wives giving care to husbands with Alzheimer's disease: A process of interpretive caring. *Research in Nursing & Health, 25,* 3, 307–316.

Rose, L., Mallinson, R. K., & Walton-Moss, B. (2002). A grounded theory of families responding to mental illness. *Western Journal of Nursing Research, 24,* 5, 516–536.

Tulviste, T. (2000). Socialization at meals: A comparison of American and Estonian mother-adolescent interaction. *Journal of Cross-Cultural Psychology, 31,* 5, 537–556.

CHAPTER 22   **Surveying: Making Use of
Research Literature**

RESEARCH UTILIZATION

The focus of this chapter is on searching and using relevant research literature. Surveying literature and incorporating research findings into clinical practice are two central aspects of **research utilization,** a process by which research findings are incorporated into clinical practice. The goal of research utilization is to foster and provide justification for clinical practices, with the ultimate aim of improving patient outcomes (Nicoll & Beyea, 1999). Research utilization skills have been identified as a core competency for evidence-based advance practice nursing (Hamric, 1996). These skills include the following:

- The ability to evaluate the quality and clinical significance of research findings
- The ability to find and disseminate research findings
- The ability to incorporate research findings into practice in various ways (McGuire & Harwood, 1996)

Several models of nursing research utilization have been proposed to promote the use of nursing research findings.[1] Table 22-1 (adapted from Stetler, 1994) presents the phases of research utilization according to one widely cited model, showing the contribution of literature surveys and the use of

[1]See Nicoll and Beyea (1999, pp. 265–267), for a comprehensive annotated list of nursing research utilization models.

TABLE 22.1	Adapted Description of the Stetler Model (1994) of Phases in Research Utilization
Phases in the Stetler Model	**Description***
1. Preparation	The researcher refines and focuses the clinical or research question of interest in preparation for surveying the literature. Especially for unfamiliar topics, this phase may involve some preliminary reading and literature searching in preparation for phases 2 and 3.
2. Validation	The researcher surveys the literature in terms of: (1) what is known, (2) what is not known, and (3) what needs to be known about a particular topic. Surveying the literature involves the use of analytic and synthetic critique skills, especially when evaluating the scientific quality and potential applicability of the findings for a particular clinical practice situation.
3. Comparative evaluation	The researcher assesses the potential usefulness of particular research findings for a given clinical practice situation. This phase involves analytic and synthetic critical thinking skills to assess the particular situational factors that may hinder or foster the adoption of research findings into practice. Comparative evaluation is an essential step in using research findings in practice.
4. Decision-making	Decision-making can result in four different outcomes: (1) The use of research findings, instrumentally, conceptually, or symbolically (2) A delayed decision that requires further consideration of the research findings or other situational variables that affect the adoption of research findings; this often occurs when additional, *existing* information is needed to make a decision (3) A decision to delay the use of the research findings because of the need for additional information about the validity of the findings or the feasibility of adopting the findings in practice; this often occurs when there is insufficient scientific evidence to support a change in practice based on the findings, *or,* when the timing or other situational variables are not favorable for incorporating the findings into a change in clinical practice (4) A decision to reject or otherwise not use the findings; this may occur for either scientific *or* feasibility reasons
5. Translation and application	The researcher casts the results of the literature review, which represent a synthesis of what is, is not, and needs to be known about a topic, in terms of the specific implications for a given clinical practice situation. The researcher takes specific action steps to implement the use of research findings.
6. Evaluation	The researcher formally evaluates the use of research findings in practice, with reference to expected outcomes. Both scientific and feasibility factors are considered in evaluating the effect of changes in clinical practice.

*Adapted for this chapter. (Adapted from Stetler, C. (1985). Research utilization: Defining the concept. *Image: Journal of Nursing Scholarship,* 17, 40–44.)

research findings in practice. As shown in Table 22-1, research utilization is a complex process that involves multiple elements that both precede and follow literature reviews and the use of research findings in practice. Surveying the literature is part of the validation and comparative evaluation phases. These phases occur after a *preparation* phase, in which the clinical or research question is refined and focused for searching a particular body of literature. The use of research findings occurs as part of the *decision-making* and *translation and application* phases. We will discuss these phases later in this chapter. Now, we turn our focus to tools and criteria for literature searches.

LITERATURE SEARCHES: TOOLS AND CRITERIA

The Goal of a Literature Search

Many research studies are designed to provide empirical evidence about questions that are of interest to both clinicians and researchers. Research findings from such studies have often been referred to as "POEMS": Patient Oriented Evidence that Matters (Shaughnessy, Slawson, & Bennet, 1994). To design a research project that can make a meaningful and useful contribution to scientific knowledge, a researcher must be familiar with the existing state of knowledge about the phenomena of interest. Similarly, clinicians engaged in state-of-the-art clinical practice must be familiar with existing research findings that address the problems that they encounter. Thus, both researchers and clinicians must approach a literature survey with the goal of maximizing their chance of summarizing the current state of knowledge in a particular area.

However, there are some differences between the goals of clinicians and those of researchers. Although both groups have an interest in empirically accurate findings and, thus, must be able to evaluate the strength of the evidence presented, researchers also approach literature with a view toward learning, and improving on, the techniques of investigation. In contrast, clinicians usually examine the study methods and procedures to understand the relevance of the assembled evidence to their clinical practice. For instance, clinicians should ask themselves to what extent the study samples in research reports resemble the clinical populations (mirror the important patient characteristics) with which they work. Although the focus of research utilization for clinical purposes differs somewhat from the approach to literature taken by a researcher, these differences in emphasis are matters of degree. As we have emphasized

throughout this book, substantive findings can never be completely divorced from the methodologic and procedural questions that support them.

A **literature search** is the formal process of locating existing information about a topic, with the goal of being able to summarize the state of knowledge. The key sources for a literature search include published literature, such as original articles (reporting the results of individual studies), review articles (evaluative summaries of an existing body of studies or other literature on a given topic), books, reports, web sites, other media, and sometimes even personal communications and other unpublished data. As will be addressed later in this chapter, assessing the quality and validity of various sources of data requires critical skills and attention to the intended use of the information. In increasing numbers and types, source materials for literature searches are now available electronically, and accessing this information requires computer and technology skills. A **literature review** is a written summary and evaluation of the information gleaned from literature searches. Such summaries may be published as extended, stand-alone review articles. More commonly, they appear as an integral part of a research report or published article.

Regardless of the specific use of the results of a literature search, to obtain an adequate understanding of the state of knowledge about a given topic, the researcher must consider three key dimensions:

1. *What is known about the topic*. A description of the current state of knowledge in an area provides the opportunity to differentiate secure, generally accepted "facts" from less secure or contested propositions. For example, literature review sections of research reports often contain summary statements of findings without detailed discussions, such as: "Several general barriers to adherence to medical therapies have been identified and extensively studied over the last 40 years. They include characteristics of the patient, provider, health care system, and sociocultural context." Reporting findings in this summary fashion is appropriate when there is a general consensus in the research community about the accuracy of the findings. In addition, as part of research reports, formal literature reviews commonly include more detailed discussions of specific prior studies, usually to highlight specific findings relevant to the current study.
2. *What is not known about the topic*. What is not known about a phenomenon is often referred to as a **research gap,** or **gap in knowledge**. In research articles, knowledge gaps are typically set in contrast to statements of what is known about a topic, because explicit identifi-

cation of the knowledge gaps provides a "natural" lead-in to, and justification for, the current study. Sometimes specific research questions and hypotheses that appear in a research article are designed to address the gaps in knowledge identified in the literature review. For example, a gap in knowledge about treatment adherence might be expressed in a research report as follows: "Although general factors in treatment adherence are well documented, by contrast, relatively little is known about cultural variables in nonadherence to antituberculosis therapy. Therefore, a key research question addressed in this study was the extent to which a socioculturally tailored intervention would be effective in increasing adherence to antituberculosis therapy."

3. *What needs to be known about the topic.* As noted above, research aims, questions, and hypotheses in a particular research study can be, and often are, based on gaps in knowledge that need to be filled. In addition, they may also be derived from "statements of need" that reflect the clinical significance and priority of the research. For example, a statement of need may provide the impetus and rationale for a research study, as expressed in the following statement: "Because drug-resistant tuberculosis has been identified as an important national public health priority by leading health agencies, the key aim of this study was to assess sociocultural factors in nonadherence to tuberculosis therapy among an identified high-risk population."

Almost all research journals require the authors of a research report to provide at least a brief and accurate review of the existing state of knowledge in a substantive area in terms of these three dimensions. Furthermore, methodologic discussions that address past difficulties with measurement, study design, or sampling in a chosen area of study are also common components of research reports. A clinician who surveys the literature in a particular area must be able to understand the limitations in the available evidence and must also be able to summarize the existing state of substantive knowledge in terms of what is known, what is unknown, and what needs to be known,[2] with an eye to the usefulness of the findings for clinical practice.

Tools for Literature Searches

With the overall goal and key dimensions of literature searches in mind, we turn now to describing the specific tools for conducting literature searches. Researchers and clinicians alike rely on these tools to obtain information about existing studies that address their questions of interest. The search process must be **systematic,** rather than haphazard, and **inclusive,** rather than arbitrarily exclusive, so that in the end, one can have confidence that the search turned up studies that are representative of the current state of knowledge in a given field. In many fields, it is impossible to conduct an **exhaustive literature search** simply because the existing literature is too vast to survey. However, a researcher should use multiple means, tools, or approaches to search the literature on a given topic until he or she reaches the point at which the likelihood of uncovering new information about a topic declines substantially. The term *exhaustive* refers to searching the literature until little significantly new information is being located. Depending on the nature of the topic, this can be a time-consuming process. Fortunately, however, some standard approaches to conducting a literature search maximize the likelihood of locating the key studies within a given area in a timely and efficient way. Many of these approaches rely on electronic resources, which are increasingly accessible in many clinical settings and require only minimal computer skills. In addition, library resources have evolved rapidly over the last decade, leading to a substantial improvement in the efficiency of search engines and other information technologies.

In the next section, we provide an overview of key tools for literature searches, followed by a discussion of practical strategies for literature searches and research utilization in clinical practice. Readers who wish to conduct in-depth literature searches, especially on highly specialized clinical topics, should consult additional resources, as suggested in the list of suggested readings, as well as qualified librarians with a specialized focus on the health sciences. Key tools for literature searches include the following:

- Computerized or electronic database searches of published research
- Searches through reference lists in key journals, books, and published articles
- Reviews of other technical information, such as reports, conference proceedings, and clinical care guidelines
- Internet (web site) searches
- Key informant information, such as personal communications, unpublished manuscripts, and unpublished data

Electronic Databases

Over the last decade, computerized databases have become the main tool for obtaining published research reports on various topics. Table 22-2 shows an annotated list of key databases that are used to locate research literature relevant

---

[2]As mentioned earlier and addressed in nursing research utilization models, additional factors apply in the effective use of research findings in practice, such as the generalizability of the study findings to specific clinical populations. More will be discussed about these issues later in this chapter.

| TABLE 22.2 | Selected Electronic Databases for Conducting Literature Searches |

Database	Description
Cumulative Index of Nursing and Allied Health Literature (CINAHL) www.cinahl.com	The major electronic database that indexes almost all nursing research that is published in English. The electronic version of CINAHL is available from 1982 to present, and currently includes 350,000+ records.
CANCERLIT	Focuses on cancer literature, and is sponsored by the National Cancer Institute (NCI). Includes electronic coverage from 1976 to present, with more than 1.4 million database records.
CATLINE	Includes books and serials at the National Library of Medicine.
Educational Resources Information Center (ERIC)	Includes the largest collection of educationally focused literature. Electronic materials are available from 1996 to present, and there are nearly 1 million records included in the database.
Health Services, Technology, Administration, and Research (HealthSTAR)	Includes published clinical and nonclinical literature on health services, technology, administration, and research. Includes 3 million+ records, and is available electronically from 1975 to present. This database is pulled from records in MEDLINE, the Hospital Literature Index, and additional journals and other source materials in key topic areas.
MEDLINE (MEDlars online)	The major electronic database that includes biomedical research reference materials. Includes electronic coverage of more than 3,800 journals from 1966 to present, and currently has 9 million+ records.
PsycINFO	An electronic database containing material from 1967 to present with 1 million+ records. This database is focused on psychological literature and is considered the major electronic database for psychology-related literature searching.

to nursing or medical practice. The main electronic databases used by researchers and clinicians are CINAHL, MEDLINE, and HEALTHSTAR. In addition, we have listed some other databases that often turn up useful references. Although the lists of resources given in this chapter are selective and are not comprehensive, they should provide researchers with a good start in accessing literature electronically and also should provide a basis for locating other relevant resources.[3]

Although computerized databases have become the main means for obtaining published research information, these databases are limited and do not necessarily cover a given type of literature exhaustively. In addition, for some topics, the indexing of key words in frequently used databases may be inadequate for identifying all of the information that has been published. This is particularly the case when key words used in the article, including the article title and text, are not matched well with standard medical subject (MeSH) headings (key search terms) that are used in MEDLINE and HealthSTAR, for example. Also, the contents of electronic databases are usually limited to the published literature or literature that is otherwise accessible at a given time to the

database developers. There is also a "lag time" between the publication of an article and the appearance of the citation in an electronic database, although this lag time has become ever shorter, especially for articles published in journals that are routinely covered by the database.

For some purposes, such as **meta-analytic reviews,** it may be desirable to have access to unpublished manuscripts or data.[4] For example, Kleiber and Harper (1999) conducted a meta-analysis to determine the size of the effect of distraction interventions on distress behavior and pain experienced by young children. The analysis was based on published and unpublished reports and data sources. In other instances, important sources of information needed for practice may not be available at all through formal publication venues (e.g., quality improvement data for a particular health care setting, unpublished reports). In these areas, existing electronic databases fall short of what is, at least in principle, available. However, such formally "unpublished" reports are increasingly available through web searches (discussed later). With these caveats mentioned, it is

---

[3]The URLs for online sites may change frequently, and new electronic resources are developed all the time.

[4]**Meta-analysis** is a quantitative approach to integrating the results of studies that have been done on a particular phenomenon. Both published and unpublished studies may be used to calculate the effect size (or magnitude of) the association between key independent and dependent variables. See chapter 17.

nonetheless becoming easier to search the literature with relative efficiency. However, the usefulness of databases still depends, to some degree, on the skills of the user, even though only limited prior knowledge and computer experience is required.

Reference List Searches

Despite the improving quality and availability of computerized search methods, it is important to remain alert to the usefulness of traditional searches of reference lists. For example, a researcher may review the reference lists in key articles that were already accessed to locate additional literature that was not identified electronically. In addition, personal files on literature pertaining to the topics of interest can provide a valuable resource for information that may not be available through computerized searches. These files are likely to contain references to reports, data, or conference proceedings that are not covered by most electronic databases.

Other Technical Information

For research utilization to occur "locally" in specific practice settings, the clinician often needs more than access to relevant research findings in the published literature. It is important for clinicians to have access to other sources of information that speak to the feasibility of implementing a change in practice, based on research. For example, suppose a clinician, who works at a primary care clinic that serves predominantly elderly, low-income clients, is considering a recommendation to change the medication-prescribing algorithms for primary hypertension. In this situation, it would be important for the clinician to consult both published clinical care guidelines, such as those developed by the U.S. Preventive Health Services Task Force or other reputable professional organizations, and "local" clinic data about how hypertension has been managed and the effectiveness of various approaches in the clinic population. There is a vast, mostly unpublished, body of literature of direct clinical relevance, often in the form of local agency or clinic reports. The quality of this information varies from poor to excellent. Accessing the relevant literature and evaluating its quality and usefulness for clinical practice issues are important and useful skills.

Internet (Web) Site Searches

Online Internet information sites have proliferated in recent years. Although they have vastly expanded our ability to access information, postings on many web sites share an important property with the previously mentioned agency reports and unpublished research: they do not necessarily go through a thorough review process. Given that almost anyone with access to the Internet can post information, the quality of online resources must be very carefully assessed for credibility and quality. A key issue in the use of web sites as sources of information is the user's ability to evaluate the credibility of the sites. Box 22-1 shows some key criteria for assessing the quality of Internet sites. Table 22-3 presents a list of selected credible health-related sites. In general, sites that were developed by federal and state health organizations, such as the many comprehensive sites

---

BOX 22.1   Key Questions for Critiquing the Adequacy of Web Site Resources

- Can the author and contact information be located on the web site and validated? For example, can the author of a survey actually be contacted for additional information?
- Is the information authored by persons with appropriate credentials? For example, are health recommendations made by persons who have appropriate academic and professional credentials, such as R.N., or M.D.?
- Are the contributors and the web site affiliated with or sponsored by a credible, known institution, such as a library, an academic institution, or a health care organization?
- Are high-quality references for statements of fact included?
- Does the information reflect the content of cited references?
- Are obvious and potential conflicts of interest (monetary and otherwise) noted in a disclaimer? For example, for-profit business (.com) websites, such as those of pharmaceutical companies, may not necessarily include balanced information about therapeutic interventions. Likewise, web sites of nonprofit organizations (.org) espousing certain missions may not necessarily include balanced information.
- Is there evidence that the information is current? For example, does the web site provide current references or the date of the last update?
- If the web site makes health-related recommendations, do the references take into account information that is both consistent and inconsistent with the recommendations?

TABLE 22.3	Selected Health-Related Search Engines, Internet Sites, and Listservs
HealthFinder *www.healthfinder.gov*	Search engine
Internet Grateful Med (IGM) *www.igm.nlm.nih.gov*	Search engine
Medical Matrix *www.medmatrix.org*	Search engine
Medscape *www.medscape.com.*	Search engine; it is also possible to register at this site to receive weekly e-mail updates and links for current research that is applicable to APN practice
National Library of Medicine (NLM) *www.nlm.nih.gov*	Search engine and comprehensive web site with many government and other publications
PubMed *www.ncbi.nlm.nih.gov*	Search engine
Journal of Family Practice (JFP) online *www.jfponline.com*	Excellent source of POEMs-type research reports
Agency for Health Care Quality and Research (AHRQ) *www.ahrq.gov*	Contains a wealth of information about clinical care guidelines and evidence-based practice
HealthWeb *www.healthweb.org*	A comprehensive health information web site for use by health care providers and users of health care
National Center for Health Statistics (NCHS) *www.cdc.gov.nchs*	Web site for the main federal agency in charge of collating public health statistics for the U.S.
National Committee on Vital Statistics (NCVHS) *http://aspe.os.dhhs.gov/ncvhs*	Web site for the advisory committee to the U.S. Secretary of Health and Human Services
National Information Center on Health Services Research and Health Care Technology (NICHSR) *www.nlm.nih.gov/nichsr.html*	Web site for a federal agency that collates and disseminates information about health services research and clinical practice guidelines
Sigma Theta Tau International *www.stti.iupui.edu*	Web site for an international honor society for nursing; includes an online library of nursing research
State Search *www.nasire.org/ss/*	Web site to locate state web sites that include links for state-level community and public health information
U.S. Preventive Health Services Task Force *www.ahcpr.gov/clinic/uspstfix.htm*	Includes recommendations and practice guidelines for primary health care screening and treatment of common health problems seen in primary care settings by APNs
McMaster University Center for Evidence-based Medicine *http://hiru.mcmaster.ca/cochrane/default.htm*	Includes links to summaries of research for evidence-based clinical practice
Oxford University Center for Evidence-based Medicine (Cochrane Library) *http://cochrane.co.uk*	U.K.-based electronic library focused on evidence-based practice; four databases are available: (1) Systematic reviews database, a good source of integrative and meta-analysis reviews of various clinical practices based on current research evidence; updated regularly (2) Abstracts of reviews of effectiveness database (3) Controlled trials registry (4) Review methology database
Doctor's Guide Publishing, Ltd. *weekly edition@docguide.com*	Provides a weekly e-mail synopsis indicating the most frequently read general medicine news, together with web-based links to articles; includes a diverse collection of citations, many of which represent POEMs-type articles
British Medical Journal *www.bmj.com* Evidence-based Nursing *www.bmjpg.com/data/ebnpp.htm*	Provides a variety of e-mail services related to evidence-based practice, including a weekly e-mail listserv with the table of contents for the *British Medical Journal;* many articles are relevant to APN practice, and individual subscribers can register for e-mail notification of specific content areas.

of the National Institutes of Health, and nonprofit organizations affiliated with academic institutions are recognized as among the most credible. However, institutional affiliation is only one factor in evaluating the quality of Internet resources. Additional criteria are presented in Box 22-1.

Key Informants

When published information about a given topic is limited or does not directly address the specific questions of interest, researchers sometimes consult experts or other colleagues who are knowledgeable about a particular topic, are likely to work on similar problems, or already have relevant data or unpublished reports. Similarly, before implementing a new intervention or clinical practice, a clinician may consult other clinicians who already have experience with it. For example, a clinician who has surveyed the literature on telephone systems used to remind patients to keep appointments may consult experienced clinicians and clinic administrators to learn about the advantages and disadvantages of various telephone reminder systems. Very often, these sources of information are important to consider, especially when planning specific changes in clinical practice based on research findings. However, it is important to remember that both the cited research and the clinical situation are examples of evidence that may not yet have gone through a rigorous review process and must be considered untested. Essentially, reliance on key informants is a form of reliance on authority and is a rational strategy in the absence of any better empirical evidence. In the spirit of science, however, it remains a preliminary strategy until better evidence comes along.

Criteria for Literature Searches

Keyword Selection

Beyond the use of specific tools to gather information, a successful literature search requires a clear understanding of the goals and purposes of the search. Nowhere is this more important than when using one, and often more than one, of the electronic databases. An electronic literature search usually starts by using keywords, including standardized words or phrases (e.g., MeSH terms) to search the database.

Suppose you want to find "intervention studies" that are designed to improve "adherence to therapeutic regimens." First, there is the question as to which database is most likely to include the journals that publish such intervention studies. For example, MEDLINE, CINAHL, and PsychINFO (for behavioral interventions) would be good starting points. Next, you may need to experiment with keyword terminology. For instance, the preferred, but certainly not exclusive,

term used in the nursing literature is "intervention studies." In the medical literature, these studies are more often referred to as "clinical trials" or "randomized clinical trials," whereas the behavioral and social science disciplines tend to prefer such terms as "experimental studies" and "behavioral experiments," and so forth. Similarly, studies of "adherence to therapeutic regimens" may also be found under the heading of "treatment compliance," whereas the use of the terms "compliance" and "adherence" without qualifiers will lead to the inclusion of many studies of purely physiologic processes. Again, the multidisciplinary nature of health-related research requires careful attention to the selection of keywords that will maximize the likelihood of finding the relevant literature. Electronic databases, such as MEDLINE and HealthSTAR, use standardized keywords (e.g., MeSH vocabulary). The use of MeSH vocabulary and the thesaurus located within these database search programs will increase the likelihood of finding useful information, especially when compared with relying exclusively on one's own intuition to find synonyms for keywords. The thesaurus subprogram that is part of the CINAHL and MEDLINE electronic databases is strongly recommended because it helps researchers to quickly locate synonyms for the different terms that are used to refer to the same topic in various types of literature.

Narrowing the Search

An initial search with an electronic database may turn up hundreds, and sometimes thousands, of references. Just reading the abstracts of this many papers could be an overwhelming task. Fortunately, most electronic databases include tutorials within the search programs that provide instruction in the use of **tree structures** or hierarchies of keywords in the databases as well as the use of **Boolean operators,** which are standardized "connecting" words for keywords, such as "and," "or," and "not," for maximizing the yield of literature searches. Although it is important to spend some time getting acquainted with these more advanced search features that are available in many electronic databases, these tools are useful only insofar as the person using them knows how to separate pertinent from less pertinent literature. Even if you do not perform the search yourself and have a librarian or professional service perform this task, you would still need to make decisions about the goals of your information search. For instance, you may decide to narrow a search from wanting to know everything there is to know about the pharmacology of antibiotic therapy to wanting to know what specific type of antibiotic should be prescribed for a particular infection in a person who has certain characteristics. Likewise, if you use one of the major electronic databases to search for literature on "depression," it will turn up tens of thousands of references. A search for literature on "depression among cancer patients" will narrow the field, but still may return an unmanageably large number of titles. Further specifications may include particular diagnoses (e.g., patients with newly diagnosed lung cancer), narrowly defined target populations (e.g., Hispanic rural residents), or specific treatments (e.g., pharmacologic interventions for depression).

Literature searches typically proceed from a general, broad search to narrower searches that focus on the subset of literature that is most relevant to the research question. However, this process of working from broad to narrow is not strictly one way. In reality, until the optimal subset of literature has been located, it is often necessary to go back and forth between broadly and narrowly defined search strategies. Searches also may be narrowed using other criteria, which may or may not be intrinsically related to the topic. At the outset, both researchers and clinicians often confine searches to publications of, say, the last 2 to 5 years. A time limitation such as this makes particular sense in a rapidly changing field. Yet, on the other hand, you might miss the best study in a field because it was published a few years earlier than the year limit you set in your search. The English language is also a common basis for literature selection, even though there is a large body of state-of-the art clinical literature published in French or German, for instance. Yet another strategy is to select articles only from journals of a particular discipline. When the point is to find literature that is relevant to a particular discipline-specific problem or theoretic concern, this approach can make sense. Yet, particularly in the health-related literature, authors from many different disciplines, publishing in a wide variety of journals, have made and will continue to make contributions that are relevant beyond their own discipline.

One important strategy for narrowing a search is to select studies based on study design or sampling procedures. When the researcher's primary concern is to understand the causal efficacy of a clinical intervention, he or she would naturally prefer to obtain evidence based on experimental studies or clinical trials. When the concern is to understand patterns of disease distribution or to obtain accurate information about access to certain kinds of health care services, a researcher would likely prefer to select population-based studies that use some form of probability sampling. When the researcher's main goal is to develop a questionnaire instrument to measure a new concept, both theoretic and exploratory qualitative studies are relevant. In such cases, one would begin the search with studies that use designs that are most relevant to the problem and would move to other studies only if the initial search yields limited results. See the list of suggested readings at the end of this chapter for references that include more comprehensive information about strategies for searching the literature.

Avoiding "Unsuccessful" Searches

Finally, the two most common causes of "unsuccessful" literature searches are:

1. Inadequate specification of the goal or question of the literature search
2. Improper or inadequate use of the database search features

When working with people who are new to conducting reviews of literature on health-related topics, we often hear a claim that nobody has published anything on a particular topic, when, in fact, there is a lot of literature available. Almost always, this problem occurs because the searcher did not use a sufficient number of keyword synonyms and alternative phrases to capture the existing literature (see the earlier discussion in this chapter regarding the use of the thesaurus subprogram). As emphasized earlier in this chapter, these types of skills are easily and quickly learned, and assistance is often readily available from librarians who are trained in state-of-the-art information technology.

READING RESEARCH REPORTS

Assuming that a literature search has been successful, a person who is seeking to become familiar with a topic will often be overwhelmed by the number of seemingly relevant research reports. With each passing year, the volume of information relevant to most health-related topics continues to expand rapidly. Given time and other constraints, it has become more and more essential for clinicians and researchers alike to "get real" (Brown, 1999) about strategies for reviewing all of this new information. Brown (1999) addressed three key tasks for clinicians who read research with the goal of informing their evidence-based clinical practice:

1. Assess the scientific quality of the research findings.
2. Determine the clinical significance of the research findings.
3. Decide whether the findings are applicable to the advance practice nurse's clinical setting and patient population.

These tasks must be accomplished without spending hundreds of hours reading scores of articles from start to finish. In this section, we provide an overview of general strategies for reading research reports, including lists of key assessment questions adapted on the basis of Brown's key three tasks (see Table 22-4).

TABLE 22.4	Key Questions in Assessing the Quality, Clinical Significance, and Applicability of Research Findings in Clinical Practice

Experimental Studies	Nonexperimental Studies
Quality	**Quality**
What blinding procedures were used? Could bias in the results have occurred as a result of awareness of the study conditions?	It is clear that the key study variables were adequately conceptualized and measured?
	How representative of the target population is the sample?
Were appropriate intervention checks carried out to ensure that the intervention was implemented faithfully?	Are the measures that were used psychometrically valid for the population that was sampled?
Is the "treatment" or "exposure" in the control group meaningfully different from that in the intervention group? Are the differences described adequately?	Did the researchers collect data on (most of) the important confounding variables so that they can be "statistically controlled" in the analysis?
How well did the random assignment process work? What were the rate and effect of study attrition?	How adequate or appropriate were the analyses for addressing the study questions?
Could anything other than the intervention itself account for the pattern of results that was found?	Were appropriate multivariate statistical procedures used to control for identified confounding variables?
What evidence was there that the random assignment process actually worked to produce preintervention equivalence?	How sound were the interpretations of the study findings?
Were appropriate statistical procedures used to compare groups on outcomes measures and to examine the effect of study attrition?	
Clinical significance	**Clinical significance**
Are the key results meaningful or substantial enough to support or result in a change in existing clinical practice?	Are the key results meaningful or substantial enough to support or result in a change in existing clinical practice?
Are any group-level differences that were found clinically significant?	Are any group-level differences that were found clinically significant?
Applicability	**Applicability**
What is the generalizability of the study findings for a given practice setting and population?	To what groups of patients would the study findings be applicable?
Did substantial risks, inconvenience, side effects, or other adverse effects occur as a result of the intervention?	How feasible in terms of time, money, and other resources would it be to change existing clinical practice on the basis of the study results?
How feasible in terms of time, energy, money, convenience, and palatability was it to implement this intervention? How feasible would it be to implement this intervention for a given clinical practice setting and population?	Could there be potentially significant risks to patients or others by changing practice based on the study results?
Could there be potentially significant risks to patients or others by changing practice based on the study results?	Would it be ethical to implement a change in practice? Based on the study findings, would it be ethical to defer implementation of a change in clinical practice?
Would it be ethical to implement a change in practice? Based on the study findings, would it be ethical not to implement a change in clinical practice?	Would there be a practical way to evaluate the results of a change in practice based on the study findings?
Would there be a practical way to evaluate the results of a change in practice based on the study findings?	

As mentioned earlier, the literature on many clinically relevant topics is often voluminous. For example, consider the topic of "treatment nonadherence," with its 40+ years of research history and literally thousands of associated reference materials in the form of articles, books, and other literature. It would be unrealistic to expect that anyone could read all of the published research in this area, so approaches to reading must be efficient while providing an effective review of the current state of knowledge. We have already seen that the first step in the process of quickly evaluating a particular set of research literature is an efficient literature search. A well-designed search will result in a more limited subset of articles and other materials that are most directly relevant to the question. This point relates to the *preparation phase* of Stetler's research utilization model, in which the clinical or research question is refined and focused as a requisite step to a formal literature search.

Assume that you decided to conduct a literature search on a topic of interest to you and that your search resulted in the selection of 80 to 100 research reports, all of which appear to be directly relevant to your specific questions. Should you obtain printed versions of all of the articles and other source materials? For the sake of efficiency, before you decide to expend resources on copying, you should consider making preliminary selections, this time based on the information provided in the abstract or summary. Fortunately, many professional journals have begun to standardize the formats of the abstracts that accompany articles. In addition to information about the research questions, hypotheses, or problems and the major empirical findings, abstracts now often include information about the type of study design and the sampling and recruitment techniques used.[5] Scanning the abstracts for references to specific study features of interest can lead to the elimination of many articles with titles that sounded promising, but do not fit your selection criteria. For instance, in the abstract, you should learn the following:

- Whether the study sample comprises N = 30 or N = 300 subjects
- Whether the study design is longitudinal or cross-sectional
- The specific target population for a particular intervention

For example, if a clinician wants to know the current state of knowledge about randomized clinical trials of telephone reminder systems for primary care patient appointments, scanning the abstracts should allow him or her to identify articles that describe the results of observational studies, so that these types of nonexperimental studies can be set aside.

Reviewing Individual Documents

Based on this preliminary work, you should now be in possession of only the most relevant research articles. The next step is to review each of the individual documents, with the overall goal of understanding the key content. See Box 22-2 for the standard format of a research report. Although not all research articles include all of the specific elements mentioned in Box 22-2, most articles have similar elements in approximately the order noted, with slight variations, depending on the formatting guidelines of the specific journal. As noted by Brown (1999), understanding what is read depends very much on being an "active reader," which means being engaged in the content at a level that is sufficient to critique the quality of the material. The material presented in this book should go a long way toward providing you with the skills needed to become an active reader. However, readers who may lack some of the skills necessary for reading research reports may find it helpful to read the abstract, introduction, and discussion sections of an article first, to gain an understanding of the overall project (aims and results) as reported in the article. Only then is it helpful to review the specific methods used, with an eye to critiquing the adequacy of what has been done in the study. Particularly for the methods section, it is important to note what information is and is not provided. Refer

---

BOX 22.2   Standard Elements in Research Reports

- Abstract
- Introduction: background, review of prior studies, statement of purpose, statement of research questions or hypotheses (as relevant)
- Methods: sample and participants, research setting, measures, procedures
- Results, including data analysis
- Discussion and conclusions
- References
- Tables, figures, appendices (as relevant)

(Adapted with permission from Brown, S. J. (1999). *Knowledge for health care practice: A guide to nursing research evidence*. Philadelphia: Saunders.)

---

[5]Any recent issue of, for example, *Nursing Research* or the *New England Journal of Medicine* will provide good examples of informative abstracts.

to Table 22-4 for key assessment questions that can be used to evaluate research reports. Also see the chapters in this book on study design, measurement, and sampling (chapters 3–21). For a formal literature review, most people find it useful to compile a summary of each article in a table with the use of index cards or another organizing system.

A critical reviewer and user of research studies always considers the **levels of research evidence** as part of the evaluation process. Thus, in a particular research report, the question should never be simply: "What are the findings?" It is also important to ask: "How good is the evidence?" Levels of research evidence are used explicitly in the development of evidence-based clinical care guidelines and other recommendations for health care developed by groups such as the U.S. Preventive Health Services Task Force. Thus, when summarizing evidence from multiple studies, one would normally differentiate among studies based on the strength of the research evidence. In this book, we have often emphasized that single studies, even if well executed, are unlikely to provide definitive answers to most research questions. In science, across-study **replicability** of findings ultimately gives us confidence in the correctness of a conclusion. Assessments of the replicability of study findings across different studies may be complicated by the use of differing types of research designs, differences in the content and delivery of interventions, and differences in outcomes and outcome measurement. Even so, more faith can usually be placed in the validity of study findings if they have been replicated in several studies. When findings are seemingly inconsistent in two or more study reports, it is important to discover the source of this inconsistency. In the final analysis, when different studies do not agree, the reader must make a reasoned judgment based on his or her knowledge of research design, measurement, sampling, and analytic strategies. When a clinician wishes to apply study findings to clinical practice, ideally, the study results should refer to settings and populations that are quite similar to those of the clinician. In practice, again, the reader must use his or her judgment, based on the most relevant evidence available.

THE USE OF RESEARCH FINDINGS IN CLINICAL PRACTICE

Beyond familiarity with the state of knowledge in a given field and the ability to assess the quality of existing research findings, there are several other considerations for using research findings in clinical practice. Foremost among these is the use to which the research findings are put (Caplan & Rich, 1975).

Instrumental Use

One of the most important aspects of research utilization is the **instrumental use** of research findings. This involves the concrete application of research findings to clinical practice. For example, several recent clinical care guidelines for preventive health screenings have included recommendations that differ from previous screening practices. Thus, the use of routine urinalysis as a screening tool for healthy adult populations is no longer recommended because recent research has shown that it is not useful.

Conceptual Use

The **conceptual use** of research findings promotes changes in understanding or worldview that may result in a change in clinical practice. For example, a student nurse may experience changes in his or her beliefs or attitudes about the mentally ill and begin to interact in different ways with mentally ill patients as a result of gaining additional knowledge about the causes and manifestations of mental illnesses.

Symbolic Use

Finally, the **symbolic use** of knowledge, addressed by Stetler (1985), involves the use of research findings to legitimize or increase the level of attention given to a current issue, without necessarily directly changing current clinical practice.

When are research findings actually "ready" for use in clinical practice (i.e., to be instrumentally implemented in concrete changes to practice)? Polit and Hungler (1999) emphasize that the dissemination of research findings into practice historically has been difficult in nursing. Much of the published research literature has been inaccessible to busy clinicians, and other approaches are needed to help reduce the gap between research published in academically oriented journals, such as *Research in Nursing & Health* or *Nursing Research,* and the world of clinical practice. Journals such as *Clinical Nursing Research* and *Applied Nursing Research* are designed for use by clinicians, but sometimes lack the level of information needed to critique the validity of the research methods. What possibilities are there for an "in-between" position?

Recent advances in information technology have made high-quality summaries of information on various health-related topics readily accessible to clinicians. Refer to Table 22-3 for examples of Internet sites. A current trend is the use of e-mail listservs, which send summaries of research or tables of contents to individual e-mail accounts. These messages usually include URLs that the recipient can click on to go directly to a given article or report of research results. In addition, centers for evidence-based medicine, such as the Cochrane Collaboration, provide easily accessible integrative reviews of key clinical topics that are updated as new information becomes available.

These newer approaches to research dissemination show promise for enhancing access to information based on empirical research. Nonetheless, the usefulness of these forms of research dissemination still depends on the reader having a basic understanding of research terminology, standards for practice, and logic. In addition, the availability of time and the necessary skills for accessing information can be problematic. Another problem is the recognition that change in clinical practice typically requires energy and commitment. Lekander, Tracy, and Lindquist

(1994) described types of barriers to research utilization, together with suggested strategies to overcome the barriers (Table 22-5). Although the strategies listed are quite general, they can serve as a basis for further discussion and consideration within a given clinical setting.

►CLINICAL RESEARCH IN ACTION
Conclusion: Two Examples of Using Empirical Evidence to Improve Clinical Practice

We conclude this chapter by describing two examples of how evidence can be used in clinical practice. The first example refers to the implementation of a small-scale change in clinical practice, and the second example refers to the use

TABLE 22.5 Obstacles and Strategies for Research Utilization	
Obstacles	**Strategies**
Lack of perceived value of nursing research	Support role modeling by nursing leadership Provide explicit sanction for research utilization activity Provide support through rewards and incentives Analyze how the organizational environment can support research utilization Link research utilization to institutional goals and objectives
Lack of access to resources	Circulate research journals, abstracts, and summaries Establish clinician access to health sciences libraries Provide education about performing literature searches Develop joint programs between schools of nursing and hospital departments of nursing Increase funding specifically for research utilization
Lack of preparation	Establish journal clubs and unit-based research councils Develop a curriculum focus on implementing research findings into practice Implement mentoring by graduate nurses in research critique and innovation
Lack of availability of research findings	Publish research results in clinical and research journals Promote teleconferences and satellite conference to disseminate findings rapidly Sponsor newsletters, presentations, and conferences devoted to research utilization
Lack of authority to autonomously change patient care procedures	Target influential leaders to lead the change process Identify stakeholders in change and involve them in the change process Collaborate with other disciplines Develop education programs to promote individuals' roles and responsibilities
Lack of motivation to change practice	Provide rewards and recognition for implementing innovations
Insufficient methods for implementation and dissemination	Promote careful preplanning for the successful implementation of research utilization Develop realistic time frames for implementation Develop appropriate evaluation programs to document results of research utilization Sponsor face-to-face communication and telecommunication as possible alternatives to print media
Lack of communication between clinician and researcher	Promote active, reciprocal exchange of ideas and information Encourage unit-based clinicians with research skills to communicate with peers

(Adapted with permission from Lekander, B. J., Tracy, M. F., Lindquist, R. (1994). Overcoming the obstacles to research-based clinical practice. *AACN Clinical Issues, 5,* 115–123.)

of prior research to implement a larger-scale change in clinical practice. Based on several studies that described the use of patient restraints in extended care facilities, Stratmann, Vinson, Magee, and Hardin (1997) implemented staff education and policy changes, with the goal of reducing the use of restraints, and then evaluated the effect of their interventions. They found almost a 50% reduction in the use of restraints after implementation of the interventions. This study is a classic example of how research utilization occurs in a clinical practice setting, starting with a clinical question (i.e., "Can restraint use be reduced?"), and extending through the evaluation phase to determine the effect of the interventions (i.e., "Were the interventions shown to be effective?").

Perhaps the most widely recognized larger-scale example of a research utilization project is the Conduct and Utilization of Nursing Research (CURN) Project that was conducted by the Michigan Nurses' Association from 1975 to 1981 (Horsley, Crane, & Crabtree, 1983). The main goal of the CURN project was to implement approaches to improving the utilization of research by registered nurses, such as the dissemination of research findings, fostering research collaboration, and effecting needed organizational changes to foster research utilization. A key conclusion of the project concerned the essential need for organizational-level support of research utilization activities. More recently, other large-scale projects of this scope have been carried out with similar types of conclusions.

Suggested Activities

1. Read a research article on a topic of interest to you. Note how well the authors present what is currently known, what is not known, and what needs to be known. Provide specific suggestions for how the authors could improve their presentation, as appropriate.

2. Read a research article on a topic of interest to you, and critique it in terms of the quality, clinical significance, and applicability of the study findings to a setting and population with which you are familiar.

3. Try a literature search strategy or investigate a computerized resource (see Boxes 22-1 and 22-2 for suggestions) that is unfamiliar to you on a topic of interest to you. Critique the quality and ease of use of the resource.

Suggested Readings

Brown, S. J. (1999). *Knowledge for health care practice: A guide to using research evidence.* Philadelphia: Saunders.

Coiera, E. (1997). *Guide to medical informatics: The Internet, communication and information technologies in health care.* New York: Chapman & Hall.

Edwards, M. (1998). *The Internet for nurses and allied health professionals.* New York: Springer-Verlag.

Fain, J. A. (1999). *Reading, understanding, and applying nursing research: A text and workbook.* Philadelphia: F. A. Davis.

Gibbs, S., Sullivan-Fowler, M., & Rowe, N. (1996). *Medical safari: A guide to exploring the Internet and discovering top health care resources.* Boston: Mosby.

Hancock, L. (1996). *Physician's guide to the Internet.* Kansas City, MO: Lippincott-Raven.

Hogarth, M. (1996). *An Internet guide for the health professional* (2nd ed.). Davis, CA: New Wind.

Locke, L. F., Silverman, S. J., & Spirduso, W. W. (1998). *Reading and understanding research.* Thousand Oaks, CA: Sage.

Norwood, S. L. (2000). *Research strategies for advanced practice nurses.* Upper Saddle River, NJ: Prentice Hall.

Peteva, R. J. (2001). *A cross section of nursing research.* Los Angeles: Pyrczak.

Pyrczak, F. (1999). *Evaluating research in academic journals: A practical guide to realistic evaluation.* Los Angeles: Pyrczak.

Report of the U.S. Preventive Services Task Force. (1996). *Guide to clinical preventive services* (2nd ed.). Baltimore: Williams & Wilkins.

Rosser, W. W., & Shafir, M. S. (1998). *Evidence-based family medicine.* Hamilton, Ontario: B. C. Decker.

Sparkes, S., & Rizzolo, M. (1998). World Wide Web search tools. *Image: Journal of Nursing Scholarship, 30,* 167–171.

References

Brown, S. J. (1999). *Knowledge for health care practice: A guide to using research evidence.* Philadelphia: Saunders.

Caplan, N., & Rich, R. F. (1975). The use of social science knowledge in policy decisions at the national level. Ann Arbor, MI: Institute for Social Science Research, University of Michigan.

Hamric, A. (1996). A definition of advanced nursing practice. In Hamric, A., J. Spross, & C. Hanson (Eds.), *Advanced nursing practice: An integrated approach* (pp. 42–56). Philadelphia: Saunders.

Horsley, J. A., Crane, J., & Crabtree, M. K. (1983). *Using research to improve nursing practice: A guide.* New York: Grune & Stratton.

Kleiber, C., & Harper, D. C. (1999). Effects of distraction on children's pain and distress during medical procedures: A meta-analysis. *Nursing Research, 48,* 44–49.

Lekander, B. J., Tracy, M. F., & Lindquist, R. (1994). Overcoming the obstacles to research-based clinical practice. *AACN Clinical Issues, 5,* 115–123.

McGuire, D., & Harwood, K. (1996). Research interpretation, utilization, and conduct. In Hamric, A., J. Spross, & C. Hanson (Eds.), *Advanced nursing practice: An integrative approach* (pp. 184–211). Philadelphia: Saunders.

Nicoll, L. H., & Beyea, S. C. (1999). In Fain J.A. (Ed.), *Reading, understanding, and applying nursing research: A text and workbook* (pp. 261–280). Philadelphia: F. A. Davis.

Polit, D. F., & Hungler, B. P. (1999). *Nursing research: Principles and methods* (6th ed.). Philadelphia: Lippincott.

Shaughnessy, A. F., Slawson, D. C., & Bennet, J. H. (1994). Becoming an information master: A guidebook to the medical information jungle. *Journal of Family Practice, 39,* 484–499.

Stetler, C. (1985). Research utilization: Defining the concept. *Image: Journal of Nursing Scholarship, 17,* 40–44.

Stetler, C. (1994). Refinement of the Stetler/Marram model for application of research findings to practice. *Nursing Outlook, 42,* 15–25.

Stratmann, D., Vinson, M. H., Magee, R., & Hardin, S. B. (1997). The effects of research on clinical practice: The use of restraints. *Applied Nursing Research, 10,* 39–43.

CHAPTER 23 Designing and Implementing Small-Scale Clinical Studies

APPROACHES TO SMALL-SCALE CLINICAL STUDIES

The focus of this chapter is on the design and implementation of small-scale clinical research studies on topics of interest to advance practice nurses (APNs). In contrast to chapter 22, which focused on the skills needed to use existing research findings, this chapter highlights the skills necessary to develop new knowledge in relation to research questions. The information in this chapter is an extension of the information covered in chapter 22 because the design and implementation of clinical research projects depends on having completed the first three phases of research utilization referred to in chapter 22 (adapted Stetler [1994] model; see Table 22-1): (1) preparation, (2) validation, and (3) comparative evaluation.

In this chapter, we start by offering a clinical research scenario that shows how existing knowledge is used selectively and adapted in the design of a small-scale clinical study. This example shows how existing information necessarily becomes the basis for planning and implementing new studies. Although the early stages of planning rely heavily on research utilization skills, these stages are essential in designing a sound study that both achieves its research goals and is feasible within the constraints of clinical practice. See Research Scenario 23-1.

With this example in mind, we turn to describing key steps in the process of designing and implementing a small-scale clinical study to provide the "flavor" of such a clinical research project. We will elaborate further on the clinical example presented in Research Scenario 23-1 to

RESEARCH SCENARIO 23.1

Using and Adapting Existing Information in the Design and Implementation of a Small-Scale Intervention Study: Example of a Diabetes Self-Management Program

Health care providers at a rural primary care clinic that serves primarily a low-literacy patient population are interested in improving the quality of type II diabetes care by implementing a formal patient self-management program. For several months, they have been meeting as a group at the biweekly provider meeting. The team consists of two APNs, three physicians, the clinic office manager, a medical student, a graduate nursing student, and a medical resident. Under the leadership of the APNs, the clinic providers have refined and focused their clinical question (preparation phase), have performed a thorough review of the existing literature on diabetes self-management programs (validation phase), and have carefully critiqued and summarized the results of their literature review (comparative evaluation phase).

At today's group meeting, a summary of the work completed to date is presented. There is a solid consensus among the providers that they should avoid wholesale implementation of an existing program that everyone is quite intrigued by, because evidence about its efficacy and cost savings may be misleading. The concern is that there is insufficient information about how well such a program works with populations of patients who have low literacy levels (less than sixth grade reading level). The providers decide to "keep in mind" the results of two published and well-designed intervention studies of the program with higher-literacy populations while designing their own small-scale pilot study to test an adaptation of the program for use with their lower-literacy population.

Based on informal discussions, the providers also recognize that the administration of their agency is quite concerned about the likelihood of higher short-term costs to implement the program. The providers recognize the need to deal with an important situational variable that affects the feasibility of the program by incorporating a **cost description*** into the design of their project. They decide to adapt certain aspects of the program, such as printed patient materials, for use with their lower-literacy patient population, while retaining other features of the original program, such as nurses providing patient coaching by telephone. However, they are uncertain as to whether the **empowerment**† aspects of the intervention will be culturally appropriate, so they also decide to incorporate focus groups with patients as part of the intervention design.

---

*A **cost description** is the most basic level of economic cost analysis in which the costs are determined in terms of adding all expenditures connected with the implementation of the program. For additional reading on types of costs analyses, see Drummond, O'Brien, Stoddart, & Torrance (1999).

†**Empowerment,** in this example, refers to patients having enough knowledge, control, and resources to implement decisions as well sufficient experience to be able to evaluate the effectiveness of their decisions (Anderson & Funnell, 2000).

illustrate the key steps in conducting a clinical research project, including a discussion of feasibility considerations.

RESOURCES: AN OVERARCHING CONSIDERATION

Good research designs do not simply follow textbook blueprints of "ideal" study designs without regard to an assessment of the available resources. The availability of adequate resources is a major part of designing and planning research. If resources are limited, it is better to scale down the expectations of what can be studied or to try to accomplish a "doable" piece of research than to try to meet study goals that are clearly unrealistic. Thus, when designing and implementing a research project, the researcher must consider and plan for resource needs. The next section details the resources that every researcher must consider because inadequacies in these areas may become substantial barriers to the successful implementation of a study.

Time

Clinical research almost always seems to require more time than anticipated during the planning stage. Many research studies have complex, highly structured research protocols that require significant time commitments from key personnel in the clinical setting. One example is the recruitment of patients in clinical settings. In today's hospital environment, in which early discharge is the norm, it is easy to miss patients who are admitted with a diagnosis of myocardial infarction, because they may have been discharged before the recruiter had the opportunity to contact them. Relying on office personnel in a primary care practice to recruit and refer eligible patients can also be problematic because of the many competing clinical and administrative demands for staff time. Even though the providers in such offices initially may have endorsed the recruitment effort, they often realize too late how time-consuming recruitment activities can be.

During the planning stages of a study, it is necessary to make a list of all major activities involved in the study, to identify the key members of the research team responsible for carrying out these activities, and to budget realistic amounts of time to accomplish the tasks. Even in clinical settings in which the researcher may anticipate an "inside advantage" as a result of working in that setting as a clinician, it is unwise to assume that clinical contributors and collaborators will be able or willing to provide "free" or contributed time to the research effort, even if they enthu-

siastically endorse the research goals. "Release time" must often be formally negotiated, and may require some form of compensation. Early in the process of research design, a timeline of project steps, with associated time frames, should be drafted, and the resource implications should be considered in the context of the timeline.

Money

Even a small-scale study can be expected to require at least some money.[1] The development of a preliminary project budget should go hand in hand with research design decisions. Researchers sometimes decide to forego certain features of research design because of budget implications. For instance, a researcher who is interested in patient satisfaction with hospital services might settle for postdischarge recruitment of surgical patients via telephone contact because the personnel time for monitoring and recruiting surgical patients while they are still in the hospital is not affordable. For inpatient recruitment of study participants, the researcher may have to pay a percentage of the salaries of the hospital staff recruiters and also face the possibility of paying additional, nonsalary costs associated with the use of staff time. Of course, while reducing recruitment costs, the likely tradeoff for recruiting patients after their discharge from the hospital is a lower response rate (Minnick & Young, 1998). Box 23-1 shows an example of cost categories to be considered by an APN who conducts a patient satisfaction survey of consecutive primary care patients.

Clinical and Research Expertise

A small-scale clinical study usually involves at least one person who is responsible for the overall study project, usually referred to as the "principal investigator," as well as several other people who are instrumental to the research process. The most common situation in clinical practice is the use of a small research team to accomplish a specific project. The roles and contributions of each team member must be assessed and specified in relation to the research goals. Adjustments often must be made to ensure that all relevant expertise is represented on the team. For example, an APN who is the principal investigator for a research project may have the needed clinical expertise for a given research topic, but may need to partner with others who have expertise in research design, sampling, and data

---

[1]See chapter 25 for an in-depth discussion of funding sources for clinical research.

BOX 23.1   Examples of Costs Associated with Conducting an In-person Patient Satisfaction Survey

- Recruitment costs, including release time for the recruiter, plus small stipends, incentives, or gratuities for the research participants (such as cash, pens, or refrigerator magnets)
- Paper for survey copies
- Pens, pencils, and printer cartridges
- Photocopies
- Interviewer time
- Computers and software, including word processing, spreadsheet, and specialized statistical software, such as SPSS SAS, STATA, etc.
- Data entry time or services
- Statistical consultation and data analysis services
- Release time for research activities
- Costs associated with the presentation and dissemination of the study findings

Although some of these costs may be covered through an institutional support agreement, they nonetheless remain costs. All researchers, especially newer researchers who have not previously sought monetary support for conducting a research project, should have their study budgets reviewed by administrators who have expertise in the preparation of research budgets as well as by experienced researchers.

---

analysis. It is also useful to identify collaborators who are at least minimally facilitative of research efforts in the needed areas. These needs should be considered early in the research design process.

Motivational Climate

Motivation refers to a variety of individual and situational factors that create a *climate* that is favorable for conducting a given research study. A researcher should think of the motivational climate as a vital resource that contributes to the success or failure of a research project. For example, the individual research team members must be sufficiently interested in the project and motivated to carry out their tasks, despite competing demands on their time and expertise. Likewise, an institutional culture that is not supportive of clinical research efforts may represent a substantial barrier to success. In this setting, the tasks associated with the research project are likely to be considered of low priority compared with nonresearch tasks. Thus, the institution plays a very important, even essential, role in at least neutralizing key barriers to research.

Space and Other Physical Resources

Very small-scale projects may be accomplished with existing resources, but larger projects typically require additional physical resources. For example, existing computers

to be used for a research project may not have the software required for data entry and analysis, or may need to be upgraded to run newer software. A special area may need to be dedicated for use during private interviews with research participants, and secure storage space may be needed to store the hard copy data. Furthermore, hardly any project can succeed without such equipment as telephones, photocopiers, and fax machines. It is in these areas where negotiating and securing institutional support is vital. Monetary compensation for usage should be included the budget, especially for larger, more resource-intensive projects.

Access to Study Participants

Access to study participants is one of the primary institutional resources *potentially* available to clinicians. However, working as a clinician in a certain setting does not necessarily improve access to potential study participants. Clinician researchers who approach patients for research purposes should keep in mind that they must comply with institutional rules and federally mandated ethical and legal requirements for accessing subjects and obtaining consent (see chapter 24). As indicated earlier, recruitment of subjects sometimes requires substantial expenditure of resources, which may include hiring special recruitment personnel who have certain language skills or clinical expertise. In some instances, it may be either unethical or unfeasible to recruit study participants from certain target populations. Also, payments are sometimes made to providers to offset the costs associated with recruiting and referring eligible subjects.[2] In short, the resource implications of subject recruitment must be considered early in the study design phase because they are often a major component of the cost of the overall study project.

In many studies, researchers make compromises in design and execution because of resource constraints. In these situations, it is important to know which resource requirements can be modified without compromising the overall quality of the study and which resource deficits would prove "fatal" to the planned research. Above all, researchers must be "imaginative realists" who are aware of specific and feasible strategies to overcome resource constraints. As emphasized earlier, planning for needed resources should begin early in the design of a research project. With the overarching role of resources in mind, we turn now to describing the major steps in research project design.

STEPS IN PROJECT DESIGN

The project design phase is critical to the success of any project. Although the practical activities associated with carrying out a research project (e.g., data collection, data analysis) often feel like the most critical part of a study, if insufficient attention is paid to creating a sound conceptual and methodologic base for the research, the study will be flawed from a scientific perspective. Of course, the practical details of implementation are important to the success of a study, but the aspects of a study that speak to its scientific validity are largely determined in the project design or planning phase. Thus, we spend some time in this section describing the major steps in project design, including the key decisions that must be made at each step.

Project Design Step 1: Refining the Question and Using Existing Literature[3]

When planning a study, it is essential to have a clear grasp of the specific research questions. For both clinicians and researchers, this aspect of project design is not as straightforward as it might seem. For instance, referring back to the type II diabetes example in Research Scenario 23-1, numerous clinically focused research questions could address "knowledge gaps" in clinical practice. An informal survey of the clinicians on the research team might show some of the following variations in research questions, all of which are related to the topic of type II diabetes self-care:

- How difficult is it for patients to manage their diabetes adequately?
- Are HgA_1C levels and the level of diabetes control correlated?
- What types of patients do well versus not well with self-care programs?
- Are older or younger patients more likely to be successful in managing diabetes?
- Is a patient's level of education related to his or her ability to manage diabetes?
- What format works best for educating patients about diabetes self-care?
- Are patients completely open when telling their health care providers how things are going with diabetes self-care management?

These illustrative questions (a true subset of dozens of questions that could be posed) differ in both focus and level of specificity. They would also need to be studied using a variety of approaches, ranging from observational to experimental study designs, and including a variety of data collection methods, such as interviews or biophysiologic tests. The study design team must come to agreement about what specifically will be studied, starting with a broad array of options and narrowing their focus to perhaps one or two specific key questions that can be addressed within the limited scope of a single study (see Box 23-2 for comments on the necessary "process" aspects of working relationships among research team members). The refinement of what specifically will be studied should be guided, in part, by existing literature as well as feasibility considerations. For example, team members may have formulated research questions that are already answered in the literature. In this case, a review of the relevant literature would show that it is already well documented that HgA_1C levels are a good predictor of, and are well correlated with, diabetes control. Thus, there is no need to conduct a new study to address this issue.

The remaining research questions generated by the team members must be pared down and given focus. One way to do this is to ask what data collection efforts or study designs would be required to answer them. For example, the first question in the previous list could be studied by doing a

---

[2]Payments made on the basis of "in-kind" reimbursements for costs are usually ethically justifiable, for example, in exchange for costs associated with time that a health care provider spends recruiting study participants, or other institutional costs. However, monetary or other types of resource payments to health care personnel or others as "incentives" to recruit study participants are increasingly controversial from an ethical perspective because of the potential for conflicts of interest and the possibility of undue coercion of potential study participants to agree to participate in research. See chapter 24 for additional information about ethical considerations for monetary payments for the recruitment of study participants and compensation of study participants.

[3]The practical aspects of literature searching are addressed in chapter 22.

BOX 23.2   The Process of the Research Project Experience

Particularly in research teams that include at least some people who have not worked together before, it is often necessary to spend some initial meetings discussing ideas before the group can rally behind a clearly understood and agreed-on focus for the project. Insufficient attention to this step may result in significant conflicts among group members and other problems in successfully implementing the study.

To build effective working relationships and define and refine the various roles in a research project, agreement on the goals of the project is essential. The success of research project implementation depends pivotally on the working relationships that develop during the design phases. Well-functioning teams in which complementary roles and mutual respect are developed facilitate the successful computation of the research project.

Beginning at this phase and extending through the remaining design steps, team members are often defining their roles within the group and also deciding for themselves whether the project holds sufficient benefit for them. At this point, some team members may decide not to continue their involvement with the project. Other team members may be added during this and other design steps, as the project ideas and research design take shape.

---

chart audit of HgA_1C levels (a serum marker of long-term diabetes control), surveying patients about perceived barriers to effective self-care management of diabetes, or surveying the health care providers of patients with diabetes. The third question might be studied by choosing a specific self-management program and using it as the basis for an experimental study in which the self-care program is compared with usual care. Records audits and patient surveys might be used to collect data about variables (e.g., age, disease severity, literacy level, motivation level) that are hypothesized to affect how well patients do. Because available resources may allow for only one type of data collection, the research team may decide which research questions should be tackled first through a discussion of study design and implications for data collection and measurement.

It is also necessary to cull, or at least reformulate, questions that are not researchable or are unlikely to be amenable to study in a small-scale clinical study. As discussed in chapter 2, questions that require a moral judgment are not directly amenable to empirical study (e.g., "Is it right to deny a liver transplant to an alcoholic as long as persons without an alcohol problem need one too?"). More common is the problem of having to turn broad, unwieldy questions into well-focused, limited-scope questions that can be researched within the available resources. For example, consider how a question could be focused from very broad to very specific, as illustrated in the list below:

- Why do people not take their medications as prescribed?
- What barriers are there to adults taking their medications as prescribed?
- Is lack of insurance or lack of purchasing power a ma-

jor reason why patients treated at a particular primary care clinic do not buy prescribed medications or "stretch out" their purchases?
- Beyond affordability, does compliance with medication regimens vary, even among patients with the same insurance access and financial means?
- What economic, social, and psychological characteristics of patients predict substantial noncompliance with medication regimens?
- Are depressed patients less likely to comply with medication regimens?

In the above list, the research question is progressively refined by first focusing on the question of barriers and then specifying particular sources of barriers. Similarly, in the first three questions, the target populations have been narrowed from "people," to "adults taking their medication," to "patients treated at a particular primary care clinic."

It is often difficult to find the right level of specificity for a study that provides insights that are useful to others, but is narrow enough to be feasible as a study project. When refining the research questions, the research team should also consider the available information on the topic.

As discussed in more detail in chapter 22, the literature review not only should be concerned with the current state of knowledge in a given area, but also should provide key information about the methods used in previous research (e.g., specific research designs, measures, and data collection approaches), as well as gaps in existing research methods. For example, the review of literature could show that provider and patient surveys are often used to gather data about barriers to diabetes self-care and that chart audits of certain measures (e.g., HgA$_1$C levels) are most often used as markers for control of a patient's diabetes. Likewise, a review of literature might show few controlled experimental studies of interventions for diabetes self-care.

Refinement of the research questions and achievement of consensus among the research team members about the main goals of the research project can be challenging. In addition, this process almost always takes significant time (at least several weeks or months). The research team should have a clear understanding of the focused set of questions that will be addressed in the study and should know why other questions were excluded from the project, even though they may have been of interest to team members. In the end, the time that is spent refining the research questions and building consensus can significantly increase the likelihood of successful project implementation.

Project Design Step 2: Selecting Theoretic and Conceptual Frameworks

As part of the literature review process, special attention should be paid to theoretic and conceptual frameworks or concepts that seem to be influential and useful in guiding research. For example, consider the topic of adherence behavior in relation to the research example in Research Scenario 23-1. Suppose that the study in this example is designed such that one of the key outcome measures is "level of adherence to diabetes self-care management plans." If an aspect of the research involves understanding why patients vary in their level of adherence, one or more of the influential conceptual frameworks focused on health behaviors could be useful to guide the study.[4]

The use of existing theoretic frameworks to guide new research is important for several reasons. First, frameworks help to organize research questions and to specify what relationships to look for among the major concepts or variables. They also help to highlight research gaps and relate the results of new studies to the existing stock of knowledge. For example, the concept of "barriers" to behavior is an important concept in studies that focus on personal health behaviors, and barriers are often incorporated into frameworks concerned with health behaviors. Reference to such a framework allows ideas to be explained in terms of what has been relatively well studied and understood. At the same time, some social or psychological cognitive–behavioral frameworks used to predict health-related behaviors have been criticized for neglecting the contribution of other potentially important types of variables, such as socioenvironmental and cultural contexts. It is in explaining the shortcomings of existing theoretic frameworks that new, fruitful questions for empirical study emerge.

One of the important benefits of using conceptual and theoretic frameworks is that they help to organize our thinking about a particular subject area. Most health-related research is concerned with relationships among variables (i.e., understanding and explaining how and why certain phenomena vary together and establishing cause-and-effect relationships among them). To the extent that a theoretic framework allows us to paint an "integrated picture" of how variables are related, it is an important *simplification* of the problem. In many cases, a research team should be able to sketch a **logic diagram** of the key study variables, in which relationships among the independent and dependent variables are identified.

We do not claim that all research, to be fruitful, must be guided by an explicit theoretic framework. For some questions, theoretic frameworks do not appear to be essential in shaping ideas. In some situations, as in certain types of qualitative research, they may actually be contraindicated. Sometimes there is not an existing, suitable theoretic framework available for conceptualizing a research problem. At other times, research is designed to answer questions of practical use that do not require any "long-winded" theoretic justification. An example can be found in the question posed by Brown et al. (2000): "Is arm span an accurate measure of height in young and middle-aged adults?" Such questions may be "a-theoretical," but are nonetheless clinically important. However, the search for relevant theoretic frameworks is an important component of all empirical research, and helps to enrich and focus the research. In the final analysis, researchers must be able to justify their research questions, in terms of either a larger theoretic context or a practical clinical problem.

Project Design Step 3: Selecting the Research Design

After considering alternative versions of the research question and settling on a theoretic framework, the researcher must contemplate the selection of a research design. Usually, it is not difficult to decide whether a study will use an observational design or entails the implementation of an intervention (experimental or quasi-experimental design). This decision rests on the emphasis given to establishing causal relationships and the feasibility of manipulating the independent variable. However, after this decision is made,

---

[4]Examples of health behavior frameworks that have been influential in nursing research on treatment adherence include the health belief model (Rosenstock, 1990), the transtheoretical model (Prochaska, Redding, et al., 1994), and the social cognitive theory (Bandura, 1977).

many details must be spelled out (e.g., Will the research design be a crossover design with 12 repeated measures or a between-groups design comparing three groups of randomly assigned study participants?). In this section, we briefly discuss some of the major considerations that affect the selection of specific research designs. Readers should also refer back to chapters 3 through 12 for a more detailed discussion of the strengths and weaknesses of various study designs.

Experimental or Nonexperimental Design

A key design decision that is made early in the planning phase is whether to use an experimental or a nonexperimental design. As mentioned earlier, the selection of the major research design category is largely driven by the specific goals of the study that are incorporated into the research question. However, it also involves feasibility and ethical considerations. With regard to the goals of the study, the key question is to consider whether the study focuses primarily on examining or testing a cause-and-effect relationship. If it does, the immediate follow-up question is whether the independent variable that is considered in the research question can be manipulated by the researcher, in terms of both feasibility and ethical acceptability. For example, to study the effects of depression on the annual frequency of primary care visits, it is clear that one can select and *observe* depressed and nondepressed adults, but cannot "make" people depressed or not depressed.[5] Furthermore, it would not be ethically defensible to deliberately induce study subjects to adopt risky behaviors (e.g., studying the physiologic effects of smoking by using a research design in which nonsmokers would be asked to begin smoking).

As we saw in chapters 6 and 7, when researchers can devise interventions, but random assignment of subjects to alternative intervention protocols is not feasible, a quasi-experimental design is the logical choice.

In all other situations—where the primary goal is to describe "what is" or the researcher is interested in establishing a cause-and-effect relationship, but cannot devise a feasible intervention—an observational research design must be chosen.

Key Questions

After this initial design decision, the "real work" begins in designing the specific details of the study. Box 23-3 shows a few key questions that a researcher must consider when planning and designing a study. This list is not intended to

be exhaustive of all relevant considerations, but represents a good starting point and contains questions for evaluating key aspects of research designs. Answering these questions will help you to think through many concrete and specific design features of a study.

Project Design Step 4: Identifying the Target Population and Choosing a Sampling Design

The adequacy of the sampling plan and recruitment strategy depends on the goals of the study as well as on feasibility and resource considerations. Recruitment of subjects for clinical studies is often limited to a few sites to which an investigator has or can gain access.

As discussed in more detail in chapter 19, it is always advisable to investigate possible differences between the *accessible study population* and the *ideal target population* addressed in the research questions. Not all studies require samples that are "representative" of large population segments, but a substantial part of nursing and other clinical research involves behavioral and psychological variables that are often correlated with the social characteristics (e.g., sex, ethnic group, socioeconomic group) of the study participants.

To the extent that is possible, sampling and recruitment plans for clinical studies must take variation in social background characteristics into account because of the potential for the generalizability of the study results to be limited.[6] The choice of a specific type of sampling design[7] is constrained by practical considerations in accessing study participants, such as the flexibility to carry out alternative sampling plans in the settings available to the researcher, the ability and willingness of members of the target population to participate,[8] and the availability of sufficient resources. Because the cost of doing research increases in direct relation to the size of the study sample and the complexity of the sampling plan, realistic sampling plans must always take into account the budgetary implications of alternative sampling schemes. Box 23-4 shows a list of questions that a researcher must consider before choosing a recruitment and sampling plan.

As the widespread use of convenience samples in clinical research attests, more ambitious sampling designs are

---

[5]See chapter 3 for a discussion of attribute variables.

[6]Representativeness is *not* always a key consideration in certain types of qualitative research. See chapters 12 and 21 for additional discussion.

[7]See chapters 19 and 20 for the major alternative sampling strategies that are available.

[8]People who are sick or recovering from a major illness are often difficult to enroll in studies.

BOX 23.3   Key Questions to Guide Study Design Decisions

- Will the study use an experimental, quasi-experimental, or observational design?
- Will the study be retrospective (relying on past data records) or prospective (relying on new data to be collected)?
- What are the specific eligibility criteria for subjects to participate in the study?
- Will the recruitment of study participants occur at a single site or at multiple sites?
- How many study groups are being compared?
- If two or more groups are compared, will study participants be assigned randomly to the comparison groups?
- What procedures will be used to monitor the (random) assignment process?
- Which potential confounding variables are so important to control that they must be "built into" the study design via stratification or matching?
- Will the study sample be stratified along some other major characteristics of interest?
- In quasi-experimental studies, what design efforts are undertaken to ensure a semblance of "equivalence" between intervention and control (both statistically and clinically)?
- For all study designs, are there plans in place to collect data on known, important confounding variables, so that they can be statistically controlled for in the analysis?
- For experimental and quasi-experimental studies, does the planned intervention represent a clinically meaningful change over current practice or "usual care" in the control group?
- How feasible in terms of time, energy, money, convenience, and acceptability will it be to implement this intervention? How feasible would it likely be to implement the intervention for a given clinical practice setting and population?
- Is the study design cross-sectional (a single observation on study subjects) or longitudinal?
- If it is longitudinal, how many observations or data collection points will be implemented?
- Will the study be a trend study, or will the same subjects be observed repeatedly (panel on cohort study)?
- For intervention studies, will pretests be included among the observation points?
- Is subject attrition likely to be a major threat to the validity of the study? If so, what study features can be built in to minimize it?
- What special personnel skills are needed for recruitment, intervention, data collection, and analysis? What training is needed?

---

often difficult to implement under "real-world" conditions. As a first step, researchers must be thoroughly familiar with the kinds of constraints that they will encounter in drawing a sample from the target population. The best starting point is the experience of other researchers who have worked with the same target population or one that is similar. A thorough review of the research literature that is based on studies done with the same target population is a good beginning. In addition, the researcher may decide to do small pilot studies to identify the types and strengths of constraints or barriers to study participation, especially if the research involves a target population that has not been well studied. This is often the case for populations identified as experiencing *health disparities* (inequality in health status compared with the mainstream U.S. population). In recent years, these subpopulations have been identified as priority research targets for the National Institutes of Health because information and research involving these

groups has been limited.[9] Researchers may need to conduct a few focus group sessions with members of the target population to identify key barriers to study participation and possible ways to reduce the barriers.

Sometimes such preliminary efforts lead to the identification of barriers that are not readily modifiable within the given resource constraints. For instance, it may not be possible to offer transportation to many study participants, if resources for conducting the research are insufficient to support this service. Another example is the need to limit post-discharge interviews to patients who have a telephone. These resource-based decisions affect sampling designs and generalizability, and must be made explicit in later reports or papers that describe the study results.

---

[9]See *www.nih.gov* for additional information about health disparities and health-related research funding priorities.

Finally, the researcher or research team should evaluate the need for statistical assistance or consultation (see chapter 20). Decisions about the research design, sampling plan, and sample size always involve statistical considerations and expertise. In some instances, the principal investigator or another member of the team has the needed expertise to make these decisions. However, in many cases, outside consultation is needed. The team statistician should possess the relevant expertise in research design, sampling, and statistical analysis for the particular type of research that is planned. The specific arrangements for collaboration can vary considerably. In some cases, the statistician may be a co-investigator on the research team, or he or she may be compensated for consultation in another way, such as through salary support or the opportunity to participate in publications by the research team. Because collaborative arrangements typically take time to

identify and develop, and require agreed-on expectations as well as adequate resources, they must be considered early in the planning process, starting at least after the research team has formulated its first set of research questions. In addition, the discussion with a statistician or methodologist may lead to further modifications in the research questions.

Project Design Step 5: Selecting Measures

The final major design step is the selection of the specific measures that will be used to gather the data. Box 23-5 lists some key questions concerning measurement issues. As mentioned earlier, the most common methods for data collection in small-scale clinical research studies are surveys (to obtain new self-report data) and medical record audits (to gather existing data). In addition, depending on

---

BOX 23.5   Key Questions about Measurement Issues

- Have the key study variables been adequately conceptualized?
- Are the measurement tools valid measures of the key concepts?
- Are the measures that are proposed for use in the study psychometrically valid for the population that will be sampled?
- Have the major measures used in the study been pretested?
- Are the laboratories used to analyze specimens and other physiologic test samples reliable? Do they follow accepted state-of-the art procedures?
- Can a blinding procedure be used for patients, interveners, the research team, or all three groups?
- If a full blinding procedure is not possible, what are the credible threats to design validity that result from awareness of the study conditions?

---

the goals of the study, researchers may use biophysiologic measures (e.g., temperature, blood pressure, serum assays).[10] At this point, researchers must consider three key issues:

1. Can the research be conducted with existing scales and measurement tools for all of the major variables that are considered in the research project, or do some variables require the development of new measurement instruments?
2. If new measurement instruments or tools must be developed, are sufficient time and resources available to test the new tools adequately before they are used in the study?
3. If existing measurement tools are used, are there specific problems with or concerns about the *application* of these measurement tools?

When conducting substantive clinical (and nonclinical) research, it is almost always advisable to rely as much as possible on *existing* measurement tools and instruments. If the reliability and validity of the key measures in a research project are in doubt, or at least require further empirical support, then it is particularly difficult to interpret negative findings or the absence of hypothesized relationships.[11] When searching for measurement tools, researchers must evaluate the known psychometric characteristics of the measures and consider whether past applications of these

measures involved target populations similar to the ones envisioned in the research project.[12]

Suppose that, even after an extensive search of the literature, no suitable measurement tool of adequate quality can be found for one or more key concepts in the planned study. At this point, researchers must either postpone their original research plan or at least plan for a pilot study to test one or more newly developed measurement scales in terms of feasibility (e.g., level of understanding of the scale items by the study participants) and face or content validity. Some type of preliminary psychometric testing, such as exploratory factor analysis[13] and internal consistency tests, is also in order. One or more pilot studies may be needed to obtain the needed information before implementing a larger-scale study. Pilot studies are essential "building blocks" to larger studies. For example, during a pilot study, the researcher may recognize that some of the measures used to collect data "do not work well" (i.e., there is evidence that they lack sufficient reliability and validity). It is best to find this out in a smaller-scale study than to expend the resources needed for a larger-scale study, only to be frustrated by the results. This discussion underscores the importance of selecting (whenever possible) a measure that has been well validated with the target population of interest. However, sometimes the development of more adequate measurement tools is unavoidable.

Finally, even if good measurement instruments are available, their application might require special skills on the part of the observers. Thus, when a research team selects measurement instruments, the team must also con-

---

[10]See chapter 17 for details on other information sources, particularly for large-scale studies. The clinical studies considered here typically involve study samples for which recruitment takes place at a few sites or a single site. These studies typically include less than a few hundred, and often less than 100, subjects. Refer also to chapter 16 on data collection techniques.

[11]In such situations, lack of a positive finding may be the result of unreliability and lack of validity of some of the measurement instruments.

---

[12]Refer to chapters 14 and 15 for a detailed discussion of reliability and validity issues in the evaluation of measurement tools.

[13]Use of this technique requires a sufficient sample size.

sider the implications for the skill requirements of data collectors or the need for special training. Particularly in intervention studies, researchers must use, as far as possible, data collectors who are blind to the treatment status of the observed study subjects. In such cases, the choice of measurement tools and their application or implementation will have direct implications for the study design, and must be considered from the start. If blinding of staff, patients, or interveners is not feasible, the team needs to discuss other procedures that help to limit the potential for bias resulting from awareness of study group assignment. This type of discussion could lead back to key design decisions about the level at which to apply random assignment to study conditions (e.g., at the institutional, health care provider, or patient level).

STEPS IN PROJECT IMPLEMENTATION

Project implementation refers to the steps involved in "actually doing" the research project. It entails four major steps, all of which involve resource considerations, as reviewed earlier in this chapter. We emphasize the importance of developing specific timelines for the major project activities. A list of specific tasks to be accomplished, with associated time frames for their completion, is an indispensable management tool for any study project.

Project Implementation Step 1: Data Collection Procedures

Data collection refers to the gathering of all information that is relevant to the research questions or hypotheses.[14] Whether the clinical study uses an observational design, is an intervention study (randomized clinical trial), or is concerned with program, outcome, or process evaluation, APNs are increasingly involved in such data collection efforts. As mentioned earlier, in clinical studies, most data are obtained through the following means: (1) record audits (i.e., abstraction of data from medical or patient insurance records), (2) self-report data (i.e., data obtained through personal interviews or written questionnaires), (3) biophysiologic measures and laboratory tests, and (4) direct observation of patients. Our discussion will focus on these four most common approaches to data collection for research projects in clinical settings.

Record Audits

Record audits are a specific type of data collection that involves "abstraction" ("pulling," or recording) of usually *selected* data from existing medical or insurance records. In clinical studies, the most common uses of record audits are to identify study subjects who meet certain eligibility criteria and to monitor study subjects on a relevant outcome variable over the observation period of the study. Almost all nurses are familiar with monitoring through daily clinical practice activities. Examples of record audits for research projects include: (1) monitoring medication prescriptions in relation to clinical guideline recommendations, (2) monitoring patient outcomes in response to interventions, and (3) using billing or insurance records to examine trends in the use and associated costs of health services among selected patient populations.

Self-report Data

Self-report data[15] include information about people's perceptions, attitudes, experiences, and (unobservable) behaviors. Such data are obtained through face-to-face interviews, telephone interviews (if patients are at home), or written questionnaire responses. For example, an APN may survey patients about their level of satisfaction with health care services and the amenities of the clinical setting, or clinical care providers may be surveyed about the need for structural and procedural improvements to enhance patient care services. Along with record audits, survey studies are probably the most common approach to gathering data in nursing research.

Biophysiologic Measures, Laboratory Tests, and Direct Observation of Patients

Finally, nurses are often responsible for collecting information on **biophysiologic measures** and **laboratory tests.** In addition, because of their relatively close and prolonged contact with patients, they are often able to perform **direct patient observations.** Increasingly, clinical studies use several, and sometimes even all, of these data collection procedures. Such *mixed* data collection efforts pose special challenges for implementation.

Because substantial amounts of patient data are routinely collected at clinical sites, one of the initial decisions during the study design process is to determine which, if any, of the ongoing clinical data collection efforts can be used for study purposes and which, if any, additional data collection efforts must be undertaken to measure key study variables. Most clinical studies rely on a mixture of new

---

[14]This section of the chapter is concerned with some of the management considerations involved in data collection. See chapter 16 for in-depth information about techniques for data collection.

[15]See the discussions of surveys (chapter 11) and data collection (chapter 16).

and existing information to address the study goals. For example, think about the data collection approaches that could be used in the hypothetical study that is described in Research Scenario 23-1. Suppose that the health care providers decided to use the following types of data collection: (1) HgA$_1$C levels from medical records, (2) patient questionnaire data on empowerment and knowledge of diabetes self-care, and (3) medical records of complications of and exacerbating factors for type II diabetes (e.g., progress notes and hospital summaries regarding diabetic neuropathy, vascular complications, and monthly weight data). Information on HgA$_1$C levels, medical complications, and exacerbating factors is obtained before, during, and after the intervention, and patient survey data are obtained before and after the intervention. This example shows the use of both existing and newly gathered information to evaluate the effects of an intervention.

Given the complexity of data collection in many clinical studies, even small-scale studies, successful implementation requires the development of a formal *data collection plan*. A **data collection plan** is a formalized, written, and well-communicated plan that specifies the procedures for data collection in precise detail. A major purpose of these plans is to provide continuity in the data collection effort in the event of turnover among personnel during the data collection phase. The plan also provides safeguards for data handling and confidentiality. Data collection plans should also specify *timelines* for all activities involved in data collection. These activities include some or all of the following:

- Setting up the physical and electronic storage facilities for all consent forms and data according to the required standards for data safety[16]
- Developing the data collection forms
- Printing the hard copies used for data collection
- Programming and formatting the data entry files, including files that record the scheduling and implementation of all contacts with patients or study participants
- Programming the interview schedules to be used for either computer-assisted telephone interviewing or computer-assisted personal interviewing
- Developing manuals or procedures to train data collectors
- Hiring data collection personnel
- Conducting training sessions with data collection personnel, including interviewers, record abstractors, and observers[17]

- Developing and testing recruitment procedures
- Selecting or purchasing gifts or other forms of compensation for study participants
- Scheduling reminders for upcoming contacts with study participants in longitudinal studies
- Setting start and end dates for various data collection activities[18]
- Specifying monitoring efforts for sample accrual
- Specifying monitoring efforts for successful assignment of subjects to various study arms in intervention studies

As this list shows, the implementation of data collection procedures may require substantial managerial skills, especially in large, multisite clinical studies. In real-world research, it is unusual for just one person to have all of the skills required for the successful implementation of a clinical study. Because of the many skills required, it is not surprising that successful clinical research is most often the result of a team effort.

Project Implementation Step 2: Data Management

After the data are collected, they must be stored securely in a way that meets all of the legal and ethical requirements for maintaining confidentiality and limiting access.[19] *Except* for consent forms and records to identify and keep track of study participants (which are often kept in a study *log book*), data are usually stored as computer files. For most clinical research, computers have become an indispensable tool for both data management and data analysis, and our discussion of data management is predicated on the assumption that readers of this text will use computer software to manage and analyze research data.[20] Box 23-6 shows some of the major steps in data management and data analysis. We will discuss these steps now.

Data Entry

Data entry involves entering "raw" (i.e., unexamined) data into a computer file. Unless the data consist of narrative texts, as in qualitative research, they are stored in numerical formats that require an explicit coding scheme. **Coding** is the process of transforming observations, test re-

---

[16]See chapter 24 for additional details about informed consent procedures and standards for record keeping.

[17]For more details on the training of data collectors, see chapter 16.

[18] From the beginning, successful data collection efforts allow for some "slack time" because subject accrual often takes more time and effort than anticipated.

[19]See chapter 24 for more details.

[20]Even the storage and analysis of qualitative or text-based data can be greatly facilitated with the use of computer software such as ETHNO-GRAPH, NUD-IST, or QUALPRO.

BOX 23.6   Key Steps in Data Management and Data Analysis

Data Management

- Performing data entry and coding
- Verifying data entry
- Performing initial analyses to check for missing values, outliers, and anomalies in codes
- Performing analysis to check for consistencies in data
- Handling missing values: logical imputations, mean substitutions, and regression substitutions

Data Analysis

- Identifying descriptive statistics and frequency distributions for all variables
- Exploring single variable distributions for skew
- Establishing and testing for multidimensionality and reliability of all major scale variables that are based on multiple items or variables
- Computing composite scale scores, using established algorithms for existing scales
- Conducting major analyses, using statistical models that address the major study questions and hypotheses

---

sults, or responses to structured questionnaire instruments into numerical information. The rules or conventions for assigning numerical values to specific bits of information are detailed in the **study code book.** For instance, in a numerical data file, responses to a survey question about the respondent's sex may be coded "0" for "male" and "1" for "female." These numbers ultimately make up the body of the computerized data file. Table 23-1 shows how a code book should be organized so that an analyst can use and make sense out of the numerical information in the data file. The major pieces of information contained in a code book include the names and locations of variables in the data file, the labels used for the variables, detailed descriptions, value codes, value labels, and information on various codes used for "missing values." Numerical data files are usually entered in spreadsheet format. In other words, they are arranged in a *rectangular* format, with rows containing information on *cases* and columns containing information on *variables*[21] (see Table 23-2). The body of the data file contains the coded *values,* which are defined with reference to the code book.

Verifying Data Entry

Even modest-sized studies easily generate data files with thousands of entries—a study involving 60 cases and 70 variables generates at least 4,200 data entry fields. For this reason, **data entry verification** and checking is an essential, although time-consuming, task. One standard procedure in large-scale studies is the use of double data entry when information from hard copies and records must be typed into the electronic data fields. After two persons have entered the data independently, it is easy to use the software to compare the files and detect inconsistencies, which can be corrected by checking the originals.[22]

With the advent of computer-aided interviewing, hard copies of study participants' responses may not be available. Especially in clinical studies that use laptop computers for patient interviews, the data files on the laptop are the only record of the responses. The software can be programmed to minimize mistakes (e.g., by disallowing "illegal" responses).[23] It can also be programmed to convert the responses on the screen automatically into verbal codes, eliminating common data entry errors. On the other hand, programming errors occur occasionally and may magnify

---

[21]All of the major statistical software packages (e.g., SPSS, SAS, STATA, BMDP, SYSTAT) have data entry windows in spreadsheet format. Data also may be stored in spreadsheet software, such as MS EXCEL or QUATTRO PRO, or database programs, such as MS ACCESS or DBASE IV. In recent years, it has become much easier to transfer data files from any of these formats into any other format, in part because many software programs accept files that are formatted in a different program, and in part, because of the availability of specialized conversion software, such as STAT-TRANSFER.

[22]The **double data entry procedure** that is described is the procedure that is recommended by the National Institutes of Health for validating data entry.

[23]An "illegal" value is one that is not defined in the code book. Assume, for example, that the primary diagnosis categories in a study of patients with cancer include breast cancer (1), colon cancer (2), and prostate cancer (3). In this case, any other value, except for the designated "missing value" code, would be "illegal."

TABLE 23.1		Sample Section of a Study Code Book	

Variable Name	Variable Column Position	Variable Description	Value Codes and Labels
ID	1–4	Study participant ID	Values: 1–1000
INTDATE	5–10	Interview date	Date format: mo/dy/yr Missing value: blank
PSEX	11	Interview date Patient sex	Male (1) Female (2) Missing values: (9)
PBDATE	12–17	Patient birthdate	Date format: mo/dy/yr Missing value: blank
PAGE	18–19	Patient age (years)	21–98 Missing value: blank
PEDUC	20	Patient education	No formal education (1) Completed grade school (2) Completed some high school (3) Completed high school (4) Completed some college (5) Completed college (6) Completed graduate degree (7) Missing values: (9)
AUDIT	21	Medical record audit sources	No audits available (0) Surgery only (1) Radiation only (2) Chemotherapy only (3) Surgery + radiation (4) Surgery + chemotherapy (5) Radiation + chemotherapy (6) Surgery + radiation + chemotherapy (7) Missing values: (9)
SURGERY	22	Occurrence of surgery	Yes (1) No (2) No audit available (3) Missing on audits (9)
SURGDATE	23–29	Surgery date	Date format: mo/dy/yr Missing value: blank
INTSURGD	30–32	Days between interview and surgery	Values: 1–69 Missing value: blank

problems.[24] In addition, no records are available to verify that the interviewer typed in the correct response. For computer-assisted telephone interviewing, such records are often available because interviews are routinely taped and

listened to by supervisors for spot-checking the quality and accuracy of interviewers. Such verification checks are resource-intensive and require adequate allocation of time and funds.

After the last bit of data has been entered, the researcher will have obtained a final **master data file.** This file contains all study-relevant variables with only numerical identifiers of study participants. *Keys that translate subject identification numbers into concrete subject identification information must be stored securely and separately, and*

---

[24]One of the authors of this book once received a data file from a computerized telephone survey in which 92% of all respondents were coded as "Black/African American," even though the target population did not contain a high proportion of minority members. A simple programming error had led to a reversal of the codes for "White/European American" and "Black/African American."

TABLE 23.2			Illustration of Data File in Spreadsheet Format*						
ID	INTDATE	PSEX	PBDATE	PAGE	PEDUC	AUDIT	SURGERY	SURGDT	INTSURGD
001	07/04/99	1	01/12/34	65	5	7	2	.	.
002	07/05/99	1	11/03/21	78	4	4	1	06/10/99	25
003	07/05/99	2	08/08/39	59	6	0	3	.	.
. . .	. . .		. . .		. . .	. . .	. . .	. . .	. . .
342	05/12/00	1	12/11/19	80	4	5	1	03/17/00	56
343	05/14/00	2	12/01/28	70	4	7	2	.	.
344	05/15/00	1	07/27/32	67	3	5	1	05/04/00	11
Etc.									

*See code book in Table 23–1 for interpretation.

should be accessible only to a very limited number of study personnel.[25] During data analysis, there will be many occasions on which variables will be recoded (see the next section). After many iterations of recoding, it is sometimes difficult to trace one's steps back to the original. For this reason, and because of the requirement that all data transformations must be open to inspection, actual data analysis should always proceed from a *copy* of the master file. *The master data file must be stored on a secure medium, such as a write-protected CD, and should never be changed.* The researcher should retain a copy of the file at each step of data management. In the event of an audit or a question about data validity, this "trail" allows the file to be checked to locate errors or verify decisions that were made about managing and coding the data.

Data Quality Checks, Consistency, and Recoding

The first task in exploring the master data file and preparing it for analysis is to run frequency distributions on all variables. Inspection of frequency tables serves several purposes. It can show:

- "Illegal" values that may still be contained in the data set
- The proper exclusion of all "missing value" categories
- "Outliers" and other "unusual" or "suspicious" values
- Variables that have unusually high numbers of missing values
- Variables that have highly skewed distributions

Many of these common problems in data sets can be addressed at this stage. Sometimes the solution involves intelligent guesswork (e.g., the recoding of a value of "55" to "5" for a variable with Likert-type response categories

numbered from "1" to "5"). Such repetitive number entries are a common problem in data entry.[26] The failure to exclude missing values from subsequent analyses is an amazingly common error in data analysis. Unless the software is specifically instructed that "8" or "9" or "99" is a code for a missing value rather than a valid response, it will include the cases with missing codes in the analysis. This can cause severe distortion in the reported results.

Outliers or extreme values in any variable distribution should be noted. Sometimes they may be the result of data entry errors, such as a reported patient age of 123 years. Even when they are not due to errors, outliers should be noted because they tend to have a disproportionate effect on the parameter estimates in statistical modeling. For instance, suppose that 10 households report the following household incomes: $10,000; $20,000; $20,000; $30,000; $30,000; $40,000; $40,000; $40,000; $50,000; and $300,000. The mean household income for this group is $58,000, which does not seem to be a valid indication of the "central tendency" or the location of the "bulk of the cases."[27]

Unless a skipping pattern is involved,[28] a variable with an unusually high number of missing responses should arouse suspicion and reflection on the source of the problem. If most variables in a given study have a missing response rate of 1% to 2%, but one variable has a missing

[26]Before proceeding with recoding to a legal value, such as "5," instead of a missing value, other clues should be pursued, such as the consistency of responses on adjacent scale items. Handling missing values is discussed later in this chapter.

[27]In this case, a better measure of central tendency would be the median (i.e., the value that cuts the distribution into a bottom 50% and a top 50%). The median for this subsample would be $35,000, at the midpoint between the two most central values.

[28]A skipping pattern typically involves information that applies only to a subgroup of the study sample (e.g., information obtained on the *amount* of smoking would apply only to current smokers).

[25]See chapter 24 for more on these confidentiality requirements.

response rate of 15%, the information in this variable may involve sensitive material, or there may be problems with question formatting, illegible records, and so forth. Some suggestions about how to handle variables with large numbers of missing responses are given below. Just as outliers can pose problems in data analysis, so can highly skewed variables. Skewed responses to categorical variables usually require some form of recoding, as when separate categories for "African American" and "Hispanic" are collapsed into a single "minority" category because not enough cases are available in either subcategory to be useful in analysis.[29]

Handling Missing Values

As discussed in chapter 16, obtaining high-quality data involves the use of conscientious data collection procedures with built-in quality control systems. However, even with the best efforts, item nonresponse inevitably occurs in any data collection effort of even moderate size. Item nonresponse can be a vexing problem during analysis because it can lead to a substantial reduction in the analyzable sample. For instance, assume that for each of the 20 questions that make up the Center for Epidemiologic Studies Depression Scale (CES-D), 1% of the responses are missing because study participants disliked the question, could not relate to it, or simply did not mark any response on a paper-and-pencil questionnaire. Further assume that the responses are missing randomly. That means that only 81.8% ($0.99^{20} = 0.8179$) of the study participants would have responded to *all* 20 items. If we insisted on computing the CES-D scale scores only for study participants who had a complete set of responses, we would lose more than 18% of the sample. That seems far less than desirable, especially when we consider that many of the study participants answered 18 or 19 of 20 questions, so we should have a pretty good overall sense of how they responded to the CES-D questions. In a situation like that, we can confine our analysis to the complete responders, which could lead to a substantial sampling bias,[30] or we can impute values for the missing responses, which may or may not result in a measurement error.

For large-scale survey studies, such as those conducted by the National Center of Health Statistics (see chapter 11),

it is a routine practice to impute values for many missing responses before the data are released for public use (Cox & Cohen, 1985; Korn & Graubard, 1999). Some of the major options are:

- *Logical imputations.* Other available subject information is used to "fill in" missing responses. For example, information about a family relationship (such as "niece") implies that the respondent must be female; being in "fourth grade" implies a likely age of 9, 10, or 11 years; and so forth.

- *Mean value imputations.* This technique refers to the replacement of missing *scale* items by the mean response for available items from the same subject. For instance, if a respondent answers 19 of the 20 CES-D questions and his or her *average* response is 0.9, this value would be substituted for the missing 20th response. Mean value substitutions make sense *only* if the predictor items are highly correlated with the missing item. This correlation can be assumed for internally consistent scales, such as the CES-D, but should not be assumed for unproven measures. Also, some statistical software programs automatically perform such mean value substitutions, even when only a few valid responses are available to predict a larger number of missing responses.[31] However, when used conservatively, such mean substitutions are preferable to dropping a case from analysis.

- *Regression imputations.* A more sophisticated form of imputation involves finding a regression prediction equation with sufficient accuracy in predicting missing values. Suppose a respondent refuses to report household income in a study of barriers to accessing health care services. However, the respondent is willing to provide information about his or her educational level, occupation, and other sources of income (e.g., rental property). If a sufficient number of study participants who responded to the household income question also answered these additional questions, it would be possible to estimate a regression equation to predict household income on the basis of this other information. The accuracy of this prediction could be tested by comparing predicted values with obtained values among the respondents who provided complete information. If the prediction is highly accurate, substitution for missing values among

---

[29]The collapsing of categories should never be simply a "mechanical" process. If there are good theoretic reasons to believe that the two or more groups that are combined behave very differently with respect to the outcome variable considered in the study, preliminary comparisons are needed before proceeding.

[30]Sampling bias is a very likely occurrence in this situation. Its magnitude can be examined by comparing complete responders with partial responders in terms of their socioeconomic characteristics or other criteria variables of interest.

[31]The SPSS "compute mean" and "compute sum" commands use a default that computes or imputes scale scores as long as one valid item response is present. Although the default can easily be overridden, careless analysis can result in substantially "fabricated" data. For example, when substantial amounts of data are missing, the imputation and substitution of the mean for missing data can substantially and significantly affect the study results.

study participants who refused to answer the income question is preferable to the sampling bias that would result from the exclusion of such respondents.

Other, more sophisticated techniques for value imputation are discussed in the relevant literature.[32] Many of the data "cleaning" efforts are necessary and are essentially common sense approaches to data management that can and must be performed for every study before the main analysis is undertaken. Ensuring that the data are as complete and error-free as possible is a prerequisite for good analysis.

Finally, the importance of good record keeping in data management cannot be overemphasized. In addition to reminding the analyst of all key decisions that went into the generation of the analyzable data set, record keeping has become the focus of heightened scrutiny by human subjects protection committees that review research projects.[33] The data collection plan and the training manual for research staff should state exactly how the data are to be tracked, stored, and otherwise managed.

Project Implementation Step 3: Data Analysis

Unless the purpose of the study is to explore the measurement properties of some of the measures used in the study, constructing scale scores on the basis of responses to multiple indicator items is another preliminary, although clearly analytic, task. For any measurement instruments used, even if they are as well established as the CES-D or the SF-36, the first step is to reconfirm the known measurement properties with the data at hand (e.g., to perform the necessary reliability analysis). Well-established measurement scales use a standard algorithm to compute total scale scores as well as subscale scores, if they exist. These algorithms should be followed unless the analyst has compelling reasons and the necessary analytic skills to deviate from the established algorithms. For less-well established scales, particularly if they are multidimensional, it is advisable to call on scaling experts to assist with the requisite factor analytic models to explore scale properties.

It is beyond the scope of this book to go into detail about statistical and other analytic strategies that allow one to answer the research questions. The appropriateness of any analytic strategy depends on the specific purposes of the project and the type of data that have been collected. For instance, narrative transcriptions obtained from open-ended interviews would require different strategies for analysis than biophysiologic data. Likewise, in some studies, simple descriptive summaries answer all of the research questions. In others, sophisticated statistical modeling is needed (and an appropriate expert should be consulted). In this section, we include a general discussion of the goals of data analysis.

Whatever the specific strategies for analysis and whatever your philosophic orientation to research, in the most general sense, data analysis involves finding interpretable *patterns* in the data. This process always involves two steps: (1) in some form, information is *summarized* (an analysis report is shorter than the actual data), and (2) during the analysis or interpretation, *concepts or categories* are used to *order* the data into meaningful *patterns*. Thus, *data never just speak for themselves or give automatic, self-evident answers*. Rather, the questions asked by the researcher guide what types of answers are obtained through analysis.

It is useful to distinguish between *exploratory* and *confirmatory* analysis. In exploratory analysis, a researcher is looking for patterns that are not fully anticipated and is, in a sense, willing to be *surprised* by unanticipated results. In confirmatory analysis, researchers test specific hypotheses (i.e., they already have firm expectations about what to find). This type of analysis is best suited to data obtained from experimental studies. However, a good researcher and analyst should always be open to the discovery of unanticipated results, which often form the basis for fruitful new research.

Data analysis often involves three steps. The first set of analyses is typically *descriptive* and provides background information on the study sample, possibly comparing it with known characteristics of the target population. For example, a sentence in a research report might read: "The sample was 60% female, 25% African American, and 75% White, with an average age of 64 years (age range, 55–76 years)." Or it might say: "The 1-year mortality rate in the sample was 4.5%, compared with 3% for the entire state and 2.5% for urban counties."

The second set of analyses is *substantive* (i.e., it is designed to address the research questions or hypotheses).[34] These *main* analyses should be clearly linked to, and appropriate for, answering the research questions or hypotheses

---

[32]The National Center of Health Statistics web site (*www.nih.gov/cdc/nchs*) provides a good starting point for more information.

[33]For additional details about institutional review board requirements for the protection of human subjects, see chapter 24.

[34]Refer to the research design chapters in this book (chapters 3–5 and 7–10) for specific examples of statistical approaches that are used to analyze data obtained from experimental, quasi-experimental, and observational study designs.

that guided the study. If the article includes tables, they should present these main findings.[35]

Finally, it is not unusual to see a series of ancillary, additional, or follow-up analyses that go beyond the analyses planned *a priori* on the basis of the research questions or hypotheses. Such analyses are usually suggested by an unanticipated finding. For example, a researcher might note a relationship between two variables that could be accounted for by another variable that was measured in the study. However, such analyses are essentially *exploratory*, and must be confirmed with other studies before being considered more "solid" evidence.

Box 23-6 provides a summary of the usual sequence of key tasks involved in quantitative data analysis. The first two steps include essential preliminary tasks and also familiarize the analyst with the data set. The next two steps involve data reduction (i.e., their goal is to convert a large number of individual indicator variables into fewer, more manageable scale scores). The final step tends to be of greatest interest to the researcher or analyst because it involves the actual testing of the research hypotheses against the data. Statistical modeling and testing should be the last step in the analytic process. Hastily executed statistical tests performed by someone who is not thoroughly familiar with the data set will only lead to errors of inference.

Project Implementation Step 4: Dissemination and Use of Study Results

The final step in project implementation is the dissemination and use of study results. This step occurs through a variety of mechanisms, including presentations and publications. Research dissemination involves skills that go beyond the basic steps of conducting research and involves establishing an explicit agenda for change based on the research findings. Dissemination of research findings to promote changes in clinical practice and health care policy is discussed in more detail in chapter 26.

CONCLUSION

The main purpose of this chapter has been to alert readers to the many considerations (including challenges to research design and implementation) that must be addressed

in carrying out clinical research. Good clinical research is not necessarily complex or highly theoretic, and many challenges can be dealt with effectively via common-sense solutions. Nurses often excel in this area as a function of their experiences in clinical practice. However, it is important to understand when it is necessary to draw on the expertise of others to accomplish the goals of a research project. It is also important to know how to access the needed expertise. As noted in our discussion of resource considerations, careful planning helps to prevent wasting resources on projects that are not designed or implemented appropriately to provide answers to the research questions.

Achieving success as a researcher involves excellent analytic thinking and problem-solving skills. Experienced nurses usually possess these strengths already. Conducting research builds on these strengths and offers the opportunity to engage in creative problem solving because no two clinical research projects are exactly alike. In addition, research projects often appeal to nurses who are curious, enjoy new challenges, and question why "standard" practice is necessarily the best practice.

►CLINICAL RESEARCH IN ACTION
A Pilot Study of a Nursing Intervention

We conclude this chapter with an illustration of a small-scale pilot intervention study, such as could be designed and implemented by an APN in a clinical practice setting. To study the effects of music and a personal message from the patient's physician on patient anxiety and the side effects of chemotherapy, Sabo and Michael (1996) conducted a pilot study with adult patients (N = 97) who were undergoing cancer chemotherapy. An intact-groups, quasi-experimental design was used, in which the patients of two different physicians who practiced in different locations were assigned, respectively, to a usual care group that received chemotherapy, but no other intervention (n = 50), and an experimental intervention group that received the intervention (n = 47). The patients in the experimental group received the intervention over the first four consecutive chemotherapy sessions. A pretest–posttest study design was used to compare the groups on the outcomes of anxiety level and side effects of chemotherapy. A significant decrease in anxiety, but not in the side effects of chemotherapy, was found for the experimental group.

The background literature review showed evidence of careful preparation, validation, and comparative evaluation. A specific gap in knowledge was identified regarding the unknown benefits of an intervention to reduce anxiety and the side effects associated with chemotherapy. The intervention would require relatively little time and money. The limitations of existing research were well described and were used to articulate the need for the study. Neuman's systems model

---

[35]Some articles contain elaborate tables that provide supporting and descriptive information (e.g., information about the sociodemographic background of study subjects), but no tables that summarize the main results. In our opinion, this approach can be less than helpful in "bringing home" or highlighting the key findings of the research.

was used as a conceptual framework to guide the research. Chemotherapy was viewed as a stressor, and the intervention was conceptualized as strengthening "flexible lines of defense." Although the linkage of the key study variables with Neuman's systems model was well described, it could be questioned how much a "grand-level" theoretic framework such as this (compared with a middle-range theory) actually "guided" the research project.

An intact-groups, quasi-experimental design was used with a convenience sample of patients who were undergoing cancer chemotherapy. The authors addressed the limitations of their study design and measurement approach in the interpretation of the study results, including extraneous variables of multiple types of chemotherapy and variations in the quality of audiotapes. In addition, bias could have been introduced by the use of an intact-groups design as opposed to random assignment of the study participants to experimental versus control study conditions. They suggested alternatives to address these limitations in future research. In summary, the study is a very good example of a small-scale clinical study that could be implemented in a number of clinical practice settings.

Suggested Activities

1. Read Sabo and Michael (1996), and critique the adequacy of the planning steps of the study, as presented in the article.
   a. Is there additional information that you would want (be specific), if attempting to replicate this study?
   b. Consider a specific setting where you have worked or currently work as a clinician. What specific changes would need to be made in the study design to make it both scientifically sound and feasible for implementation in this setting? Explain why you would recommend these specific adaptations.
2. Using the steps outlined for designing and implementing a small-scale clinical study, outline a brief proposal for a study of a topic that is of interest to you. In developing your ideas, be sure to justify both the scientific and feasibility considerations, as outlined in this chapter.

Suggested Readings

Hulley, S. B., Cummings, S. R., Browner, W. S., Grady, D., Hearst, N., & Newman, T. B. (2001). *Designing clinical research* (2nd ed.). Philadelphia: Lippincott Williams & Wilkins.

Norwood, S. L. (2000). *Research strategies for advanced practice nurses.* Upper Saddle River, NJ: Prentice Hall.

Sabo, C. E., & Michael, S. R. (1996). The influence of personal message with music on anxiety and side effects associated with chemotherapy. *Cancer Nursing, 19,* 283–289.

References

Anderson, B., & Funnell, M. (2000). *The art of empowerment: Stories and strategies for diabetes educators.* Alexandria, VA: American Diabetes Association.

Bandura, A. (1977). Self-efficacy: Toward a unifying theory of behavioral change. *Psychological Review, 84,* 191–215.

Brown, J. K., Whittemore, K. T. & Knapp, T. R. (2000). Is arm span an accurate measure of height in young and middle-aged adults? *Clinical Nursing Research, 9, 1,* 84–94.

Campbell, D. T. (1969). Reforms as experiments. *American Psychologist, 24,* 409–429.

Cox, B. G. & Cohen, S. B. (1985). *Methodological Issues for Health Care Surveys.* New York and Basel: Marcel Dekker, Inc.

Drummond, M. F., O'Brien, B., Stoddart, G. L., & Torrance, G. W. (1999). *Methods for the economic evaluation of health care programmes* (2nd ed.). Oxford, UK: Oxford University Press.

Korn, E. L. & Graubard, B. I. (1999). *Analysis of Health Surveys.* New York, NY': John Wiley & Sons.

Minnick, A., & Young, W. B. (1998). Comparison between reports of care obtained by postdischarge telephone interview and predischarge personal interview. *Outcomes Management for Nursing Practice, 3, 1,* 32–37.

Prochaska, J. O., Redding, C. A., Harlow, L. L., Rossi, J. S., & Velicer, W. F. (1994). The transtheoretical model of change and HIV prevention: A review. *Health Education Quarterly, 21,* 471–486.

Rosenstock, I. M. (1990). The health belief model: Explaining health behavior through expectancies. In Glanz, K., F. Lewis, & B. Rimer (Eds.), *Health behavior and health education* (pp. 39–62). San Francisco: Jossey-Bass.

Sabo, C. E., & Michael, S. R. (1996). The influence of personal message with music on anxiety and side effects associated with chemotherapy. *Cancer Nursing, 19,* 283–289.

Stetler, C. (1994). Refinement of the Stetler/Marram model for application of research findings to practice. *Nursing Outlook, 42,* 15–25.

CHAPTER 24   Ethical Issues in Research Involving Human Subjects

INTRODUCTION TO ETHICS IN RESEARCH

Throughout this book, we have referred to ethical issues in research, with reference to this chapter for additional reading. The main objective of this chapter is to extend shorter treatments in previous chapters by providing a more indepth discussion of applied ethical issues in nursing research involving human subjects. "Ethical" situations have to do with questions of morality, including issues of right and wrong. **Ethics** is an academic discipline based in the philosophic and social sciences that is concerned with both descriptive and prescriptive questions of morality. Ethics focuses on concepts and principles of how human beings do and should think and behave. In a research context, ethics is concerned with the moral concepts and principles that underpin socially recognized and sanctioned professional and legal obligations. Ethical codes, guidelines, and standards underpin the legal regulations for the ethical conduct of research.

We start our discussion with the observation that ethical issues are intrinsic to everyday clinical practice and research activities. Although ethical dilemmas (conflicts between ethical principles), as experienced on a daily basis, may not be highly dramatic, they are nonetheless quite important to practice and research activities. Central to all ethical dilemmas is the need to balance the possible benefits and harms of intervention or research participation. For example, in daily clinical practice, advance practice nurses (APNs) routinely balance the desire or need to do good for the patient (beneficence principle) against issues such as patient autonomy (respect for persons principle) and working within resource limitations (justice principle). Suppose that an APN wishes to provide a patient with a newer, more expensive medication that he or she believes may benefit the patient more than the older, less expensive medication that the patient is currently taking. However, the APN faces limitations in terms of what he or she can prescribe, based on the medication formulary and the patient's ability to pay for the medication. Likewise, a clinical researcher is concerned with how to best provide participants with full disclosure of the risks and benefits of research (respect for persons and right to freedom from harm), in addition to a number of other key ethical issues that we will address in this chapter. For example, how should a researcher communicate with study participants about risks and benefits in a way that is fully understandable, so that a given participant can make an informed choice about study participation, yet is unlikely to cause undue alarm or provide false reassurance?

Before reading further, look at the examples of ethical considerations that are associated with conducting health research (shown in Box 24-1). Each example shows one or more possible benefits of research participation as well as possible harms. In some cases, the research design can be adapted to reduce the risks, thereby providing a better balance of benefits and risks and allowing research to be conducted in a way that is both scientifically and ethically acceptable. In other cases, it may not be possible to research certain questions because of ethical considerations. The examples included in Box 24-1 are not intended as a complete list, but are provided to give a "flavor" of the issues that we will address in this chapter.

The focus in this chapter is on human subjects, who constitute the majority of participants in applied clinical nursing research studies. However, some nursing and medical research studies investigate physiologic processes for which researchers may use **animal models** (research using animal subjects) to study topics such as cognitive function (e.g., see Davis, Gimenez, & Therrien, 2001; Holden & Therrien, 2000) and anorexia and acute inflammatory processes (e.g., see Lennie, Wortman, & Seeley, 2001; Lennie, 1998). Animal models are used for research that may be considered too risky or unethical to perform with human subjects.[1]

THE EVOLUTION OF PRINCIPLES TO PROTECT HUMAN SUBJECTS IN RESEARCH

Health care professionals often think of ethical principles and ethical behavior in research as natural or "obvious." After all, health care providers and clinical researchers are expected to behave ethically at all times. However, unfortunately, the history of ethics in health care and clinical research has shown otherwise. Recent history is fraught with examples of both intentional and unintentional ethical

---

[1]For those who are considering the ethical aspects of animal model research, research with animal subjects is controversial. Especially during the last decade, attention to the rights of animals has increased. Before becoming involved in animal research projects, it is essential to become familiar with the key positions of various stakeholders in the controversy. We recommend reviewing the American Psychological Association "Guidelines for Ethical Conduct in the Care and Use of Animals" (available at: *http://www.apa.org/science/anguide.html*), U.S. Department of Agriculture guidelines (available at: *http://www.usda.gov/*), and standards and rules published in the Federal Register (available at: *http://www.archives.gov/federal_register/*) as well as selected articles in the reference and suggested reading lists for this chapter. Researchers can find additional perspectives on the use of animal subjects in research by visiting the web sites and reviewing the publications of social advocacy groups for animals.

BOX 24.1   Examples of Ethical Considerations Associated with Selected Research Questions

Research Question

What position fosters optimal blood circulation in hospitalized patients with cardiac disease?

Ethical Considerations

The answer to this research question could help improve clinical practice within the target population. Suppose that a nurse researcher wanted to test the research question by using an experimental design in which patients are randomly assigned to a position (supine vs. side-lying). The researcher would also need to consider the potential for harm. For example, patients who are placed in a particular position may do worse physiologically compared with the other patients, or individual patients within either comparison group may do worse than they would if they were placed in the other position. For ethical reasons related to balancing benefits and risks, it may not be possible to retain random group assignment if an individual patient needs to be placed in a different position based on physiologic needs.

How satisfied are primary care patients with their health care providers?

This research question seems relatively innocuous because little or no physical risk is associated with completing a satisfaction survey in a clinic waiting area. However, because of the potential risk for patients to be treated differently (either worse or better) by their health care providers on the basis of responses to the survey, it would be very important for the researcher to carefully consider how the study would need to be designed to protect the confidentiality of patient responses. For example, patient surveys would need to be identified by a subject identification number only, with no names included. Care would also need to be taken to protect patient confidentiality in collecting survey data, for example, by providing patients with unmarked, sealable envelopes in which to place their computed surveys before submitting them.

Do depressed patients benefit from participating in Internet chat room discussions with other depressed patients?

The possible benefit to the patients needs to be weighed against the possibility of loss of confidentiality or worsening of patients' depression in response to the intervention. For example, even if patients are using chat room names (and not their real names), if patients inadvertently reveal personal information that could make their identities known to others, they may experience adverse consequences associated with the social stigma of mental illness. Likewise, some patients could experience a worsening of depressive symptoms, either in response to the intervention itself or as a result of other factors. For both issues, the researcher would need to think carefully about the development and pretesting of specific research protocols to minimize these risks. For example, as part of the informed consent process, at the outset of the study, the researcher may need to counsel patients about the potential risks of disclosing personal information to other study participants and also to provide study participants with specific strategies for protecting their confidentiality. Likewise, the researcher would need to build in a safety monitoring plan as part of the intervention research design (see the discussion of protecting human subjects in original research studies) in which the level of depressive symptoms is monitored throughout the study. Depending on the specific patient population, it may be important to include a protocol for crisis intervention for patients who experience thoughts of harming themselves or others.

misconduct involving a variety of health care professionals, such as nurses (see Benedict & Kuhla, 1999). At perhaps no other point in history have ethical issues in health care and research received the current level of attention, including the legal regulation that is now increasingly evident in Western societies. Especially during the last decade, there has been a rapid proliferation of publication in nursing and other health-related disciplines regarding ethical issues in clinical practice and research. A literature search using the keyword "ethical" or "ethics" will result in thousands of citations. Publications devoted to ethical issues have also greatly expanded; some of the newer national-scope journals devoted to research issues involving human subjects include *Bioethics, IRB: A Review of Human Subjects Research, Nursing Ethics, Research Nurse,* and *Human Research Report.* Almost all research-intensive academic institutions and health science centers now have extensive information available on research using human subjects, including web sites devoted to providing ethical and legal guidance. In addition, there are numerous national ethics web sites (Box 24-2). Guidelines and regulations for the ethical conduct of research (and ethical behavior standards in general) are evolving rapidly.

Why are ethical issues currently receiving so much attention? Several historical factors, based on events that have occurred over the last 70+ years, account for the recently heightened attention to ethical issues. Some of the most important factors are:

- Societal awareness of relatively recent "landmark" events in the early to mid-20th century, in which severe disregard for standards of ethical conduct occurred. Examples include Nazi medical experiments conducted during World War II, the U.S. Public Health Service Tuskegee Syphilis Study, radiation experiments conducted by the Atomic Energy Commission, and certain psychological experiments involving the deception of study participants. These landmark events will be briefly described, including a discussion of the major international codes of ethics that were developed in response to them.
- A large increase in research involving human subjects in the post–World War II era. This increase in research multiplied the opportunities for mistreatment of human research subjects.
- Media attention to "high-profile" ethical dilemmas in the context of advanced technology health care development, such as the ability to sustain or prolong life under circumstances that would not have been possible at an earlier time. Examples include the Nancy Cruzan life support case, which involved a right-to-die ethical

dilemma; life support of very premature infants who otherwise would not have survived; and resuscitation of near-drowning and severely injured accident victims.
- Rapidly developing biotechnologies, for which ethical standards are unclear or debatable. Examples include cloning and genetic manipulation.
- Rapid growth of computer technology and information systems. These developments led to much easier access to information, including computerized health information, and growing public concern about compromise of the privacy of health and other personal information (e.g., employer discrimination based on knowledge of health information, criminal use of Social Security numbers in "identity theft"). More will be discussed later in this chapter about recently enacted regulations that affect privacy and other evolving regulations for research (see the discussion of federal rules and requirements that protect human research subjects.)
- Increasing societal awareness of, and concern with, unethical conduct in various segments of society, including (but not limited to) health care. Examples include business accounting scandals in major corporations and research on integrity issues in various areas of society, such as education and business.
- Media attention to contemporary "high-profile" cases of ethical misconduct or questionable practices in clinical research. Examples include the well-publicized 2000 death of an 18-year-old research participant in a University of Pennsylvania genetic therapy research study and controversial direct marketing practices of the pharmaceutical industry. Other recent high-profile cases will be discussed later in this chapter.

History of Ethical Violations and Relevance to Major Codes of Ethics

During the Nazi regime in Germany in the 1930s and 1940s (World War II era), members of certain racial and religious minority groups, especially Jews and Gypsies, were used as involuntary research subjects in medical experiments that were conducted in concentration and death camps. These experiments included deliberate exposure of people to diseases, drugs, and other tests of the ability to bear stress or hardship. Persons who were used as experimental subjects were exposed to cruel physical or psychological "treatments," and most died as a result of the experiments. These experiments aroused justified international condemnation after World War II. Yet, experimentation without adequate concern for the protection of human subjects had also occurred in the United States. For example, the U.S. Public

BOX 24.2 Web Sites Concerning Research Ethics

Web Site	Description
Office for Civil Rights *http://www.hhs.gov/ocr/hipaa/*	Information about privacy regulations, including the current DHHS proposal, "National Standards to Protect the Privacy of Personal Health Information." Includes links to privacy regulation legislation and legislative updates.
Administrative Simplification *http://aspe.hhs.gov/admnsimp/Index.html*	Index for various federal administrative simplification news and legislative updates. Includes information about privacy, data standards, and transactions pertaining to health-related research regulation.
U.S. Department of Health and Human Services (DHHS) Office for Human Research Protections (OHRP) *http://ohrp.osophs.dhhs.gov/irbasur.htm*	Information about the National Institutes of Health commitment to protection of the welfare and rights of human research participants. A key link in this web site is the federal Common Rule (45 CFR 46), available at: *http://ohrp.osophs.dhhs.gov/humansubjects/guidance/45cfr46.htm*. The Common Rule describes federal requirements for the protection of human subjects in research. See also the National Institutes of Health (NIH) "Human Participant Protections Education for Research Teams" online tutorial at *http://cme.nci.nih.gov/*.
Institutional review boards (IRBs) of academic research institutions (various) *Example:* Michigan State University, University Committee on Research Involving Human Subjects (UCRIHS): *http://www.msu.edu/unit/ucrihs/*	Most academic research institutions now have one or more web sites with information about the protection of human subjects. These web sites can be very useful for gathering information about local IRB requirements as well as national issues. For example, the UCRIHS web site includes a "News and Resources" link available at: (*http://www.msu.edu/unit/ucrihs/ucrihsnews.html),* This site provides frequent updates about both local IRBs and evolving national regulations. In addition, these links often provide information about other resources for learning, such as selected key readings and links to other web sites.
National Institutes of Health Bioethics Resources on the Web *http://www.nih.gov/sigs/bioethics/.*	A comprehensive clearing house web site with news and links to related web sites, such as DHHS requirements for the protection of human subjects and the ethical conduct of research.
The President's Council on Bioethics *http://www.bioethics.gov/sites.html*	This Council was created by President George W. Bush in 2001 (Executive Order 13237), to "advise the President on bioethical issues related to advances in biomedical technology. This web site includes drafts of a number of staff working papers related to biotechnology, cloning, reproductive cloning, and therapy vs. enhancement interventions.
National Reference Center for Bioethics Literature *http://www.georgetown.edu/reaserach/nrcbl*	Contains comprehensive resources for literature searches on bioethics; online bioethics resources; a National Bioethics Advisory Commission digital archive (this commission expired in 2001); bibliographic, educational and teaching, and library resources; and links to other bioethics organizations and web sites. See also the Library and Information Services Gateway, Kennedy Institute of Ethics, Georgetown University, available at: *http://www.georgetown.edu/research/nrcbl/index2.htm*. There is a link at this site to the "National Information Resource on Ethics & Human Genetics." Library services are publicly funded by the National Library of Medicine and National Human Genome Research Institute.
The Federal Register Online *http://www.archives.gov/federal_register/*	Standards and rules (regulations), including final rules and updates as well as commentary and discussion on evolving regulations.

Health Service Tuskegee Syphilis Study (1932–1972) was a 40-year study of the effects of untreated syphilis among indigent, rural African American men in the South. Men who had syphilis were monitored medically to assess the effects of disease progression; however, information about the diagnosis, the course of the disease without treatment, and medical treatment for the disease was withheld. Likewise, during the Cold War years, federally sponsored radiation experiments took place in the United States and other Western countries. These experiments involved tests of the effects of radiation on prisoners and hospitalized patients whose ability to provide valid informed consent could be in question. These experiments were often justified on the basis of the societal need to understand, for example, what levels of radiation could safely be used in diagnostic imaging. Other instances of violations of informed consent have occurred in psychological experimentation involving the use of deception. For example, in the Milgram electric shock experiments (Milgram, 1963; Milgram, 1964), research participants believed that they were responsible for inflicting physical pain on other study participants by administering electric shocks in response to "disobedient" behavior.

As a result of the World War II war crimes trials, the **Nuremberg Code** (1947) was developed via the International Scientific Commission on Medical War Crimes (Weindling, 2001). The Nuremberg Code is important both because it was the first major international-level code of ethics and because it provided a basis for modern standards for appropriate experimentation on human research subjects, including the requirement for voluntary informed consent for study participation (Katz, 1996).[2] The second major international code of ethics was the **Declaration of Helsinki** (1964; revised in 1975), which highlighted the importance of individual needs over the needs of science and society. Both the Nuremberg Code (informed consent concept) and the Declaration of Helsinki (concept of risk minimization to individuals) have served as the foundation for subsequent U.S. federal regulations that guide research (Woodward, 1999). In addition to these two major international codes of ethics, many other disciplines, including nursing, have developed their own codes of ethics. For example, the American Nurses Association (1975) published *Human Rights Guidelines for Nurses in Clinical and Other Research,* and various other regional and specialty nursing organizations have published codes of ethics. For example, the Midwest Nursing Research Society (1996) published

Guidelines for Scientific Integrity. Most codes of ethics in various disciplines are quite similar regarding the basic concepts of ethical behavior, but also include content that is specific to the discipline or area of study (Polit & Hungler, 1999).

More Recent Examples of High-Profile Research Misconduct Cases

The landmark ethical cases that we described earlier were important to the development of major ethical codes, including the exposition of key ethical principles (beneficence, respect for human dignity, and justice) that underpin the legal regulations for research in the United States. More recently, certain high-profile research misconduct cases, as well as other factors related to societal changes (e.g., technology, privacy issues), have spurred the development of additional research regulations. We review a few more recent landmark cases here, including their implications for ethical research regulations. The full effect of these and future cases remains to be seen. See Research Scenario 24-1.

In terms of ethical standards for research conducted with human subjects, these recent cases share the allegation that researchers violated the standards for informed consent by failing to provide sufficient information about risks (respect for persons) and failing to disclose potential financial conflicts of interest. These and other recent cases have resulted in changes in the conduct of research at academic institutions and health centers. For example, researchers who submit grant applications for funding must now complete a declaration of potential or actual conflicts of interest. Likewise, researchers must declare potential or actual conflicts of interest in the informed consent form used with research participants. We now elaborate on key ethical principles in the conduct of research.

The Belmont Report and Key Ethical Principles

The **Belmont Report** (1978) merits special mention because of its role in identifying the three main ethical principles on which contemporary standards for research ethics are based. The content of the Belmont Report became the foundation for research regulations in federally sponsored research in the United States. The three principles are as follows:

1. *Beneficence* refers to the principle of at least doing no harm (freedom from harm), or refraining from exploitation of study participants, and promoting both

---

[2]Some historical scholars have argued that informed consent issues were recognized and regulations for human experimentation were in effect much earlier than is often reported (Sass, 1983; Vollman & Winau, 1996).

RESEARCH SCENARIO 24.1

Recent Cases of Alleged Violations of Research Ethics

In *Gelsinger v. University of Pennsylvania* (2000) and *Alderman v. University of Pennsylvania* (2001), researchers at the University of Pennsylvania were sued based on allegations that the defendants did not provide sufficient information about the risks associated with participation in a gene therapy experimentation program and that they did not disclose the researchers' and the University's financial interests in the research. Jesse Gelsinger, an 18-year-old research participant, died as a result of participation in a gene therapy clinical trial. Delores Alderman, another research participant in the same clinical trial, also alleged that the principle of respect for human dignity (see the next section of this chapter) was violated because insufficient information was provided about risks and financial interests. Similar issues have arisen in other recent clinical trials court cases. For example, in *Wright v. Hutchinson Cancer Research Center* (2001), allegations of inadequate informed consent for experimental cancer treatment and undisclosed financial conflicts of interest were cited. In *Aller v. University of California at Los Angeles* (1992; outcome pending in 2002), a lawsuit was filed against the UCLA institutional review board, alleging that the university contributed to misleading study participants about the risks of participation in a study (suicide in the context of medication changes) that involved withdrawing medication from people who were being treated for schizophrenia.

---

individual and societal benefits that are directly related to participation in research.

2. *Respect for persons* encompasses both the right to self-determination (autonomy) and the right to full disclosure (fully informed consent for research participation).

3. *Justice* concerns the right to privacy and the right to fair treatment in the context of research participation.

Next, we elaborate on each principle and discuss its implications for research. As previously mentioned, **ethical dilemmas** involve significant conflicts between two or three of the key principles in which the correct or preferred course of action is not clear.

Beneficence and Risk–Benefit Balance

Health care providers, including nurses, are usually well acquainted with the principle of beneficence as a central value in clinical practice. In this chapter, we discuss the application of this principle in clinical research. Beneficence has both passive (do no harm) and active (promote good) aspects. Research is ethically acceptable only when it is based at least on the first concept of avoiding harm. Obviously, research is considered unethical if it results in significant or permanent harm to the research participants (e.g., disability, death, severe distress, psychological trauma). To minimize the likelihood of harm, the following safeguards must be in place. These safeguards are formally assessed by human subjects research review committees, most often known as **institutional review boards (IRBs)** in organizations that receive federal funds. For institutions that receive federal funds, IRBs are organizationally based (local) ethics committees that are legally mandated to review research protocols for compliance with the following established ethical standards:

- *Use of appropriately credentialed and trained personnel.* This includes the principal investigator and all research staff who will handle any aspect of the study that involves contact with study participants, data, or other project management issues.
- *Use of appropriate study monitoring procedures or protocols.* This refers not only to the oversight role of the IRB (see the discussion of the role and function of IRBs), but also to adherence of the research team to the established protocols for collecting data, interacting with study participants, and monitoring the effects of the study on the study participants. The principal investigator and research team must know if, and when, a study should be suspended or stopped because of concerns that continuation might harm the study participants. For example, if a principal investigator discovers that an experimental drug may have severe side effects that were not previously known, he or she must be prepared to suspend the study immediately and take the necessary steps to ensure that the study participants will receive the appropriate care. In intervention studies that are federally sponsored, this is a regulatory requirement and is formally referred to as a "Data and Safety Monitoring Plan." See also the U.S. Department of Health and Human Services (DHHS) web sites (see Box 24-2).
- *Use of appropriate review, pilot testing, and study debriefing procedures.* In survey studies, especially if they involve personally sensitive topics, researchers should be careful and thoughtful when developing

questions. They should also use experienced consultants and research team members to review and pilot test ("test run") interviews and role-play actual interview situations. In most cases, research teams will discover that some adjustments must be made to the protocol before pilot testing can be performed with actual research subjects. In addition, researchers have often underestimated the psychological impact (distress potential) of exploring personally sensitive topics. The utmost care must be taken to ensure the comfort and well-being of study participants, including being willing to stop an interview at any time, to counsel a distressed study participant, and to arrange for appropriate follow-up care or treatment. For example, a researcher who is interviewing victims of domestic assault must be attuned to the distress level of the study participants, who are recalling assault experiences. In addition, the researcher should refer study participants to additional resources as needed for psychological assistance. The information to be gained (benefit) must be carefully weighed against the potential risk to the research participant (possible increased psychological distress).

- *Use of the least vulnerable study population possible.* Different study populations may be chosen based on the risk level of the research. For example, in experimental drug trials, animal test subjects are usually exposed first to new drugs to determine their safety before experimentation is performed with human subjects. Likewise, tissue cultures may be used to test the effects of various new interventions before tests are done using living tissue of human subjects.

Nonexploitation means not putting the needs of others, including the needs of the researcher or society, ahead of the needs of the individual research participant. We have mentioned some allegations of exploitation from recent court cases, including failure to disclose financial interests and sufficient information about research risks to research participants. Exploitation can take many forms, most of which are not fully intentional. For example, a researcher who is strongly invested in having complete data for each study participant may train her or his research staff to focus on obtaining full answers for each question. Such emphasis may lead a member of the research team to disregard a study participant's reluctance or unwillingness to answer certain questions (e.g., questions about household income, use of illicit substances, or history of mental health problems). Likewise, a researcher may be engaging in exploitation by failing to obtain active consent for study participation and instead choosing to obtain passive consent

through an "opt out" process. An example is mailing potential study participants a letter of invitation to participate in a study, with instructions to sign and return the letter only if they do *not* wish to participate.

Other forms of exploitation include failing to correct a study participant's misconceptions about the role of the researcher or the goal of a study. For example, a patient may agree to participate in a research project because he or she believes that doing so will result in better clinical care for a health problem. In some instances, the demand for research participation may exert undue pressure, if power differences between researchers and subjects are involved. For example, college students who are enrolled in introductory psychology courses and participate in the research of faculty members for extra credit points in class must be offered time- and effort-equivalent options other than research participation for obtaining extra class credit. More overt forms of exploitation include taking personal advantage of the trust relationship between the researcher and the research participant for personal gain (e.g., a physician or an APN who uses his or her clinical relationship with patients to encourage them to enroll in a study). Likewise, to encourage patients who have a certain health problem to enroll in a research study, a clinician may create a mailing list of patients for another researcher, who can then contact these patients and "drop the name" of their treating clinician.

Finally, the "active" form of beneficence involves tangible benefits as a result of research participation to either the individual research participant or to broader society. People consent to participate in research for a variety of reasons, including altruism, a belief in possible personal benefit, or simply a wish to help a researcher. As noted earlier concerning nonexploitation, the researcher must be open and direct with people about the benefits (or lack thereof) of study participation. For example, study participants should not be led to believe that completing a survey about desired amenities (e.g., parking, lighting, furniture) at a new clinic site will guarantee that these amenities will be included.

Direct benefits to individual research participants must be provided at a level that is consistent with compensation for time, travel, and other expenses or inconveniences associated with study participation. A research participant may receive a small token of appreciation (e.g., key chain, refrigerator magnet, coffee mug) in exchange for the time and effort required to complete a brief survey. Likewise, as compensation for his or her time and other expenses, a research participant who travels to a data collection site for a 1-hour interview may receive reimbursement for mileage, a stipend for gasoline, or a small payment ($10 or $20). The level of direct benefits from study participation should be kept at a compensation level, as opposed to a high level of incentive. Excessive incentives or gratuities (e.g., monetary payments, special treatment) are potentially exploitative, especially for vulnerable populations (e.g., students, low-income people). Likewise, undue or excessive incentives provided for others to recruit study participants should be avoided. For example, paying clinic staff to recruit research study participants from clinic waiting rooms is very controversial because of its potential for exploitation. In general, other means of obtaining informed consent are preferred. For example, the patient's health care provider or another clinic staff member who has been adequately trained in the ethical conduct of research should provide potential study participants with the initial information about the research study.

Beneficence is usually considered in relation to the risk–benefit balance of a research project (**risk–benefit ratio**). Standards for the ethical conduct of research require minimizing the risks of research participation. At the same time, the benefits must be at least neutral (passive, or at a "do no harm" level). In the planning phases of the research project, the researcher and research team must give careful consideration to attaining the appropriate risk–benefit balance. In some instances, decisions about research design may result in unacceptably high risks to potential study participants. For example, conducting an in-depth interview for research purposes within 10 minutes of a victim's presentation to the emergency department after a sexual assault, to minimize "recall bias," would be considered unduly exploitative of severely traumatized patients. Polit and Hungler (1999) suggested a useful "reality check" for researchers who are considering the risk–benefit balance of a research project: researchers might wish to consider their comfort level with having a family member participate in the research. This "real-person" standard is often used informally to evaluate the quality of nursing and health care in general (e.g., "Would you want yourself or your family to be cared for in this setting?").

A general criterion used by IRBs to evaluate the risk–benefit balance of research is whether the benefits and knowledge that are to be gained justify the potential risks to study participants. For example, in a research study of an experimental cancer chemotherapy protocol, the potential benefits to the research participants and the scientific knowledge to be gained must outweigh the risks of the experimental treatment. The patient must be fully informed of the risks and benefits (see the next section) to make an informed choice about whether to participate in the experimental trial.

In describing the potential risks of a research study, researchers should note that there is no such thing as a "risk-free" study (i.e., all research studies carry at least some risk, however minimal). **Minimal risk** (see information later in this chapter and at the web sites listed in Box 24-2 for federal guidelines and regulations) is defined by federal criteria as equivalent to or less than the risks that are encountered in everyday life or while performing include many routine daily activities. Examples of minimal risk include physical or psychological examinations or procedures, such as a patient history and physical. In some instances, when risks are greater than minimal (e.g., experimental cancer chemotherapy), the utmost care must be taken in the research design and study protocols to ensure an optimal balance of risks and benefits. In certain types of studies, it may not be possible to accurately estimate all risks in advance. For example, an experimental drug may have adverse effects that were previously unknown. When the risks of study participation outweigh the benefits (e.g., an experimental cancer chemotherapy is less effective than conventional care), the study should be stopped (if it has started), redesigned (if feasible), or otherwise permanently discontinued.

Respect for Persons

Respect for persons is a key ethical principle that involves the right to full information (disclosure) and the right to self-determination (autonomy) with regard to decision-making about research participation. To make a fully informed decision, a potential research participant must have adequate information about the potential and known risks and benefits of study participation. The person also must be able to decide freely whether to enroll in the study or to continue participation. More specifically, people have the right to **full disclosure** of the specific risks and benefits that could occur as a result of research participation as well as the right to decline or discontinue study participation at any time and for any reason. Failure to provide full disclosure can result in a legal basis for a lawsuit. Disclosure occurs through a formal process of **informed consent,** which is described in more detail later in this chapter. Likewise, as part of the informed consent process, people must be notified that they can freely decide whether to participate in the study, that they can discontinue their participation at any time, and that declining or discontinuing study participation will not result in the loss of benefits to which they are otherwise entitled. In addition, study participants should be informed that they do not have to answer any questions that they do not want to answer. For example, a research participant who declines to provide information about household income or illicit substance use should not be penalized in any way, not even by way of disapproval or pleading (unduly coercive behavior) of an interviewer with regard to obtaining the information. Examples of this type of coercion include the following statements: "Well, okay, it would really help us to have the information, but you don't *have* to provide it." "We can't use your data unless we have answers to all of the questions." "Since we're paying you by the time you spend, you will receive less money if you don't answer all of the questions.")

It is important to mention some special issues regarding the standards of full disclosure and self-determination. First, the specific level at which disclosure of risks and benefits should occur continues to be debated by ethicists and researchers. Various standards have been proposed, but in general, the researcher should follow a "reasonable person" standard by disclosing the major and most common risks (together with specific benefits, if any), and also provide an explicit risk–benefit analysis of study participation in the consent form for the study. For a review of these issues and recommendations for shared treatment decision-making, see Holmes-Rovner and Wills (2002). Second, certain **vulnerable populations** (as defined by federal criteria) may be compromised in their ability to make fully informed, fully free choices about study participation. These populations include:

- Minors
- Pregnant women
- Women of childbearing age
- Institutionalized persons (e.g., prisoners, people in health care institutions)
- Students
- Low-income persons
- Minorities
- Incompetent persons or those with diminished capacity to give consent

When vulnerable populations are sampled for research purposes, the level of study review and monitoring is usually greater, including scrutiny of the risk–benefit balance.

When study participants' knowledge of the study aim may affect the results, researchers have used one or both of two controversial approaches to obtain valid data: (1) deception of the study participants regarding the goals of the study and (2) covert observation for data collection purposes. **Covert data collection,** including audits of existing records that have been stripped of individual identifiers (e.g., hospital patients' names and addresses), may be ethically acceptable (see the discussion of ethical issues in the use of clinical and administrative data), but even research that ultimately may be "exempt" from the need for in-

formed consent *must* be reviewed by the appropriate IRB. As a general principle, researchers should never independently decide whether IRB approval is needed for a particular data collection procedure, including covert data collection procedures. The appropriate IRB should always be consulted about any procedure that a researcher proposes to use to collect data.

Anthropologic research often involves covert data collection in the form of observing people in social situations. For example, anthropologists may be interested in how people interact in public places under crowded and less crowded conditions, driving habits of people in urban versus rural areas, or the cultural practices of indigenous populations in remote areas. In contrast to research in which the participants are fully informed of the study goals, risks, and benefits, with a study that involves covert data collection, the researcher must provide the IRB with a well-justified explanation as to why this type of data collection is needed and justifiable. In recent years, there has been considerable controversy about how "covert" certain types of data collection in anthropologic research have been, and as in high-profile clinical trials, questions have arisen about possible exploitation of study subjects. Like other disciplines, anthropologic research has codes of ethics that outline the researcher's responsibilities to protect the rights of human subjects.

Of the two approaches, **deception** (active misinforming) of study participants is the most controversial. Deception most commonly involves misinforming the study participants about the goals of the research to study the effects of human behavior unaffected by knowledge of the study hypotheses. Perhaps the best-known example of deception occurred in a series of controversial psychological studies that were conducted in the 1960s on "obedience" behavior, in which the study participants falsely believed that they were administering electric shocks to other study participants who had been "disobedient" (Baumrind, 1964; Baumrind, 1985; Milgram, 1963; Milgram, 1964). Many study participants were severely emotionally distressed by their participation in the research and had not been informed in advance of the potential risks of participation.

The research community continues to be somewhat divided in opinion about the use of deception, with many researchers (especially in the last decade or so) feeling that few, if any, circumstances justify deception. For example, there has been a recent controversy about the use of "sham" surgery in clinical trials, in which study participants are randomly assigned to receive "real," or actual, surgery versus "sham," or fake, surgery (Dekkers & Boer, 2001; Macklin, 1999). These studies are not without significant risks to study participants (i.e., risk of surgical infection, adverse effects of anesthesia), and it could be argued that the benefits of the research would not outweigh the risks for the patients who have the sham surgery. Some researchers, especially psychologists, continue to believe that deception can be acceptable, provided that the risks are truly minimal and are well outweighed by the benefits of the research (see The American Psychological Association's 1982 Code of Ethics regarding the use of deception, available at: *http://www.apa.org*). The final decision about the appropriateness of a study design involving the use of deception (or any other type of study design) resides with the IRB, and is *never* a decision that is made independently by a researcher.

Justice

Justice concerns the rights to privacy and fair treatment in the context of research participation. Privacy concerns are currently receiving a great deal of attention, and regulations are developing rapidly for the control of personal information (see the web sites listed in Box 24-2 for information updates). Almost all clinical research studies involve collecting and examining data about health and other personal information. People are understandably concerned about how this information will be used, including the specific

safeguards that will be used to ensure that the information remains confidential. As a result of new federal regulations, IRBs are now mandated to provide routine audits of study procedures for research projects. A major emphasis in these audits is to ensure that the privacy of human subjects is protected. Box 24-3 shows a list of specific privacy safeguards that are routinely examined by auditors as well as other issues in the ethical conduct of research (e.g., maintenance of informed consent records).

When researchers obtain informed consent for study participation, they must explain (in the study consent form) whether the data that are collected will be considered confidential or anonymous. **Anonymous** data collection means that the researchers have no way to link the identifying information for study participants with the data provided. For example, a researcher may ask patients in a waiting room to complete anonymous surveys about their satisfaction with clinic health care services. The survey contains no identifying information about the study participant (e.g., name, mailing address, telephone number). In contrast, **confidential** data collection means that the researcher potentially or actually can link the identifying information for study participants with the data. In this situation, the researcher must provide assurances, including

---

BOX 24.3	Data Management and Storage and Informed Consent Safeguards that May be Audited by IRB Staff

- Separation of study participant names from ID numbers (consent forms stored separate from data, data identifiable only by study participant ID number on paper and computer records)
- Locked and otherwise secure access to study participant data and other project records, including paper and computer records
- Adequacy of records for tracking gratuities provided to study participants for study participation (specific dates for when participants received payments, what specific payment they received)
- A count of signed consent forms (at least as many consent forms as study participants from whom data have been collected)
- Review of each consent form for a study participant signature and date of signature (to confirm consent as well as that the date recorded on the consent form was not before IRB approval for starting data collection)
- Page-by-page review of the content of study materials actually being used for the project (interview packets, consent forms) against what is actually on file in the grant IRB project folder
- Review and discussion of general work procedures for the research staff related to maintaining the confidentiality and integrity of records (locking of doors when out of the office, logging off of computers when they are not in use, compliance with DHHS-required ethics training)
- Review and discussion of the contents of the grant IRB project folder with the principal investigator for any reports of adverse incidents
- Dated and detailed records of the specific training of research staff in research ethics and study procedures
- Witness of an informed consent process taking place in "real time" on-site with a researcher and a study participant as part of the research audit process

specific information about the methods used to safeguard confidentiality, to the study participants. For example, "Your interview will be audiotaped, but no names or other information that could identify you to others will be included on the tapes," or "The master list that includes your name and mailing address will be stored separately from your data in a locked file cabinet that is accessible only to designated members of the research team." Any potential limits to the confidentiality of the research data and the identities of study participants must be clearly described in the study consent form. An example is specific emergency circumstances, such as severe suicidal or homicidal ideation that would require research staff to contact emergency services for assistance.

Three other general principles for data collection foster privacy safeguards and are standard procedure in research projects:

1. *Collect identifying information only when necessary for the purposes of the research.* For example, it would be necessary to collect the telephone numbers of study participants only if the research design involved contacting the study participants for additional data via telephone. The proposal that is submitted for IRB review and the study consent form must provide a sound rationale for collecting identifying information.
2. *Identify research data only by study participant identification numbers.* For example, "Study participants 112, 165, and 203 indicated a strong preference for the health care provider to make the treatment decision." Generally, however, research results should be reported in aggregate form only, and in a way that preserves the confidentiality of the identities of individual participants. This assurance of confidentiality should be included in the study consent form. In qualitative case report studies, where narratives from individual participants are often included, care should be taken to disguise the identity of individuals (e.g., by referring to the participant by a fictitious first name and avoiding the use of potentially identifying descriptive information). Thus, a case description could refer to a patient by the name of "Mary" (not her real name), but should avoid an overdescription of "Mary" as ". . . a 101-year-old, upper-middle-class White woman living in the Sunset Retirement Community on the west side of West Keys, Florida," because such specific information could make the true identity of "Mary" known to others.
3. *Destroy identifying information whenever feasible and as soon as possible.* This process should be included in the research proposal for IRB review and outlined in the study consent form. For example, a researcher might

link three surveys from the same patient from different time points on the basis of identifying information, such as the participant's name. Once the survey data are linked and data collection is complete, it would no longer be necessary to retain the participant's name in association with the data.

The principle of justice includes the right to fair and equitable treatment in research. Simply put, this means that all research participants must have equal access to the benefits and equal exposure to the risks associated with the research. Fair treatment also means that people who decline to participate, do not participate fully, or decide to withdraw from a study are treated in the same way as other study participants. Research participants should be treated with respect and civility at all times, and should have access to research staff at any time, as needed. They should also be able to receive any services that are required in the context of research participation, including emergency services or treatment for injuries that occur as a result of research participation. These assurances must be included in the research proposal that is submitted for IRB review and outlined in the study consent form.

FEDERAL RULES AND REQUIREMENTS TO PROTECT HUMAN SUBJECTS IN RESEARCH

Thus far in this chapter, we have referred to "standards" and "regulations" for the ethical conduct of research. We now turn to describing the specific federal rules and requirements that are designed to protect human subjects in research. Ethical guidelines and legal regulations for the ethical conduct of research are evolving rapidly. As a result, at least some of the text of this chapter is likely to be out of date by the time of publication. Researchers should consult the appropriate Internet sites regularly to keep abreast of the rapidly changing information on ethics. Box 24-2 shows an annotated list of key web sites to help readers to "stay current" with regard to research ethics. These online references are intended to supplement and, in some instances, particularly for evolving regulations, update the text of this chapter with new developments. Review of these web sites will be useful in conjunction with reading the following sections.

The Code of Federal Regulations and Multiple Project Assurances

The Code of Federal Regulations (45 CFR 46), also known as the "Common Rule," is the main legal guideline for research requirements (see the link to this document in Box 24-2). It is conceptually based on and derived from the codes of ethics that were described earlier in this chapter. IRBs, which evaluate and make recommendations for research proposals, are guided by the requirements of the Common Rule (see the discussion in this chapter of the role and function of IRBs) and are legally required to uphold these requirements via the institutional agreement referred to formally as the *"Multiple Project Assurance (MPA) of Compliance with DHHS Regulations for Protection of Human Research Subjects."* An example of an MPA for a selected academic research university is available at: *http://www.msu.edu/unit/ucrihs/Assurance.html.* The core requirements outlined in this sample MPA are the same for other institutions. *The Common Rule applies to all federally funded research and all other research on human subjects, regardless of sponsorship.* The outlines the specific responsibilities of the institution, the administration at the research site, the IRB, the investigators, and the affiliated institutions and investigators.

Final Privacy Rule: Standards for Privacy of Individually Identifiable Health Information

All researchers should also be familiar with the evolving standards for the protection of personal privacy, including personally identifiable health information (refer to Health Insurance Portability and Accountability Act [HIPAA] online resources in Box 24-2). The Privacy Rule (Standards for Privacy of Individually Identifiable Health Information), which took effect in April 2001, ". . . creates national standards to protect individuals' personal health information and gives patients increased access to their medical records" (see the Health and Human Services Fact Sheet, available at: *http://www.hhs.gov/news/press/2002pres/20020321.htm).* Most covered entities, including health plans, health care clearinghouses, and health care providers who use certain electronic transactions, must comply with the Privacy Rule by April 2003. Proposed modifications of the Privacy Rule were implemented in April 2003 (see Box 24-2 for links to updates on the Privacy Rule). Key requirements of the current version of the Privacy Rule include:

- Patients must be informed about their privacy rights and the institutional practices regarding privacy rights.
- Informed consent and authorization must be obtained to use and disclose information for purposes other than treatment, payment, and health care (e.g., informed consent and authorization are required for research uses of patient health information).

- Covered entities must obtain a patient's specific authorization before sending him or her marketing materials (e.g., pharmaceutical products).

The specifications of the Privacy Rule are still being developed with regard to researchers' needs, but are already affecting access to research participants and research data. A current proposal for modification of the Privacy Rule is for "limited disclosure" of patient health information to researchers. This would not include information that would allow the participant to be identified, and the researcher would need to seek authorization from the participant to use the data. The authorization would be limited to contacting the individual for the specified research purpose. Recontacting the individual for future research studies would require specific authorization.

The net effect of the Privacy Rule for research is that access to patient health information is expected to become more strictly regulated in the near future. In particular, the standards for the need for informed consent are becoming more stringent, and authorization by the patient is required for the use of personal health information. Health entities and IRBs are currently implementing key aspects of the Privacy Rule. Researchers should consult IRBs and key web sites for new developments.

THE ROLE AND FUNCTION OF INSTITUTIONAL REVIEW BOARDS

As mentioned earlier, IRBs are legally mandated to review research proposals and make recommendations about the ethical status of the research. An IRB performs objective reviews of the merits and risks of proposed research and provides guidance to both institutions and researchers about the ethical conduct of research. The fact that the IRB is external to the research team is quite important in terms of protecting human subjects from possible exploitation by researchers, who may carry biases about their research, despite usually good intentions. For example, sometimes IRBs find that the materials submitted for review lack sufficient disclosure of risks or that the protocol does not contain adequate protections for possible exploitation of research participants. In addition to performing external oversight, the IRB has the legal authority to:

- Approve the proposed research plan and procedures as submitted
- Require revision of any aspect of the research plan that concerns the protection of human subjects
- Reject the proposed research plan as unethical and

not capable of revision to meet established ethical standards

Within this overall role, the IRB performs a number of functions in the review and monitoring of research. According to the Code of Federal Regulations (Common Rule), IRBs must evaluate research proposals and provide ongoing monitoring of research that uses human subjects in terms of the following specific federal requirements:

- *The risk–benefit balance is appropriate.* Potential or actual risks to the research participants must be minimized, and the risks must be considered reasonable in relation to the benefits to either the individual subjects or society.
- *The selection of participants is fair and consistent with the aims of the research.* Under federal criteria, investigators must provide specific and sound scientific and ethical rationale for the inclusion or exclusion of:
  - Women
  - Children
  - Minorities
  - Other vulnerable populations
- *Informed consent is obtained and documented appropriately.* See also the discussion of informed consent in this chapter. In most instances, written consent is required to be on file, but exceptions may be made in special circumstances (e.g., when obtaining written consent could be culturally inappropriate or offensive to potential study participants from some target populations). The researcher must justify and obtain IRB approval for any variations that are considered nonstandard.
- *An appropriate data and safety monitoring plan is in place.* For federally funded intervention studies, a formal, written Data and Safety Monitoring plan is required. However, the development of such a plan is desirable for all research, regardless of whether an intervention is being tested, and would be an expected part of any research proposal reviewed by the IRB.

IRB review of a research proposal occurs at one of three levels. Box 24-4 summarizes the specific types of research that are included within each level of review.

- *Exempt from review.* The proposed research involves no more than minimal risk. "Exempt from review" refers specifically to exemption from *full board review. Researchers should never decide independently that their research is exempt from IRB review.* All research must be submitted for IRB review. If the IRB concurs that the research meets the criteria for exemp-

tion, the IRB issues an "exemption approval" letter to the researcher.
- *Expedited review.* The proposed research involves no more than minor risk. If there is any question about the level of risk involved in a proposed research project, the proposed project should undergo full board review.
- *Full board review.* All research that cannot be categorized as "exempt" or "expedited" must undergo full review.

For research projects that involve the collection of socially sensitive information or that involve significant actual or potential risks, full IRB review is usually required. Many types of studies, especially if they involve minimally invasive survey questions or biophysiologic measures, may be exempt from full review and subject to expedited review. The levels of review differ in terms of the number of reviewers involved and the need for a full committee vote (as with full board review). The membership, qualifications, and credentials of IRB committees are currently under scrutiny. In addition, recommendations have been made for the certification of IRB committees in the future to provide a level of quality control and standardization to the review of research. There is wide variability in the judgments of IRBs, even within the same geographic region, and some IRB committees may not be well equipped to deal with the increasing complexity of evaluating ethical standards in research.

IRBs are federally mandated to conduct procedure audits of in-process projects. Local IRBs and the federal Office for Protection of Research Subjects are legally authorized to inspect any materials or resources associated with a research project at any time, with or without prior notice. Audit procedures may be set in motion on a routine basis, or for alleged due cause or concern about violations of ethics standards. In instances of severe ethics violations, the IRB or federal oversight office is empowered to suspend the research project, or even all of the research projects at a given institution, until the ethical deficiencies are remediated. Box 24-3 shows aspects of informed consent and study procedures that are the focus of routine IRB audits.

THE PROTECTION OF HUMAN SUBJECTS IN ORIGINAL RESEARCH STUDIES

Thus far in this chapter, we have discussed the basic principles and procedures for protecting human subjects in original research studies. In this section, we elaborate on two protection issues: (1) standards for informed consent and (2) safety monitoring plans.

BOX 24.4 Summary of Types of Research within Levels of IRB Review

Level of Review	Types or Categories of Research
Exempt from full board review	Research conducted in established or commonly accepted educational settings, involving normal educational practices, such as: (1) research on regular and special education instructional strategies or (2) research on the effectiveness of or the comparison among instructional techniques, curricula, or classroom management methods.

Research involving the use of educational tests (cognitive, diagnostic, aptitude, achievement), survey procedures, interview procedures or observation of public behavior *unless:* (1) the information taken from these sources is recorded in such a manner that subjects can be identified, directly or through identifiers linked to the subjects; and (2) any disclosure of the human subjects' responses outside the research could reasonably place the subjects at risk of criminal or civil liability or damage the subjects' financial standing, employability, or reputation. (See also Expedited review.)

Research involving the use of educational tests (cognitive, diagnostic, aptitude, achievement), survey procedures, interview procedures or observation of public behavior if the human subjects are elected or appointed public officials or candidates for public office.

Research and demonstration projects that are conducted by or subject to the approval of the DHHS and are designed to study, evaluate, or otherwise examine: (1) public benefit or service programs, (2) procedures for obtaining benefits or services under those programs, (3) possible changes in or alternatives to those programs or procedures, or (4) possible changes in the methods or levels of payment for benefits or services under those programs.

Taste and quality evaluations and consumer acceptance studies, if wholesome foods without additives are consumed or if a food is consumed that contains a food ingredient at or below the level, and for a use, found to be safe or an agricultural chemical or environmental contaminant at or below the level found to be safe by the Food and Drug Administration or approved by the U.S. Environmental Protection Agency and Department of Agriculture.

Note: If using voice, video, digital, or image recordings, the review category is automatically raised to Expedited.

Expedited review	Clinical studies of drugs and medical devices may be expedited only if: (1) an investigational new drug application is not required; research on marketed drugs that significantly increases the risks or decreases the acceptability of the risks associated with the use of the product is not eligible for expedited review; or (2) (i) an investigational device exemption application is not required or (ii) the medical device is cleared or approved for marketing and the medical device is being used in accordance with its cleared or approved labeling.

Expedited reviews may pertain to the following means of data collection:

Collection of blood samples by finger stick, heel stick, ear stick, or venipuncture as follows: (1) from healthy, nonpregnant adults who weigh at least 110 lb. For these subjects, the amounts drawn may not exceed 550 mL in an 8-week period, and collection may not occur more frequently than 2 times per week; or (2) from other adults and children, considering the age, weight, and health of the subjects; the collection procedure; the amount of blood to be collected; and the frequency with which it will be collected. For these subjects, the amount drawn may not exceed the lesser of 50 mL or 3 mL/kg in an 8-week period, and collection may not occur more frequently than 2 times per week.

Prospective collection of biologic specimens for research purposes by noninvasive means. Examples: (1) hair and nail clippings obtained in a nondisfiguring manner; (2) deciduous teeth obtained at the time of exfoliation or if routine patient care indicates a need for extraction; (3) permanent teeth if routine patient care indicates a need for extraction; (4) excretions and external secretions (including sweat); (5) uncannulated saliva collected either in an unstimulated fashion or stimulated by chewing gumbase or wax or by applying a dilute citric solution to the tongue; (6) placenta removed at delivery; (7) amniotic fluid obtained at the time of rupture of the membrane before or during labor; (8) supragingival and subgingival dental plaque and calculus,

BOX 24.4   Summary of Types of Research within Levels of IRB Review (continued)

Level of Review	Types or Categories of Research
	provided the collection procedure is not more invasive than routine prophylactic scaling of the teeth and the process is accomplished in accordance with accepted prophylactic techniques; (9) mucosal and skin cells collected by buccal scraping or swab, skin swab, or mouth washings; (10) sputum collected after saline mist nebulization.
	Collection of data through noninvasive procedures (not involving general anesthesia or sedation) routinely used in clinical practice, excluding procedures involving x-rays or microwaves. Where medical devices are used, they must be cleared or approved for marketing. (Studies intended to evaluate the safety and effectiveness of the medical device are not generally eligible for expedited review, including studies of cleared medical devices for a new indication.) Example: (1) physical sensors that are applied either to the surface of the body or at a distance and do not involve input of significant amounts of energy into the subject or an invasion of the subject's privacy; (2) weighing or testing sensory acuity; (3) magnetic resonance imaging; (4) electrocardiography, electroencephalography, thermography, detection of naturally occurring radioactivity, electroretinography, ultrasound, diagnostic infrared imaging, Doppler blood flow, and echocardiography; (5) moderate exercise, muscular strength testing, body composition assessment, and flexibility testing where appropriate given the age, weight, and health of the individual.
	Research involving materials (data, documents, records, or specimens) that have been collected or will be collected solely for nonresearch purposes (such as medical treatment or diagnosis).
	Collection of data from voice, video, digital, or image recordings made for research purposes.
	Research on individual or group characteristics or behavior (including, but not limited to, research on perception, cognition, motivation, identity, language, communication, cultural beliefs or practices, and social behavior) or research using survey, interview, oral history, focus group, program evaluation, human factors evaluation, or quality assurance methodologies.
	Continuing review of research previously approved by the convened IRB as follows: (1) where (i) the research is permanently closed to the enrollment of new subjects; (ii) all subjects have completed all research-related interventions; and (iii) the research remains active only for long-term follow-up of subjects; or (2) where no subjects have been enrolled and no additional risks have been identified; or (3) where the remaining activities are limited to data analysis.
	Continuing review of research, not conducted under an investigational new drug application or investigational device exemption, where categories 2–2 through 2–8 do not apply, but the IRB has determined and documented at a convened meeting that the research involves no greater than minimal risk and no additional risks have been identified.
Full board review	All other research that cannot be categorized as "exempt" or "expedited."

Adapted with permission, Michigan State University.

Standards for Informed Consent

Informed consent is most appropriately viewed as a process by which the researcher and a potential study participant communicate about the goals, benefits, and risks of the research. The goal of informed consent is to allow the person to make an informed decision about whether to participate in the research. Procedures for informed consent should support the intent of the three key ethical principles (beneficence, respect of persons, justice). To recap our discussion about ethical principles, informed consent is an important mechanism to ensure that people have the rights to:

- Remain free from harm and undue exploitation
- Receive any benefits to which they are entitled as a result of research participation
- Receive fair treatment that ensures the protection of personal privacy
- Be fully informed of the risks associated with research participation

- Freely decide whether to participate or to continue to participate in research at any time, without forfeiture of benefits to which they would otherwise be entitled

Box 24-5 lists key information that, according to federal law, must be included in consent forms for research studies. Local IRBs may require different specific wording for some of these elements. Some IRBs leave the wording of consent forms to the discretion of the researcher as long as they contain all of the information elements. Other IRBs are more restrictive, providing researchers with a standardized "boilerplate" or form template that allows less flexibility in adapting the wording for the specific purposes of the research project.

Increasingly, **process consent** procedures are used when the researcher will have repeated contact with study participants and for time-limited projects that may involve "high-stakes" decisions (e.g., experimental trials of treatments for serious or potentially terminal conditions). Process consent procedures are also used when the researcher may not be able to anticipate "how the study will evolve" (Polit & Hungler, 1999) in terms of the specific activities of the research participant and the risks, benefits, and time commitment. Finally, process consent is useful in situations in which there are reasonable questions about the person's preference for participation versus nonparticipation (e.g., a patient whose mood varies widely from day to day).

Process consent has the advantage of allowing study participants to formally revisit their decision to participate in the study at intervals that are appropriate to the nature of the research. For example, a person who is undergoing experimental chemotherapy for cancer may be asked to sign a consent form before each chemotherapy session. Time in the session must be allocated for the patient to discuss his or her perceptions of the treatment experience. Process consent most often involves personal discussion and interactive review of consent forms with the data collector and the study participant. Process consent increases the autonomy of study participants by giving them repeated formal opportunities to ask questions and discuss their perceptions. However, in any research situation, the researcher should take the utmost care to ensure that study participants fully understand the risks and benefits of participation and freely choose whether to participate.

Safety Monitoring Plans

Increased safeguards must be implemented for research projects that involve more than minimal risk or involve the use of vulnerable populations (see the list of federally defined vulnerable populations earlier in this chapter). As dis-

cussed earlier, a well-specified and pretested data and safety monitoring plan is required for all federally funded intervention studies. This type of plan is also applicable to research in which there are any risks to the research participants. For example, suppose that a nurse researcher plans to interview victims of domestic assault about their experiences with recovery from trauma. The researcher would need to propose specific safeguards to protect the privacy of the study participants as well as the confidentiality of the data. In addition, the researcher would need to develop a safety plan to ensure the well-being of the study participants, who may experience emotional distress when recalling their assault experiences. In this kind of research, all interviewers should be trained and experienced in crisis intervention, and specific arrangements should be made in advance to refer study participants to mental health resources for treatment, as needed. More extensive ("full" reviews) of research proposals and safeguards are normally required for any research in which the subjects are drawn from federally defined vulnerable populations. The researcher must give careful consideration to how the rights of these study participants will be fully protected.

ETHICAL ISSUES IN THE USE OF CLINICAL AND ADMINISTRATIVE DATA SETS

In contrast to what we just said about the need to protect human subjects in original research studies, the use of clinical and administrative data sets may appear more straightforward with respect to protecting human subjects. The analysis of large-scale data sets that are available at the state or federal level has long been a mainstay of important research on health services. However, major ethical issues regarding the use of clinical and administrative data sets involve concerns about the privacy of personal information, including health information, and the lack of informed consent. Analysis of already collected data is a type of "covert" research in the sense that individual participants do not necessarily provide informed consent for their personal information to be used in research (see also the section of this chapter that discusses the Privacy Rule). As mentioned earlier, the analysis of existing data may be ethically acceptable if the existing records have been stripped of individual identifiers (e.g., hospital patients' names and addresses).

For example, a health services researcher might use an existing data set collected by a state department of community health to analyze trends in infant births and mortality rates over a 10-year period. The data set contains no

BOX 24.5	Key Information Elements of a Consent Form*

Information Element	Description
Title and summary explanation of research	The title of the research project must appear across the top of the consent form. A reasonable summary explanation of the research, with its purposes and procedures stated in language that can be understood by the research subject, should appear in the first paragraph.
Risk and benefits	The study participants should be fully informed of all potential or actual risks and benefits associated with their participation in the research. Risks include possible psychological, physical, social, or economic harms that may be associated with research participation. Specific benefits to the study participant should be described; e.g., "To compensate for your interview time and transportation costs, you will be paid $20 in cash."
	For clinical trials in which the consent forms may be quite lengthy, a short summary version of the consent form may be developed for reference by the research participant, in addition to review of the longer consent form. It is always advisable to review the key risks and benefits of study participation at the outset of data collection and again as needed during the course of the study. If a participant's ability to provide valid consent is in question (e.g., a patient who is temporarily cognitively impaired while recovering from general anesthesia), data should not be collected from that participant until the ability to provide valid consent is documented.
Estimate of subject's Time; study Procedures	Study subjects must be given an estimate of the total amount of time required (e.g., number of sessions, frequency of testing). The participant's specific activities should also be described; e.g., "You would complete two telephone interviews, each approximately 30 minutes long."
Voluntary participation; refusal to participate; discontinuing participation without penalty	Study participants must be informed that participation is voluntary and that they may choose not to participate at all, may refuse to participate in certain procedures or to answer certain questions, or may discontinue the experiment at any time without penalty or loss of benefits to which the subjects are otherwise entitled.
Confidentiality and anonymity	Data gathered from human subjects must be treated with strict confidence on the part of the investigator, except in special circumstances approved by the IRB. Subjects shall not be identifiable in any report of research findings; on request and within these restrictions, results may be made available to subjects. Information on disposition of data, including who will have access to the data, should also be included.
	Consent forms should include the following statement about confidentiality: "Your privacy will be protected to the maximum extent allowable by law."
	All drug or medical device study consent forms should include a notice that the U.S. Food and Drug Administration, the study sponsor, and the IRB may inspect all records, including subject records.
Researcher conflicts of interest	The potential for conflict of interest occurs when the researcher or a member of the researcher's immediate family receives financial or other rewards (e.g., computers, software, laboratory equipment) from the sponsor of the research. If a potential conflict of interest is disclosed, the sponsor and the researcher's relationship with the sponsor should be briefly described on the consent form. Some sample statements:

(1) "The research described is supported by a grant from Company X to Institution Y for which Dr. Z is a principal investigator."
(2) "The research is sponsored by Company X. Dr. Y is serving as a consultant to the company on this project."
(3) "The researcher is sponsored by Company X. Dr. Y discloses that he owns stock in the company (serves on the board of the company)," etc.

(box continues on page 390)

BOX 24.5 Key Information Elements of a Consent Form* (continued)

Information Element	Description
Contact person for subjects	The form must include instructions on how to contact study personnel (name, phone number, and e-mail) with any questions or concerns that are raised by participating in the study. IRB contact information should also be provided.
Minor subjects	If the subject is a minor, provisions should be made for obtaining a parent's or guardian's informed consent (signature) *and* the minor's signed consent or verbal assent whenever feasible.
Debriefing procedure	When appropriate, a procedure for debriefing the subjects should be included. This is required when experiments involve deception.
Consent in cover letter, face sheet, or via phone	If the investigator incorporates the elements of consent in a cover letter, a face sheet to a written questionnaire, or as part of a telephone contact, the consent statement must include the following: "You indicate your voluntary agreement to participate by completing and returning this questionnaire." Or, "You indicate your voluntary agreement to participate by beginning this phone interview."
Experimental procedures	The form must identify any procedures that are experimental; include a description of any reasonably foreseeable risks or discomforts to the subject; and contain a statement to the effect that the experiment has been explained to the subjects, including any inherent risks or discomforts. *Note:* Alternatives to the proposed medical study therapy should be described in the consent form before the section that describes the study therapy and research.
If a treatment is involved	If a treatment is involved, no beneficial effects may be guaranteed; in the case of experimental treatment, subjects must be informed of alternative or standard treatments available and their record of success.
Risk of physical injury to the subject	If there is a risk of injury to the subject, one of the following statements must appear on the consent form:
Note: The National Bioethics Advisory Commission Report (August, 2001) asserts: "Participants who are harmed as a direct result of the research should be cared for and compensated."	If the research is performed at [name of institution] facilities or by [name of institution] employees or students: (1) "If you are injured as a result of your participation in this research project, [institution] will provide emergency medical care if necessary. You will not be held responsible for any medical expenses incurred as a result of this injury. All such medical expenses incurred by you as a result of this injury shall be paid by [name of payee]." *or* (2) "If you are injured as a result of your participation in this research project, [institution] will provide emergency medical care if necessary. If the injury is not caused by the negligence of [institution], you are personally responsible for the expense of this emergency care and any other medical expenses incurred as a result of this injury." If there is risk of injury to the subject, but the research is not performed at [name of institution] facilities and is performed by persons who are not [name of institution] employees or students and who do not identify themselves as associated with [name of institution], a statement must appear in the consent form that indicates: who will be responsible for providing emergency medical treatment in the event of injury and who will be responsible for payment for this treatment.
Placebo-controlled studies	The University Committee on Research Involving Human Subjects (UCRIHS) requires that the following paragraph be placed in the consent form of placebo-controlled studies. It may be modified as necessary for the terms of your study: "This is a placebo-controlled study. There will be two (or more) groups of patients; one or more groups will receive the active drug that is being studied; the other(s) will

BOX 24.5   Key Information Elements of a Consent Form* (continued)

Information Element	Description
	receive a placebo. A *placebo* is an inactive substance that will have no direct effect on your illness. The patients in the study will be assigned at random, that is, by a method of chance, to one of the groups. You will have an equal chance of being in a placebo group or an active drug group. Neither you nor your physician will know which group you are in."
Economic costs to subjects	This section applies only where subjects are paying some kind of fee for service and there is a need to distinguish fees for ordinary care or service from fees that might result from the subject's participation in research.
	Investigators must incorporate one of the following three paragraphs into the consent form.
	(1) Your participation in this research project will not involve any additional costs to you or your health care insurer.
	or
	(2) Your participation in this research will necessitate additional procedures [indicate procedures, e.g., obtaining medical tests and examinations] that will be discussed with you. The cost may be covered by your insurance. Those costs not covered by insurance will be provided by research funds. However, you will still remain responsible for insurance deductibles and copays.
	or
	(3) Your participation in this research project may involve additional costs to you for [indicate source of cost, e.g., drug, device, diagnostic procedure, therapeutic procedure]. Your health insurance probably will not pay for all of these additional costs. We [or your health care providers] estimate that the additional, unreimbursed costs to you will not exceed [$ amount]. If the actual costs exceed this estimate, you are still responsible for them.

*(Adapted from the Michigan State University, Committee on Research Involving Human Subjects.)

information that could be used to identify individual people (i.e., the database includes no names, addresses, telephone numbers, or Social Security numbers). Usually, in this situation, the IRB would require the department of community health information systems staff to remove all of the potential identifiers before giving the researcher a copy of the data for analysis. In addition, the researcher would prepare an application for IRB review as usual, proposing a specific plan to safeguard the transfer and storage of data (e.g., computer files will be password-protected and data will be stored in locked file cabinets). In the application, the researcher would indicate why he or she believes that the research is exempt from full board review. If the IRB committee agrees that the research is exempt from full review, the researcher would receive an approval letter that reflects this decision. To meet ethical standards for research, the research proposal must be reviewed and approved by the IRB before the researcher obtains and ana-

lyzes the data. A common area of confusion for researchers is the term *exempt,* which some have understood to mean that the researcher can decide whether his or her research proposal is exempt from review. All research *must* undergo IRB review, and the IRB (not the researcher) is legally responsible for deciding whether the research is exempt from full board review.

In addition, covert data collection, including the use of existing medical records, should *never* be used as a substitute for obtaining informed consent, when implementing an informed consent procedure would be more appropriate. For example, IRBs increasingly decline to approve certain types of quality assurance studies done in health care settings, in which a *post hoc* analysis of patient medical records is done without the consent of the patients, even though it would have been possible (in terms of both time and resources) for the researcher to obtain informed consent. Thus, if an APN collects survey data from patients in clinic waiting rooms regarding their level of satisfaction "for internal quality assurance purposes," the APN may not publish the results of the research because informed consent was not obtained from people who, in effect, functioned as research subjects. Likewise, researchers who propose to analyze medical records without an appropriate IRB review *in advance* of data collection and analysis are in violation of ethical standards for research.

CONCLUSION

In summary, ethical principles and the legal regulations that guide research have been largely driven by historical experiences with the unethical treatment of human subjects. The ethical principles of beneficence, respect for human dignity, and justice, together with their specific implications for the ethical conduct of research, have been derived in large part from this historical experience. These principles have been adopted as part of several major international and numerous discipline-specific codes of ethics. Ethical codes underpin the legal regulations that guide research, including specific, standard steps that are taken to ensure the protection of human subjects.

___

Suggested Activities

1. Review the research questions and considerations shown in Box 24-1. For each research question, outline answers to the following questions:
   a. Can the research design be adjusted so that the research question can be addressed in an ethically appropriate way? Be specific about the design adjustments you would recommend, and explain how the research question can be answered if the suggested changes are implemented.
   b. If you do not believe that the research question can be addressed based on the adjustments to the research design that you would recommend, state how the research question could be altered to allow the study to be conducted ethically. If you believe that the research question would need to be altered, provide a rationale for whether you think that adjustments to the question could be scientifically and clinically justifiable.
2. What specific ethical considerations (if any) would need to be taken into account when conducting research with the following populations?
   a. Children younger than 18 years of age
   b. Adults older than 65 years of age
   c. Pregnant women

d. Adults with advanced stages of cancer
e. Adults with mood or anxiety disorders
___

Suggested Readings

Anderlik, M. R., & Rothstein, M. A. (2001). Privacy and confidentiality of genetic information: What rules for the new science? *Annual Review of Genomics and Human Genetics, 2,* 401–433.

Anonymous. (1996). Research ethics and the medical profession: Report of the Advisory Committee on human radiation experiments. *Journal of the American Medical Association, 276,* 403–409.

Baumrind, D. (1964). Some thoughts on ethics of research: After reading Milgram's 'behavioral study of obedience.' *American Psychologist, 19,* 420–423.

Baumrind, D. (1985). Research using intentional deception: Ethical issues revisited. *American Psychologist, 40,* 165–174.

Benedict, S., & Kuhla, J. (1999). Nurses' participation in the euthanasia programs of Nazi Germany. *Western Journal of Nursing Research, 21,* 246–263.

Byrne, G. (2000). Participant-observer data collection. *Professional Nurse, 16,* 912–915.

Cassell, E. J. (2000). The principles of the Belmont Report revisited: How have respect for persons, beneficence, and justice been applied to clinical medicine? *Hastings Center Report, 30,* 12–21.

Cerinus, M. (2001). The ethics of research. *Nurse Researcher, 8,* 72–89.

Committee on Animal Research and Ethics (CARE). (2002). Guidelines for ethical conduct in the care and use of animals. American Psychological Association. Available at: *http://www.apa.org/science/anguide.html*

Coy, K. L. (2001). The current privacy environment: Implications for third-party research. *Journal of Continuing Education in the Health Professions, 21,* 203–214.

Ernst, E. (1994). Unethical behavior of Nazi doctors. *Journal of the Royal Society of Medicine, 87,* 246.

Evans, M. (2000). Justified deception? The single blind placebo in drug research. *Journal of Medical Ethics, 26,* 188–193.

Faden, R. R., Lederer, S. E., & Moreno, J. D. (1996). U.S. medical researchers, the Nuremberg Doctors Trial, and the Nuremberg Code: A review of findings of the Advisory Committee on human radiation experiments. *Journal of the American Medical Association, 276,* 1667–1671.

Faraone, S. V., Gottsman, I. I., & Tsuang, M. T. (1997). Fifty years of the Nuremberg Code: A time for retrospection and introspection. *American Journal of Medical Genetics, 74,* 345–347.

Haggerty, L. A., & Hawkins, J. (2000). Issues in clinical nursing research: Informed consent and the limits of confidentiality. *Western Journal of Nursing Research, 22,* 508–514.

Harkness, J. M. (1998). The significance of the Nuremberg Code. *The New England Journal of Medicine, 338,* 995–996.

Herrera, C. D. (2001). Ethics, deception, and 'those Milgram experiments.' *Journal of Applied Physiology, 18,* 245–256.

Holmes-Rovner, M., & Wills, C. E. (in press). Improvements in informed consent from research in behavioral decision making and communication. *Medical Care.*

Katz, J. (1996). The Nuremberg Code and the Nuremberg Trial: A reappraisal. *Journal of the American Medical Association, 276,* 1662–1666.

LaVaque, T. J., & Rossiter, T. (2001). The ethical use of placebo controls in clinical research: The Declaration of Helsinki. *Applied Psychophysiology and Biofeedback, 26,* 23–37, 61–65.

Lutz, K. F., Shelton, R. C., Robrecht, L. C., Hatton, D. C., & Beckett, A. K. (2000). Use of certificates of confidentiality in nursing research. *Journal of Nursing Scholarship, 32,* 185–188.

Michigan State University, University Committee on Research Involving Human Subjects. Home page URL: http://www.msu.edu/unit/ucrihs/.

Milgram, S. (1963). Behavioral study of obedience. *Journal of Abnormal Psychology, 67,* 371–378.

Milgram, S. (1964). Group pressure and action against a person. *Journal of Abnormal and Social Psychology, 69,* 137–143.

Milgram, S. (1964). Issues in the study of obedience: A reply to Baumrind. *American Psychologist, 19,* 848–852.

Miller, A. G. (1986). *The obedience studies: A case study of controversy in social sciences.* New York: Praeger.

Miller, F. G., Rosenstein, D. L., & DeRenzo, E. G. (1998). Professional integrity in clinical research. *Journal of the American Medical Association, 280,* 1449–1454.

National Commission for the Protection of Human Subjects of Biomedical and Behavioral Research (1978). Belmont report: Ethical principles and guidelines for research involving human subjects. Washington, DC: US Government Printing Office.

Nicks, S. D., Korn, J., & Mainieri, T. (1997). The rise and fall of deception in social psychology and personality research, 1921 to 1994. *Ethics and Behavior, 7,* 69–77.

Nicoll, L. L., & Beyea, S. C. (1998). Research corner: The ethical conduct of research. *AORN Journal, 67,* 1237–1238, 1240, 1243.

Redsell, S. A., & Cheater, F. M. (2001). The Data Protection Act (1998): Implications for health researchers. Methods used in two studies to obtain access to subjects. *Journal of Advanced Nursing, 35,* 508–513.

Reverby, S. M. (1997). History of an apology: From Tuskegee to the White House. *Research Nurse, 3,* 1–9, 15–18.

Roff, S. R. (2000). Human radiation experiments: What price informed consent? *Medicine, Conflict, and Survival, 16,* 291–301.

Rogero-Anaya, P., Carpintero-Avellaneda, J. L., & Vila-Blasco, B. (1994). Ethics and research in nursing. *Nursing Ethics, 1,* 216–223.

Rollin, B. E. (1990). Animal welfare, animal rights and agriculture. *Journal of Animal Science, 68,* 3456–3461.

Samei, E., & Kearfott, K. J. (1995). A limited bibliography of the federal government-funded human radiation experiments. *Health Physics, 69,* 885–891.

Sass, H. M. (1983). Reichsrundschreiben 1931: Pre-Nuremberg German regulations concerning new therapy and human experimentation. *Journal of Medicine & Philosophy, 8,* 99–111.

Sears, J. M. (2001). The payment of research subjects: Ethical concerns. *Oncology Nursing Forum, 28,* 657–663.

Sieber, J. E., Iannuzzo, R., & Rodriguez, B. (1995). Deception methods in psychology: Have they changed in 23 years? *Ethics and Behavior, 5,* 67–85.

Soskolne, C. L. (1997). Ethical, social, and legal issues surrounding studies of susceptible populations and individuals. *Environmental Health Perspectives, 105,* (Suppl 4), 837–841.

Steinbok, P. (1995). Ethical considerations relating to writing a medical scientific paper for publication. *Child's Nervous System, 11,* 323–328.

Steneck, N. H. (1997). Role of the institutional animal care and use committee in monitoring research. *Ethics & Behavior, 7,* 173–184.

Striefel, S. (2001). Ethical research issues: Going beyond the Declaration of Helsinki. *Applied Psychophysiology and Biofeedback, 26,* 39–59, 67–71.

Tadd, W. (2000). The Helsinki Declaration: Why all the fuss? *Nursing Ethics, 7,* 439–450.

Taylor, H. A. (1999). Barriers to informed consent. *Seminars in Oncology Nursing, 15,* 89–95.

U.S. Department of Health, Education, and Welfare. (1979). Protection of human subjects: Belmont Report.

Ethical principles and guidelines for the protection of human subjects of research. *Federal Register, 44*, 23192–23197.

Vollman, J., & Winau, R. (1996). Informed consent in human experimentation before the Nuremberg Code. *British Medical Journal, 313*, 1445–1449.

Weindling, P. (2001). The origins of informed consent: The International Scientific Commission on Medical War Crimes, and the Nuremberg Code. *Bulletin of the History of Medicine, 75*, 37–71.

Woodward, B. (1999). Challenges to human subject protections in U.S. medical research. *Journal of the American Medical Association, 282*, 1947–1952.

References

Baumrind, D. (1964). Some thoughts on ethics of research: After reading Milgram's 'behavioral study of obedience.' *American Psychologist, 19*, 420–423.

Baumrind, D. (1985). Research using intentional deception: Ethical issues revisited. *American Psychologist, 40*, 165–174.

Benedict, S., & Kuhla, J. (1999). Nurses' participation in the euthanasia programs of Nazi Germany. *Western Journal of Nursing Research, 21*, 246–263.

Committee on Animal Research and Ethics (CARE). (2002). Guidelines for ethical conduct in the care and use of animals. American Psychological Association. Available at: *http://www.apa.org/science/anguide.html*

Davis, A. E., Gimenez, A. M., & Therrien, B. (2001). Effects of entorhinal cortex lesions on sensory integration and spatial learning. *Nursing Research, 50*, 77–85.

Dekkers, W., & Boer, G. (2001). Sham neurosurgery in patients with Parkinson's disease: Is it morally acceptable? *Journal of Medical Ethics, 27*, 151–156.

Holden, J. E., & Therrien, B. (2000). The effect of familiarity on distraction and single cue use after hippocampal damage. *Biological Research for Nursing, 1*, 165–178.

Holmes-Rovner, M., & Wills, C. E. (2002). Improvements in informed consent from research in behavioral decision making and communication. *Medical Care, 40*(9), V30–V38.

Katz, J. (1996). The Nuremberg Code and the Nuremberg Trial: A reappraisal. *Journal of the American Medical Association, 276*, 1662–1666.

Lennie, T. A. (1998). Relationship of body energy status to inflammation-induced anorexia and weight loss. *Physiology & Behavior, 64*, 475–481.

Lennie, T. A., Wortman, M. D., & Seeley, R. J. (2001). Activity of body energy regulatory pathways in inflammation-induced anorexia. *Physiology & Behavior, 73*, 517–523.

Macklin, R. (1999). The ethical problems with sham surgery in clinical research. *The New England Journal of Medicine, 341*, 992–996.

Milgram, S. (1963). Behavioral study of obedience. *Journal of Abnormal Psychology, 67*, 371–378.

Milgram, S. (1964). Group pressure and action against a person. *Journal of Abnormal and Social Psychology, 69*, 137–143.

Polit, D. F., & Hungler, B. P. (1999). *Nursing research: Principles and methods* (6th ed.). Philadelphia: Lippincott.

Sass, H. M. (1983). Reichsrundschreiben 1931: Pre-Nuremberg German regulations concerning new therapy and human experimentation. *Journal of Medicine & Philosophy, 8*, 99–111.

Vollman, J., & Winau, R. (1996). Informed consent in human experimentation before the Nuremberg Code. *British Medical Journal, 313*, 1445–1449.

Weindling, P. (2001). The origins of informed consent: The International Scientific Commission on Medical War Crimes, and the Nuremberg Code. *Bulletin of the History of Medicine, 75*, 37–71.

Woodward, B. (1999). Challenges to human subject protections in U.S. medical research. *Journal of the American Medical Association, 282*, 1947–1952.

CHAPTER 25 Sources of Funding for Clinical Studies

INTRODUCTION TO FUNDING SOURCES AND GRANT PROPOSALS

In this chapter, we focus on sources of funding for clinical studies that are of interest to advance practice nurses (APNs) and other health care professionals as well as on the principles of successful grant writing. Although many APNs intend to engage mainly in clinical practice, in which they are primarily users of research findings (see chapter 22), skills in proposal writing for funding are nonetheless an excellent asset, especially for APNs who are interested in research or other clinical projects that may require outside funding (e.g., see Nash & Marcott, 1999; Rohrbach & Kinney, 1996).

As noted in chapter 23, resources play an overarching role in the success of a research project (i.e., the success of a research project rests not only on the knowledge and skills associated with project design and implementation, but also on the accessibility of the necessary resources).

Box 25-1 summarizes general resource considerations (adapted from chapter 23) for the initial planning phase of a research project.

A **grant proposal** (or **grant application**) that is submitted to a funding source can be thought of as a "marketing" document, in which specific resource needs for conducting a research project are described and linked to requests for specific amounts of money. The focus of this chapter is on two aspects of effective resource acquisition: (1) identifying appropriate funding sources or agencies and (2) writing grant proposals. APNs may be involved in writing grants, either as principal investigators (PIs) or project directors or as members of project teams in various other capacities. This chapter provides an overview of this process, with the goal of providing readers with a good starting point for applying for research funding. We have also included information about a variety of resources (see Boxes 25-1 through 25-4 and the list of suggested readings) for further exploration.

OVERVIEW OF FUNDING SOURCES

Although researchers in the health professions often express concern about the lack of available funding,[1] compared with some other professions, there are many public

---

[1]Concerns about funding also show the increasingly competitive nature of grants funding in which, over time, relatively more researchers are seeking funding in relation to the available funds (e.g., see Streiner, 1996). Attaining funding is not impossible for novice researchers who submit a sound proposal that is well matched to the priorities of a funding source, but many grant review processes tend to favor more experienced researchers.

BOX 25.1   Overall Resource Considerations for Initial Planning of a Grant Proposal

Time
Is there sufficient time, including institutional support for "release time" for the PI and other key study personnel from other activities, to carry out the research project activities? Aside from time allocations for personnel, will the research project itself actually be doable within the established timetable of project activities?

Money
How much money will be needed to carry out the project? Budget considerations should include costs for personnel; space, equipment, and supplies; travel; consultation; and other expenses specific to the project. What are the potential sources of internal and external funding?

Clinical and Research Expertise
Who is best qualified and otherwise able to be the principal investigator? What other expertise is needed in the form of co-investigators, project managers, collaborators, and consultants? Is the needed expertise readily available?

Motivation Level and Institutional Support
Is the climate favorable for successfully conducting the research? Are key research team stakeholders and the institution positively and sufficiently invested in the success of the project?

Access to Target Population
What barriers exist to gaining access to the target population? To what extent could these barriers feasibly and ethically be overcome, so that the research can be carried out successfully?

and private funding sources available for clinical research. In this section, we provide a brief overview of the major public and private sources of funding in the United States and discuss sources of funding at the local, state, and national levels. Box 25-2 highlights information about selected funding sources.[2]

Public Funding Sources

Public funding sources are also referred to as "government-sponsored funding." Public funding is available for clinical research at the state and federal levels, in the form of contracts and grants. **Contracts** involve a formal agreement between a researcher and a funding agency. The researcher conducts agency-initiated (as opposed to researcher-initiated) research within a particular budget allocation, often in response to a legislative mandate concerning some aspect of public health. Contracts are usually less flexible than grants because the researcher is bound to certain preconditions for the study questions and methods, as determined by the funding agency. Information about contract opportunities is made available publicly via **requests for proposals (RFPs).** Although opportunities for contracts have increased in recent years, most researcher-initiated research continues to be funded through **grants.** For grant-funded research, the researcher independently develops a research project and an associated budget for submission to a funding agency. Some "hybrid" approaches to contracts and grants have evolved in recent years; however, the distinction between *agency-initiated* and *researcher-initiated* projects continues to be useful.

At the federal and state levels, funding opportunities are publicized through postings of **program announcements (PAs)** and **requests for applications (RFAs).** PAs are broad topic areas that reflect an agency's funding priorities, for which investigator-initiated grant applications are solicited, usually over a period of 2 to 5 years. RFAs are more focused requests for investigator-initiated grant applications, which are typically limited to less than 2 years. (RFAs are also colloquially referred to as RFPs, although the RFP designation is technically used to refer to requests for proposals associated with contracts, as discussed earlier.) Within PAs and RFAs, various **funding mechanisms,** or specific types of grant application processes, are used. These processes shape the required focus and scope of the application or proposal as well as the specific research budgets that are allowable. Especially at the federal

level, funding mechanisms are quite diverse in terms of project scope, length of time for funding, and required level of experience of the PI. Information about PAs and RFAs sponsored by the National Institutes of Health (NIH) is published in the "NIH Guide for Grants and Contracts," available at: *http://grants1.nih.gov/grants/oer.htm.* Other federal agencies also post information about PAs, RFAs, and RFPs on their web sites. Information about state-level PAs and RFPs can often be found by visiting the home page of the web site for a given state or contacting key staff listed on the state web site.

State and Local Funding

States and localities are often interested in forming partnerships with clinical agencies to study questions of relevance to public health. Most state funding occurs through contracts, rather than through grants, and funded research projects focus on state-identified health priorities. As a result, these research projects are often less flexible in terms of research questions and methods. Successful contract partnerships involve "win–win" agreements that require negotiation and compromise on the part of both the agency and the researchers. Projects may involve collection of original data or analysis of public domain databases. For example, based on prioritized community health needs, a state department of community health may be interested in research on such topics as:

- A needs assessment of urban communities regarding mental health care services
- Interventions to improve knowledge of healthful nutritional practices for preschool-age children in rural, low-income families
- An evaluation of a mandated mental health preadmission screening process for nursing home placement
- Strategies to reduce teen pregnancy in index counties that have higher-than-average teen pregnancy rates

Many other topics could be identified. These examples are just a few that we selected based on our knowledge of research projects in Michigan.

In contrast to the federal level, for which well-organized and standardized information exists about funding through contracts and grants, specific state and local public funding opportunities can be more challenging to locate and access. Locating state funding opportunities typically takes time (sometimes months), especially if the researcher is not involved in work or other civic activities that facilitate regular communication with key sources of information. In addition, state funds for research may be less secure during times of crisis, such as during fiscal shortfalls. If budget cuts occur, state funds that are provisionally earmarked for re-

---

[2]As noted in earlier chapters, the URLs for web sites are subject to change. However, updated information about resources can often be found by doing a keyword search using an Internet search engine.

BOX 25.2 Public and Private Funding Sources

Public Sources

National Institutes of Health (NIH): *http://www.nih.gov/.* The grants home page is available at: *http://grants1.nih.gov/grants/oer.htm.* Information about specific grant funding opportunities is available at: *http://grants1.nih.gov/grants/funding/funding.htm.* To view information about the 27 institutes and centers comprised by the NIH, see *http://www.nih.gov/icd/.*

National Institute of Nursing Research: *http://www.nih.gov/ninr/.* Specific information about grants is available at: *http://www.nih.gov/ninr/research/dea.html.* Also, Medscape provides a free e-mail listserv for nurses, which includes summaries of NINR-sponsored nursing research projects (see *http://www.medscape.com/nurseshome*).

Agency for Healthcare Research and Quality: *http://www.ahcpr.gov./* Specific information about grant opportunities is available at: *http://www.ahcpr.gov/fund/*

Veteran's Health Administration: *http://www.va.gov/*

Substance Abuse and Mental Health Services Administration (SAMHSA): *http://www.samhsa.gov.* Specific information about grant opportunities is available at: *http:www.samhsa.gov/news/click1_grants.html.*

Centers for Disease Control and Prevention (CDCP): *http://www.cdc.gov*

Healthfinder: *http://www.healthfinder.gov*

MEDLINEplus: *http://www.medlineplus.gov*

U.S. Consumer Gateway: Health: *http://www.consumer.gov/health.htm*

Private Sources

Sigma Theta Tau International: *http://www.nursingsociety.org/.* See *http://www.nursingsociety.org/research/research_grants.html* for information about small grant opportunities administered by Sigma Theta Tau International as well as a variety of joint partnership grants with other nursing professional organizations.

For a resource list of family foundations see *http://fdncenter.org/learn/topical/family.html.* Also see the main web site for the Foundation Center at *http://fdncenter.org,* for information about the Foundation Center Foundation Grants Index, which is updated each year and contains subject headings for 28 different topic areas, including health-related topics. University libraries may carry an online subscription to the CD-ROM database, which is updated twice a year with current information on more than 54,000 foundations and corporate sources of grant funding.

Oryx Press Online Grants Database: *http://207.66.110.169/gs/cgi-bin/welcome.pl.* Provides information about more than 10,000 funding opportunities and 3,400 sponsoring organizations.

The Michigan State University Libraries web site contains a compilation of web pages and books that are of potential interest to nonprofit organizations seeking health-related funding, available at: *http://www.lib.msu.edu/harris23/grants/2health.htm#w.* The Michigan State University Libraries web site also has a nursing-specific compilation of web pages, books, databases, and announcements of grant funding opportunities in nursing for individuals, available at: *http://www.lib.msu.edu/harris23/grants/3nursing.htm.* The nursing-specific site contains extensive information about professional organizations in nursing that sponsor small-scale research projects. Grant opportunities at these Michigan State University web sites can be searched by academic level of the investigators, by the target population of interest, and by research subject (e.g., health, nursing). The web sites are updated yearly.

Health Organization Web Sites

The following health organizations (mostly nonprofit) are of interest to nurses and include information about sources of funding for research:

Health Web: *http://healthweb.org*

MayoClinic.com: *http://www.mayoclinic.com*

Medem: *http://www.medem.com*

New York Online Access to Health: *http://www.noah-health.org*

American Cancer Society: *http://www.cancer.org*

American Society of Clinical Oncology: *http://www.asco.org*

Children's Defense Fund: *http://www.childrensdefense.org*

World Health Organization: *http://www.who.org*

Robert Wood Johnson Foundation: *http://www.rwj.org*

American Botanical Council: *http://www.herbalgram.org*

BOX 25.2	Public and Private Funding Sources (continued)

American Diabetes Association: *http://www.diabetes.org*
Juvenile Diabetes Foundation: *http://www.jdf.org*
National Coalition Against Domestic Violence: *http://ncadv.org*
American Association for Retired Persons: *http://www.aarp.org*. See also the web site on research on health and
   long-term care at: *http://www.aarp.org/health/list.html*.
American Heart Association: *http://www.americanheart.org*
National Headache Foundation: *http://www.headaches.org*
American Academy of Pain Management: *http://www.aapainmanage.org*
American Academy of Sleep Medicine: *http://www.aasmnet.org*
National Sleep Foundation: *http://www.sleepfoundation.org*
National Spinal Cord Injury Association: *http://www.spinalcord.org*
American Stroke Association: *http://www.strokeassociation.org*
National Stroke Association: *http://www.stroke.org*
National Women's Health Network: *http://www.womenshealthnetwork.org*
National Women's Health Resource Center: *http://www.healthywomen.org*
Society for Women's Health Research: *http://www.womens-health.org*
American Association for Home Care: *http://www.aahomecare.org*

search may be reallocated for other needs. In contrast, federal budgets tend to be somewhat more stable from year to year. In addition, state-level research priorities may shift from year to year, depending on which public officials are in office at a given time, whereas federal research priorities tend to be more predictable over approximately 5-year intervals. Community organizations that receive and disburse public funding for research purposes are likely to be even more diverse in terms of funding opportunities and processes.

Useful starting points for identifying public funding opportunities include the following: (1) review web sites to identify state and local organizations, and (2) visit the research resources section of the library of a local university. As with many other professional situations in which a networking strategy is needed to attain a "toehold" to move forward, it is often useful to use a "snowball" technique to develop contacts to obtain needed information and access to funding opportunities. Often, it is useful to look for someone in your place of employment who has or has had research funding from a state or local organization and work outward from there, through phone calls and e-mails to identified points of contact.

Federal-Level Funding: The National Institutes of Health

The **NIH,** which comprises 27 institutes and centers, provides most federal-level funding for clinical research (see

Box 25-2 for online links).[3] Within the NIH, the National Institute of Nursing Research (NINR) is dedicated to funding nursing research. However, most of the other NIH institutes and centers also fund applied clinical research projects that are of interest to nurses. Opportunities for both grants and contracts are available from the NIH. A researcher who is considering applying for NIH funding should carefully read the detailed information on grants and contracts (available at the NIH web site), including information about the various institutes and centers, funding mechanisms, specific PAs and RFAs that may be well-matched with a research idea, and steps involved in preparing an application.[4] Within the last few years, the NIH grants web site has been greatly expanded, and now provides all of the basic information that is needed to understand NIH funding, including frequently asked questions about preparing grant applications. Additional strategies for applying for grants are discussed later in this chapter.

---

[3]Other federal agencies within the Department of Health and Human Services, such as the Substance Abuse and Mental Health Services Administration and the Agency for Healthcare Research and Quality, also fund clinical research, but most federally funded nursing research is funded through NIH. Readers who are interested in funding via other federal agencies should consult the links for web sites provided in Box 25-2. Many of the points that we discuss for NIH funding also apply to these agencies, including the standard forms that are used to apply for grants and contracts as well as overall application considerations.

[4]The NIH web site provides extensive information about individual NIH institutes and centers. Therefore, except for NINR, we have not listed these institutes or centers in Box 25-2.

BOX 25.3　　Summary of Steps in the NIH Grant Review Process

1. The application is received by the NIH Center for Scientific Review and reviewed for compliance with application guidelines before it is assigned to an institute and study section for scientific review. An application may be returned without review because of serious deviations from application guidelines.
2. Reviewers critique the application for scientific merit at a study section meeting and assign a priority score (average of priority scores assigned by individual reviewers). Reviewers may decline to score an application if there are serious deviations from application guidelines (such as serious ethical concerns about the proposed research).
3. The application is reviewed for funding by the advisory council of the institute based on its priority score.
4. For most (but not all) NIH funding mechanisms, the PI may revise and resubmit the application up to two times.*

*There are certain exceptions, such as the NIH B/START (R03) funding mechanism that is used for pilot research studies, in which the PI may revise and resubmit the application one time only.

To serve as a PI for an NIH grant (other than the F-series predoctoral fellowships), the researcher usually must have doctoral-level academic credentials.[5] With the exception of K-series (career development), some R-series (research investigator), and F-series (traineeship) funding mechanisms (see the NIH web site for additional details), most NIH funding mechanisms are designed for applicants who already have done at least some research, intend to incorporate clinical research as a significant part of their daily work activities, and are ready to move to larger projects that require more funding than can be obtained from most private sources. Thus, most small-scale clinical research projects that represent first efforts at research, but require external funding, are likely to be funded by private sources or a combination of private and intramural sources.

Because the NIH approach is so often referred to and used in modified form by other professional organizations and foundations, we provide an overview of the NIH process (Box 25-3) as a point of reference (also see the NIH web sites listed in Box 25-2). When a grant application is mailed to NIH, it is first reviewed administratively by staff at the Center for Scientific Review to verify that it complies with the grant preparation guidelines and is matched with the appropriate institute and study section. Then it is assigned to a **study section** (a group of experts in the content area) and institute for scientific review. The PI normally includes a cover letter with the application, indicating the PI's suggestions for institute and study section assignments. The CSR staff members often concur with the PI's suggestions, but in some cases, a different assignment is made.

The study section reviewers perform the first level of review of the application for scientific merit. These reviewers discuss the application and assign it a **priority score.** Most NIH applications are reviewed at a study section meeting, presided over by a **Scientific Review Administrator (SRA),** who represents the administrative staff of the funding institute, as well as a member of the study section, who chairs the meeting. Priority scores range from 1.0 (best) to 5.0 (worst). The priority score that is assigned to an application is the average of scores assigned by individual reviewers. In most instances, a primary reviewer and several secondary reviewers are assigned to provide written critiques and commentary for a study section meeting. Others attending the study section meeting may also participate in the discussion, after the assigned reviewers have presented their comments. The second level of application review is for funding merit and is performed by the advisory council of the institute. Applications are funded in rank-order of priority scores, with lower-scored applications receiving higher priority for funding, based on the available funds. Note that NIH applications usually receive **dual level review.** The first level of review is based on scientific merit, as reflected in the application priority score. The second level of review is fiscal, as based on the application priority score and the **funding line** (the threshold between applications that receive funding and those that do not receive funding in that review cycle).

From the time of submission to NIH, even if the original application is funded without need for revision, resubmission, and re-review, almost a full calendar year (also referred to as the length of the **review cycle**) will have

---

[5]Exceptions are sometimes made based on the experience level of the researcher and the availability of excellent research resources, such as a well-experienced research team that has at least some doctoral-level investigators and consultants.

elapsed. For most applications that are submitted to NIH, a funding award is not made for the first version. Even experienced investigators who have substantial track records of funding sometimes must revise and resubmit their applications, based on feedback from reviewers, before receiving funding.[6] Thus, the process of obtaining NIH funding is quite competitive and typically involves 1 to 2 years, even for an original application that is very well prepared and rated as scientifically sound by the reviewers.

Private Funding Sources

Many private funding sources are available for clinical research. Compared with even 5 years ago, the ease of locating information about private funding opportunities has been greatly facilitated by the Internet. Most research university libraries have a section that includes materials related to grant funding opportunities (e.g., see the Michigan State University Libraries web site examples in Box 25-2). Likewise, there are increasingly comprehensive and useful compilations of online clearinghouses of resources for funding opportunities (see Box 25-2). A variety of new nursing books are appearing in print as annotated compendiums of online sites (e.g., for a recent example, see Fitzpatrick, Romano, & Chasek, 2001). Many of these resources are available to the public without charge, and reviewing these web sites is one of the most efficient approaches to locating a large amount of information on funding opportunities. Nursing journals associated with specialty areas and organizations also publish articles on funding opportunities for nursing and clinical research.[7]

Private funding sources include both nonprofit foundations and for-profit entities. Relative to the broad scope of NIH priorities, most private funding sources fund a narrow range of research related to their priority missions. For example, the American Cancer Society funds clinical research that pertains to the prevention and cure of cancer as well as interventions to assist people who have cancer. Likewise, the American Heart Association funds research related to the prevention and cure of cardiovascular disease, and so forth. Also, compared with NIH funding, much less funding is available from most private sources, with some notable exceptions (e.g., because of its revenue base, the Robert Wood Johnson Foundation can make multimillion dollar awards to teams of researchers). Foundations most often focus on small grants programs that are specifically designed to meet the needs of researchers who are not yet applying for larger-scale NIH funding.

Professional (usually nonprofit) organizations use a wide variety of review processes for grant applications. In many instances, foundations request a short letter of intent or a brief (often 2–3 pages) initial **concept paper**[8] that outlines the major ideas for the research proposal, together with **biographical sketches** of the investigators (including credentials, professional background, grants experience, and publications; see the NIH grants forms link for the most widely used biosketch template), a research timeline, and an estimated budget. Foundation staff review the initial materials submitted by the researcher. If there is sufficient interest in what is proposed, the researcher may be asked to submit a more detailed application for funding. In some instances, the application is reviewed by the foundation staff, but in many other instances, the review process more closely resembles the NIH approach, such as that used by the Alzheimer's Association small grants program. Increasingly, professional organizations are using online review procedures; for example, Sigma Theta Tau International and the Alzheimer's Association small grants programs have recently moved to confidential online review of grant applications. For private funding sources, the researcher may have an opportunity to revise a grant application based on the written comments of reviewers.

For-profit funding agencies for clinical research include pharmaceutical and medical device companies. Corporate funding is probably the most controversial source of research funding because the proprietary interests of the funding entity can create conflicts of interest for the researcher. For example, a pharmaceutical company that is funding a clinical trial of an investigational drug may be invested (often in subtle ways) in the researcher whose results are most favorable to the drug. A clinical researcher who would like to obtain future funding from a drug company may be pressured (again, often in subtle ways) to produce results in a way that suits industry needs. These potential conflicts of interest are not always problematic, but safeguards for scientific integrity must be carefully considered and planned for in the design of research that is funded by a for-profit interest. For example, the contract should clearly specify the conditions under which the results will be reported in ways that ensure compliance with

---

[6]Resubmissions of NIH grants are usually limited to two, but there are certain exceptions.

[7]See the list of suggested readings in this chapter for recent examples of articles that address funding sources and principles of grant writing.

---

[8]When the concept paper includes information about the project aims and background or significance, the paper may also be referred to as a **statement of specific aims.** See the description of key elements of statements of specific aims in this chapter.

standards of scientific integrity. In addition, the level of autonomy of the research team in conducting the research, including any proprietary limits to autonomy, should be specified in detail.

Regardless of the type of funding source, reports of research that are publicly disseminated always must meet established standards for scientific integrity. These standards include reporting the funding source and any other potential conflicts of interest. Most professional organizations that sponsor research, including nursing organizations, have established guidelines for scientific integrity. Information and guidelines for researchers about conflicts of interest are available at the NIH web site.

Intramural Resources

Most small-scale clinical studies that are done within a single clinical setting are likely to be supported by **intramural** (internal, or within-agency) **resources.** Even a small-scale, agency-based research project should be expected to have some expenses (see chapter 23 for examples). Because internal funds or other resources are typically quite limited, the scope of the study must match the available resources. For example, an APN may want to test the effectiveness of follow-up telephone calls made by nurses on outcomes in patients who are seen in primary care settings for significant symptoms of depression. The APN may be able to obtain administrative support for dedicated time of clinic nurses to make follow-up telephone calls to patients, including infrastructure costs (e.g., telephone lines, costs of telephone calls). He or she may also be able to obtain administrative support for obtaining limited research and statistical consultation as well as the use of an existing clinic computer to conduct data analyses. A clinic-based study such as this does not have an "official" budget, but the costs of the study are incorporated within the existing infrastructure by reallocating some resources that are essential to the implementation of the project. As noted in Box 25-1 and discussed in more detail in chapter 23, assessing the level of support (such as administrative time, climate, and motivation) for a research idea is an essential step in assessing the feasibility of a research project.

BASIC PRINCIPLES OF GRANT WRITING

Review of the considerations listed in Box 25-1 and refinement of the focus of a specific research project within resource constraints are the initial steps in the development of a grant proposal or application. The time needed to develop a grant application for a funding agency varies; however, especially for first-time or larger-scale projects, the process can be expected to take an average of 6 months of planning and preparation, from project inception to application submission. Steps in the process of application development include:

- *Identify a potential source of funding.* As part of the initial planning process, the researcher should review web sites and other materials to identify funding agencies that provide a good match for the research proposal. Reviews of written materials should be followed up with e-mails and telephone calls to key contact persons in the funding agencies to clarify the agencies' interest level in the research proposal as well as to obtain more specific guidance for application development. Brief concept papers or statements of specific aims developed by the research team often serve as the expected basis of discussion with funding agency staff. Funding agencies differ considerably in their processes and requirements for applications, and it is very important to understand these rules so that a competitive application can be submitted. Usually, researchers identify first- and second-choice funding sources, so that the application can be efficiently submitted to another funding source if the first choice source does not accept the proposal.

- *Organize the research team and refine the aims of the study.* See also the discussions of developing research teams and clarifying the aims of research in chapter 23. A PI (or co-PIs) must be identified, and the needs for and roles of other team members must be identified, together with interested and qualified individuals who can fill those roles. Whenever possible, a new researcher should identify one or more mentors with substantial experience in grant writing and a track record of obtaining research funding. Research teams for small-scale clinical studies may consist of a PI, a project manager or research assistant, and a statistical consultant. However, the composition of the research team depends on the specific nature of the research project. The specific aims must be clearly articulated in writing, preferably with the participation or input of all key research team members and funding agency staff, and the final draft of the aims should be mutually agreeable to all members of the team.

As described in chapter 23, the refinement of study aims and the specific study questions or hypotheses is normally an iterative process that requires an investment of time. However, the quality of the future application is usually well worth the investment of time.

- *Review at least one successfully funded application.* The researcher should obtain at least one application that has been recently (within the last few years) funded by the funding source of interest. The research team should review and discuss this application. Such a discussion can show key approaches in the "model" application that could maximize the likelihood for funding of the application that is being developed. Ideally, the funded application should be similar in topic focus to the application that is being developed, but this is not as essential as obtaining at least one funded application on any topic that could show a successful approach for obtaining funding. The NIH Computer Retrieval of Information on Scientific Projects (CRISP) online database (available at: *http://crisp.cit.nih.gov/)* is a valuable source of information on federally funded research projects. CRISP includes information about projects funded by the NIH, the Substance Abuse and Mental Health Services Administration, the Health Resources and Services Administration, the Food and Drug Administration, the Centers for Disease Control and Prevention, the Agency for Health Care Research and Quality, and the Office of Assistant Secretary of Health. The database is available to the public without charge, and users can search the database by keywords, or by specific projects and study investigators. CRISP can be used to good advantage to locate possible consultants and mentors for a grant application, and researchers who have received federal funding may also have useful information to share about private funding sources.
- *Manage the work of the research team and address the personal and situational barriers to writing.* Successful grant applications and research projects are strongly underpinned by the ability to work well within groups as well as the ability to overcome personal and situational barriers to writing. See McGuire (1999) for a discussion of strategies for building and maintaining interdisciplinary research teams. See Wills (2000) for a discussion of strategies to manage personal and situational barriers to the writing process.
- *Follow the funding agency's guidelines and procedures for grant application development.* This point cannot be overstated. Otherwise sound grant applications often fare poorly in the review process because of noncompliance with important agency requirements. For example, researchers sometimes submit applications for funding to NIH that do not include key required elements. Examples include failure to discuss safety monitoring plans or safeguards for human subjects in an application for funding of a clinical intervention study

with a vulnerable population, ignoring format guidelines for margins and font size of the text of the application, and failing to submit the required number of copies of the application. Any errors of this sort, however minor or inconsequential they may seem to a researcher at the time, may result in return of the application without review or consideration for funding, or at least a serious penalty of the application priority score by the application reviewers. Before submission to the funding agency, applications should be read multiple times by the PI and other proofreaders and also checked against a list of requirements for the application to identify content, typographical, and format errors. In addition, the written materials regarding the requirements and priority foci of the funding agencies usually are not sufficient to guide the development of a grant application. Additional discussion with designated agency staff is usually needed to fully understand how the research proposal must be articulated and to ensure that the application is maximally competitive. Contacts with project staff offer an opportunity to cultivate a relationship that will be useful in the development of an application that is maximally "responsive to," or is an effective marketing document for, the agency's funding priorities.
- *Allow sufficient time near the end of the application development process to complete administrative tasks.* This consideration involves determining the time frames needed for the collection of the required signatures (usually multiple) on the application, for obtaining secretarial assistance with placing the necessary grant materials on the required forms, and for photocopying and collating the grant materials. It is wise to allow at least a week or two longer than what the PI or research team thinks is necessary to accommodate unanticipated delays, such as illness or equipment (e.g., photocopy machine, computer) breakdowns.
- *Develop a well-specified timetable of key activities.* The timetable should be cross-referenced against the sections or requirements of the application, and specific tasks and due dates should be included for various members of the research team. The timetable should be viewed as a dynamic document that is updated at least once a week, in response to team needs, or more often, as needed, by the PI or project manager.
- *Use writing outlines.* Many writers find it helpful to first develop an outline of key ideas, especially if multiple members of the research team will be involved in writing the grant application. For example, a statistician who is asked to contribute a section on sampling design,

power analysis, and statistical analysis should have specific guidance (in outline or "bullet point" form) from the PI or research team about the key points to address in relation to the specific aims of the grant application. Other members of the research team may be asked to contribute sections on procedures for data collection, protection or safety monitoring plans for human subjects, intervention protocols, and so forth. Although the PI ultimately assumes responsibility for the final content of the application, communication can be greatly facilitated by the use of a writing outline that is also linked to the specific tasks of the team members as specified in the project timetable.

- *Seek outside review.* Throughout the process of grant application development, critical reviews of draft materials should be sought from members of the research team as well as from other qualified people. A grant application must never be submitted "cold" to the funding agency without preapplication review by at least one qualified reviewer who is not a core member of the research team. This is particularly important as the time for submitting the grant application nears, when the research proposal is well developed, but there is still time to make changes. Arrangements for outside review should be made well in advance. Qualifications that should be sought in one or more application reviewers include:
  - The ability to provide timely, balanced, and constructive critical feedback in a fashion that could be expected from the reviewers at the funding agency
  - Knowledge of the key requirements of the funding agency
  - Insight into the review process that is used by the funding agency (i.e., for an NIH grant application review, ideally, the reviewer should have experience serving as an NIH study section reviewer)
  - Scientific expertise in the content area of the research proposal, including the associated concepts and methods

New researchers, in particular, often must work on developing the ability to respond in a positive, nondefensive manner to critical feedback on their work. The ability to use feedback to improve the quality of one's work is necessary for achieving success in obtaining research funding and in other scholarly activities. When applying for funding, the researcher should recognize the benefit of receiving critical comments in a less "public" forum (e.g., from one or two reviewers selected by the PI rather than the very public forum of a research funding agency review process). However, despite their best efforts, all researchers eventu-

ally experience harsh criticism or outright rejection. Researchers should be persistent and learn how to avoid taking criticism or rejection personally (see Wills, 2000, for a detailed discussion of strategies for overcoming personal barriers to scholarship).

Typical Elements of a Grant Application

Successfully funded grant applications have both high scientific quality and a clear, concise, and compelling style of writing in support of the proposed research. As mentioned earlier, a grant application can be thought of as a "marketing" document with which the researcher convinces the reviewer that the proposed project is worth the funds requested. The presentation should be both balanced and truthful with regard to the potential limitations of the proposed research, and should discuss possible alternatives to address the identified limitations. The writer must think as a reviewer would, providing a clear rationale for decisions and anticipating and addressing potential questions about the quality of the research proposal. Box 25-4 lists the most typical elements of a grant application. It is based on the format used by NIH for many research investigator (R-series) types of awards. We provide additional suggestions below for each key element.

Cover Letter to the Funding Agency

As already mentioned, grant applications should not arrive at a funding agency "out of the blue," without prior discussion with the funding agency project staff. In the case of a funding agency that has multiple divisions, such as NIH, the cover letter can also include suggestions for which particular institute, study section, or division might be most appropriate to review the application. This letter also should provide the project staff with any other special information that is not included in the grant application.

Title

Good titles are short, but adequately describe the research, allowing the reviewers or agency project staff to quickly grasp the key concepts. The use of unnecessary words and modifiers should be avoided. In some instances (e.g., for NIH grants), a limited number of characters may be allowed in the project title.

Abstract

The abstract for a grant application, if included, provides a brief (usually no more than _- to 1-page) summary of the research problem and the significance, key concepts, design, sample, measures, analyses, and expected outcomes.

BOX 25.4   Typical Sections of a Grant Application Based on the NIH Format

Cover letter to funding agency
Title
Abstract
Table of contents
Budget and budget justification, including a description of the research team and consultants
Biosketches for the research team members and consultants
Description of the research facilities, equipment, and other resources
Specific aims of the research (usually 1 page long), including the key research questions and hypotheses
Significance and background of the research problem (what is and is not known, what needs to be known and what
 gap in knowledge the proposed research will fill)
Results of preliminary studies
Proposed research design, linked to the research questions and hypotheses
Sample (including the target sample size and power calculations, study inclusion and exclusion criteria, sampling
 design, and recruitment plan)
Measures, linked to the independent and dependent variables described in the research questions and hypotheses,
 including psychometric information
Plans for pilot testing
Statistical analyses (overall approach and specific analyses to address major research questions and hypotheses)
Study and data management procedures
Timeline for study activities
Human subject considerations (see Chapter 24), including applicability of a safety monitoring plan
Inclusion of children
Inclusion of women or minorities
Data safety monitoring plan (required for intervention studies and should be addressed under human subject
 considerations for research with any vulnerable population; see chapter 24 for federal definitions of vulnerable
 populations)
References
Appendices

The abstract plays an important role in summarizing the key aspects and providing a compelling case for the importance of the research. Importantly, it helps the reviewers to remember the key points of the research as they review the main body of the application. Because of its central role in orienting the reviewers, the abstract should be very well polished. It is usually written in final form after the rest of application, including the research proposal section, has been written.

Table of Contents
The table of contents is a very useful organizing aid, both to help the research team to double-check that all required items are included in the grant application and to help the reviewers to locate items of interest quickly. The application should use any standard headers that are part of the instructions for application preparation, and the headers in

the text of the application should correspond to those used in the table of contents.

Budget and Budget Justification
The budget includes categories of expenses and requested amounts of funds for each itemized category. The budget section for NIH grants (and grant applications that use a similar format) includes "thumbnail" descriptions of each research team member and consultant. Providing a clear, adequate description of research team members and consultants in the budget is very important. Similar to the abstract and table of contents, many reviewers will use the thumbnail descriptions of key personnel as a reference point. Therefore, the descriptions must be polished and succinct, and provide a clear rationale for how each person provides a meaningful contribution to the research project. For complex organizations or research team configurations, it

may be useful to include a small organizational chart that shows the relationships among key personnel.

Work on the budget section should be started early in the application development process. Normally, it takes time to locate all of the specific budget information that is needed for the application, especially if there is not a designated administrative budget contact person to consult regarding costs and preferred ways to describe and account for various expenses. The proposed budget usually must be justified on a line-by-line basis and linked to the specific activities that will be performed within the grant. The NIH has a standardized process for preparing the budget and justification, but other funding sources are likely to vary considerably in the format and level of detail required. The final budget must be appropriate, neither underestimating nor significantly overestimating project costs. Administrative consultation should be sought throughout the budget development process, including advice about items that may be either inaccurately estimated or missing. Reviewers notice the percentages of time allocated to key personnel (i.e., too low, about right, too high), and they also pay attention to budget estimates for specific items that seem too high or too low, based on their own experiences.

Biosketches

A **biosketch** is usually included for each key research team member and consultant who will be involved with the project. The format and length of biosketches vary by specific funding agency, but biosketches are often 2-page summaries of a person's job title, academic degrees and other credentials, employment history, research grants and relevant experience, publications, and professional honors. In effect, the biosketch is a streamlined résumé or curriculum vitae that focuses on specific credentials and experience related to research. Especially if some team members have limited research experience, it is quite important to be clear and convincing in the budget justification about the specific contributions that each person will make. Reviewers compare biosketches with the budget justification, and they often downscore (penalize) a grant application because a team member does not appear to have the appropriate credentials or experience for the role that he or she will perform.

Description of Facilities, Equipment, and Other Resources

Key resources for performing the research should be described, including:

- The physical location in which the research will take place, including space for data collection and analysis
- Computer resources and other equipment

- Other facilities that will promote efficient and adequate performance of the proposed research (e.g., access to library facilities, journals, back-up equipment)

An efficient strategy for writing this section is to obtain a copy of this section from another grant application. This information can then be adapted for use in the new grant application. The final description must be tailored to the specific needs of the grant. As with the budget justification, this description should convince the reviewers that the resources are adequate for carrying out the proposed research. If specific resources are not mentioned or are not adequately described, reviewers may assume that the resources are not available, and may penalize the grant application score on that basis.

Specific Aims

The specific aims are a statement of the main objectives of the research. The aims derive from a clear, concise statement of the research problem, including a statement of its health significance and a clear description of the gap in knowledge that the proposed research will address. The aims should be written in simple, nontechnical language. The descriptions of the research questions and hypotheses that are included with the broader statements of the main objectives should be clear and brief. The specific aims should clearly state the concepts (independent and dependent variables) to be addressed in the research, including a concise statement of what important new knowledge will be developed on the basis of the proposed research. As mentioned earlier in this chapter, research proposals can be thought of as marketing tools. In particular, the specific aims are a key part of the proposal, in which the research ideas must be "sold" in a compelling way to the application reviewers. Thus, although short, the specific aims are probably the most important part of the research proposal section of the grant application.

Significance and Background

As discussed in chapter 22, the goal of a literature review is to determine what is known, what is not known, and what needs to be known about a topic of interest.

In writing the significance and background section of a grant proposal, the researcher must communicate these dimensions of the state of the science in a clear and concise manner. What is known, what is not known, and what needs to be known must be linked explicitly to the specific aims of the proposed research. For example, if a nurse researcher has identified a critical gap in knowledge about the effectiveness of reminder interventions for keeping primary care appointments, this gap should be identified, along with a statement of what new knowledge the proposed research will contribute to the current deficit. The space available in a proposal for this section can vary greatly, from less than 1 page to multiple pages, so the amount of elaboration will depend on the specific guidelines of the funding source.

Results of Preliminary Studies

This section includes a summary of relevant prior research done by the researcher. The results should be described, and specific statements should be included about the importance of the findings and what additional research needs to be done, as linked with the proposed research. For example: "The pilot testing of the intervention with 30 subjects (n = 15 experimental group; n = 15 control group) showed that tailored reminder interventions (using the subject's preferred mode of reminder versus a standard telephone reminder) increased appointment keeping among those in the experimental group. However, the sample size was very limited for drawing substantive conclusions about the efficacy of the experimental intervention, and the study participants were disproportionately well-educated and upper middle class. Therefore, these preliminary results must be replicated in a larger-scale trial and with a more representative sample of primary care patients." For small-scale clinical studies, there may not be earlier study results to be reported. If this is the case, it should be stated, but the researcher can include information about the clinical observations or experiences that led to the decision to do the proposed research, including (if available) information about the prevalence or incidence of the phenomenon in the target population.

Study Design

The statement of specific aims and the methods section (including study design, sample, measures, data analysis, data management, and study timeline) are the most important parts of the proposal, in terms of where the reviewers are likely to focus their attention.[9] The research design to be used should be clearly identified by name and linked explicitly to the specific aims and research questions or hypotheses. For example: "To assess the efficacy of the appointment reminder system, a preintervention–postintervention design will be used, including a 1-year preobservation period and a 1-year postobservation period." Specific details about the design follow a general orienting statement such as this, including the number and timing of observations and inter-

vention points. Care should be taken to remind the reviewer of the questions or hypotheses to be tested and to link the discussion to how the design will address these questions or hypotheses. Overall, the most important principle is to state clearly what will be done and to provide clear rationales for the decisions that are made. It is often very useful to provide a figure or table in the text to show the number and timing of observations and the measurements or data to be obtained at each observation point. It is important to remember, however, that figures or tables should *simplify* the discussion in the text. If they are overly complex, they may be difficult for a reviewer to understand easily.

Sample

The discussion of the sample identifies the specific target population from which the sample will be drawn and describes the key characteristics of the population (e.g., age, sex distribution, geographic location). Sample inclusion and exclusion criteria also should be included, together with a justification for the criteria. The specific sampling design and the plan for recruiting study participants should be described. For federally funded research, researchers must provide a discussion and a justification of the rationale for the inclusion or exclusion of certain groups, such as women, children, and minorities. The specific sample size that will be used should be identified, and the reviewer should be referred to the section of the proposal that includes the power calculations that show that the sample size estimates are adequate to perform the major analyses.

Measures and Pilot Testing

The specific measures to be used should be identified by name, and key references for the measures should be cited. The selected measures should be explicitly related to the measurement of the previously identified independent or dependent variables, and a rationale should be provided for why the researcher considers the measures adequate or the best available. Relevant psychometric information about measures (e.g., reliability, validity) should be included (see chapter 14). Where appropriate, justification should be included for why a given measure was selected instead of others. A discussion of plans to pilot test the measures should be included, particularly if the researcher is using measures that have not been validated or assessed for feasibility of use with the target population.

Data Analysis

The overall approach to statistical analysis should be described, together with the specific analyses that will be performed to address the major research questions or

---

[9]Research design issues were covered extensively in chapters 3 through 12. Refer to those chapters for specific design considerations.

hypotheses. As with other sections of the grant application, it is important to be explicit about the rationale for decisions. The researcher should consult a statistician for the development of this section of the proposal, including power calculations that guide decisions about sample size.

Study and Data Management Procedures

The specific steps for gathering data and the day-to-day management of the research project relevant to grant activities should be described. Long descriptions of specialized procedures (e.g., a complex procedure for tissue preparation and sectioning for analysis) can often be placed in an appendix for the reviewer to refer to later. However, the key information that is necessary for the reviewer to evaluate the soundness of the approach should be placed in the text of the proposal. Data management procedures (e.g., recording, storage, cleaning) should be clearly described in enough detail so that the procedures can be replicated in another study (see also chapter 16).

Study Timeline

A clear study timeline should be presented. The research team should carefully consider the timeline, and it should be a realistic depiction of when each project activity will occur. A common mistake is to underestimate the length of time required for certain activities, particularly preparation of the proposal for review by an institutional review board (see chapter 24), recruitment of research participants, and data collection. It is useful to summarize the study timeline in the form of a figure or table. Finally, the timeline should allow time for data analysis and dissemination of the study findings, even if these activities will take place after the grant funding has ended.

Research Conducted with Human Subjects (Including Applicability of a Safety Monitoring Plan)

The ethical issues involved in conducting research with human subjects, including safety, informed consent, and privacy, should be described (see chapter 24). The safety considerations should take into account the applicability of a safety monitoring plan. A safety monitoring plan is required for federally funded intervention studies. This type of plan is also appropriate for any research performed with vulnerable populations (see chapter 24 for a list of groups that meet federal criteria for vulnerable populations). The inclusion or exclusion of minorities, children, and women should be addressed in proposals for federal funding as well as in proposals for other types of grants as applicable

and required. See the NIH web site for further information about specific federal requirements for the protection of human subjects.

References

The references should show that the researcher has an excellent command of both the current information and the methods that are the focus of the proposed research. Because of the space limitations associated with most grant proposals, the cited literature should include key works, but not a comprehensive compendium of work that is relevant to the focus of the proposed research. In research proposals for clinical studies, most references (except for citations of certain seminal or classic references) should be from within the last 5 years.

Appendices

Appendices are used to provide supporting data or other detailed technical information. Items that are often included in appendices include publications or manuscripts written by the research team, detailed algorithms for project management or data preparation and management, questionnaires, and other forms.

CONCLUSION

A wide variety of funding sources and mechanisms are available for clinical research projects. The specific eligibility criteria and review processes vary, depending on the source and type of funding, but some general principles of grant writing apply to most situations. A well-written grant is responsive to the instructions of the funding agency and is an effective marketing tool for a research idea.

Suggested Activities

1. Review the resources listed in Box 25-2 and in the list of suggested readings to learn more about funding opportunities that are of interest to you.

2. Arrange to meet with someone who has been or is currently funded as a PI for a research grant. Talk with him or her about his or her perceptions of the benefits and challenges of obtaining a grant.

3. Review the research priorities described on the NINR web site (www.nih.gov/ninr/).

   a. To what extent do these priorities reflect your research interests?

   b. Do you agree with the NINR priorities? Provide a rationale for the priorities that you think should or should not be included.

Suggested Readings

Alvarez, M. E. (1998). Granting writing in the home health arena: Getting started. *Home Healthcare Manager, 2,* 19–20.

Alvarez, M. E. (1999). Granting writing in the home health arena: The proposal. *Home Healthcare Nurse Manager, 3,* 24–27.

Beyea, S. C., & Nicoll, L. H. (1998). Research corner: Finding research funding sources. *AORN Journal, 68,* 462, 464, 466.

Camarena, J. (2000). A wealth of information on foundations and the grant seeking process. *Computers in Libraries, 20,* 26–31.

Cohen, M. Z., Knafl, K., & Dzurec, L. C. (1993). Grant writing for qualitative research. *Image: Journal of Nursing Scholarship, 25,* 151–156.

Fitzpatrick, J. J., Romano, C., & Chasek, R. (Eds.) (2001). *The nurses' guide to consumer health web sites.* New York: Springer.

Foundation Center. (2001). *Foundation yearbook: Facts and figures on private and community foundations.* New York: Foundation Center.

Hester, S. H. (2000). Strategies for successful grant acquisition. *Journal of the New York State Nurses Association, 31,* 22–26.

Jones, L. L. (1999). Research, publication, and funding sources: Part I. *Journal of Trauma Nursing, 6,* 61–66.

Kachoyeanos, M. K. (1997). Keys to research: Research funding sources. *Maternal Child Nursing, 22,* 323–324.

Kachoyeanos, M. K. (1997). Research funding sources. *Maternal Child Nursing, 22,* 323–324.

Kachoyeanos, M. K. (1997). Granting writing. *Maternal Child Nursing, 22,* 267.

Kemp, C. (1991). A practical approach to writing successful grant proposals. *Nurse Practitioner, 16,* 51, 55–56.

Lawrence, S., Camposeco, C., & Kendzior, J. (2000). *Foundation giving trends: Update on funding priorities.* New York: Foundation Center.

Locke, L. F., Spirduso, W. W., & Silverman, S. J. (1993). *Proposals that work: A guide for planning dissertations and grant proposals* (3rd ed.). Thousand Oaks, CA: Sage.

Madden, V. (1998). Funding sources for nurse researchers. *Practice Nurse, 15,* 180.

Malone, R. E. (1996). The research column: Getting your study funded: Tips for new researchers. *Journal of Emergency Nursing, 22,* 257–459.

McGuire, D. B. (1999). Building and maintaining an interdisciplinary team. *Alzheimer's Disease and Associated Disorders, 13,* (Suppl 1), S17–S21.

McIlnay, D. P. (1998). *How foundations work: What grantseekers need to know about the many faces of foundations.* San Francisco: Jossey-Bass.

Nash, K., & Marcott, R. T. (1999). Funding a school-based health center. *Nurse Practitioner, 24,* 142–146.

National Committee for Responsive Philanthropy. (2000). *Grants: Corporate grantmaking for racial and ethnic communities.* Wakefield, RI: Moyer Bell.

Rasey, J. S. (1999). The art of grant writing. *Current Biology, 9,* R387.

Richards, D. (1990). Ten steps to successful grant writing. *Journal of Nursing Administration, 20,* 20–23.

Ries, J. B., & Leukefeld, C. G. (1995). *Applying for research funding: Getting started and getting funded.* Thousand Oaks, CA: Sage.

Rohrbach, S., & Kinney, R. (1996). Grant writing rewards the community and the home care team. *Home Care Provider, 1,* 306–309.

Smith, S. H., & McLean, D. D. (1988). *The ABC's of grantsmanship.* Reston, VA: American Alliance for Health, Physical Education, Recreation, and Dance.

Stange, K. C. (1996). Primary care research: Barriers and opportunities. *Journal of Family Practice, 42,* 192–198.

Steinecke, A., & Ciok, A. E. (1997). Aging research and education centers in the United States: A compendium. *Academic Medicine, 72,* 863–874.

Streiner, D. L. (1996). While you're up, get me a grant: A guide to grant writing. *Canadian Journal of Psychiatry, 41,* 137–143.

Wells, N., & Hurley, A. C. (1999). Idea to application: You are in charge. *Alzheimer's Disease and Associated Disorders, 13,* (Suppl 1), S111–S116.

Wills, C. E. (2000). Strategies for managing barriers to the writing process. *Nursing Forum, 35,* 5–13.

Wittstock, L. W., & Williams, T. (1998). *Changing communities, changing foundations: The story of diversity efforts of twenty community foundations.* Minneapolis, MN: Rainbow Research.

Zagury, C. S. (1997). Funding: Other funding sources/suggestions for obtaining grants. *Alternative Health Practitioner, 3,* 133.

References

Fitzpatrick, J. J., Romano, C., & Chasek, R. (Eds.). (2001). *The nurses' guide to consumer health web sites.* New York: Springer.

McGuire, D. B. (1999). Building and maintaining an interdisciplinary team. *Alzheimer's Disease and Associated Disorders, 13,* (Suppl 1), S17–S21.

Nash, K., & Marcott, R. T. (1999). Funding a school-based health center. *Nurse Practitioner, 24,* 142–146.

Rohrbach, S., & Kinney, R. (1996). Grant writing rewards the community and the home care team. *Home Care Provider, 1,* 306–309.

Streiner, D. L. (1996). While you're up, get me a grant: A guide to grant writing. *Canadian Journal of Psychiatry, 41,* 137–143.

Wills, C. E. (2000). Strategies for managing barriers to the writing process. *Nursing Forum, 35,* 5–13.

CHAPTER 26 Dissemination of Research Findings to Promote Changes in Practice and Policy

INTRODUCTION TO RESEARCH DISSEMINATION

The final phase of the research process is the dissemination (publicizing) of research findings to selected audiences. **Research dissemination** is a key step in the research utilization process (translation and application; see chapter 22, Figure 22-1), in which the research findings are presented in terms of specific implications for a given situation (e.g., practice, policy) and specific recommendations or action steps are included for how to use the research findings. The research process is not truly completed until the effects of knowledge dissemination can be assessed.

Attention to research dissemination has increased in recent years, and federal funding has been awarded to research centers in nursing and other health-related disciplines that focus on research dissemination.[1] At the same time, the lack of nursing research publications relative to other disciplines has become of greater concern, as evidenced by the editorials that have appeared in many recent issues of research-oriented nursing journals (also see Winslow, 1996). All practice disciplines, including nursing, are dependent on a unique base of knowledge to guide clinical practice and other activities. In applied fields, such as nursing, there is little point in doing research for the sake of acquiring knowledge, without some ultimate application to practice. There is general consensus in the nursing research community that researchers have a responsibility to disseminate the results of their studies, including working to overcome barriers to the communication of research findings and other ideas of benefit to nursing (Norwood, 2000; Wills, 2000). Advance practice nurses (APNs) who engage in research activities share this obligation.

Because research dissemination is the culmination of the research process, strategies to foster research utilization are the focus of this final chapter. As in the other chapters in Part VII, the goal is to provide the reader with a good starting point for embarking on research dissemination. We have also provided an extensive list of suggested readings for further investigation of various approaches to research dissemination.

---

[1]For a nursing example, see the web site for the Gerontological Nursing Interventions Research Center at the University of Iowa School of Nursing (available at: *http://www.nursing.uiowa.edu/gnirc/dissemin.htm*). This center has disseminated more than 26 evidence-based nursing practice protocols for health issues that affect older adults (see *http://www.nursing.uiowa.edu/gnirc/rddc_protocol-May2002.htm*).

GENERAL CONSIDERATIONS IN RESEARCH DISSEMINATION

Effective research dissemination involves paying careful attention to key conditions that must be created to maximize the effect of the findings for a given purpose (e.g., bringing about a change in clinical practice or broader policies). The first step in the dissemination of research findings is **audience analysis** (Norwood, 2000), in which the researcher thinks carefully about the following questions:

- What particular audience should hear about the findings?
  - Professional colleagues in clinical practice, research, or education?
  - Health care users?
  - Policy makers or legislators?
  - Administrators?
- Based on the audience, how should the findings be communicated?
  - In writing?
  - Verbally?
  - Visually?

Going beyond the broad categories of audience and type of communication approach, Box 26-1 presents key considerations for disseminating research findings. Effective communication is based on careful consideration of the challenges to communication and implementation of effective strategies to overcome the identified challenges.

SPECIFIC APPROACHES TO RESEARCH DISSEMINATION

Written Publication

The key advantage of disseminating research findings through written publication is that a lasting record will be created that is potentially (and increasingly) accessible worldwide. Written publication is the most prestigious form of communication for both the writer and the profession, and it is often the most useful mode of communicating research findings. Although successful publication in scholarly journals requires a certain level of knowledge as well as writing skills, APNs who have not previously published, but are participating in research, have an excellent opportunity to develop the necessary skills. Although there are dozens of readily accessible articles and books on writing for publication in nursing and other health-related fields (see the list of suggested readings), the best way to develop these skills is to write for publication. In addition, there are many potential personal and situational barriers to writing

BOX 26.1   Considerations in Choosing an Appropriate Communication Mode for Research Dissemination

- What are the most important "take home" messages (up to three key points) that should be conveyed to the selected audience, and why? This analysis helps to frame the key outcomes of the communication.
- What is the background of the target audience?

Existing knowledge about the topic (very knowledgeable/not at all knowledgeable)

Interest level in the topic (interested/not interested)

Expectations for information vs. other needs, e.g., being "engaged" or entertained by the communication process

Preferred mode of interaction, e.g., lecture, written materials, group interaction

Other issues that may "compete" with effective delivery of the message, including audience time constraints, fatigue level, and differences in values, language, and culture

- For any background issues that you identify that could interfere with optimal communication, how can communication be adapted accordingly?

(Wills, 2000). Boxes 26-2 and 26-3 show suggested strategies for overcoming personal and situational barriers, respectively. In addition to professional journals, opportunities to publish include other printed media, lay publications, letters, and other advocacy efforts. Each type of **publication outlet** (source of printed information) reaches a particular audience. Depending on the specific goal or goals of the researcher, more than one outlet may be used.

Professional Journals and Other Printed Media

Professional journals, books, reports, and other printed material are the main media used to communicate research findings to a professional audience. Journal articles are usually used to report the results of single research studies, whereas research findings reported in books are most often based on the results of multiyear programs of research. Standalone reports and other printed materials may be used for a variety of purposes (e.g., an annual executive summary prepared for a funding agency as part of a progress report for a multiyear grant or contract). In this chapter, we focus primarily on journal articles because they are the most common means of communicating research findings from individual studies (see the discussion of publishing in professional journals later in this chapter). First, we turn to less prestigious, yet vitally important, forms of dissemination that provide a more direct link between the "expert" and the broader public.

Lay Publications

Many people obtain at least some health information via one or more types of lay (nonprofessional) publications.

Most experienced APNs know that patients often bring information from lay sources to health care visits to seek professional input for their personal health care decisions. For this reason, APNs must be familiar with the key sources of information that are used by patients in particular populations (e.g., teenagers, women, men, older adults). The dissemination of research findings and conclusions in lay publications can help to promote broad changes in public policy. In addition, by offering patients advice on obtaining specific information during health care visits with busy clinicians, lay publications encourage people to participate actively in their own health care. Lay publications may also influence legislative efforts that benefit health care users. For example, patients who are empowered by information on how to evaluate and contest the decisions of health maintenance organizations (HMOs) to deny certain health care services may foster a "groundswell" of public support for national and state reform of HMO policies (e.g., required coverage for a minimum length of hospital stay for postpartum patients) and other mechanisms to balance the decision-making authority of HMO utilization review panels.

APNs can provide high-quality information to a wide range of health care users by publishing nontechnical reports of research findings and commentary on other topics on web sites as well as in journals, newsletters, newspapers, magazines, and other media. To succeed in publishing in these types of media, the APN must understand the needs of specific audiences and tailor the information to fit these needs. The APN also must be able to write in a nontechnical and culturally and socially acceptable manner. To determine the appropriate level and style of writing, the

BOX 26.2 Strategies for Personal Barriers to Writing

Type of Personal Barrier	Strategies
Thoughts and feelings	
Low motivation for writing; dearth of ideas for what to write	Regularly read widely in areas of clinical and research interest
	Write about clinical issues of personal interest
	Do not assume that findings or techniques are already known to others
	Cultivate a sense of writing as an urgent priority
	Partner with others and share writing tasks
Viewing self as an "imposter"; low confidence in ability to publish because of perceived lack of knowledge or skills	Understand key gaps in knowledge for practice needing research
	Read articles and books in writing for publication
	Find a mentor or writing partners with complementary skills
	Seek out classes, continuing education offerings, or workshops
	Remember that knowledge and skills develop with practice
Fear of negative feedback or rejection	Allow time for emotional reactions to feedback
	Avoid taking feedback personally
	Seek support for feelings, but avoid dwelling on catastrophic fears
	Ask objective colleagues to provide input before submitting material
Managing anxiety and frustration during writing	View work *progress* as more important than work *pace*
	Take frequent breaks and reward self for meeting due dates
	Recognize perfectionism and unrealistic expectations as pitfalls
	Balance writing with other activities that are restorative
Understanding the writing and publication process	
Unrealistic view of the writing process as too challenging or very straightforward	Map out a comprehensive work plan according to the parts of the paper
	Team with experienced writers or mentors and share writing tasks
	Expect writing to take time, effort, and many drafts
	Understand that ideas rarely flow smoothly at the outset
	Don't expect class papers or theses to be publishable "as is"
Inaccurate views of the review and publication process	Understand that critique is a normal part of the review process
	Remember that rejection can be avoided only by not writing
	Keep in mind that expert writers often have papers rejected
	Consider submitting the paper to another journal if it is not accepted
	Understand that rejection occurs for many reasons other than quality
	Refuse to give up; persistence usually pays off
Personal work habits	
Getting started	Write whatever comes to mind first, no matter how unpolished
	Plan to write for only 10 to 15 minutes per session at first
	Establish a realistic writing schedule, and adhere to it
	Work first on the parts of the project that seem easiest to do
	Start by writing the title to focus on the key concepts
	Polish the first paragraph and the purpose statement to provide focus
Procrastination	Recognize personal patterns of procrastination
	Schedule writing times regularly and frequently, at least weekly
	Schedule writing sessions at times of best performance and when there are no distractions
	Set due dates for each part of the writing project
	Plan a personal reward for meeting each due date
	Discuss weekly writing plans with supportive friends and colleagues

(Adapted with permission from Wills, C. E. (2000). Strategies for managing barriers to the writing process. *Nursing Forum, 35*, 5–13.)

BOX 26.3   Strategies for Overcoming Situational Barriers to Writing

Barrier	Strategies
Time and personal energy	
Lack of time for writing	Schedule regular weekly writing times on the calendar
	Protect writing time by being assertive with others about priorities
	Keep in mind that *priorities* matter more than *time*
Lack of uninterrupted or quality time to write	Find a place to write that is free from distractions
	Schedule frequent, brief writing sessions
	Reorganize calendar to protect the most productive writing times
	Match work to the best times for a given type of work
Lack of energy for writing	Rank-order priorities daily and weekly
	Decide what can be put aside to prioritize writing
Other resources	
Lack of emotional support; institutional culture that does not support research or publication; lack of mentorship for writing	Regularly discuss goals and progress with supportive others
	Avoid individuals who are negative about writing progress and goals
	Contact local academic institutions to find interested others
	Contact staff education department and nursing school resources
	Explore the feasibility of establishing a writing group at work
	Contact local schools of nursing to aid in finding interested others
Lack of appropriate work space, computer, financial support	Explore the feasibility of resources through work
	Negotiate for resources in exchange for other services
	Form partnerships with others who have the needed skills and resources
	Reevaluate personal resources that could be allocated for writing

(Adapted with permission from Wills, C. E. (2000). Strategies for managing barriers to the writing process. *Nursing forum, 35,* 5–13.)

APN should read sample articles from publications in which he or she wishes to publish. Although professional journal articles typically use specialized technical and statistical language (e.g., "RCT or Type I error"), material written for lay audiences must be presented in a more conversational and personally engaging style, without jargon. For example, compare the style of the initial sentence of a hypothetical article about the public health significance of menopausal symptoms in a professional research journal versus a similar article in a lay health magazine targeted at women:

- *Professional research journal:* "Several recent large-scale studies have shown that 60% to 75% of women older than 50 years of age experience clinically significant symptoms of menopause, particularly hot flashes and symptoms of depression and anxiety (Smith, Brown, Johnson, et al., 1997, 1999; Levatis, Jones, & Hemkis, 2000, 2001; Tricost, Adkins, Brown, et al., 2002)."
- *Lay health magazine for women:* "Lately, research is showing that most women (up to three in four women) over the age of 50 who are going through the change of

life ("menopause") have hot flashes (unpredictable spells of feeling overly hot and perspiring a lot) and can feel much moodier and more nervous than usual. If you're one of these women, this news story is for you."

Both examples provide the same overall message, namely, that research has replicated the finding that certain menopausal symptoms (effects of hormonal changes on the autonomic and central nervous systems) occur in most women. The examples differ in the style of writing (technical versus nontechnical) and the level of engagement of the reader (nonengaged and objective versus individually focused). The sentence written for the professional journal is presented in a style that is appropriate for a professional audience, including the use of references to studies as part of statements of fact, to meet scientific standards for the credibility of information sources. In contrast, the sentence written for the women's magazine is presented in nontechnical language and addresses a selected audience of women who may be experiencing menopausal symptoms.

Despite the differences in writing style, however, the scientific standards for the quality of the information conveyed should be the same in both types of publications. Just as when writing for scientific audiences, APNs must provide complete, balanced information when writing for lay publications. In the example given for the women's magazine, it would also be quite important to provide a list of scientifically validated resources for readers who wish to obtain additional information. This resource information allows the material presented in the lay publication to be relevant for a much broader audience, including readers who are not necessarily health care researchers, but want to review original research articles, web sites, and so forth.

Letter Writing and Other Types of Advocacy

Letter writing and other advocacy efforts via printed materials usually involve focused attempts to influence either local or broader public policy. Such advocacy often refers to the results and implications of research (in the context of this chapter). For example, an APN may write a letter, citing specific research, to request a policy change in a health care organization or may write to a legislator to request support of legislative efforts to reform health care policy. Like writing for lay publications, the style of this kind of letter must be nontechnical, but accurate, with reference to specific research findings, as appropriate. To be effective as a form of policy advocacy, letter writing must be well focused in terms of both the issue at hand and the requested steps for action. A careful assessment is needed to identify the key public policy stakeholders (i.e., specific legislators or other opinion leaders in the community who are in a position to generate constructive change). For example, consider the scenario in Box 26-4 regarding an APN's approach to statewide change in school policies with respect to snack machines in school cafeterias. In this example, the APN first gathered data about a problem that had important public health implications and then used the research findings to garner additional resources to support policy change.

"Podium" Presentations

The image that many people have when thinking about research presentations is that of a professional presentation at which an individual, standing at the front of a room behind a podium, addresses a group of people about a certain topic. Of course, talks can be given in a variety of settings other than to a professional audience. When research findings are presented to nonresearcher audiences, the same considerations apply as discussed for written publications, including the importance of good audience analysis. The ability to present oneself and one's ideas in a clear, professional, and credible manner is an essential skill for an APN,

regardless of role. Thus, APNs should be well versed in and very comfortable with effective, well-polished techniques of professional speaking, regardless of whether the focus of the presentation is research findings.

An advantage of the podium presentation or "talk" is that the researcher has a "captive" audience with which to share research results or other ideas. When a researcher is interested in obtaining audience feedback to stimulate his or her thinking about preparing a research report, giving talks can be quite useful. For example, members of an audience may raise points about the analysis of the results or the interpretation of the findings that the researcher had not previously considered. Of the various forms of presentations, talks at professional meetings offer the greatest visibility for the researcher because the audience is composed of a select group of professionals who are interested in the research topic. However, the select nature of the audience is also the key limitation of oral presentations relative to written publication of research findings. However, when preparing for a talk, the researcher must organize the research results in a way that facilitates writing for publication. Many researchers who publish regularly use the preparation for conference presentations as an opportunity to write a draft of the material for publication.

Talks or poster presentations given at professional conferences usually undergo a formal review process that is normally spelled out in the conference brochure. The most common approach is for a presenter to submit a written **abstract** of the presentation that is reviewed for acceptance by the program committee or selected peer reviewers.[2] The instructions provided as part of the call for abstracts include the focus or scope of the conference, the guidelines and requirements for writing an abstract, a description of the abstract review process, and the due date. The content and style of the abstracts will vary, depending on the particular conference. For example, the word limit can vary considerably. However, overall, abstracts for conferences that focus on research findings have much in common. The common elements of an abstract that reports the results of research (in order of appearance) are:

* *Significance of the clinical problem.* This statement explains why the clinical problem is important and why the audience should care about the topic. Such a discussion is not always required.

---

[2]For some types of conferences, presenters may be asked to provide a fully developed manuscript for review. Accepted manuscripts may then be published as a set, either as conference proceedings or in a special supplement to a journal.

BOX 26.4   Example of a Public Health Policy Change Based on Research Findings

An APN practicing in a school-based primary care clinic became interested in the nutritional habits of school-age children in reference to the food options provided within local school systems. It was her informal observation that the children at the school in which her clinic is located selected less nutritious, high-fat, high-sugar food from cafeteria vending machines for lunch rather than waiting in line for more nutritionally balanced and healthful hot school lunches. This informal observation was confirmed by the APN's questioning of children who came to the clinic for health services.

The APN was curious about the extent to which this issue occurred beyond her local school district, and asked the state department of community health (SDCH) about the availability of funding to conduct a study on the extent of the issue. With the support of a $20,000 contract that she obtained through a request for proposals via the SDCH, the APN designed and conducted a survey of all school districts in the state to find out the answers to the following general questions:

1. Does [name of specific school] have one or more vending machines in the school cafeteria? If yes, what types of items [checklist] are stocked in the vending machine(s)?
2. How many children (proportion of school population) buy a school lunch, select food from a vending machine, bring lunch from home, or forego lunch, for an index period of 3 months?
3. What factors influence children's preferences for school cafeteria food, vending machine food, home-packed food, or no food at lunchtime?

The results of the study showed that a large majority of children (> 70%) selected vending machine food over school cafeteria food during the 3-month index period. Children who selected vending machine food indicated that they wanted to avoid long waits in cafeteria lines, that they liked the vending machine food better anyway, and that they did not believe that the vending machine food was ". . . all that bad for you." A portion of the survey done with school administrators showed that they were generally aware of the poor nutritional value of vending machine foods, but saw vending machines placed in school cafeterias as a "necessary evil" because of the large amount of revenue generated by vending machine sales to support various school activities that are not covered by general budgets.

The APN wrote a report of her research findings and presented it at a meeting of SDCH administrators and public health officials. She also implemented a focused letter-writing campaign (via e-mail) to selected state legislators who had voiced an interest in public health issues. Through the letter-writing campaign and the research report, the APN gained the support of two legislators and several community organizations, including a majority of the local Parent–Teacher Organizations, to sponsor legislation to eliminate vending machines in school cafeterias statewide and to earmark a limited amount of additional funds for support of school activities that previously had been supported by revenues from school vending machines. She was also invited by the SDCH to develop a proposal for a model intervention program for the public school system, focusing on nutrition education interventions for children and targeted changes to school lunch menus to better incorporate children's food preferences.

- *Purpose of the study.* The purpose is often stated in one sentence. Information about specific research questions or hypotheses also may be required.
- *Theoretic framework, approach, or perspective used to guide the research.* Although this information is not always required, professional nursing organizations tend to request it, and some conference calls include a requirement or preference to identify a nursing theoretic framework.

- *Methods*
  - *Sample and sampling design.* This discussion may require only one or two sentences.
  - *Data collection procedures.* The procedures used to collect the data are described (e.g., "Patients were interviewed via telephone at 3 and again at 6 months after the intervention. . .").
  - *Research design.* The design is described in one sentence, using standard scientific terms (e.g., "A

pretest–posttest design was used to evaluate the effects of the intervention. . .").

- *Measures*. The measures are identified, and information about their reliability and validity are provided, as appropriate.
- *Data analysis*. The types of analyses used to address the key research questions are identified.
- *Results*. The results are described in enough detail to allow the reviewer to evaluate how the research findings support the conclusions.
- *Conclusions*. This section provides a specific summary of the meaning or interpretation of the results, as related to the purpose of the study and the study questions or hypotheses.

In addition to these standard elements, abstracts are also reviewed with regard to their relevance to the conference objectives. They also may be judged on the basis of originality, creativity, or unique contribution to nursing knowledge. Abstracts may be penalized for typographical errors or problems with the presentation of the material. As with other types of professional writing, for the best chance of acceptance, it is important to follow the guidelines and requirements for abstract preparation and submission.

The time allocated for a professional talk is usually 15 to 30 minutes, and 15 to 20 minutes is the most common length of time allowed. Time frames also vary depending on the format of the presentation. For example, more time may be allowed for presentations that involve interaction with the audience, with less time allotted for conference formats that provide quick updates about research projects that are in progress. A very large body of nursing literature is dedicated to the topic of preparing for professional presentations (see the list of suggested readings), and researchers who have limited experience with presenting at conferences should refer to these articles. A novice might find it helpful to ask colleagues to critique a "practice" version of the talk, so that he or she can use the feedback to improve the presentation. Even an experienced researcher should rehearse the presentation at least individually to ensure that the talk can be presented within the time limits. Careful attention should be paid to the quality of visual aids, such as slides or overheads. To be most effective, visual aids should not contain an excessive amount of information. Judicious use of color is best; colors should contrast well, but should not be too bright or otherwise distracting. The researcher also should ensure that all visual materials can be clearly seen by the members of the audience who are seated farthest from the podium. It is helpful to test the presentation equipment beforehand to be sure that it works adequately as well as to become familiar with its operation.

Poster Presentations

Poster presentations are visual displays of key research findings. Typically, posters are shown on display boards, usually in a room set aside at a conference to allow for interactive discussion between the poster presenter and poster viewers. Poster presentations are less formal than spoken presentations, and they allow the researcher to interact with other individuals and address their specific interests in the research. In contrast to a podium presentation or talk, in which there is usually little time for interaction between the presenter and the audience, a poster session maximizes the opportunity for interaction. In addition, many people are able to view a poster if it is displayed for several hours; in contrast, relatively few people can attend a talk that is scheduled concurrently with other talks.

The guidelines for preparing visual materials for a poster presentation are similar to those for preparing visual aids for a podium-based talk (also see the articles included in the list of suggested readings). The researcher should be careful to follow the guidelines for poster preparation that are provided by the conference organizers. Usually, key research results are presented in graphic and textual form on cardboard, poster board, laminated paper, or a computerized display. The requirements for size and format may differ according to the specific conference guidelines. Guidelines for poster presentations also indicate the appropriate methods for affixing printed materials to display boards (e.g., thumbtacks, Velcro brand hook and loop tape).

PUBLISHING IN PROFESSIONAL JOURNALS

Selecting a Journal

In thinking about publishing a research article, an early step is to consider which journals best match the article in terms of topic and professional audience. For example, a researcher who has completed a study on the effectiveness of tailored interventions for reminding patients about primary care appointments can choose from a wide variety of journals. If the researcher is interested in reaching a nursing audience, he or she might select a key nursing research journal, such as *Nursing Research, Research in Nursing & Health,* or the *Western Journal of Nursing Research,* which have the largest nurse researcher readerships.[3] If the re-

---

[3]In our discussion, we do not endorse any particular journal. The selected examples are used only for the purpose of illustration.

searcher is interested in reaching a specialty nursing audience (e.g., primary care clinical nurse specialists), he or she might select a journal such as *Nurse Practitioner*. Likewise, if the researcher wants to reach a broader professional audience, such as health services researchers (including nurses, physicians, health psychologists, and social workers), he or she might select a major interdisciplinary journal, such as *Health Services Research* or *Journal of Family Practice,* or a journal such as the *Journal of the American Medical Association,* which has a broader and substantially interdisciplinary readership.

To determine which journal might be a good match for a planned article, one should review representative issues of several journals, including the current author guidelines. Tables of contents and author guidelines for many journals are available online via the journal publishers' web site or through research university libraries. Some questions to consider are:

- *What do the author guidelines indicate about the key foci and scope of the journal?*
- *What types of articles and topics seem to receive the most coverage in the journal?*
- *How sophisticated are the sampling methods, research designs, and statistical analyses that appear in the articles that are published in the journal?*
- *What audiences do the published articles appear to target?*

In addition to reviewing the author guidelines and published articles, prospective authors can contact the journal editor via a **query letter** (these days, more appropriately referred to as a **query e-mail**) with questions about the appropriateness of a particular manuscript topic and other issues. Before sending a query, however, the researcher should consult the author guidelines to determine the editorial policy for queries. Some guidelines recommend sending a query before submitting a manuscript, whereas others recommend against a query letter. Because of the increased online availability of author guidelines and other information for most major journals, queries are best reserved for questions that cannot be addressed via review of the author guidelines.

Researchers often identify first- and second-choice journals for the submission of a completed manuscript. The first-choice journal is usually the one that is the best match with regard to topic, methods, and target audience. The second-choice journal provides a "back-up" plan if the manuscript is rejected by the first-choice journal. In the scientific community, as a standard of scientific integrity, it is understood and expected that a manuscript will be submit-

ted to *only one* journal at a time, as a professional courtesy to the journal editor.

Authorship Standards and Manuscript Review Procedures

Other standards for scientific integrity concern the authorship of publications. Everyone who is listed as an author should have provided significant input into the manuscript, in terms of developing and writing the ideas. "Developing" means having conceptual input into one or more aspects of the research (e.g., literature review, methods, data analysis, conclusions). "Writing" is the process of recording ideas, and involves drafting and revising sections of the manuscript. This participation in the development and writing of the manuscript distinguishes people who are eligible for authorship from those who have provided technical assistance in conducting the research. Although data collectors and study participants play essential roles in the research process, they do not qualify as authors solely on the basis of their technical assistance. Although those who provide technical assistance do not qualify for authorship, their contributions can be acknowledged in the article.

By convention, the first author is the person who made the largest contribution to the article, followed by the second author (who made the second largest contribution), and so forth.[4] If two or more authors shared equal responsibility and made equal contributions, this can be indicated in the article, usually as an author note. An **author note** is a brief note that is set apart from the main body of the text, usually on the first or last page of the article. Author notes often list credentials, academic positions, and acknowledgment of research funding sources, as well as contact information for the author.

Most nursing and other health-related journals are **refereed.** This means that manuscripts submitted to the journals are reviewed for appropriateness for publication, and a decision is made about the disposition of the manuscript on that basis. Manuscripts that are submitted to a journal may be accepted for publication "as is" (very rare, especially for high-quality research journals), accepted on the condition that required revisions are made satisfactorily, or rejected. Communication with the editors of journals about the status of a manuscript that was submitted for review almost always occurs in writing. Journals that focus on the

---

[4]This convention applies to all nursing research journals and to most other publications in the applied life sciences. However, in certain basic, nonapplied sciences, there is a convention for the most senior author to be listed as the last author. The journal editor should be consulted about the specific conventions for a given journal.

publication of research reports are typically more competitive (i.e., they reject manuscripts more often) than clinical journals that include many types of articles. Manuscript reviewers usually include experts who are knowledgeable about the topic and methods (**peer reviewers**). In addition, manuscripts undergo **editorial review** by journal editors or editorial board members. There is a general consensus in the scientific community that research publications should appear in peer-reviewed journals because reports in these journals are critiqued by other experts before they appear in print.

The processes used for reviewing manuscripts vary. A **blinded** review is one in which the reviewers of the manuscript receive a copy of the paper with the identifying information (e.g., author name, address, professional affiliation) removed. The most prestigious journals follow this blinding process in the belief that it helps to foster the reviewer's objectivity in performing a scientific review of the work. It is the policy of other journal editorial boards to forego blind review on the basis that many reviews are not truly "blind" (i.e., reviewers recognize the identity of the author, despite removal of obvious identifying information) and the further belief that reviewers should be expected to be objective, regardless of whether they know the identity of the author.

Content of a Research Report: General Considerations[5]

Many primers have been published in nursing and other health-related fields about the mechanics of writing for publication. See the list of suggested readings for examples. A reader who is considering writing for publication for the first time should review a few articles from the list to get started. Personal and situational barriers can be major challenges for busy clinicians (see Boxes 26-2 and 26-3). In this section, we review key considerations for the content of a research report.

Background: Setting the Stage

The introductory section of a research article (i.e., abstract, significance of the clinical problem, research problem, purpose of the study, theoretic framework or model if applicable, and research questions or hypotheses) should lay a sound conceptual foundation for the description of the research methods, results, and conclusions (i.e., "set the stage" for the description of the research in a way that shows how the research fits with existing work). The title

should concisely and accurately describe the key problem addressed in the research study. The abstract should be a clearly written, concise summary of the research project, and should provide a basis for readers to decide whether they want to read the text of the article. Readers should be able to see clearly how the clinical problem and an identified gap in knowledge have driven the need for the research study. In addition, they should be able to understand how the researcher conceptualizes the research project within broader conceptual frameworks or theories, as applicable. One of the most common difficulties experienced by writers vying for publication is an initial inability to "spell out" what they are thinking in nontechnical language. Technical concepts must be added as appropriate and clearly defined the first time they are used. The purpose of the study and the particular research questions or hypotheses should be stated clearly and explicitly (see earlier chapters). Most journals have specific guidelines for the format of these sections, including standard headings for paragraphs. These guidelines should be carefully followed. As mentioned earlier, sample articles from recent issues of the journal to which the manuscript will be submitted can be used as models for writing an article.

Methods

The methods section should be written in a way that will allow a reader to replicate or otherwise evaluate the study findings, based on the level of information presented in the article.[6] The key characteristics of the sample should be described, and the inclusion and exclusion criteria should be addressed. In addition to describing the sampling strategy used to select study participants, the researcher should state the rates of agreement to participation, the actual number of study enrollments, and the numbers and percentages of people who discontinued study participation. Ethical issues in the protection of human subjects should be addressed as applicable and as required by journal policy. Relevant analyses of missing data and study dropouts should be included, especially if attrition or missing data account for a substantial portion of the initial study sample. The description of the study design should include standard research design terminology, clearly identified de-

---

[5]Refer to chapter 22 for additional details.

[6]Because the space allocations for journal articles are typically quite limited, details that were initially provided by the researchers may be edited so that the manuscript meets the journal page restrictions. In general, 15 to 20 pages of double-spaced, typewritten text for a manuscript submitted to a journal is standard, and sometimes there are more stringent page requirements, depending on the type of article. The most common areas in which information is "streamlined" to meet space requirements are the background and measures sections.

pendent and independent variables, the number and timing of measurement points, and other relevant information about control of extraneous variables.[7] For these descriptions and others included in the methods section, explicit rationales should be provided so that readers can understand why particular decisions were made. Methods used to collect data should be clearly described, including the steps taken in data collection, computer entry, and data cleaning. Space limitations normally preclude publication of the measures used, but adequate information should be provided to allow the reader to understand how and why variables were measured in the way they were. In addition, relevant psychometric information about the measures (reliability and validity results from previous studies or the current study) should be included. The development and testing of measures that were newly developed for the study should be described, and basic information should be provided about the scoring of various measures (e.g., summated scores involving adding scores for individual items, weighted average scores). The statistical procedures used to analyze the results can be described in this section or incorporated into the discussion of the results (see the next section). The specific procedures that were used should be identified by name, and appropriate references should be cited for techniques that may not be familiar to some readers. The researcher should give the reason for using particular statistical procedures and relate them to the study questions or hypotheses.

Results

The research findings are reported in the results section. Often, authors incorporate the discussion of statistical procedures into this section, but this depends on the journal guidelines and the writing style of the authors. Descriptive findings, such as characteristics of the sample and scores on key measures, are usually reported first, followed by a discussion of the results that address the key study questions or hypotheses. The description of the results of inferential statistics should include the test value, relevant degrees of freedom, sample size (as relevant), and significance level of the test result.[8] Additional or follow-up analyses, done as elaborations or to answer additional questions that arose on the

basis of the main results, are usually reported after the key questions or hypotheses are discussed. Tables and figures should be used judiciously[9] to show key results and data patterns. Tables and figures can be used to show the main points and patterns in the data simply and clearly, while using space economically. For example, in a study that involves three comparison samples, the researcher might summarize the characteristics of each sample in a single table. Statistically significant differences in the general characteristics of the groups or the measures central to the study questions or hypotheses can be highlighted in the text. Figures can be used to show complex relationships between variables (e.g., a statistically significant interaction between two variables).

Discussion

The final section of a research article contains a brief recap of the study results, followed by the conclusions and implications of the findings for clinical practice, further research, and health care policy, as applicable. The conclusions should be as specific as possible and should be tailored to the interests of the readership and the focus of the journal. For example, the discussion of the results of a nursing research study prepared for an applied clinical audience should be heavily weighted in terms of the implications for nursing practice. Likewise, an article prepared for a theoretically oriented nursing research journal should emphasize the implications for additional theoretically based research. The discussion section highlights the importance of the study findings for the development of knowledge, but also should include a discussion of potential limitations of the study design and results. In addition, particularly for studies that involve cause-and-effect relationships, this section should include alternative explanations that could be reasonably considered in relation to the study findings. The discussion section should also address potential extraneous variables, together with a statement about the plausibility of the alternative explanations. If the alternative explanations are reasonable, this should be stated. Likewise, if the researcher believes that his or her study design has greatly reduced or ruled out certain alternative explanations, this should be stated, along with the rationale for this position. The researcher should identify important limitations (actual or potential) to the sampling and study design and suggest alternatives for improvement. If there do not appear to be reasonable alternatives to the approach that was used, the researcher should state this.

---

[7]Refer also to chapters 12 and 18 for a discussion of qualitative research methods. There are some important differences in the conventions for qualitative and quantitative research approaches.

[8]In addition to following the specific author guidelines for a given journal, readers who are preparing research manuscripts for publication should consult the *Publication Manual of the American Psychological Association* (American Psychological Association, 2001) for more specific information on the conventions for reporting statistical results.

---

[9]Refer to the *Publication Manual of the American Psychological Association* (American Psychological Association, 2001) for more information and helpful suggestions for the format and content of tables and figures.

CONCLUSION

In conclusion, writing data-based research reports and articles is an art that requires practice and judgment in addition to the specific technical skills needed to interpret the results. Only actual practice improves one's skills. All authors should attempt to write as clearly as possible. The difficulty associated with reading many articles in professional or scientific journals rarely has to do with not knowing the specific analytic techniques that were used. Usually, the difficulty stems from the need to understand ideas and empirical evidence that are not presented clearly.

Suggested Activities

1. Select several articles from the list of suggested readings that are of interest to you to read for further information about the topics covered in this chapter.
2. If you are considering writing for publication for the first time, review the personal and situational barriers to writing that are listed in Boxes 26-2 and 26-3. Perform a self-assessment to identify which of these challenges to writing might pertain to you. Identify some specific strategies for how you would reduce or eliminate these challenges to writing for publication.
3. Read a report of research that is of interest to you in a current issue of a nursing journal. Review the content and style of writing in relation to the content of this chapter. Identify the strengths and limitations of the presentation of the article.

Suggested Readings

Ament, L. A. (1994). Strategies for dissemination of policy research. *Journal of Nurse Midwifery, 39,* 329–331.

Anthony, D. (2000). Distance learning and research dissemination using online resources. *Nurse Researcher, 8,* 53–64.

Ashworth, P. (1996). Writing and submitting abstracts for conference presentation. *Nurse Researcher, 4,* 39–48.

Bell, J. M. (2000). Transforming your conference presentation into a publishable article. *Journal of Family Nursing, 6,* 99–102.

Beyea, S. C., & Nicoll, L. H. (1998). Research corner: Developing and presenting a poster presentation. *AORN Journal, 67,* 468–469.

Beyea, S. C., & Nicoll, L. H. (1998). Research corner: Writing an integrative review. *AORN Journal, 67,* 887–890.

Biancuzzo, M. (1994). Developing a poster about a clinical innovation: Part II. Creating the poster. *Clinical Nurse Specialist, 8,* 203–207.

Butts, J. (1998). Finding the right fit: Podium, poster, paper or publication? Part I. *Mississippi RN, 60,* 9, 14.

Byrne, M. (2001). Research corner: Disseminating and presenting qualitative research findings. *AORN Journal, 74,* 731–732.

Carroll-Johnson, R. M. (1999). New benefit to writing for publication. *Oncology Nursing Forum, 26,* 669.

Cronenwett, L. R. (1995). Effective methods for disseminating research findings to nurses in practice. *Nursing Clinics of North America, 30,* 429–438.

Dexter, P. (2000). Tips for scholarly writing in nursing. *Journal of Professional Nursing, 16,* 6–12.

Dougherty, M. C. (1999). Electronic research dissemination. *Nursing Research, 48,* 239.

Evans, M. L. (2000). Polished, professional presentation: Unlocking the design elements. *Journal of Continuing Education in Nursing, 31,* 213–218.

Fain, J. A. (1998). Research update: Writing an abstract. *Diabetes Educator, 24,* 353, 355–356.

Fitzpatrick, J. J. (1999). The joys of publishing. *Applied Nursing Research, 12,* 59.

Forbes, D., & Phillipchuk, D. (2001). The dissemination and use of nursing research. *Canadian Nurse, 97,* 18–22.

French, B. (2000). Networking for research dissemination: Collaboration and mentorship. *Nurse Researcher, 7,* 13–23.

Garity, J. (1999). Creating a professional presentation: A template for success. *Journal of Intravenous Nursing, 22,* 81–86.

Grady, P. (2001). News from NINR: Making a difference. *Nursing Outlook, 49,* 257.

Grant, J. S. (1998). Writing manuscripts for clinical journals. *Home Healthcare Nurse, 16,* 813–822.

Hegyvary, S. T. (2000). Standards of scholarly writing. *Journal of Nursing Scholarship, 32,* 112.

King, C., McGuire, D., Longman, A., & Carroll-Johnson, R. (1997). Peer review, authorship, ethics, and conflict of interest. *Journal of Nursing Scholarship, 29,* 163–167.

Krawiec, P. A. (1995). The use of tables, illustrations, and graphs for effective research presentation. *Journal of Vascular Nursing, 13,* 92.

McCann, S., Sramac, R., & Rudy, S. (1994). The poster exhibit: Planning, development, and presentation. *Orthopaedic Nursing, 13,* 43–49.

Mee, C. L. (2002). 10 lessons on writing for publication: Confidence, patience, and attention to detail will put you well on your way. *Nursing, 22,* 25–26.

Mohr, W. K. (1999). Op-ed: Reflections on writing. *Nursing Outlook, 47,* 198–199.

Montgomery, K. S., Eddy, N. L., Jackson, E., Nelson, E., Reed, K., Stark, T. L., & Thomsen, C. (2001). Global research dissemination and utilization: Recommendations for nurses and nurse educators. *Nursing and Health Care Perspectives, 22,* 124–129.

Moore, L. W., Augspurger, P., King, M. O., & Proffitt, C. (2001). Insights on the poster preparation and presentation process. *Applied Nursing Research, 14,* 100–104.

Morin, K. H. (1996). Practical hints: Poster presentations. Getting your point across: effective use of color, typography, and basic design principles. *American Journal of Maternal Child Nursing, 21,* 307–310.

Muscari, M. E. (1998). Do the write thing: Writing the clinically focused article. *Journal of Pediatric Health Care, 12,* 236–241.

Nemcek, M. A. (2000). Getting published online and in print: Understanding the publication process. *AAOHN Journal, 48,* 344–348.

O'Connor-Bruchak, K. (1994). Publishing in lay journals. *Communication How-Tos, 9,* 1–2.

Pattinson, M. (1998). Presentation of self: Being heard. *Advanced Practice Nursing Quarterly, 3,* 10–13.

Plawecki, H. M., & Plawecki, J. A. (1998). Writing for publication: Understanding the process. *Journal of Holistic Nursing, 16,* 23–32.

Robinson, D., Collins, M., & Monkman, J. (1997). A practical guide to writing for publication. *Nurse Researcher, 5,* 53–64.

Robinson, K. R. (1997). Issues in clinical nursing research: You + research = nursing practice program. *Western Journal of Nursing Research, 19,* 265–269.

Sandelowski, M. (1998). Writing a good read: Strategies for representing qualitative data. *Research in Nursing & Health, 21,* 375–382.

Sedhom, L. N., Gerardi, T., King, K. B., Kelleher, C., Cesta, T. G., Conahue, R. D., Bove, A. F., & Oboyski, A. K. (2000). Disseminating nursing research to the consumer. *Journal of the New York State Nurses Association, 31,* 21–24.

Selby, M. L., Tornquist, E. M., & Finerty, E. J. (1989). How to present your research: The ABCs of creating and using visual aids to enhance your research presentation: Part 2. *Nursing Outlook, 37,* 236–238.

Silva, M. C., & Ludwick, R. (2000). Ethics of electronic publishing. *Online Journal of Issues in Nursing* (May 5). Available at http://www.nursingworld.org/ojin/

Straka, D. (1996). Making powerful presentations: How to get a "10" from your audience. *Advanced Practice Nursing Quarterly, 2,* 65–67.

Strickland, T. (1999). Conference presentations with confidence. *Case Manager, 10,* 68–70.

Sullivan, E. J. (2002). Top 10 reasons a manuscript is rejected. *Journal of Professional Nursing, 18,* 1–2.

Taggart, H. M., & Arslanian, C. (2000). Creating an effective poster presentation. *Orthopaedic Nursing, 19,* 47–52.

Thomas, S. P. (1998). The long journey to publication: Some thoughts on the journal review process. *Issues in Mental Health Nursing, 19,* 415–418.

Wildman, S. (1998). Publishing your work in nursing journals. *Professional Nurse, 13,* 419–422.

Wills, C. E. (2000). Strategies for managing barriers to the writing process. *Nursing Forum, 35,* 5–13.

Windle, P. E. (2001). Celebrating successes through poster presentation. *Journal of Perianesthesia Nursing, 16,* 337–39.

Zotti, M. E., Selby-Harrington, M. L., & Riportella-Muller, R. (1994). Communicating research findings to readers of clinical journals: Guidance for prospective authors. *Journal of Pediatric Health Care, 8,* 106–110.

References

American Psychological Association. (2001). *Publication manual of the American Psychological Association* (5th ed.). Washington, DC: American Psychological Association.

Norwood, S. L. (2000). *Research strategies for advanced practice nurses.* Upper Saddle River, NJ: Prentice Hall.

Wills, C. E. (2000). Strategies for managing barriers to the writing process. *Nursing Forum, 35,* 5–13.

Winslow, E. (1996). Failure to publish: A form of scientific misconduct? *Heart and Lung, 25,* 169–171.

Appendix A

Computation and Interpretation of Common Univariate Descriptive Statistics

INTRODUCTORY COMMENTS

Statistical summary measures can be divided/classified depending on how many variables are involved in the summary measure and whether or not they serve the purpose of describing sample data or inferring to population values ('parameters') beyond the sample.

Concerning the number of variables involved, we typically distinguish among univariate, bivariate, and multivariate statistics. Univariate statistics summarize information from a single variable (examples are means or standard deviations), bivariate statistics consider the joint variation of and relationship between two variables (examples are correlations, odds-ratios, regression coefficients in simple regressions), and multivariate statistics combine information from at least three variables (examples: multiple regression coefficients, factor scores, Cronbach's alpha, etc.).

The distinction between descriptive and inferential statistics cuts across the distinction based on number of variables. Statistics usually serve two purposes: to summarize information about the sample data at hand, and to make inferences beyond the particular sample to a target population from which the sample is drawn. The first task is accomplished using descriptive statistics, the second task is accomplished using inferential statistics. In fact, every statistic should be thought of as fulfilling a descriptive and an inferential purpose, with the latter usually being the more important function.

In particular, this means that descriptive and inferential statistics should NOT be thought of as referring to different statistical measures. Thus, a mean or a median can be calculated from sample data to describe the particular sample, or the sample mean or median can be used to make inferences about the population mean or median from which the sample was drawn. This principle applies to all statistics: a correlation, a regression coefficient, and an odds-ratio all provide descriptions of particular sample data and can be used to estimate population parameters.

Here, we first show how some basic descriptive statistics are calculated from sample data.

In Appendix B, we briefly consider statistical inference based on sample data, using the t-test.

UNIVARIATE DESCRIPTIVE STATISTICS

In the following, we consider only univariate descriptive statistics (i.e., statistical summary measures that describe single variables from a single sample/data set).

(A) Measures of Central Tendency:

To summarize information contained in sample data, we often use measures of central tendency. Such measures serve the purpose of indicating the 'typical' score on a variable of interest, in other words a measure of central tendency is supposed to give a shorthand description of the scores obtained by the 'bulk' of the cases.

If a variable is measured at the interval or ratio level

(i.e., the distances between scores are defined), then the arithmetic mean is the most commonly used measure of central tendency. It is defined as follows:

(1) The (arithmetic) mean is defined in the following way:

$$\bar{X} = (1/N)(\Sigma\ X_i) = (\Sigma\ X_i)/N = (X_1 + X_2 + \ldots + X_N)/N$$

In words, the arithmetic mean '$\bar{X}$' (read: "X-bar") is the sum of all (valid) scores divided by the number of cases (with valid responses). The Greek symbol 'Σ' is used as the summation operator (i.e., it symbolizes the instruction that one should add all 'X_i' scores before dividing by the number of cases).

'X_i' stands for any possible score on the variable 'X', where 'i' refers to the i-th case. Thus, in a sample of $N = 4$ cases, we would add/sum the individual scores X_1, X_2, X_3, X_4. Thus, in this case, $\Sigma\ X_i = X_1 + X_2 + X_3 + X_4$. See the following table containing four hypothetical diastolic blood pressure scores:

TABLE A-1. Computation of Sample Mean

Subject	Variable	Actual Diastolic BP Score
1	X_1	78
2	X_2	86
3	X_3	82
4	X_4	90
$N = 4$		$\Sigma\ X_i = 336$
		$\bar{X} = (\Sigma\ X_i)/N = 336/4 = 84$

Note the two (completely equivalent) ways of computing the sample mean. In the table we used $\bar{X} = (1/N)(\Sigma\ X_i) = (X_1 + X_2 + \ldots + X_N)/N$, but we could also have used $\bar{X} = \Sigma\ X_i/N = (1/N) \times X_1 + (1/N) \times X_2 + \ldots + (1/N)\ X_N$. Substituting the numbers from the table, we get: $\bar{X} = 1/4 \times 78 + 1/4 \times 86 + 1/4 \times 82 + 1/4 \times 90 = 19.5 + 21.5 + 20.5 + 22.5 = 84$.

(2) Another measure of central tendency is the median, which represents the value that cuts the sample in half, such that the lower half of the scores lie below the median and the upper half above the median. To find the median, first rearrange the distribution from lowest to highest score. For the four diastolic BP measures, we would rearrange them as follows: 78, 82, 86, 90. It is clear that the median must lie somewhere between 82 and 86, since a value between these two would cut the distribution into a lower and upper half. By convention, when the median lies between two numbers, we choose

the arithmetic mean of theses two numbers as the median value. In the current example, that would be $(82 + 86)/2 = 84$. If a distribution has an odd number of scores, we choose the one in the middle as the median value.

(3) The third—and simplest—measure of central tendency is the mode. It refers to the most frequently occurring value in a distribution. In the current diastolic BP example, every value occurs only once, so either all should be considered a mode or none of them. However, in many distributions there is a most frequently occurring value, and the mode is easily picked, counting the cases in each category.

These frequently encountered measures of central tendency serve different purposes and convey different information. As already mentioned, the mean can only be computed for interval- or ratio-level variables. The median presupposes at least an ordinal-level of measurement, since the assumption is that the variable scores can all be rank-ordered from the smallest to the largest value. The mode makes no assumptions about measurement level and is the only measure of central tendency available for nominal-level/categorical variables. On the other hand, measures of central tendency that make fewer assumptions can always be applied to variables with higher levels of measurement, as the following table shows:

Measures of Central tendency and Levels of Measurement in Variables

Measurement	Acceptable Measures of Central Tendency		
Nominal/categorical	mode		
Ordinal/rank-order	mode	median	
Interval/ratio	mode	median	mean

(B) Measures of Dispersion or Spread:

Sample means as measures of central tendency may or may not be informative about the 'central tendency' among the variables scores, depending on the distribution of the scores. In addition to considering central tendency, it is also important to consider various measures of dispersion or spread of values around some central value.

(1) For interval- and ratio-level variables, the most important measure(s) of dispersion are the variance and the standard deviation. Consider again the diastolic BP example:

TABLE A-2. Computation of Sample Variance and Sample Standard Deviation:

Subject	Variable Symbols:			Actual Diastolic BP Scores:		
	X_i	$X_i - \bar{X}$	$(X_i - \bar{X})^2$	X_i	$X_i - \bar{X}$	$(X_i - \bar{X})^2$
1	X_1	$X_1 - \bar{X}$	$(X_1 - \bar{X})^2$	78	$78 - 84 = -6$	$(-6)^2 = 36$
2	X_2	$X_2 - \bar{X}$	$(X_2 - \bar{X})^2$	82	$86 - 84 = 2$	$(2)^2 = 4$
3	X_3	$X_3 - \bar{X}$	$(X_3 - \bar{X})^2$	82	$82 - 84 = -2$	$(-2)^2 = 4$
4	X_4	$X_4 - \bar{X}$	$(X_4 - \bar{X})^2$	90	$90 - 84 = 6$	$(6)^2 = 36$

$$\text{Sum of Squared Deviations} = \Sigma(X_i - \bar{X})^2 = 80$$
$$\text{Variance} = \Sigma(X_i - \bar{X})^2/(N-1) = 80/3 = \underline{26.67}$$
$$\text{Standard Deviation} = \sqrt{\Sigma(X_i - \bar{X})^2/(N-1)} = \sqrt{26.67} = 5.16$$

In order to compute the sample variance, we must already know/have computed the sample mean. From each score or value, X_i, we subtract the sample mean, $X_i - \bar{X}$, square these differences, $(X_i - \bar{X})^2$, and sum them for all sample values, $\Sigma(X_i - \bar{X})^2$. The latter measure is referred to as the sum of squared deviations or the total sum of squares (TSS). In order to obtain the sample variance, we divide this total sum of squares by its degrees of freedom: $\Sigma(X_i - \bar{X})^2/(N-1)$. This measure is called the sample variance and represents the *mean squared deviations* of observed sample values/scores from their mean. It can be shown that in order to obtain an unbiased sample estimate of the population variance, the calculation of the sample variance involves the division of the TSS by its degrees of freedom $(N-1)$ and not the sample size (N) (Snedecor & Cochran, 1989). The standard deviation (SD) is obtained by taking the square-root of the variance (VAR): $SD = \sqrt{VAR}$. The advantage from a descriptive point of view is that the SD measures the deviations from the mean in the original metric: it is a measure of the average deviation from the sample mean.

(2) The most common measure of dispersion for ordinal-level data is the inter-quartile range. As with the median, we first rearrange the distribution from lowest to highest score and then carve out the middle 50% of the distribution, with 25% of the values below the lower bounds (=25% percentile) and 25% of the distribution above the upper bounds (=75% percentile).

(3) In health care research, measures of dispersion for nominal/categorical data are rarely, if ever, used. We mention the Gini concentration coefficient for interested readers (Agresti, 1990).

(4) An additional measure of dispersion is the range. It refers to the difference between the largest and smallest score/value in the distribution.

(C) Description of Sample Variables:

Consider the following distributions of diastolic blood pressure scores in three samples, each of size N=10:

TABLE A-3. Hypothetical Diastolic Blood Pressure Scores From Three Samples of Size N=10

Sample 1: X_i	Sample 2: Y_i	Sample 3: Z_i
$X_1 = 73$	$Y_1 = 70$	$Z_1 = 67$
$X_2 = 74$	$Y_2 = 70$	$Z_2 = 70$
$X_3 = 74$	$Y_3 = 70$	$Z_3 = 74$
$X_4 = 75$	$Y_4 = 71$	$Z_4 = 76$
$X_5 = 75$	$Y_5 = 71$	$Z_5 = 76$
$X_6 = 75$	$Y_6 = 79$	$Z_6 = 77$
$X_7 = 75$	$Y_7 = 79$	$Z_7 = 77$
$X_8 = 76$	$Y_8 = 80$	$Z_8 = 77$
$X_9 = 76$	$Y_9 = 80$	$Z_9 = 78$
$X_{10} = 77$	$Y_{10} = 80$	$Z_{10} = 78$
Sum = $\Sigma X_i = 750$	Sum = $\Sigma Y_i = 750$	Sum = $\Sigma Z_i = 750$
Mean = $\bar{X} = (\Sigma X_i)/N = 750/10 = 75$	Mean = $\bar{Y} = (\Sigma Y_i)/N = 750/10 = 75$	Mean = $\bar{Z} = (\Sigma Z_i)/N = 750/10 = 75$
Median = 75	Median = 75	Median = 76.5
Mode = 75	Mode(s) = 70, 80	Mode = 77
Variance = $(\Sigma X_i - \bar{X})^2/(N-1) = $ 12/9 = 1.33	Variance = $(\Sigma Y_i - \bar{Y})^2/(N-1) = $ 214/9 = 23.78	Variance = $(\Sigma Z_i - \bar{Z})^2/(N-1) = $ 122/9 = 13.56
Standard Deviation = $\sqrt{(\Sigma X_i - \bar{X})^2/(N-1)} = \sqrt{1.33} = 1.15$	Standard Deviation = $\sqrt{(\Sigma Y_i - \bar{Y})^2/(N-1)} = \sqrt{23.78} = 4.88$	Standard Deviation = $\sqrt{(\Sigma Z_i - \bar{Z})^2/(N-1)} = \sqrt{13.56} = 3.68$
Range of X_i: $77 - 73 = 4$	Range of Y_i: $80 - 70 = 10$	Range of Z_i: $78 - 67 = 11$

Frequency Distribution of Diastolic BP Scores in Sample 1

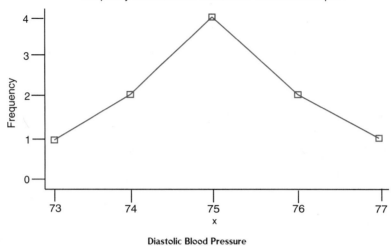

Diastolic Blood Pressure

As the table values and the summary statistics indicate, all three distributions have the same mean, but the medians and modes are not consistent across the three samples. The reason is that only in a completely symmetric, unimodal distribution, as in Sample 1, are the mean, median, and mode identical. In Sample 2, the distribution is still symmetric, but it is bimodal with the most frequently occurring values at either the low extreme (70) or the high extreme (80). Finally, the distribution of scores in Sample 3 is skewed to the left: while the bulk of the distribution (7 out of 10 values) lies between 76 and 78 inclusive; three out-

liers to the left 'drag down' the mean to 75. In this situation of a skewed distribution, the median is clearly a better measure of central tendency, in the sense that it gives a better indication for how the bulk of the cases score.

Note the large differences among the variances (and standard deviations) of the three sample distributions: The standard deviations in Samples 2 + 3 are more than 4 or 3 times larger than the standard deviation in Sample 1. Clearly, the values in the latter samples are much more dispersed. The range also indicates the differences in dispersion; however, since it is entirely determined by the two most extreme val-

Frequency Distribution of Diastolic BP Scores in Sample 2

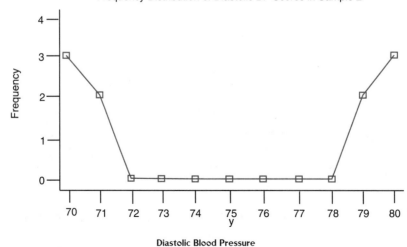

Diastolic Blood Pressure

Frequency Distribution of Diastolic BP Scores in

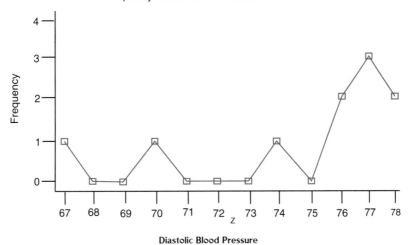

Diastolic Blood Pressure

ues, the range can sometimes be a misleading indicator. For instance, notice that the range for Sample 2 is a little smaller (10) than for Sample 3, yet the variance and standard deviation indicate that Sample 2 has the greatest dispersion among scores. The latter assessments are better reflections of the prevailing pattern, since both variance and standard deviation take all values into account and show the average (squared or linear) deviations from the mean.

Appendix B Estimating the Standard Error of a Mean Difference

Table B-1 is a reproduction of Table 3-4 in Chapter 3 and presents the results from an independent-sample t-test. Descriptively, it shows an observed sample mean of 80.33 in the treatment group and a mean of 84.48 in the control group.

In order to test whether or not the observed mean difference of 4.15 is "statistically significant," we need a test statistic that incorporates the null-hypothesis. For the independent sample t-test, the test-statistic is as follows:

(1) $T = [(\bar{X}_t - X_c) - (\mu_t - \mu_c)] / [\sqrt{s_t^2/n_t + s_c^2/n_c}]$

This looks complicated, but becomes much simpler if we look at its parts. In the numerator of the test-statistic, we see two differences: the difference between the observed sample means of the treatment group and the control group, $\bar{X}_t - \bar{X}_c$, and the true difference between treat-

ment and control group, $\mu_t - \mu_c$. However, according to the *null-hypothesis*, we expect that the intervention has *no* effect, thus we hypothesize that the true difference will be equal to zero: $\mu_{t - \mu c} = 0$.

This leads to a simplification of the numerator of the test statistic as follows:

(2) $T = (\bar{X}_T - \bar{X}_c)/[\sqrt{s_t^2/n_t + s_c^2/n_c}]$

The denominator of this expression provides the *sample estimate* of the standard error of the *mean difference* depicted in the numerator. In other words, we are evaluating the observed mean difference in relation to its standard error. In a two-sample comparison, there are two means to be estimated and two associated standard error estimates: $s_t/\sqrt{n_t}$, i.e., an estimate of the standard error of the mean in

---

Table B-1. Mean Diastolic BP Scores in Treatment (N=50) and Control (N=50) Groups after Intervention

Comparison Groups	Observed Sample Means	95% CI for Group Means	Observed Mean Difference	Standard Error of Mean Difference	95% CI for Mean Difference	t-value	Two-tailed Significance Level (p-value)
Treatment Group (N=50)	80.33	77.71 − 82.95					
			4.15	1.908	.35 − 7.95	2.175	.032
Control Group (N=50)	84.48	81.68 − 87.28					

the treatment group and $s_c/\sqrt{n_c}$ (i.e., an estimate of the standard error of the mean in the control group). Both of these standard error estimates enter into the standard error estimate of the *mean difference*.

If we can assume that the two standard errors are essentially the same, we can combine or pool them into a single estimate by taking the weighted mean of the two separate standard error estimates: $\sqrt{s_t^2/n_t + s_c^2/n_c}$. This expression equals the square-root of the variance in the treatment group (s_t^2) divided by its size (n_t) and the variance in the control group (s_c^2) divided by its size (n_c). This formula is completely analogous to the situation of estimating the standard error of a single mean, which involves taking the square-root of the sample variance (s^2) from a single sample divided by its size (n).

Note that we assumed the equality of the standard error (and variances) in the two comparison groups. There is a statistical test, known as the Levene's test, that can be used to test this assumption. Most introductory statistics texts cover this test (e.g., Munro, 2001).

For the independent-sample *t*-test in Table B-1, the test-statistic is as follows:

$$T = (\bar{X}_t - \bar{X}_c)/[\sqrt{s_t^2/n_t + s_c^2/n_c}]$$

$$T = (80.33 - 84.48) / [\sqrt{9.49^2/50 + 9.59^2/50}] =$$
$$-4.15/\sqrt{90.06/50 + 91.97/50} =$$
$$-4.15/\sqrt{1.801 + 1.839} =$$
$$-4.15/\sqrt{3.64} =$$
$$-4.15/1.908 =$$
$$-2.175$$

The resulting *t*-value tells us that the observed difference between the means in the treatment and control groups (-4.15) is equivalent to -2.175 standard errors. As the significance level (*p*-value) in Table B-1 indicates, the probability of observing a mean difference of 2.175 standard errors or larger is 0.032, or in only 3.2% of all random assignments, can we expect to observe a difference of this magnitude or larger merely by chance.

Appendix C Random Numbers and Their Use

The following table shows 800 random numbers, generated by the STATA 7.0 'uniform' pseudo-random number function.

5723	3648	6587	5789	3515	5109	0542	1437	5261	5918
0117	9099	0674	2033	0271	1875	2792	0061	2082	8330
7236	0182	2923	3335	9150	0357	5920	4108	7836	6027
1917	7734	4171	8312	3833	2591	0333	3453	0386	4248
9618	1137	4549	7222	3958	5137	1991	4175	2478	7184
3755	2671	0758	3540	3688	1792	5415	7021	2008	5002
6457	7792	8528	5065	9254	7604	3530	1562	2561	8073
7766	1332	6280	8111	7604	2630	5301	1625	0039	6363
2811	8776	4586	4209	9216	6679	6431	1402	6875	4410
9287	0836	5009	1729	3277	7663	2329	1750	0756	5172
8773	0005	9255	9185	8776	7972	2879	1777	7028	1781
3125	5831	7064	3120	8999	3833	4384	7817	8108	5334
8609	1031	0188	7508	6372	2118	8958	4583	6287	9167
4772	2333	1038	9137	5897	1257	3277	0118	9074	5830
9331	1601	3208	6697	5662	7923	4494	9711	4226	3323
1376	3269	6421	1188	7799	0005	2048	1034	0068	1414
2383	3227	9413	1992	4621	5427	7579	2338	5112	8506
9222	4764	3331	0156	2251	6187	3666	1343	2624	8088
1117	6042	6330	4530	1162	0002	3926	6367	3281	1877
2645	9864	2099	7167	2363	4316	4112	3685	7543	4103

(A) Use of Random Numbers to Assign Cases to Treatment and Control Groups:

If the experiment involves only two comparison groups (= treatment or control groups), enrolled subjects can be assigned consecutively in blocks of two. Thus, the first two enrolled cases form the first block, the next two (number 3 + 4) the second block, and so forth. The random assignment to either treatment or control group proceeds as follows: Pick any row or column in the random number table, for instance, the first column. If the random number is even, the first case in the first block is assigned to the treatment group; if the random number is odd, this case will be assigned to the control group. By default, the second case in the block is always assigned to the remaining group.

Example: The first random number in the first column is '5' or odd. Thus, case number 1 in block 1 is assigned to the control group, and case number 2 in block 1 to the experimental group. The second random number in the first column is '0', which counts as even. Case number 3 in the second block will be assigned to the treatment group, and case number 4, the remaining case in the second group, will be assigned to the control group, etc.

(B) Use of Random Numbers to Sample from a Target Population Represented by a Sampling Frame:

Suppose you intend to obtain a simple random sample of 300 nurses from a state list of licensed nurses containing 9,345 names. One possibility is to assign a number from 1 to 9,345 to each nurse listed in alphabetical order. Then use four-digit random numbers from the table, starting in row 1 going from left to right, to select the cases until a sample of 300 is drawn. If the random number happens to be larger than 9345, ignore it and move on to the next number.

Example: Using the random number table in this appendix, one would first select the 5,723rd nurse from the list, followed by the 3648th nurse, etc. until a full sample of 300 selections is obtained.

GLOSSARY

Absolute risk. Probability of an adverse outcome in a population group; see also **relative risk.**

Accessible population. Study population defined in terms of geographic location, institutional affiliation, or study unit characteristics to which the researcher has access, given the available resources; see also **target population.**

Accuracy. See also **measurement reliability.**

Age-adjusted incidence or mortality rates. Recalculation of incidence or mortality rates for a particular population group based on the assumption that its age-distribution is identical to that of the standard (U.S.) population; assists in comparing rates among different population groups.

Analysis of covariance (ANCOVA). Multivariate statistical model with interval/ratio level dependent variable(s) and both nominal (= factors) and interval/ratio level (= covariates) independent variables; statistical model combining regression analysis and analysis of variance.

Analysis of variance (ANOVA). Multivariate statistical model with interval/ratio level dependent variable(s) and nominal-level (= factors) independent variables; the model focuses on predicting/estimating mean differences between the groups defined by the factor levels.

Applied research. Research designed to give answers to a specific practical/clinical problem.

Attribute variable. Variable that cannot be controlled or manipulated by the researcher, but can only be observed (e.g., age of study participants).

Attrition. Loss of study participants at any point between enrollment and completion of the study; also known as **(subject) mortality** or **dropout rate**. If attrition is non-random, it can compromise the comparison between study groups and be a threat to design validity.

Audit trail. Methodological device to improve the confirmability of qualitative data, including carefully documented records of changes or decisions concerning data collection approaches and interpretation decisions.

Basic research. Research for the purpose of generating new knowledge that may not (yet) have immediate practical application.

Between-subjects design. Experimental study design in which different groups of study participants are exposed to intervention or control treatments.

Between-subjects variation. Variation in outcome scores attributable to differences among study subjects.

Binary variable. See **dichotomous variable.**

Blinding. Technique most commonly applied in **clinical trials,** whereby observers (of outcomes) and study participants are kept ignorant about the study participants' membership in treatment or control group(s). The intent is to avoid unconscious measurement bias; see also **double-blind study** and **triple-blind study.**

Blocking. The process of grouping study participants into "blocks" of 2, 3, 4, etc. as soon as they are recruited, and then randomly assigning the study participants from within the blocks to the comparison (treatment and control) groups in a study; see also **matching.**

Case-control study. Observational (non-experimental), analytical study-design in which study participants are selected on the basis of the disease outcome being studied: cases, who have contracted the disease, and controls, who have not; the goal is to find systematic differences between these groups with respect to their exposure to suspected risk factors; see also **odds-ratio.**

Census. Data collection involving all members of a population.

Clinical trial. See **randomized clinical trial.**

Cluster sampling. A probability approach to selecting study participants that involves multiple and successive stages of sampling study units; essential, when complete listing of the population elements is not feasible or possible and the target population may be widely dispersed.

Codebook. Manual for a particular study that contains the rules or conventions for naming all variables and for assigning numeric values to the specific levels of these variables.

Coding. *In quantitative studies:* translation of information collected into variables with quantitative codes; see also **codebook;** *in qualitative analysis:* the process of subsuming particular instances of narrative information under broader conceptual categories; see also **grounded theory.**

Cohort study. Observational (non-experimental), analytical study-design in which study participants are selected on the basis of the degree of their exposure to a (hypothesized) risk factor, who are then followed to observe incidence rates for disease outcomes.

Complex hypothesis. Statement that relates more than one dependent and/or more than one independent variable to each other.

Concept. A word or term that represents a collection of phenomena considered to fall into the same category; an abstract representation of observations (e.g., blood pressure, anxiety, etc.); see also **observational concept, indirectly observable concept,** and **construct.**

Conceptual framework. A collection and model of interrelated concepts/constructs that provide a fruitful language and orientation, in which to frame substantive research problems. Such conceptual frameworks or models are sometimes also referred to as grand theories, as in role or general systems theory.

Concurrent validity. Assessment of the validity of a new measurement tool through comparison to an external criterion variable measured at the same time as the new measurement tool.

Condition-specific health status measure. Outcome measure that captures signs or symptoms associated with a particular disease; see also **generic health status measure.**

Confidence interval. The range of values within which the true population parameter is likely to fall with X% confidence; its calculation is based on standard error estimates obtained from the sample data; see also **confidence limits.**

Confidence limits. The extreme values or outer limits of a specified **confidence interval.**

Confounding variable. A variable that "distorts" the relationship between the independent and dependent variables, on which the research focuses, unless its effect is controlled statistically or through the research design; also known as *third variable, nuisance variable,* or *control variable;* see also **control variable.**

Constructs (theoretical concepts). Abstract concept invented by researchers/scientists to assist in the explanation of a constellation of issues/problems (e.g., *self-care agency* or *role*).

Content validity. The degree to which the verbal questionnaire items that make up a measurement scale actually tap into the conceptual dimensions of the concept that is purportedly measured.

Continuous variable. A variable that can take on infinitely many values or gradations (e.g., time since operation, body temperature, etc.).

Control group. Comparison group in an experimental study which does not get the treatment/intervention: it provides the benchmark against which the magnitude of the intervention effect is measured; comparison group of study participants in a case-control, who did not contract the disease or critical outcome being studied.

Control variable. A variable that is measured in a research project, although it is not the primary focus of investigation, because it is suspected to "distort" the relationship between the independent and dependent variable(s); this allows the analyst to adjust statistically the estimates of the effects of the independent on the dependent variable(s); see also **confounding variable,** and **third variable.**

Convenience sampling. A non-probability approach to selecting study participants based on their (easy) accessibility to the researcher(s); see also **non-probability sampling.**

Correlation (coefficient). Any of a number of statistical measures of association that indicate the degree to which two variables vary together; correlation coefficients are usually standardized to take on values ranging from -1 to $+1$, with 0 indicating the absence of a relationship/association between two variables and ± 1 indicating 'perfect' positive or negative associations; correlation coefficients that are widely used include: the Pearson product moment correlation (a measure of linear association between two interval/ratio level variables), Spearman's rho and Kendall's tau (measures of association between two ordinal variables), and Phi and Kramer's V (measures of association between two nominal/categorical variables).

Counterbalanced design. Cross-over design without random assignment/sequencing of treatment levels; see also **cross-over design.**

Criterion validity. Assessment of the validity of a measurement tool through examination of how well it predicts an *external* criterion variable; see also **concurrent validity** and **predictive validity.**

Criterion-referenced measurement scale/test. Measurement/test scores that rely on external criteria (usually established by experts) for judging an individual test-taker's performance; see also **norm-referenced measurement scale/test.**

Cross-over design. Experimental study design in which study participants are exposed to all randomly sequenced treatment levels and subject to repeated observations or measurements; see also **counterbalanced design.**

Cross-sectional study design. Study design (usually a survey) that calls for a single data collection point for all study participants (e.g., cross-sectional survey).

Data imputation. Substitution of values for missing information on study variables; several approaches are used in health care studies, including logical imputation, mean-value imputation, regression imputation, hot-decking, etc.

Degrees of freedom. A statistical concept relevant to the estimation of population variances based on sample data; it is generally calculated as the sample size minus the number of estimated parameters involved in the estimation of the specific statistic.

Dependent variable. A study variable, the variation of which the researcher wants to explain; the endpoint in a particular causal chain; dependent variables are always observed, never directly manipulated; also known as **outcome variable, endogenous variable, criterion variable,** etc.

Descriptive research. Research focused primarily on offering accurate "pictures" of reality (e.g., distribution of a disease in a population or reports on health-related attitudes in a subgroup of the population).

Design validity. Validity of causal inference in empirical studies; degree to which all rival hypotheses to a particular study hypothesis can be excluded in an experimental study; also known as **internal validity.**

Dichotomous variable. Variable which takes on only two distinct values/categories (e.g., sex [male vs. female] or mortality status [dead or alive]); also known as **binary variable.**

Diffusion of treatment. "Contamination" of control group(s) or control condition(s) with treatment effects. Such carry-overs or diffusion can occur in between-subjects studies, when either participants or others involved in the intervention/treatment contact the control subjects or in repeated treatment studies (*cross-over designs*), when the effects of the treatment linger on into the control phase.

Directional hypothesis. Hypothesis that indicates in which direction the dependent variable is expected to change as the independent variable changes.

Dose-response. Degree to which variations in the strength or duration of exposure generate associated variations in the incidence of the adverse outcome.

Double-blind study. Clinical trial in which neither the study participants nor the observer(s) of the outcomes know which subjects are assigned to treatment or control conditions; see also **clinical trial.**

Emergent research design. Qualitative approach to research, involving a rejection of a fixed, pre-planned research design; see also **exploratory research** and **inductive approach to research.**

Empirical evidence. Observational or experimental data that address or speak to the research problem at hand.

Empirical research. Any research that bases its claims and conclusions about how things work on empirical evidence.

Empiricism. Philosophical outlook often associated with traditional science; one major assumption of empiricism is that there is an *objective reality* that exists independently of the human observer, even though its perception might well be colored by the limitations of human abilities to observe and process information about that reality. Variants of empiricism include **logical positivism** and **falsificationism.**

Error sum of squares. See **within-group sum of squares (WGSS).**

Ethnography. Research approach rooted in anthropology focusing on understanding and describing the cultural processes of particular population groups; its primary method is **fieldwork.**

Evidence-based practice. Explicit integration of clinical/empirical research evidence into the clinical decision-making of the health provider.

Experiment. Study design that requires, at a minimum, an independent or **treatment variable** manipulated by the researcher, **random assignment** of study participants to the various treatment conditions or levels, and control over extraneous factors/environment; see also **randomized clinical trial.**

Experimental variable. See **treatment variable.**

Exploratory research. Research explicitly designed to probe reality or investigate hunches so as to obtain preliminary evidence that can serve as a basis for more formal, future research; research without theory-derived hypotheses; preliminary measurement studies with the goal to develop standardized measurement instruments; see also **inductive approach to research.**

Fact. Statement about "what is the case" that is taken to be true for the time being.

Factor analysis. A multivariate statistical technique used to assist in the establishment of construct validity; factor analysis can be used to either find groups of variables or items that correlate with each other more, but less with other variables or items (*exploratory factor analysis*); factor analysis can also be used to test for the existence of pre-determined groupings of variables (*confirmatory factor analysis*).

Factorial design. Experimental study/clinical trial in which at least two treatment variables are manipulated simultaneously.

False negatives. Cases/patients predicted by a diagnostic or screening test *not* to have a certain disease or condition, although they do have it.

False positives. Cases/patients predicted by a diagnostic or screening test to have a certain disease or condition, although they do *not* have it.

Field notes. Records containing the data for ethnographic research (e.g., descriptions of events, activities, and interaction patterns occurring in the field setting); field notes are composed on several levels, traditionally denoted as observational, theoretical, methodological, and personal notes.

Focus group interview. Group session for the purpose of conducting a semi-structured, qualitative interview in which a small group of study participants (6 to 12 people) discuss among each other a series of pre-determined focus questions provided by the researcher.

Formal definition. Definition of new concept in terms of already-known concepts (e.g., automobile = horseless carriage); see also **ostensive definition.**

Fruitfulness (or goodness) of a concept/construct. "Staying power" of a concept or construct (i.e., its ability to illuminate many research questions and problems).

Generalizability. Inference that study findings from a particular study sample can be assumed to hold in target population (within specifiable error margins); presupposes random sampling/selection of study participants.

Generalization (statistical). Using a probability calculus and information from a random/probability sample to draw inferences about the characteristics of the population from which the sample was drawn.

Generic health status measures. Self-report health status measures that cover multiple dimensions of health (e.g., physical, emotional, and social functioning, as well as pain and an overall assessment of health and well-being, as perceived by the respondent to the instrument); see also **condition-specific health status measure.**

Gold standard. Measurement procedure for a particular variable that is widely accepted as the best available; it is used as the standard against which all other/new measurement procedures are compared; see also **measurement validity** and **measurement reliability.**

Grand theory. See **conceptual framework.**

Grounded theory. A qualitative, inductive research approach that aims to develop theory based on the interpretation of qualitative data; through a series of ever-more abstract **coding** steps, the data are supposed to 'yield' the emerging concepts and theories; see also **coding.**

Historical research. Mostly qualitative research tradition focused on the reconstruction and interpretation of historical events using both primary (historical) and secondary (later) source materials.

History. Occurrence or intrusion of all events that might represent alternative causes—in addition to the major cause on which a study is focused—for observed outcomes.

Hypothesis. A statement concerning an expected empirical outcome under specified conditions; a statement about the expected relationship among two or more variables; empirical implication of a theory.

Incidence rate. A ratio of the number of new (*incident*) cases incurring a particular disease/event within a given time period to the population at risk for the disease, measured in person-time.

Independent variable. A variable in a research study that is considered a cause of other variables called dependent variables; in experimental studies, independent variables are deliberately manipulated by the researcher(s); also known as **explanatory variable, predictor variable, exogenous variable;** see also **dependent variable.**

Indirectly observable concept. Concept that refers to phenomena that must be inferred from observations (e.g., subjective experiences and mental processes, such as *anger* and *depression*).

Inductive approach to research. Any research approach that attempts to use specific, time- and locality-bound data to arrive at general patterns or theories; see also **exploratory research.**

Informed consent. Disclosure statement to be signed by each study participant that contains a clear account of all the risks and benefits involved in the participation in a particular research study.

Institutional Review Board (IRB). Research review committee of an organization (e.g., hospital, university) in which human subjects research is conducted and which receives federal funds; an IRB is legally mandated to review research protocols for compliance with established ethical standards.

Instrumentation bias. Systematic biases in the comparison of treatment and control groups (or exposed and non-exposed cohorts) that are attributable to changes/differences in measurement procedures.

Intact groups. Pre-existing social groups that are used as comparison groups in research, such as in quasi-experiments; in research involving intact groups, the researcher cannot select the individual members of the comparison groups.

Interaction effect. In a study with multiple independent variables, the joint effect of two or more independent variables on the outcome variable, which goes beyond the mere additive effect of each independent variable separately; see also **main effect.**

Interaction of selection and treatment. Limited generalizability of inferences from an experimental study due to the fact that the intervention effects apply only to the specific participants in the study sample; see also **generalizability.**

Interaction of testing and experimental stimulus. Changes in experimental effects depending on whether or not a study participant was tested prior to the introduction of the experimental stimulus/treatment.

Internal validity. See **design validity.**

Internal-consistency reliability. The degree to which responses to multiple items designed to measure the same psycho-social concept correlate; an overall measure of this reliability concept is Cronbach's Alpha.

Inter-rater reliability. The degree to which two or more observers agree when rating the same observations independently on a predetermined scale; measures include Cohen's kappa and Kendall's *W* Coefficient of Concordance; also known as **inter-observer reliability.**

Interrupted time series design. Study design which involves a series of (repeated) observations prior to implementing an intervention, followed by a series of (repeated) observations after the implementation of the intervention.

Intervening variable. Variable that is thought of as occupying an intermediate position in a causal chain (e.g., in the chain of X =>Y =>Z, Y would be considered the intervening variable).

Intervention study. Experimental or quasi-experimental clinical study in which human study participants are exposed to deliberately manipulated behavioral/medical treatments; also known as **clinical trial**.

Intervention variable. See **treatment variable.**

Interview schedule. Written instrument/form that contains all stem items and response formats for questions to be asked in a survey (personal or telephone) interview; also known as **survey instrument.**

Item-non-response. Missing responses specific to particular questionnaire items or study variables; often the result of problems with the question item.

Levels of measurement. Classification of measurement procedures based on the types of mathematical operations that can legitimately be performed on the measurement scores; the four main levels of measurement are *nominal/categorical, ordinal, interval,* and *ratio.*

Life table.   Summarizes the mortality or morbidity experience of a particular population of interest; table entrees are usually stratified by age and include, for each observation period (usually one year), the number of population members entering the observation period and the number/proportion lost due to mortality or some other event of interest; life tables contain the information for person-year/person-time exposure relevant to the construction of the denominator of incidence rates; see also **person-time** and **incidence rates.**

Logical positivism.   See **empiricism.**

Logistic regression model.   See **regression analysis.**

Longitudinal study design.   Any study that involves data collection on more than one occasion.

Main effect.   In a study with multiple independent variables, the effects of one independent variable holding the other independent variables constant; see also **interaction effect.**

Manipulation.   Change in independent or treatment/intervention variable deliberately effected by the researcher.

Matching.   The process of selecting subjects based on a common characteristic, like female vs. male or smoker vs. non-smoker, who are then assigned to the study comparison groups in fixed ratios; its purpose is to ensure equal representation of each subject group in the study comparison group; see also **blocking** and **stratified randomization.**

Maturation.   Refers to all over-time changes in study participants that are not related to any particular *external* events, but instead appear to reflect *internal* changes in the study participants themselves.

Measurement bias.   Degree to which a measurement instrument systematically over- or underestimates the true score.

Measurement error.   Any deviation of observed measurement outcomes from true state of affairs; measurement results may deviate from the true scores in a predictable or *systematic* way (=> **measurement bias**) or they may fluctuate in a more or less *random* fashion (=> lack of **measurement reliability**).

Measurement.   Assignment of numbers (numerical "scores") to attributes of objects or study participants according to a specified rule system.

Measurement reliability.   Degree to which random error is absent from a particular measurement procedure; consistency and repeatability of measurement results that use a particular measurement procedure; independence of measurement results from time, place, or person performing the measurement; ratio of true score variance to observed score variance; also known as **accuracy.**

Measurement validity.   Degree to which a particular measurement procedure or instrument captures the theoretical concept of interest.

Member checking.   Process of validation in qualitative studies whereby study participants review and validate transcripts and interpretations of qualitative data.

Meta-analysis.   A method of statistically summarizing and evaluating the *results* of many research studies on a given topic.

Middle range theory.   Theory that deliberately limits itself to a "manageable" set of problems and variables that yields testable hypotheses and can be empirically investigated in a given research project (e.g., Pender's Health Promotion Model).

Multi-trait-multi-method matrix method (MTMM). Method designed to establish the construct validity of a measurement tool, based on the examination of correlation patterns involving questionnaire items measuring at least two distinct but related concepts, administered using at least two distinct data collection techniques; see also **factor analysis.**

Multivariate statistics.   Any statistical model that involves the simultaneous analysis of three or more variables (e.g., regression analysis, ANOVA, survival analysis, factor analysis, etc.).

Narrative data.   Recordings or transcripts of verbal conversations obtained during unstructured interviews.

Network sampling.   See **snowball sampling.**

Non-equivalent control group.   Comparison group in a case-control or quasi-experimental study that, because of lack of individual random assignment, may systematically differ from the intervention or case-group; see also **intact group.**

Non-equivalent control group design.   Any intervention study design that compares study groups that have not been constituted through random assignment; see also **quasi-experiment.**

Norm-referenced measurement scale.   Measurement scale or test that has been calibrated with reference to a target population, such that individual scores can be related to the distribution of scores on the target population; see also **criterion-referenced measurement scale/test.**

Observational concept.   Concept that refers to phenomena observable through the senses.

Observational study.   Research in which the outcomes or interest are only observed after or when they occur, but no treatment or independent variable has been manipulated; also known as *ex-post-facto study, correlational study,* or *descriptive study.*

Odds.   Ratio of the probability of an event occurring to the probability of that event not occurring in a population group: p/(1−p); see also **odds-ratio.**

Odds-ratio.   Ratio of two odds; in **case-control studies,** it is the ratio of the odds of exposure to a risk factor among cases versus the odds of exposure to the same risk factor among controls; see also **relative risk.**

Open cohort study.   Cohort study, in which the exposure status of study participants will be determined or reclassified, depending on changes in their exposure to a risk factor over the observation period.

Operational definition.   See **operationalization (of concepts).**

Operationalization (of concepts).   The process that specifies and defines the empirical (measurable) phenomena to which a concept refers; measurement operations that define the procedures of how a concept is to be observed; translation of concepts into measured variables also referred to as **operational definition.**

Ostensive definition.   Implicit definition of a concept through usage; see also **formal definition.**

Outcome (variable).   See **dependent variable.**

Outcomes evaluation.   Evaluation and assessment of the overall effectiveness of an intervention or program.

Oversampling.   Use of larger sampling ratios for smaller population groups to obtain adequate representation in the study sample.

Paired-samples *t* test.   Statistical test for the comparison of two mean scores in *related* or *paired* groups. Pairing may involve linking two different samples.

Panel study.   Survey study with repeated interviews of the same study sample.

Paradigm.   Set of philosophical assumptions about the nature of reality and appropriate methods of inquiry, with which researchers approach their research, as for example in the **quantitative** and **qualitative** research traditions.

Participant observation.   Method of observing study subjects that requires the researcher or observer to become part of and actively participate in the social networks and interaction patterns that are being studied. A participant observer may sometimes conceal his or her identity as a researcher.

Periodicity effect.   Threat to validity in time series data; fluctuations in outcomes that tend to occur in fixed and repeating intervals over time (e.g., circadian rhythm).

Person-time.   The denominator in a rate measure; person-time measures the "population at risk" for the observation period, during which the incidences of new cases of mortality or morbidity are observed; for example, if 10 persons are observed for 1/2 year, 20 persons for 1 year and 30 persons for 2 years, the total population at risk for a particular outcome would be 85 person-years: $10 \times \frac{1}{2} + 20 \times 1 + 30 \times 2 = 85$; see also **incidence rate** and **life table.**

Phenomenological research.   A qualitative research approach rooted in concepts from philosophical phenomenology focused on uncovering the "true" meanings that subjects ascribe to their experiences and actions; its aim is to discover the "essence" of a phenomenon through a procedure called *bracketing one's existence;* the goal is to immerse oneself in the data in ways that allow the intended meanings to emerge.

Polytomous variable.   Variables with multiple (more than two) discrete categories, such as "smoker status" (non-smoker, former smoker, current smoker) or religious affiliation.

Population.   Any universe of subjects, cases, units, or observations containing all possible members.

Population-normed scale.   Standardized measurement scale, the scores of which are calibrated in reference to population averages (e.g., average SAT score = 1,000).

Positivism.   See **empiricism.**

Post-test only design.   Experimental design in which study participants are observed only after the treatment has been introduced.

Power (of a statistical test).   Probability that a hypothesized effect is found to be statistically significant in a study sample (i.e., the probability of finding an effect when it exists); statistical power (1-β) is the complement of a **Type II error.**

Predictive validity.   Assessment of the validity of a new measurement instrument through prediction of future scores on an external criterion variable.

Pre-test/post-test design. Experimental design in which study participants are observed both before and after the treatment has been introduced.

Process evaluation. Research that focuses on the process or activities of implementing an intervention/program in relation to the outcomes achieved.

Program evaluation research. Research designed to provide information about the success of an action program, educational program, or a particular model of practice.

Prospective study design. Study design which involves future observations of study participants; experimental studies are always prospective; among observational studies, cohort studies often employ prospective designs.

Purposive sampling. A non-probability approach to selecting study participants, so that they represent certain subject characteristics that are deemed relevant to the investigation; also known as **judgmental sampling**; most often, study participants are selected for their "heterogeneous" characteristics; commonly used in sampling for measurement studies and qualitative research.

P-value. The probability that an observed effect or relationship in a study sample is due to sampling chance. See also **significance level.**

Qualitative research. Research that eschews measurement and focuses on interpretive, non-numerical narrative interpretation.

Quantitative research. Research in which the studied phenomena are measured and scored on numerical, standardized scales, which, in turn, allows for mathematical/ statistical modes of analysis.

Quasi-experiment. Experimental study design in which the introduction and withholding of treatment(s) are under the control of the researcher, but study participants are not randomly assigned to various treatment conditions and use of pre-existing **intact groups** is common.

Quota sampling. A non-probability approach to selecting study participants based on the notion that the study sample should contain the same proportions of subjects as the target population with respect to a few salient characteristics, such as sex, race, age-groups.

Random assignment. Assignment of study participants to study comparison groups on the basis of a probability scheme (determined by chance alone); its main purpose is to avoid systematic differences between the attributes of subjects in treatment and control groups; also known as *randomization.*

Random sampling. Selection of study participants from larger target populations groups on the basis of a probability scheme (determined by chance alone); random sampling (or random selection) provides a technical means of generalizing from a particular sample to a larger target population (i.e., its purpose is to obtain an unbiased selection from the target population with the goal of obtaining a representative sample); see also **simple random sampling and stratified random sampling**.

Randomized clinical trial (RCT). Experimental study in clinical settings in which study subjects are randomly assigned to different treatment levels combined with efforts to avoid measurement bias through blinding procedures; see also **double blind study** and **triple blind study.**

Recall bias. Biased reporting of past events, activities, or emotions by study participants because of memory problems, unwillingness to answer questions, truthfulness, etc.; in case-control studies, recall bias refers to the systematic *difference* in the information remembered and reported by cases and controls.

Reductionism. The belief that complex phenomena can be analyzed focusing on explanations involving the relationships among (some) constituent parts, which, in turn, can be explained in terms of their constituent parts.

Regression analysis. Family of statistical models in which the 'best' functional form of the relationship between a dependent/outcome variable, denoted as y, and one or more independent variables, denoted as $x_1, x_2 \ldots x_k$, is estimated. Some popular regression models include the linear regression model (with a continuous outcome variable) and the logistic regression model (with a binary outcome).

Regression sum of squares. See **within-group sum of squares (WGSS).**

Regression to the mean. See **statistical regression.**

Relative risk. Ratio of the incidence rate of an adverse outcome in the group exposed to a risk factor compared to the group not exposed to the risk factor; see also **incidence rate.**

Reliability. See **measurement reliability.**

Repeated cross-sectional survey. Repeated selection of survey samples from a changing target population (e.g., selection of random samples from the civilian, non-institutionalized resident population in the United States).

Repeated measures design. Any study design in which study participants are observed more than once; repeated measures studies may be experimental (e.g., cross-over design) or observational (e.g., panel study).

Repeated-measures reliability. See **test-retest reliability.**

Replicability. Study findings that can be "replicated" or repeated/confirmed in other studies that use similar study procedures.

Research dissemination. Refers to the process of presenting research findings together with specific implications for a given practice or policy situation and recommendations for relevant action steps for using the research findings.

Response rate. The ratio of the number of persons completing a study to the number of persons eligible for the study; also known as *study participation rate*.

Retrospective study design. Non-experimental study design in which researchers draw on observations made and recorded in the past; case-control studies often employ retrospective designs.

Risk factor. Any characteristic that contributes to a higher risk of contracting a particular disease or experiencing an adverse outcome (mortality, accidents, diseases).

Salomon four-group design. An experimental study design in which study participants are randomly assigned to four groups—one treatment and one control group with only post-test measurements, and one treatment and one control group combined with pre-test/post-test measurements. This design allows one to disentangle the effects of exposure to a pre-test from the effects of exposure to the treatment.

Sample. Any subset of cases, units, or observations from a larger **population** of cases, units, or observations.

Sampling. The process of selecting a particular subset from a larger population or universe.

Sampling bias. See **selection bias.**

Sampling distribution (of a test-statistic). Frequency distribution of all possible sample outcomes of a particular test-statistic based on all possible samples drawn from a specific population; the mathematical/statistical function describing the sampling distribution is known as the probability density function and is based on the assumption that sample units were randomly drawn from the population; if the sampling distribution is known, one can estimate the probability that a particular sample value falls within any desired limits.

Sampling error. Deviation of sample estimate from true value of population parameter due to the fact that the random sampling process leads to variations in sample outcomes.

Sampling frame. List or data bank that represents all elements/units/study participants of an accessible target population; used as a basis for random sampling of study participants.

Scaling algorithm. A standardized procedure for converting observations numerically using a fixed formula incorporating weight to be assigned to each variable that is part of the scale.

Secondary data analysis. Analyzing an existing data set, gathered in a previous study, for the purpose of testing new hypotheses or relationships among variables.

Selection bias (in experimental and analytical studies). Any selection procedure that results in the selection of comparison groups (e.g., experimental vs. control groups or exposed vs. non-exposed groups), which differ in their background characteristics; also known as *differential selection*.

Selection bias (in sampling). Any selection procedure of study participants that leads to study samples that are unrepresentative of the target population.

Sensitivity. Probability that a diagnostic or screening test confirms the presence of a disease or health condition in a patient who has it. See also **true positives**.

Sensitivity analysis. A general method to determine how robust statistical estimates are in light of changing assumptions.

Significance level. The probability value set by the researchers for a Type 1 error. If the *p*-value falls below the significance level (conventionally often set at 0.05), the null-hypothesis is rejected. See also *p*-**value** and **Type I error.**

Simple hypothesis. Statement about the expected relationship between one independent and one dependent variable.

Simple random sampling. A probability approach to selecting study participants, such that each population member has the same chance of being selected into the sample.

Snowball sampling. A non-probability approach to selecting study participants that relies on early study participants for help in identifying or recruiting further study participants who meet the study criteria; also known as **network sampling;** used in qualitative research studies or with special populations difficult to locate otherwise; see **non-probability sampling.**

Specificity. Probability that a diagnostic or screening test confirms the absence of a disease or health condition in a patient who does not have it. See also **true negatives**.

Spurious relationship. Correlation that differs from zero, but does *not* indicate a causal relationship (i.e., it is due to correlations with confounding variable[s]); see also **correlation.**

Statistical regression. The tendency of extreme measurement scores to revert to the mean (average) score in repeated measures; also known as **regression to the mean.**

Strata. Division of target population into mutually exclusive subgroups based on some characteristic of interest to a research project; "strata" is a plural noun, "stratum" being the singular.

Stratified (random) sampling. Sampling plan in which random or probability sampling occurs only within predetermined homogeneous subject groups (**strata**) (e.g., separate random selection of study participants from among men and women); through the use of different sampling ratios, certain population segments may be deliberately over- or underrepresented in the study sample.

Stratified randomization. Random assignment of study participants to treatment and control groups *within* homogeneous subject groups (e.g., separate random assignment of smokers and non-smokers to comparison groups); see also **blocking** and **matching.**

Structured interview. An interview style in which most or all questions are predetermined and interview respondents are asked to make choices among fixed response categories. Interviewers follow standardized interview techniques applied to all interviewees.

Study arm. One of the comparison groups in an experimental study or clinical trial; subjects within a particular study arm are exposed to one level of treatment or treatment combination differing from all other study arms/study groups.

Systematic sampling. A probability approach to sampling in which every *n*th population member is selected from a population list or **sampling frame,** with the first member selected randomly.

Target population. Population of all potential study units that meets the study inclusion criteria (i.e., in whom or which the researcher is interested); see also **accessible population.**

Testing effects. Changes in measurement outcome resulting from re-taking the same test two or more times (e.g., the very fact of having taken an earlier test [pre-test] influences the results in subsequent test taking [post-test]).

Test-retest reliability. The degree to which repeated observed measurement scores correlate with each other; also known as **repeated-measures reliability.**

Theory. A symbolic/abstract representation of an aspect of reality, formulated verbally or mathematically; theory provides an explanatory model that specifies how and why selected concepts/variables are related to each other.

Total sum of squares (TSS). A measure of the total variation in the dependent variable in ANOVA and linear regression models: the sum of squared deviations of all sample observations on the outcome variable from the sample mean: $\Sigma\,(Y_{ig} - \bar{Y}..)^2$.

Transferability. The ability to apply local findings from a particular qualitative study to different contexts and settings; see also **generalizability.**

Treatment variable. Independent variable in an experiment or clinical trial that is manipulated by the researcher; also known as **experimental variable** or **intervention variable**.

Trend line. A line that best depicts how an outcome variable of interest changes over time, usually uninterrupted by an intervention.

Trend study. Study that follows changes in population groups; see also **repeated cross-sectional survey.**

Triangulation. The use of multiple methods to collect data for the purpose of improving the credibility of findings.

Triple-blind study. Clinical trial in which neither the study participants, the health professionals treating them, nor the persons who observe or record the outcome are aware of which subjects are assigned to treatment or control conditions.

True negatives. Cases/patients whose disease- or condition-*free* status is confirmed by a diagnostic or screening test.

True positives. Cases/patients whose *disease or condition* is confirmed by a diagnostic or screening test.

Type-I error. The error of wrongly rejecting a true null hypothesis (e.g., concluding in an experiment that an intervention is effective when, in fact, it is not); see also **significance level** or **p-value.**

Type-II error. The error of failing to reject a false null-hypothesis (e.g., concluding in an experiment that an intervention is not effective when, in fact, it is); see also **power of a statistical test.**

Unbiased estimator. Statistical estimator that has the property that the mean of its sampling distribution (or its expected value) is equal to the true population parameter; see also **sampling distribution.**

Unstructured interview. An interview style in which the flow and content of the interview are largely determined by the interactions between interviewer and interviewee; such exploratory interviews do not contain fixed response formats or predetermined questions except for directions concerning the general topic areas.

Value (held by a person). Preference for a particular course of action.

Value (of a variable). Particular score or category that a variable can take on (e.g., a study participant's age of 23; or female sex).

Value-free science. The claim that disputes over facts (what is the case) and means-ends/cause-effect relations can be separated from disputes over values.

Variable. Actual measurement outcomes or the collection of scores that represent the range of phenomena referred to in a single study concept (e.g., the concept age is represented in an empirical study by the variable age [i.e., all possible age values that the study subjects may take on]). For a study variable to vary, it must take on at least two values; otherwise, it is a constant in the study.

Within-group sum of squares (TSS). A measure of the variation in individual scores of the dependent variable in ANOVA that is *not* accounted for by the independent variable(s) or factor(s) in the model; also known as **error sum of squares** or, in regression models, as **regression sum of squares.**

Within-subjects design. Experimental study design in which study participants are exposed to more than one treatment level; see also **cross-over design.**

Within-subjects factor. Treatment variable to which study the same participants are exposed at different or multiple levels; see also **within-subjects design.**

INDEX

Page numbers followed by "f" denote figures, "t" denote tables, and "b" denote boxes